American Medical Association

Physicians dedicated to the health of America

Medicare RBRVS:
The Physicians' Guide

2002

Patrick E. Gallagher, MBA
Editor

Todd Klemp, MS, MBA
Sherry L. Smith, MS, CPA
Managing Editors

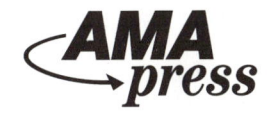

AMA press

© 2002 American Medical Association.

Coding and Medical Information Systems Group
Fifth revised edition of *Medicare Physician Payment Reform: The Physicians' Guide,* published in 1992
All rights reserved. Printed in the USA

CPT® five-digit codes, two-digit numeric modifiers, and descriptions only are © 2001 American Medical Association. No payment schedules, fee schedules, relative value units, scales, conversion factors, or components thereof are included in CPT. The AMA is not recommending that any specific relative values, fees, payment schedules, or related listings be attached to CPT. Any relative value scales or related listings assigned to the CPT codes are not those of the AMA, and the AMA is not recommending use of these relative values.

CPT is a registered trademark of the American Medical Association.

US Public Laws and federal rules and regulations if and as included in this publication are in the public domain. However, their arrangement, compilation, organization, history, and references, along with all CPT and all other materials in this publication, are subject to the above copyright notice.

Additional copies of this book may be purchased from:

Order Department: OP059602
American Medical Association
For order information, call toll-free 800 621-8335

Internet address: www.ama-assn.org/catalog

For other correspondence address inquiries to:

Medicare RBRVS
American Medical Association
515 N State St
Chicago, IL 60610

ISBN 1-57947-205-2

AC28:02-P-010:1/02

Acknowledgments

The American Medical Association (AMA) is extremely grateful to AMA staff and others who continue to make this book a reality.

The Department of Physician Payment Policy and Systems is responsible for the content of this publication and is staffed by Roseanne Eagle, MPP; Patrick E. Gallagher, MBA; Monica Horton, MPP; Todd Klemp, MA, MBA; Robin Russell; and Sherry L. Smith, MS, CPA.

Kurt D. Gillis, PhD, senior economist in the AMA's Center for Health Policy Research edited chapter 10. Thanks are also due to Sharon McIlrath, Julie Letwat, and Jean Narcisi for their comments on various chapters. Elise Schumacher, Rosalyn Carlton, Jean Roberts, Ronnie Summers, Boon Ai Tan, and Anne Serrano, shepherded the project through the editorial production process.

The AMA thanks the following individual AMA/Specialty Society RVS Update Committee members, Advisory Committee members, Practice Expense Advisory Committee Members, and the Health Care Professional and Advisory Committee members for their efforts in advocating RBRVS improvements to the Centers for Medicare and Medicaid Services (formerly the Health Care Financing Administration).

AMA/Specialty Society RVS Update Committee (RUC)

James G. Hoehn, MD
RUC Chairman

James Blankenship, MD
American College of Cardiology

James P. Borgstede, MD
American College of Radiology

Melvin C. Britton, MD
American College of Rheumatology

Neil H. Brooks, MD
American Academy of Family Physicians

John Derr, MD
American Society of Plastic Surgeons

Lee Eisenberg, MD
AMA CPT Editorial Panel

John O. Gage, MD
American College of Surgeons

William Gee, MD
American Urological Association

Meghan Gerety, MD
American Geriatrics Society

Alexander Hannenberg, MD
American Society of Anesthesiologists

James E. Hayes, MD
American College of Emergency Physicians

David F. Hitzeman, DO
American Osteopathic Association

Charles F. Koopmann, Jr, MD
American Academy of Otolaryngology – Head and Neck Surgery

Barbara Levy, MD
American College of Obstetricians and Gynecologists

J. Leonard Lichtenfeld, MD
American College of Physicians– American Society of Internal Medicine

John E. Mayer, Jr, MD
Society of Thoracic Surgeons

David L. McCaffree, MD
American Academy of Dermatology

Bill Moran, MD
Practice Expense Advisory Committee

Bernard Pfeifer, MD
American Academy of Orthopaedic Surgeons

Gregory Przybylski, MD
American Association of Neurological Surgeons

William Rich, MD
American Academy of Ophthalmology

Chester W. Schmidt, Jr, MD
American Psychiatric Association

Bruce Sigsbee, MD
American Academy of Neurology

Sheldon B. Taubman, MD
College of American Pathologists

Richard Tuck, MD
American Academy of Pediatrics

Paul E. Wallner, MD
American Society for Therapeutic Radiology and Oncology

Richard W. Whitten, MD
American Medical Association

Don E. Williamson, OD
Health Care Professionals Advisory Committee

RUC Advisory Committee

Bibb Allen, MD
American College of Radiology

Joseph L. Bacotti, MD
Contact Lens Association of Ophthalmologists

Sherry Barron-Seabrook, MD
American Academy of Child and Adolescent Psychiatry

Stephen N. Bauer, MD
College of American Pathologists

Karl E. Becker, MD
American Society of Anesthesiologists

Richard Blonsky, MD
American Academy of Pain Medicine

Frederick Boop, MD
Congress of Neurological Surgeons

Keith Brandt, MD
American Society of Plastic Surgeons

Robert L. Bree, MD
Association of University Radiologists

Joel V. Brill, MD
American Gastroenterological Association

Thomas H. Browning, MD
American Society for Gastrointestinal Endoscopy

Rhonda H. Cobin, MD
American Association of Clinical Endocrinologists

Paul E. Collicott, MD
American College of Surgeons

Thomas L. Dent, MD
Society of American Gastrointestinal Endoscopic Surgeons

Richard A. Dickey, MD
The Endocrine Society

Daniel Ein, MD
American Academy of Allergy, Asthma & Immunology

Richard E. Fine, MD
American Society of Breast Surgeons

Richard E. Fulton, MD
Radiological Society of North America

Enrico Garcia, MD
American Society of Abdominal Surgeons

Lanny R. Garvar, DMD
American Dental Association

Robert Gillespie, MD
American Burn Association

Gary Alan Gramm, MD
American Osteopathic Association

Gary Gross, MD
Joint Council of Allergy, Asthma and Immunology

Curtis W. Hawkins, MD
Society for Investigative Dermatology

M. Bradford Henley, MD
American Orthopaedic Association

George A. Hill, MD
American College of Obstetricians and Gynecologists

Stephen A. Kamenetzky, MD
American Academy of Ophthalmology

Ronald Kaufman, MD
American College of Rheumatology

Laura C. Knobel, MD
American Academy of Family Physicians

Steven E. Krug, MD
American Academy of Pediatrics

Stephen Lane, MD
American Society of Cataract and Refractive Surgery

Richard S. Lang, MD
American College of Preventive Medicine

Sidney Levitsky, MD
Society of Thoracic Surgeons

Robert Maisel, MD
The Triological Society

James D. Maloney, MD
American College of Cardiology

Scott Manaker, MD, PhD
American College of Chest Physicians

David F. Martin, MD
American Academy of Orthopaedic Surgeons

Geraldine B. McGinty, MD
American Roentgen Ray Society

Charles Mick, MD
North American Spine Society

Wayne Miller, MD
American College of Medical Genetics

Clay Molstad, MD
American College of Physicians - American Society of Internal Medicine

Daniel J. Nagle, MD
American Society for Surgery of the Hand

Harvey L. Nisenbaum, MD
American Institute of Ultrasound in Medicine

Marc R. Nuwer, MD, PhD
American Clinical Neurophysiology Society

Thomas G. Olsen, MD
American Academy of Dermatology

Tye Ouzounian, MD
American Orthopaedic Foot and Ankle Society

Emil P. Paganini, MD
Renal Physicians Association

William Perruzi, MD
Society of Critical Care Medicine

Herbert S. Peyser, MD
American Society of Addiction Medicine

John E. Pippen, MD
American Society of Clinical Oncology

Alan L. Plummer, MD
American Thoracic Society

J. Arliss Pollock, MD
American Society of Neuroradiology

Louis Potters, MD
American Society for Therapeutic Radiology and Oncology

John Queenan, Jr, MD
American Society for Reproductive Medicine

James S. Regan, MD
American Urological Association

RADM Frederic G. Sanford, MD
Association of Military Surgeons of the United States

Peter Sawchuk, MD
American College of Emergency Physicians

Gary R. Seabrook, MD
The Society for Vascular Surgery

Anthony Senagore, MD
American Society of Colon and Rectal Surgeons

Ronald A. Shellow, MD
American Psychiatric Association

Charles Shoemaker, MD
American Society of General Surgeons

Samuel Silver, MD
American Society of Hematology

J. Baldwin Smith, MD
American Academy of Neurology and American Academy of Sleep Medicine

Lee E. Smith, MD
American Academy of Facial Plastic and Reconstructive Surgery

Samuel D. Smith, MD
American Pediatric Surgical Association

Susan Spires, MD
American Society of Cytopathology

Michael L. Steinberg, MD
American College of Radiation Oncology

Charles M. Stiernberg, MD
American Academy of Otolaryngology – Head and Neck Surgery

Dennis Stone, MD
American Medical Directors Association

Mark Synovec, MD
American Society of Clinical Pathologists

Vincent Tranchitella, MD
American Association of Electrodiagnostic Medicine

Henry C. Vasconez, MD
American Association of Plastic Surgeons

Robert L. Vogelzang, MD
Society of Cardiovascular and Interventional Radiology

Ted Watson, MD
American Academy of Otolaryngic Allergy

Paul R. Weiss, MD
The American Society for Aesthetic Plastic Surgery

John C. Wheeler, MD
American Society for Maxillofacial Surgeons

John A. Wilson, MD
American Association of Neurological Surgeons

Michael A. Wison, MD
Society of Nuclear Medicine

John A. Zitelli, MD
American Society for Dermatologic Surgery

Robert M. Zwolak, MD
American Association for Vascular Surgery

Practice Expense Advisory Committee (PEAC)

Bill Moran, MD
PEAC Chairman

James Anthony, MD
American Academy of Neurology

Stephen N. Bauer, MD
College of American Pathologists

Katherine Bradley, PhD, RN
American Nurses Association

Ann C. Cea, MD, FACR
American Medical Association

Manuel D. Cerqueira, MD
American College of Cardiology

Neal H. Cohen, MD
American Society of Anesthesiologists

Thomas A. Felger, MD
American Academy of Family Physicians

Blair C. Filler, MD
AMA CPT Editorial Panel

Mary Foto, OTR
Health Care Professionals Advisory Committee

Ronald L. Kaufman, MD
American College of Rheumatology

James H. Kelly, MD
American Academy of Otolaryngology – Head and Neck Surgery

Gregory Kwasny, MD
American Academy of Ophthalmology

Alex G. Little, MD
Society of Thoracic Surgeons

James Metcalf, MD
American Association of Neurological Surgeons

Ron Nelson, PA-C
American Academy of Physician Assistants

Tye Ouzounian, MD
American Academy of Orthopaedic Surgeons

Dighton C. Packard, MD
American College of Emergency Physicians

Emil Paganini, MD
American College of Physicians – American Society of Internal Medicine

Julia M. Pillsbury, DO, FAAP
American Academy of Pediatrics

James B. Regan, MD
American Urological Association

Jeffrey I. Resnick, MD
American Society of Plastic Surgeons

Anthony Senagore, MD
American College of Surgeons

Ronald Shellow, MD
American Psychiatric Association

Daniel Mark Siegel, MD
American Academy of Dermatology

Susan E. Spires, MD
American Society of Cytopathology

Robert J. Stomel, DO
American Osteopathic Association

Craig Strafford, MD
American College of Obstetricians and Gynecologists

Neal O. Templeton, MD
American College of Radiology

Charles H. Weissman, MD
American Society of Clinical Oncology

RUC Health Care Professionals Advisory Committee

Samuel M. Brown, PT
American Physical Therapy Association

Mary Foto, OTR
American Occupational Therapy Association

James M. Georgoulakis, PhD
American Psychological Association

Emily H. Hill, PA-C
American Academy of Physician Assistants

Jerilynn S. Kaibel, DC
American Chiropractic Association

Marc Lenet, DPM
American Podiatric Medical Association

Karen Smith, MS, RD
American Dietetic Association

Walter Smoski, PhD, CC
American Speech-Language Hearing Association

Nelda Spyres, LCSW
National Association of Social Workers

Eileen M. Sullivan-Marx, PhD
American Nurses Association

Don E. Williamson, OD
American Optometric Association

Foreword

Medicare RBRVS: The Physicians' Guide is a result of the American Medical Association's (AMA) commitment to provide its members and other physicians with accurate, up-to-the-minute information on the critical issues facing the medical profession. Few changes in federal government policy toward the profession were as profound as Medicare's implementation of a physician payment schedule based on the resource-based relative value scale (RBRVS) on January 1, 1992. This new system was the first major change in how Medicare pays for physicians' services since that program's inception in 1965.

The RBRVS is now entering its 11th year. And it reflects many policy objectives that the AMA sought for a fair and equitable RBRVS payment schedule. It established the principle that payments for physician services should vary with the resource costs of providing those services, both across services and across geographic areas. It eliminates many of the old system's confusing features. Finally, the RBRVS did indeed stave off far more onerous payment approaches.

We also recognize that implementation of this system caused some disruptions for physicians and patients. Limits on physicians' charges are more restrictive and many physicians have faced often substantial reductions in revenue. In addition, Medicare patients in some areas may find that their access to care has been reduced because some physicians are limiting the number of new Medicare patients they are accepting into their practices. The AMA is committed to doing all it can to minimize the hardships physicians and their patients face and to ensure that the system is refined as quickly as possible and updated to reflect changes in medical practice and resource costs.

Since the introduction of the RBRVS, the AMA has been working together with state medical associations and national medical specialty societies to address long standing concerns about the accuracy of the RBRVS. Recently, the AMA has been working closely with the national specialty societies to respond to the Centers for Medicare and Medicaid Services' (CMS) (formerly the Health Care Financing Administration's) regulations on resource-based practice expense relative values. Specifically, the AMA has provided the staff and leadership to the AMA/Specialty Society RVS Update Committee (RUC) to play a leading role in the process to refine the underlying data used in the practice expense methodology. The AMA is committed to ensuring that practice expense RVUs are based on verifiable and accurate data for all specialties. During the refinement process, the AMA via the RUC will continue to work closely with specialty societies to ensure that the data used to calculate practice expense relative values are representative of physicians' actual practice expenses.

On January 1, 2002, several important improvements in the physician work relative values will be implemented due to the efforts of the RUC and the national specialty societies. The RUC reviewed comments on nearly 900 CPT codes and provided recommendations to CMS in October 2000. CMS has announced that it will implement more than 95% of these recommendations, including increases to vascular surgery, general surgery, cardiothoracic surgery, and diagnostic mammography.

Under a final rule published on November 1, 2001, the Medicare conversion factor would fall from $38.26 in 2001 to $36.61 in 2002, for a reduction of 5.4%. The 5.4% reduction is the result of the sustainable growth rate (SGR) system which sets a target spending rate that is tied to the performance of the national economy. The large payment cut in 2002 follows increases of 5.4% in 1999 and 4.5% in 2000 and demonstrates that despite legislative modifications in 1999, the SGR is still extremely volatile with large payment increases in one year followed by decreases the following year. The anticipated cut in the conversion factor will further exacerbate reductions that many specialties face in the final year of the phase in to resource-based practice expense values and offset the increases others had expected to see. At press time, the AMA and other physician groups were pressing for Congressional action to stop the 5.4% cut. Whether that activity is successful or not, we also intend to mount a campaign to eliminate the SGR as of 2003 as has been recommended by the Medicare Payment Advisory Commission.

The AMA remains committed to providing practicing physicians with the information they need to understand and deal with payment reform. The Physicians' Guide is both a culmination of our work over the past few years and a beginning of our efforts for the future. We sincerely hope that you find it useful. We will continue to publish annual revisions, reflecting updated Medicare policies and payment schedule components. We urge you to send questions, as well as any suggestions for or comments about this book, to:

Physicians' Guide
Physician Payment Policy and Systems
American Medical Association
515 N State St
Chicago, IL 60610

James F. Rodgers
Vice President, Health Policy
American Medical Association

Contents

ix Foreword by Robert W. Gilmore, MD

xv Introduction: A Guide to *Medicare RBRVS: The Physicians' Guide*

Part 1

The Roots of Medicare's RBRVS Payment System

Chapter 1

2 **Development of the Resource-Based Relative Value Scale**

2 The Profession's Interest in an RBRVS

5 The Government's Interest in an RBRVS

6 The Harvard RBRVS Study

8 Reaction to the Completion of Phase I

9 Medicare Reform

Chapter 2

12 **Legislation Creating the Medicare RBRVS Payment System**

12 The Prescription for Changing the Medicare Physician Payment System

13 OBRA 89 Physician Payment Reform Provisions

17 Changes in Law and Regulations

Chapter 3

20 **The Scope of Medicare's RBRVS Payment System**

Part 2

Major Components of the RBRVS Payment System

Chapter 4

24 **The Physician Work Component**

25 The Harvard RBRVS Study

28 The 1992 RVS Refinement Process

29 The AMA/Specialty Society RVS Update Process

32 Five-Year Review

Chapter 5

36 The Practice Expense Component

- 36 Data Used to Assign Charge Based Practice Expense RVUs
- 36 The OBRA 89 Method
- 39 Concerns With the OBRA 89 Method
- 40 OBRA 93 Revisions to the Practice Expense Component
- 40 Resource-Based Practice Expenses
- 46 Refinement of Resource Based Practice Expenses

Chapter 6

49 Professional Liability Insurance (PLI) Component

- 49 Data Used to Assign Charge Based PLI RVUs
- 50 Creating Resource-Based PLI Relative Values
- 52 Combining Work, Practice Expense, and PLI RVUs

Chapter 7

53 Geographic Variation in the Payment Schedule

- 53 The OBRA 89 Provision for Geographic Adjustment
- 54 Geographic Practice Cost Indexes
- 56 Evaluating the GPCIs
- 56 Medicare Payment Localities

Chapter 8

59 The Medicare Payment Schedule

- 59 The Formula for Calculating the Payment Schedule
- 61 Worksheet for Determining the Impact of the Medicare Payment System on Individual Physician Practices

Chapter 9

65 Balance Billing Under the Payment Schedule

- 65 The PAR Program
- 66 Limiting Charges
- 67 Monitoring Compliance

Part 3

The RBRVS Payment System in Operation

Chapter 10

70 Updating the Payment Schedule
70 Conversion Factor Updates
73 Updating the Relative Values
75 Updating the GPCIs

Chapter 11

76 Standardizing Medicare Part B: RBRVS Payment Rules and Policies
77 Defining a Global Surgical Package: Major Surgical Procedures
79 Minor Surgery and Nonincisional Procedures (Endoscopies)
80 Payment to Assistants-at-Surgery
80 CPT Modifiers
84 Travel
84 Telephone Management
84 Payment for "New" Physicians
84 Payment for Provider-Based and Teaching Physicians
85 Professional/Technical Component Services
88 Pathology Services
89 Payment for Supplies, Services, and Drugs Furnished Incident to a Physician's Service
91 Payment for Nonphysicians
93 E/M Codes and Other Coding Issues Under the Physician Payment Schedule
99 New Legislative Initiatives to Detect Fraud and Abuse
100 Payment Policy Changes due to Legislation
102 Other Payment Policy Changes Adopted Under the RBRVS
103 AMA Advocacy Efforts

Part 4

The RBRVS Payment System in Your Practice

Chapter 12

106 Practice Managment Under the RBRVS: Implications for Physicians
106 Bringing All the Changes Together
107 The Practice Management Audit
108 Electronic Data Interchange
110 The Participation Decision
111 Private Contracting
112 Using the RBRVS to Establish Physician Charges

Chapter 13

114 **Non-Medicare Use of the RBRVS: New Survey Data**
114 Survey Design
115 Characteristics of Respondents
115 Adoption Rate, All Payers
116 Use of RBRVS by All Payers
118 Adoption of the RBRVS Among the Four Payer Types
119 Use of the RBRVS Among the Four Payer Types
121 Opinion of the RBRVS
122 Factors That Influence Adoption of RBRVS
122 Other Uses of the RBRVS
123 Conclusion
123 AMA Position on Medicare Physician Payments and Fee-for-Service

---

Part 5

Reference Lists

126 **List of Relative Value Units, Payment Schedule, and Payment Policy Indicators**
448 **List of Geographic Practice Cost Indexes for Each Medicare Locality**
453 **RVUs for Anesthesiology Services**
455 **Anesthesia Base Units**

Appendixes

466 **A. Glossary of Terms**
471 **B. Directory of Resources**
483 **C. Temporary Codes—Splints and Casts**

Index

487

Introduction
A Guide to Medicare RBRVS: The Physicians' Guide

Medicare RBRVS: The Physicians' Guide has been developed as a comprehensive guide for physicians to Medicare's payment system for physicians' services that became effective January 1, 1992. In addition to providing detailed background information and explaining all features of the physician payment system, *The Physicians' Guide* is also a reference for physicians and their staff to use in answering particular questions about the system. This 11th revised edition of *The Physicians' Guide* reflects a more detailed discussion of Medicare's payment policies, as well as 2002 relative values. It also provides updated information on new payment rules that took effect in 2002; more details for each CPT code on applicable payment policies; recent legislative changes in the RVS for 2002; and policy actions the AMA has taken since enactment of payment system revisions. Finally, information on use of the RBRVS by Medicaid programs and the private sector is described. To assist physicians in obtaining answers to their own questions as quickly as possible, *The Physicians' Guide* is organized in five parts:

Part 1 introduces the RBRVS payment system. It provides a history and overview of the enabling legislation, explaining the efforts of the government and the medical profession that led to adoption of the RBRVS payment system and introducing its key components.

Part 2 describes these key components, explaining in detail the resource-based relative value scale, geographic adjustments, conversion factor, and limits on physicians' charges.

Part 3 explains the operation of the payment system, including calculation of payments. This part describes all of the system's payment policies, including global surgical packages, modifiers, payment for assistants-at-surgery, evaluation and management codes, and other issues.

Part 4 focuses on how the RBRVS payment system may affect physicians' practices. This part describes how private and public non-Medicare payers are changing their physician payment programs in response to the Medicare RBRVS and emerging forms of physician payment, such as capitation.

Part 5 presents all the elements that are necessary to calculate the Medicare payment schedule: 2002 relative value units and payment policy indicators for each physician's service and geographic practice cost indexes (GPCIs) for 2002 for each Medicare payment locality.

Physicians interested in understanding how and why Medicare's payment system was revised and how each of its components was established may wish to read Parts 1 through 4 in their entirety. Those interested only in understanding how payments are calculated and what the impact will be on their practice may wish to skip Parts 1 and 2 and begin with Part 3.

CPT/RVU File on CD-ROM

A must have tool for reimbursement disputes, contract negotiations, and for determining fees.

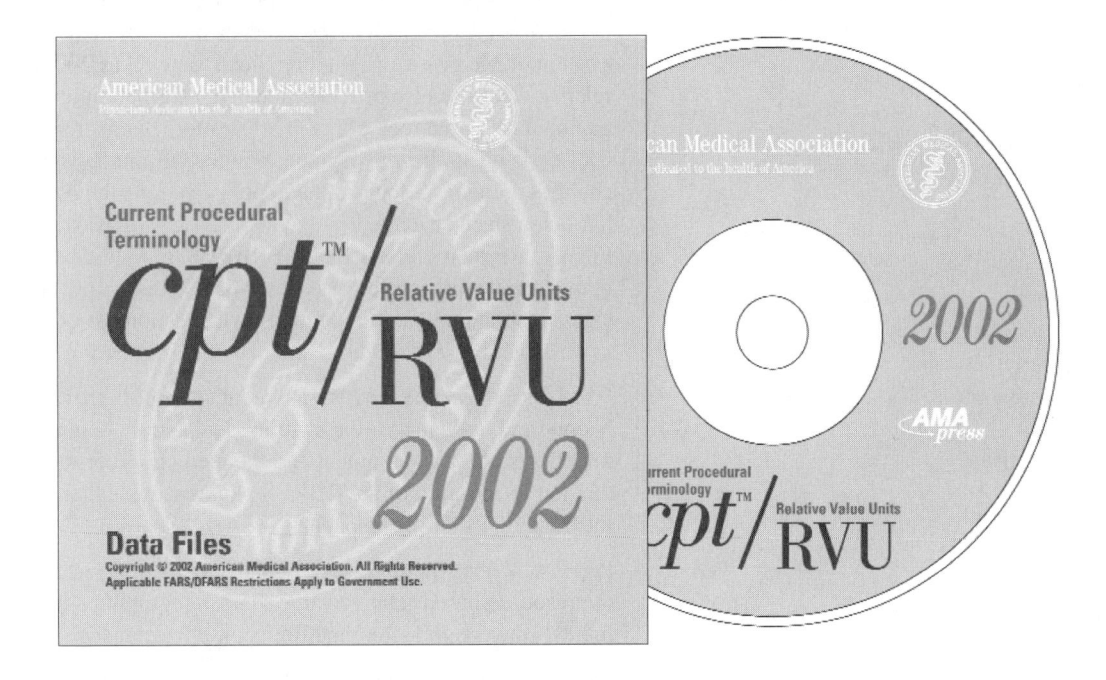

The 2002 CPT/RVU data files provide a tab-delimited and a pipe-delimited data text file containing the complete CPT descriptor package and all elements necessary to calculate the Medicare payment schedule including the 2002 relative value units (RVUs) and payment policy indicators for each physician service. The data file contains:

- 5-character CPT code
- Modifiers
- Short, medium and long CPT procedural description
- Work RVU
- Facility Practice Expense RVU
- Non-facility Practice Expense RVU
- PLI RVU
- Total Facility RVU
- Total Non-facility RVU
- Global Period covered by the payment

For more information on this product, visit the AMA Press web site at **www.amapress.org** or call 800 621-8335.

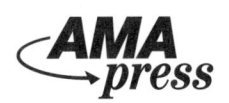

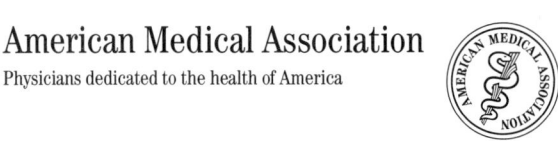

AMA press

American Medical Association
Physicians dedicated to the health of America

Part 1
The Roots of Medicare's RBRVS Payment System

Part 1 provides an introduction to and overview of the way Medicare pays for physicians' services under the RBRVS payment system. Chapter 1 reviews the history of this approach to paying for physicians' services and explains why Medicare adopted this physician payment system. Chapter 2 summarizes the development of the RBRVS payment system legislation, including an overview of its major provisions. Chapter 3 briefly defines the scope of the RBRVS physician payment system and explains which Medicare-covered services are subject to the revised laws and regulations.

Chapter 1
Development of the Resource-Based Relative Value Scale

The resource-based relative value scale (RBRVS) payment schedule was fully phased in on January 1, 1996. The system's most significant changes to Medicare physician payment occurred during 1992, the first year of implementation; however, numerous legislative and regulatory provisions have been adopted since then that have had a major effect on the Medicare RBRVS. In addition, relative payment levels have continued to shift throughout the transition to the full fee schedule. As a result, many physician practices have had to make major readjustments. This 11th revised edition of *The Guide* describes the refinements and legislative changes made to the system during these first 10 years.

The transition to Medicare's RBRVS-based physician payment system began on January 1, 1992, culminating nearly a decade of effort by the medical profession and the government to change the way Medicare pays for physicians' services. Interest in changing the payment system for Part B of Medicare, which covers physicians' services, was initially motivated by steep annual increases in Medicare expenditures. Pressure to change the Part B payment system increased following the 1983 implementation of "prospective pricing" for the hospital portion of Part A, which covers inpatient hospital and nursing home services.

Three factors combined to heighten interest in physician payment reform between 1983 and the adoption of the 1989 payment reform legislation: rising dissatisfaction with Medicare's original payment system; continued escalation in Part B costs; and the promise of a credible basis for a new payment schedule-RBRVS. This chapter describes these three factors, including the rationale for organized medicine's involvement in RBRVS development, the alternative payment reform approaches considered by physicians and the federal government, Phase I of the Harvard University RBRVS study, and the events that followed publication of the Phase I Final Report in the autumn of 1988.

The Profession's Interest in an RBRVS

In 1994, payments for physicians' services comprised about 77% of expenditures for Medicare Part B, with the remainder divided among clinical laboratory services, durable medical equipment, hospital outpatient services, drugs, managed care services, and several other Medicare benefits.[1] The move to an RBRVS physician payment schedule represented the most significant change in Part B since Medicare's inception in 1966. For 25 years, Medicare physician payment was based on a system of "customary, prevailing, and reasonable" (CPR) charges.

The CPR system was designed to pay for physicians' services according to their actual fees, with some adjustments to keep government outlays predictable. It was based on the "usual, customary, and reasonable" (UCR) system used by many private health insurers. Medicare defined "customary" charges as the median of an individual physician's charges for a particular service for a defined period of time. The "prevailing" charge for this service was set at the 90th percentile of the customary charges of all peer physicians in a defined Medicare payment area. (CPR was specialty specific.) The "reasonable" charge was defined as the lowest of the physician's actual fee for the service, that physician's customary charge, or the prevailing charge in the area.

Problems With CPR

Due to the diversity in physicians' fees for the same service, the CPR system allowed for wide variation in the amount Medicare paid for the same service. The insurance companies that process Medicare Part B claims, called Medicare carriers, added to this diversity through their own policies. For example, some carriers paid only one prevailing charge per service, while others paid a different prevailing rate for each physician specialty providing the service. As a result, wide variations in Medicare payment levels developed among geographic areas and physician specialties.

Although these variations initially caused some dissatisfaction within the medical profession, the dissatisfaction reached a crescendo between the mid-1970s and the mid-1980s when Medicare placed a series of controls on CPR reimbursement levels. Designed to stem the growth in program costs, the first of these controls progressively reduced prevailing charges from the 90th to the 75th percentile. It was followed by an extension of the federal government's wage and price freeze on payments for physicians' services.

After lifting the freeze, the government implemented a new control in 1976, when it tied increases in prevailing charges to increases in the Medicare Economic Index (MEI). The MEI is intended to measure annual growth in physicians' practice costs since 1973 (prevailing charges in 1973 were in turn based on 1971 actual charges) as well as general earnings trends in the economy.

The major effect of the price controls and the MEI limit was to make permanent the basic pattern of Medicare prevailing charges that existed in the early 1970s. This pattern remained virtually unchanged until 1992. Payments per service were, therefore, unresponsive to changes in clinical practice and technology. Although compensation levels for new, high-technology procedures were generally commensurate with their high initial cost and limited availability, many physicians believed that payment increases for visits and consultations lagged far behind increases in the complexity and cost to diagnose and manage Medicare patients. Because compensation for new procedures remained relatively high even when their relative costs declined over time and compensation for visits remained relatively low while their relative costs increased, relative payment levels were thought to have become distorted.

Payment levels also remained stable across geographic areas. Consequently, as innovations in clinical practice and technology spread to rural and suburban areas, compensation did not increase. As a result, payment differences among Medicare localities, states, and regions remained, generally reflecting charge patterns that prevailed during the 1970s, despite changes in practice or demographics. Thus, Medicare often paid physicians in neighboring regions and states with similar costs of practice at very different levels for the same service.

As the prevailing charges became increasingly outdated, physicians in primary care specialties and rural areas, in particular, began to call for change. A new set of CPR changes occurred in the 1980s. These included a second freeze on payment levels accompanied by limits on physicians' actual charges and reduced payments for surgical procedures deemed to be "overpriced." The CPR changes brought more calls for payment change to physicians in other specialties and geographic areas and accelerated interest in long-term, comprehensive physician payment reform. Because of the many constraints on CPR, Medicare's physician payment system had become complex, confusing, unpredictable, and unrelated to physicians' actual fees, producing exactly the opposite result from what CPR's architects had intended.

Options for Change

In the mid-1980s, as physician dissatisfaction with CPR continued to grow and government policymakers produced several payment reform proposals, the medical profession faced several options for change:

- modifying CPR;
- extending the new approach introduced for hospitals under Part A of Medicare, diagnosis related groups (DRGs), to physicians' services;
- mandating Medicare's health maintenance organization (HMO) program or other capitation approaches to be the dominant means of payment under Part B; and
- replacing CPR with a payment schedule based on a relative value scale (RVS).

Each option had its supporters and critics. Support was generally divided between physicians who wished to maintain the status quo by modifying CPR and those seeking to develop an indemnity payment schedule based on an RVS.

Under such a schedule, Medicare would pay a standardized "approved amount" for each service regardless of the physician's fee for the service, rather than basing payments on individual physician's fees as they originally had been under CPR. (The Medicare "approved amount" includes both the 80% that Medicare pays and the 20% patient coinsurance.) Although Medicare would pay a standardized approved amount, physicians would still be able to charge patients their full fee. The difference between the Medicare-approved amount and the physician's fee is called the "balance bill."

In an HMO-based system, HMOs receive a monthly Medicare payment for each beneficiary enrolled in the organization. The HMO pays physician and hospital services but usually limits patients' choices of physicians and hospitals.

Under the hospital DRG system, the hospital receives a standardized amount for each patient admitted with a particular diagnosis. The standardized amount represents the average hospital's cost to provide the average bundle of services required to treat patients with that diagnosis. Although a physician DRG system would vary from the hospital DRG system, the basic concept of bundling or packaging services covered by a single payment would be the same.

Of the four major payment reform options, only CPR and a payment schedule are fee-for-service systems. Many medical professionals felt that preserving fee-for-service under Medicare was critical to protecting physicians' clinical and professional autonomy. Although the AMA supported a pluralistic payment system, it believed that adopting physician DRGs or mandatory capitation for Medicare, given the program's size, would severely threaten physicians' ability to use their own professional judgment in patient-care decisions.

Historically, the AMA had also opposed policies to restrict or eliminate physicians' ability to charge patients the difference between their fee and the Medicare-approved amount. A DRG- or capitation-based system for physicians' services would, by definition, impose mandatory assignment, a policy requiring physicians to accept the Medicare-approved amount as payment in full, thereby prohibiting balance billing.

To preserve fee-for-service as a viable option under Medicare, the AMA pursued two parallel tracks. First, using lobbying efforts to influence legislation and litigation challenging the legality of various statutory provisions, it tried to eliminate or mitigate the most onerous aspects of CPR, including the fee limits, the Physician Participation Program (see Chapter 9), and the payment reductions. Second, it sought to develop a new RVS and the policy basis for its implementation, if appropriate. The first track achieved only limited success because Congress was reluctant to enact changes that would increase beneficiary expenses, and the courts upheld congressional authority to limit physicians' fees.[2]

The basis for the RVS. An RVS is a list of physicians' services ranked according to "value," with the value defined with respect to the basis for the scale. Using an RVS as a basis for determining payments and fees is a familiar concept for physicians and insurers. The California Medical Association developed the first RVS in 1956 and updated it regularly until 1974. Beginning in 1969, the California Relative Value Studies (CRVS) were based on median charges reported by California Blue Shield. Physicians used the CRVS to set fee schedules, and a number of state Medicaid programs, Blue Cross/Blue Shield plans, and commercial insurers used it to establish physician payment rates. In the late 1970s, however, Federal Trade Commission (FTC) actions raised concern that the CRVS might violate antitrust law, leading the California Medical Association to suspend updating and distributing the CRVS.

Although many possible options existed for constructing a new RVS in the mid-1980s, the medical profession favored either a charge-based or a resource-based RVS. In a charge-based RVS, services are ranked according to the average fee for the service, the average Medicare prevailing charge, or some other charge basis. For example, if the average charge for service A is twice the charge for service B, the relative value for service A would be twice that of service B.

In a resource-based RVS, services are ranked according to the relative costs of the resources required to provide them. For example, suppose service A generally takes twice as long to provide, is twice as difficult, and requires twice as much overhead expense (such as nonphysician personnel, office space, and equipment) as service B. Then the relative value of service A in an RBRVS is twice that of service B.

An RVS must be multiplied by a dollar conversion factor to become a payment schedule. For example, if the relative value for service A is 200 and for service B is 100, a conversion factor of $2 yields a payment of $400 for service A and $200 for service B. Likewise, a conversion factor of $0.50 yields payments of $100 for A, $50 for B, and so on.

Most surgical specialty societies supported development of a charge-based RVS. These groups believed that physicians' fees provided the best basis for determining relative worth because fees reflected both the physician's cost of providing the service and the value of the service to patients. In addition, with readily available data, a charge-based RVS could easily become the basis for a payment schedule, thereby improving the degree of national standardization and eliminating the wide payment variations. However, experience with portions of the Harvard RBRVS study that used charge data demonstrated that such data contained errors and often produced anomalous and unreasonable results.

Most nonprocedural specialty societies also considered these factors but reached a different conclusion, which the AMA shared. These groups believed that in a well-functioning market, physicians' relative charges would reflect their relative costs. In their view, however, Medicare payment levels did not reflect the prices that would emerge from a well-functioning market. They believed that the wide gap between payments for visits and payments for procedures, as well as the wide variations in payments for the same service between geographic areas and specialties, failed to reflect differences in the costs of the resources necessary to provide them. They also believed that the constraints on Medicare payments, including the freezes, reductions in prevailing charges, and tying annual updates to the MEI, had further distorted charges, so that Medicare charges would not provide an appropriate basis for a new RVS.

After weighing all of these factors, the AMA decided to drop a charge-based RVS, concluding that it was likely to preserve the same historical charge pattern that generated the dissatisfaction with CPR. The AMA believed that an RVS based on relative resource costs was more likely to equitably cover physicians' costs of caring for Medicare patients. In choosing to pursue development of an RBRVS, the AMA also emphasized that:

- any RVS-based payment system must reflect the often substantial variations in practice costs between geographic areas; and
- based on its long-standing policy, it would strongly oppose any newly developed payment system that required physicians to accept the Medicare-approved amount as payment in full.

The AMA proposal to develop an RBRVS. The AMA believed that organized medicine's participation in the development of an RBRVS was a key factor in physician acceptance of such a system. In January 1985, after discussing the issue with the national medical specialty societies, the AMA submitted a proposal to the Centers for Medicare and Medicaid Services (CMS) (formerly known as the Health Care Financing Administration, the government agency responsible for administering the Medicare program) to develop a new RVS based on resource costs with extensive involvement of organized medicine and practicing physicians. Responding 2 months later, CMS said that despite its desire to involve organized medicine in developing an RBRVS, antitrust considerations raised by the FTC precluded a direct contract between CMS and a physicians' organization.

Because CMS had stated its intention to contract with a university or independent research center instead of a medical organization, the AMA discussed the possibility of jointly developing an RBRVS with several major universities. After careful consideration, the AMA accepted a Harvard University School of Public Health proposal for a "National Study of Resource-Based Relative Value Scales for Physician Services." It was similar to the AMA's earlier proposal and outlined an extensive role for the medical profession. With funding by CMS, Harvard began its study in December 1985.

The Government's Interest in an RBRVS

Through 1983, efforts to curtail the growth in Medicare spending focused principally on reducing expenditures for inpatient hospital care. Although Part B expenditures had been rising steeply each year, physicians' services accounted for only about 22% of Medicare spending, while hospital services accounted for about 70%. Hospital cost containment efforts, which curbed construction, admissions, length of stay, and intensity of services, had greater potential to reduce total Medicare spending than efforts to reduce spending on physicians' services.

The prospective pricing system (PPS), introduced in 1983 to pay for Medicare patients' hospital costs, provides a standardized payment for each hospital admission, with variations to reflect geographic differences in wage rates and hospital location (urban or rural). The PPS authorized additional payment for "outlier" cases requiring exceptionally long stays or high costs. Admissions are categorized according to approximately 500 DRGs with payment based on the national average cost of hospital care for patients with a particular diagnosis.

The PPS assumes that hospitals care for patients whose severity levels range from mild to high within each DRG. While it is recognized that some patients' care will cost more than others, in the long run the cost of caring for all patients within a DRG is expected to equal the average approximate payment for the DRG. Because the DRG payment is the same regardless of the hospital's actual cost to provide care for a particular patient, prospective pricing provides an incentive for hospitals to improve their cost-efficiency.

Government policymakers view PPS as a success because the average annual growth rate in Medicare expenditures for inpatient hospital care decreased from 18% between 1975 and 1982 to 7% between 1983 and 1990. However, the extent to which PPS is solely responsible for this trend is unclear. In addition, those who believe that DRGs may adversely affect quality of care have been critical of PPS.

Governmental Options for Change

After the introduction of prospective pricing, Congress and the Reagan administration turned their attention to reducing growth in Medicare spending for physicians' services, and the CPR system came under increasing attack. However, many physicians believed that CPR payments for primary care services and services provided in rural areas were inequitable. Although many members of Congress shared that view, other government and health policy officials criticized CPR as being inflationary. They argued that fee-for-service medicine encouraged overuse of services and that CPR encouraged overpricing of services, especially invasive and high-technology services.

Buoyed by the successful implementation of DRGs for hospitals, the government began exploring the feasibility of DRGs for physicians. In 1983, as part of the same law that created the prospective pricing system for hospitals, Congress mandated that CMS study physician DRGs for Medicare and submit its report with recommendations by 1985.

In 1985, Congress also gave CMS authority to enroll Medicare beneficiaries in HMOs on a "risk-sharing" capitation basis. Previously, CMS could only enroll Medicare patients in HMOs using cost-based contracts, meaning that the HMO's capitation payment would rise or fall at year end depending on the actual cost of the services provided to Medicare enrollees. Under risk-sharing, if costs incurred by the HMO were less than the capitation payment, the HMO could retain up to 50% of the savings, but it would have to absorb 100% of any losses. *By 1988, about 3% of Medicare beneficiaries had enrolled in HMOs and by 1999 that number had increased to over 17% of Medicare beneficiaries.*

Expansion of HMOs for Medicare was partially a response to papers by health economists, published in the early 1980s, stating that the regulatory efforts of the 1970s had failed to control rising health care costs and calling instead for more competition in health care. The HMOs were viewed as the foundation of a more competitive system, in which employees and individuals enrolled in government entitlement programs could choose from a variety of HMO-type plans. Competition between these plans for enrollees would provide incentives for the plans to maintain low costs and premiums while providing high quality of care and amenities not offered by the Medicare fee-for-service program. The CMS developed a strategy for increasing Medicare enrollment in HMOs and HMO-type plans, which it called the Private Health Plan Option. Agency interest in such health plans, as well as among members of Congress, has accelerated in the current health care environment. Despite strong support in Congress and the administration for mandating either DRG or HMO options for Medicare, the potential problems these options presented were also well known. For example, DRGs for physicians would be administratively complex and could produce serious inequities. In contrast to the approximately 490 DRGs for about 6500 hospitals, more than 7000 codes describe the services that more than 500,000 physicians provide. Even if a DRG system could be developed for physicians' services, averaging DRG payments over the patient mix of a physician practice would be more difficult than it is for hospitals.

Recognizing these problems, and responding to strong pressure from the AMA and organized medicine, Congress continued to explore fee-for-service options for Medicare physician payment reform. In the Consolidated Omnibus Budget Reconciliation Act of 1985 (COBRA, Public Law 99-272), Congress mandated that the secretary of Health and Human Services (HHS) develop an RBRVS and report on it to Congress by July 1, 1987. Simultaneously, however, legislation had been introduced in Congress to establish a DRG payment system for the major hospital-based physician specialties: radiologists, anesthesiologists, and pathologists.

Establishing the Physician Payment Review Commission

To evaluate the various physician payment reform options and to advise Congress, COBRA also created the Physician Payment Review Commission (PPRC). Composed of physicians, health policy researchers, and patient representatives, the PPRC's 13 members were nominated by the congressional Office of Technology Assessment. The PPRC's first meeting took place in November 1986.

The PPRC reviewed the options for Medicare payment reform, including changes in CPR, physician DRGs, and expansion of capitation plans. It also studied international experience with physician payment, including the payment systems of Germany and Canada. The Commission's First Annual Report to Congress, submitted March 1, 1987, endorsed the concept of a payment schedule for Medicare. One year later, the PPRC recommended that the payment schedule be based on an RBRVS. A minority opinion signed by three commissioners endorsed the concept of a Medicare payment schedule, but opposed the decision to base the schedule on relative resource costs because the RBRVS study had not yet been completed.

The Harvard RBRVS Study

With Congress considering proposals for physician DRGs and the Reagan administration advocating its Private Health Plan Option for Medicare, the PPRC's 1987 endorsement of an RBRVS-based payment schedule gave a much-needed boost to the medical profession's efforts to preserve fee-for-service payment under Medicare. The other major factor that bolstered support for this payment reform alternative was the

Harvard University RBRVS study. In addition to its intense lobbying and grassroots efforts, the AMA's argument that Congress should wait for results of the study before undertaking any major reform of Medicare's payment system was a crucial element in defeating proposals for physician DRGs.

The principal investigators in the Harvard study, William C. Hsiao, PhD, and Peter Braun, MD, had conducted previous studies that provided the foundation for the CMS-funded RBRVS study. In a 1979 exploratory study, Hsiao and William Stason, MD, attempted to rank 27 physicians' services provided by five specialties according to the time each service required and the complexity of each unit of time. Study results suggested that physicians had difficulty distinguishing between duration and complexity in ranking services. Consequently, the study results were considered unreliable. In a second study conducted by Hsiao and Braun in 1984, physicians directly ranked the overall work involved in their services without distinguishing between time and complexity. Although this study produced more consistent rankings, problems developed with the scale that was used (ie, the closed numeric scale, from 1 to 100, led to unreasonably low values for lengthy procedures).

In the national study, which began in 1985, CMS initially funded the Harvard team to develop an RBRVS for 12 physician specialties:

- anesthesiology;
- family practice;
- general surgery;
- internal medicine;
- obstetrics and gynecology;
- ophthalmology;
- orthopedic surgery;
- otolaryngology;
- pathology;
- radiology;
- thoracic and cardiovascular surgery; and
- urology.

Six additional specialties were funded independently and included in the study at the request of the relevant national medical specialty societies:

- allergy and immunology;
- dermatology;
- oral and maxillofacial surgery;
- pediatrics;
- psychiatry; and
- rheumatology.

The scope of what came to be known as Phase I of the study was considerably broader than previous studies. Its objectives were to develop an RBRVS for each of the 18 specialties included in the study and to combine the specialty-specific scales into a single cross-specialty RBRVS. Although COBRA required the secretary of HHS to report to Congress on the development of this cross-specialty RBRVS by July 1, 1987, the Omnibus Budget Reconciliation Act of 1986 (OBRA 86, PL 99-509) extended the report's submission date until July 1, 1989. The following year, Congress expanded the study mandate to include an additional 15 specialties, which became Phase II of the Harvard study. Phase III refined estimates from the earlier phases and expanded the RBRVS to include the remaining services coded by the Current Procedural Terminology (CPT) system. Because Phase III was not completed by the January 1, 1992, implementation date, CMS established a process involving carrier medical directors (CMDs) to assign work relative value units (RVUs) to about 800 services for which Phase I and II data were not available. Phase III data were also used as part of CMS's refinement process for work RVUs first published in the 1992 Final Notice as part of the November 25, 1992, *Federal Register*. The study's methods and results are described in detail in Chapter 4.

The AMA's Role in the RBRVS Study

Under the terms of its subcontract from Harvard, the AMA's major role in the RBRVS study was to serve as a liaison between the Harvard researchers, organized medicine, and practicing physicians. The AMA worked with the national medical specialty societies representing the studied specialties to secure physician nominations to the project's Technical Consulting Groups. These groups studied specialty-provided advice to the researchers, helped to design the study's survey of practicing physicians, and reviewed and commented on its results.

Drawing on its Physician Masterfile, the AMA also supplied representative national samples of practicing physicians in each of the studied specialties. Throughout Phases I and II, the AMA advised the Harvard researchers, and an AMA representative attended every meeting of the Technical Consulting Groups.

The Association's liaison role ensured that the RBRVS was based on the experience of a representative national sample of practicing physicians and that the specialty societies, through representation on the Technical Consulting Groups, were involved in important aspects of the development of relative values for their specialties. Involvement of both the AMA and the specialty societies also enhanced the study's credibility with practicing physicians and helped to increase its acceptance among physicians after results became available.

One additional benefit of organized medicine's involvement in the study was the high level of communication about the study, its results, and its policy implications. From 1985 to

1991, the front page of American Medical News covered this subject at least six times each year. Articles also appeared regularly in the *Journal of the American Medical Association (JAMA)*, specialty journals such as *The Internist* and the *Bulletin of the American College of Surgeons,* state journals such as *Ohio Medicine,* and major newspapers, including the *New York Times.*

Reaction to the Completion of Phase I

On September 29, 1988, nearly 3 years after the study's inception, Harvard submitted its final report of Phase I of the RBRVS study to CMS. An overview of the study ran simultaneously in the *New England Journal of Medicine.* The entire October 28, 1988, issue of *JAMA* was devoted to the study. In addition to a series of articles on the study's methods and results, as well as simulations of the impact of a payment schedule based on the Phase I results, the *JAMA* issue included editorials by AMA, CMS, and PPRC leaders.

With completion of Phase I, the debate over whether Medicare should adopt an RBRVS-based payment schedule for Part B reached a pivotal moment. There were passionate views on all sides. Many rural and primary care physicians called for immediate adoption of a new Medicare payment system; surgeons viewed the study more cautiously. Even though CMS had funded the study, then-CMS Administrator William R. Roper, MD, expressed several reservations about continuing fee-for-service payment under Medicare:

"... we face substantial problems in controlling the overall growth in expenditures for physicians. A fee schedule based on a relative value scale, no matter how carefully constructed, cannot be expected to address the growth in the volume and intensity of services. Whatever their merits, fee-for-service systems do not provide physicians with incentives to control this growth."[3]

The AMA's reaction to the study affirmed its belief that Medicare should adopt a payment schedule based on an appropriate RBRVS, but it reserved judgment about whether the Harvard study should serve that purpose. In his *JAMA* editorial on the subject, James S. Todd, MD, then the AMA's Senior Deputy Executive Vice President, stated: "We went into this study with our eyes open. We have not wavered in our support for completing this study, or in our insistence that the AMA has no prior commitment to support its results or implementation." He went on to state:

"... there must be external review and validation of the study's credibility, reliability, and validity. No less important will be the consideration of whether and how this academic research should be translated into the cold, hard realities of Medicare policy. The medical profession must and will assume a leading role in both of these endeavors."[4]

AMA Policy on the RBRVS Study

Immediately after the study's release, the AMA began an intensive evaluation to determine whether it could support the Harvard RBRVS as the basis for a Medicare payment schedule. It conducted an internal evaluation of the study's final report and also retained the Consolidated Consulting Group, Inc, to provide an independent assessment of the RBRVS study. In November 1988, the Association convened a meeting of 300 representatives of national medical specialty societies, state medical associations, and county medical societies to solicit their views on the study. To draft the AMA's policy positions on the RBRVS and related implementation issues, the AMA Board of Trustees appointed a Physician Payment Task Force comprising members of the Board and the AMA Councils on Medical Service and Legislation.

After considering the recommendations of this task force, findings from the internal and external reviews of the study, and the views of medical society representatives, the AMA Board of Trustees prepared a 40-page report containing its recommendations on the RBRVS, balance billing, geographic adjustments, and other policy issues. These recommendations became the focus of a hearing at the December 1988 meeting of the AMA's House of Delegates at which more than 100 delegates testified.[5]

A principal theme of this testimony was the delegates' desire to maintain the AMA's leadership role in Medicare physician payment reform. Recognizing that change was coming, the key question was whether the change would be acceptable to the profession or a government-designed system without input from the medical profession. They also recognized that organized medicine would need to remain unified for the AMA's policy proposals to be politically viable.

After a committee of the delegates amended the Board's recommendations to reflect the testimony presented at the hearing, the full House of Delegates unanimously adopted the revised recommendations. Unanimity was possible only because so many groups within the House agreed to compromise on policies that might concern their own specialty or locality in order to create a new payment system that would serve the interests of the entire medical profession.

The key policy the AMA adopted at the December 1988 meeting was that the "Harvard RBRVS study and data, when sufficiently expanded, corrected, and refined, would provide an acceptable basis for a Medicare indemnity payment system." In addition, this policy specified which parts of the study needed improvement and acknowledged that specialties whose RBRVS data had significant, documented technical deficiencies needed to be restudied. The AMA committed itself to work with Harvard, the national medical specialty societies, CMS, Congress, and the PPRC to obtain the necessary refinements and modifications.

Besides these policies on the Harvard RBRVS study, the AMA's recommendations provided a blueprint for all the major features of a new Medicare physician payment system:

- Payment schedule amounts should be adjusted to reflect geographic differences in physicians' practice costs, such as office rent and wages of nonphysician personnel.
- Geographic differences in the costs of professional liability insurance (PLI) would be especially important, and these differences should be reflected separately from other practice costs. A transition period should be part of any new system to minimize disruptions in patient care and access.
- Organized medicine would seek to play a major role in updating the RBRVS.

The AMA reemphasized its long-standing policy on balance billing that physicians should have the right to decide on a claim-by-claim basis whether to accept the Medicare approved amount (including the patient's 20% coinsurance) as payment in full. The Association also stated its intention to oppose any attempt to use implementation of an RBRVS-based system as a means to obtain federal budget savings, and to oppose "expenditure targets" for Medicare—a scheme that would automatically tie the payment schedule's monetary conversion factor to projected increases in utilization of services. Finally, the AMA sought to eliminate differences between specialties in payment for the same service. Part 2 (Chapters 4–9) discusses each of these policy issues in greater detail.

The PPRC's Recommendations

Immediately after this momentous House of Delegates meeting, the Association began advocating its Medicare physician payment reform policies before the PPRC, hoping to influence the recommendations the Commission would include in its 1989 Annual Report to Congress. These advocacy efforts were largely successful, and the Commission's recommendations, with several noteworthy exceptions, closely paralleled those of the AMA. Like the AMA, the PPRC endorsed the Harvard RBRVS study as the basis for a new Medicare payment schedule. Its list of necessary improvements was similar to those identified by the Association. It also recommended using adjustment factors to reflect geographic differences in practice costs, eliminating specialty differentials, and opposing the use of the RBRVS's initial conversion factor to obtain budget savings.

The views of organized medicine and those of the PPRC sharply diverged, however, on two policies: balance billing and expenditure targets. Given the widespread support for mandated assignment, which would have required physicians to accept the Medicare approved amount as payment in full, the AMA was pleased that the PPRC did not make such a recommendation. Against strong AMA opposition, however, the Commission did recommend placing percentage limits on the amount physicians could charge above the Medicare approved amount, although it did not specify a percentage. In contrast, the AMA believed that Medicare should establish only what it would pay and allow physicians to determine what they would charge.

The Commission's recommendation for a Medicare expenditure target was essentially its response to those who criticized fee-for-service payment systems because they did not control growth in costs or utilization. The AMA believed, in contrast, that an expenditure target could adversely affect patient access, and that profession-developed practice parameters held considerably more promise for reducing unnecessary utilization. Despite these differences, the AMA and PPRC core recommendations advanced the same fundamental reform: a Medicare payment schedule based on an expanded and refined Harvard RBRVS, with appropriate adjustments for geographic differences in practice costs and PLI costs. Congress had been under increasing pressure to take action to stem the flight of physicians from rural areas and primary care specialties and to change Medicare's physician payment system rather than continue its piecemeal, budget-driven approach. In early 1989, these factors heightened congressional interest in an RBRVS-based system, prompting initial legislative proposals from three different congressional subcommittees, which eventually became the foundation for the current fee-for-service payment system.

Medicare Reform

Succeeding chapters describe the legislative and regulatory issues that arose between 1992 and 1999 affecting Medicare RBRVS implementation. Some of the most significant changes to the system were adopted in 1994 under the OBRA 93, which altered the Medicare Volume Performance Standard (MVPS) update process. The legislation sought to slow the growth in Medicare spending, in part, by restricting physician payment increases. Support for significant legislative reform of the Medicare program continued to build during 1996. Such support was driven by the program's escalating costs, which were projected to outpace the ability of the federal government to pay them. Medicare costs will continue to grow due to a swiftly growing elderly population that will further swell with the addition of the baby-boom generation; increased longevity of Medicare beneficiaries; and expanding medical technologies.

Republican-led efforts to reform the Medicare program failed in 1996, due to a presidential veto. The basis for compromise, however, was established and led to enactment of significant legislative reform in 1997. The Balanced Budget Act of 1997, signed by President Clinton in August 1997, calls for systemic Medicare program changes, including a wider array of health plan choices for beneficiaries, referred to as Medicare+Choice or Medicare Part C. It also alters the methodology for determining traditional fee-for-service payments under the Medicare RBRVS and permits physicians to furnish health care services to Medicare patients on a private fee-for-service basis. Under the Balanced Budget Act, Medicare beneficiaries may elect to receive benefits through either of two options:

1) the traditional Medicare fee-for-service program, or
2) Medicare+Choice plan.

Medicare+Choice plans include:
- Health Maintenance Organizations (HMOs)
- Private fee-for-service plans;
- Combination of a Medical Savings Account (MSA) coupled with a catastrophic insurance policy;
- Provider Sponsored Organizations (PSOs); and
- Preferred Provider Organizations (PPOs).

Until the end of 2001, Medicare beneficiaries can enroll and disenroll from Medicare+Choice plans at any time. However, beginning in January 2002, elections will be limited. This change in election period limitations is known as "lock-in." In particular, beginning in 2002, beneficiaries may only elect plans during the Annual Election Period (AEP) in November, once during the Open Enrollment Period (OEP) from January through June, or at any time during a Special Election Period. In 2003, the OEP is reduced in length and lasts from January through March. In general, at all other times during the year, a Medicare beneficiary cannot enroll in a new plan and cannot disenroll to traditional Medicare. Beneficiaries will be able to make plan changes in some circumstances, such as when they move or if their plan terminates its contract.

Under Medicare+Choice, monthly premiums are to be paid from the Medicare trust fund on behalf of beneficiaries to the health plan they select. Such payments are based on a capitation rate calculated annually for each payment area and adjusted for each enrollee based on such factors as age, disability status, gender, and institutional status. The program also initiates the concept of a defined contribution under a new MSA option. A brief description of each Medicare+Choice option follows. The number of choices varies greatly depending on where a patient lives.

Organizations that offer Medicare+Choice plans to beneficiaries are private companies that voluntarily enter into 12-month contracts and each year have the opportunity to choose whether or not to renew their contracts. Details concerning changes to the traditional Medicare program appear in the designated chapters.

Traditional fee-for-service. Physician payments under the Medicare RBRVS will be determined according to a single conversion factor of $36.1992, effective January 1, 2002. Updates to the conversion factor will be determined by a sustainable growth rate based on growth in real gross domestic product.

The sustainable growth rate methodology is described more fully in Chapter 10. Implementation of resource-based practice expenses began on January 1, 1999, and will be fully implemented on January 1, 2002. Practice expense relative values for 1999 and beyond will include separate values depending on where the service is performed. Services provided in a physician's office are assigned a nonfacility practice expense RVU while services performed in a hospital and other settings are assigned a facility practice expense RVU. These and other changes to practice expense relative values are discussed in Chapter 5.

Private fee-for-service plan. The legislation establishes a new "private fee-for-service" plan option. Such a plan will reimburse hospitals, physicians, and other health care providers at a rate determined by the plan on a fee-for-service basis without placing the provider at financial risk; will not vary such rates for physicians and other providers according to utilization rates; and will not restrict physician participation in such plans as long as they are authorized to provide the covered services and agree to accept the terms and conditions of payment established by the plan.

Provider-sponsored organization. A PSO is defined as a public or private entity that is organized and operated by a health care provider or group of affiliated providers; provides a substantial proportion of the required health care services under the contract directly through the providers; and maintains a majority interest by the affiliated providers who share substantial financial risk. Although Medicare+Choice organizations must be organized and licensed under state law as risk-bearing entities, the legislation creates an exception for PSOs. PSOs could apply to the federal government for a waiver of certain state licensing requirements, for example, if the state failed to complete action on a licensing application within a specified period of time or if the state denied such an application. Waivers will be effective only for 3 years and cannot be renewed. They also will not apply in any other state.

Coordinated care plan. Coordinated care plans include but are not limited to HMOs, with or without a point-of-service option, and PPOs. All cost contracting arrangements were eliminated effective January 1999. Many of the new requirements under Medicare+Choice most significantly affect coordinated care plans. These plans are currently widespread and, together with traditional fee-for-service, continue to be the most widely available option to beneficiaries.

Medical savings account demonstration project. A 4-year demonstration project was organized by CMS to test beneficiary enrollment in MSA plans. Up to 390,000 Medicare beneficiaries are permitted to select this option, which began in October 1998.

Private Contracting

In addition to these Medicare+Choice options, the Balanced Budget Act permits physicians and their Medicare patients to enter into private contracts to provide health care services. Private contracting arrangements are permitted only if certain conditions are met, including: 1) the physician does not receive Medicare payment for any items or services, either directly from Medicare or on a capitated basis; 2) inclusion in the contract of specified beneficiary protections, such as disclosure that Medicare balance billing requirements will not apply and the patient has the right to receive items and services offered by other physicians participating in Medicare; 3) physician agreement through an affidavit filed with CMS to file no Medicare claims for any services provided to Medicare patients for a 2-year period. Details on the new private contracting provisions are provided in Chapter 12.

New Commissions

The Balanced Budget Act established a new National Bipartisan Commission on the Future of Medicare that was charged with recommending reforms that would ensure the long term solvency of the Medicare program. The Commission disbanded in March after failing by one vote to achieve agreement on proposed reforms. However, some of its members have proposed legislation that would make Medicare reforms similar to some of those that have been suggested by the AMA, including the use of government contributions to finance individually owned coverage.

The BBA also created a new Medicare Payment Advisory Commission (MedPAC) to advise Congress on Medicare payment policies. The new Commission merged the roles of PPRC and the Prospective Payment Assessment Commission, which had been formed to advise Congress on payments to hospitals and other facilities. As part of its March 1999 report, MedPAC called for a series of AMA-backed changes in the SGR methodology and several of these changes were adopted by Congress. These include a provision that will reduce oscillation between positive and negative Medicare physician fee updates as well as one that requires that each spring CMS must provide and MedPAC must comment on the projected SGR and physician update for the following year. In addition, Congress directed the Agency for Health Care Policy Research and MedPAC to look at how the SGR could be modified to account for changes in technology, site of service, and beneficiary mix.

References and Notes

1. Committee on Ways and Means. *Overview of Entitlement Programs: 1994 Green Book.* Washington, DC: Committee on Ways and Means; 1994:1075.

2. *American Medical Association, et al v Bowen,* US Court of Appeals, Fifth Circuit, No. 87-1755, October 14, 1988. 857 FW 267 (5th Cir 1988).

   American Medical Association, et al v Bowen, US District Court, Northern District of Texas, Dallas Div, No. 3-86-3181-H, January 20, 1987. 659 FSupp 1143 (ND Tex 1987).

   Massachusetts Medical Society, et al v Dukakis, US District Court, District of Massachusetts, No. 85-4312-K, June 5, 1986. 637 FSupp 684 (DMass 1986).

   Massachusetts Medical Society, et al v Dukakis, US Court of Appeals, First Circuit, No. 86-1575, March 30, 1987. 815 FW 790 (1st Cir 1987), cert denied, 484 US 896 (1987).

   Whitney v Heckler, US Court of Appeals, 11th Circuit, No. 85-8129, January 22, 1986. 780 FW 963 (11th Cir 1986), cert denied, 479 US 813 (1986).

   Whitney v Heckler, US District Court, Northern District of Georgia, Atlanta Division, No. C84-1926, February 4, 1985. 603 FSupp 821 (ND Ga 1985).

   American Medical Association, et al v Heckler, US District Court, Southern District of Indiana, Indianapolis Division, No. IP 84-1317-C, April 18, 1985. 606 FSupp 1422 (SD Ind 1985).

   Pennsylvania Medical Society v Marconis, 755 FSupp 1305 (WD Pa), aff'd, 942 FW 842 (3rd Cir 1991).

   Medical Society of the State of New York v Cuomo, 1991 US Dist LEXIS 16405 (SDNY 1991).

3. Roper WR. Perspectives on physician payment reform. *N Engl J Med.* 1988;319:866.

4. Todd JS. At last, a rational way to pay for physicians' services? *JAMA.* 1988;260:2439-2440.

5. The AMA's House of Delegates comprises 477 voting representatives of all 50 states, as well as Puerto Rico; 124 national medical specialty societies; and representatives of special groups such as the Medical Students Staff Section, Organized Medical Staff Section, and the Young Physicians Section. The House is therefore an extremely democratic organization representing all types of physicians from all areas of the country.

Chapter 2
Legislation Creating the Medicare RBRVS Payment System

In 1989, after years of debate within the medical profession about the distortions in historical charges, battles with Congress and the administration over rising expenditures, and a 4-year wait for the results of the Harvard resource-based relative value scale (RBRVS) study, Congress finally enacted a new Medicare physician payment system. The process that led to enactment of the payment reform legislation was in many ways more historic than the law itself: the partnership forged between the medical profession, beneficiary groups, the Congress, and the Bush administration was unprecedented in the development of US health policy. The law resulting from this process gave participants a reasonable measure of what they had sought:

- an RBRVS-based payment schedule for physicians that narrowed specialty and geographic differences and retained some balance billing;
- continued balance billing limits for patients; and
- a system for monitoring expenditure increases for the government.

This chapter provides a brief history and an overview of the physician payment reform legislation and the regulations promulgated since its enactment.

The Prescription for Changing the Medicare Physician Payment System

During the spring of 1989, the AMA, the Physician Payment Review Commission (PPRC), Centers for Medicare and Medicaid Services (CMS) (formerly the Health Care Financing Administration), and others presented their recommendations at several congressional hearings on Medicare physician payment reform. As the 1989 budget reconciliation process began, all three congressional subcommittees with jurisdiction over the Medicare program presented proposals for such a reform for inclusion in what became the Omnibus Budget Reconciliation Act of 1989 (OBRA 89, PL 101-239):

- the Health Subcommittee of the House Ways and Means Committee;
- the Subcommittee on Health and the Environment of the House Energy and Commerce Committee; and
- the Subcommittee on Medicare and Long Term Care of the Senate Finance Committee.

From the outset, the process of developing the payment reform legislation was controversial. The key parties to the legislative process presented markedly different initial proposals. Accepting the consensus between the AMA and the PPRC, however, all three included a geographically adjusted payment schedule based on an RBRVS as their core.

The two most critical areas of contention for physicians were expenditure targets and balance billing limits. Although the AMA continued to oppose billing limits within Congress, balance billing limits were not an issue, only the specific percentage. Because Congress had enacted limits on Medicare balance billing under "customary, prevailing, and reasonable" (CPR) several years earlier (the maximum allowable actual charges, or MAACs), balance billing limits were considered a continuation of an existing policy rather than a completely new proposal. Moreover, balance billing limitations were necessary to obtain support for payment reform from beneficiary organizations, such as the American Association of Retired Persons.

The AMA opposed expenditure targets, believing they would simply reduce payment reform to another federal budget cutting tool. Under the Ways and Means provision, if the annual increase in Medicare expenditures exceeded a predetermined target increase, payments would automatically be reduced to recoup the overage. At the AMA's urging, the Energy and Commerce bill did not contain an expenditure target provision. Throughout the summer and fall of 1989, the AMA and the specialty societies worked closely with the three committees to forge a bill they all could support. As a result of this unprecedented joint effort by organized medicine, Congress, and the administration, the Senate finance bill emerged with a provision for a Medicare Volume Performance Standard (MVPS), which addressed the difficult issue of increases in utilization but eliminated the most objectionable aspects of the expenditure target proposal.

OBRA 89 Physician Payment Reform Provisions

In December 1989, Congress passed and President Bush signed OBRA 89, enacting the Medicare physician payment reform provisions into law. The legislation called for a payment schedule based on an RBRVS composed of three components:

- the relative physician work involved in providing a service;
- practice expenses; and
- professional liability insurance (PLI) costs.

The OBRA 89 defined most key features of Medicare's new payment system for physicians' services:

- a 5-year transition to the new system beginning on January 1, 1992;
- adjusting each component of the three RBRVS components for each service for geographic differences in resource costs;
- eliminating specialty differentials in payment for the same service;
- calculating a "budget neutral" conversion factor for 1992 that would neither increase nor decrease Medicare expenditures from what they would have been under a continuation of CPR;
- a process for determining the annual update in the conversion factor;
- tighter limits on balance billing beginning in 1991; and
- an MVPS to help Congress understand and respond to increases in the volume and intensity of services provided to Medicare beneficiaries.

Each of these key legislative provisions is described briefly below; the components of the payment system are described in greater detail in Parts 2 and 3 (Chapters 4 through 11).

The RBRVS

As the AMA and PPRC had recommended, the physician work component of the RBRVS was to be based (implicitly) on data from the Harvard study, and the 1992 start date allowed Phase II of this study to be completed and reviewed prior to implementation. Physician work refers to the physician's individual effort in providing the service: the physician's time, the technical difficulty of the procedure, the average severity of the patient's medical problems, and the physical and mental effort required. A serious shortcoming in Phase I of the Harvard study was its approach to estimating physicians' relative practice costs. The legislation therefore provided a different method to determine the relative values for this component and for the PLI component.

In the Harvard study, the practice cost relative value of a service was related to the physician work relative value. In the transition to an RBRVS-based payment schedule, such an approach would mean that if the relative work of a service would lead to a reduction in its Medicare payment level, the relative practice costs would reduce the payment for the service even more. Both the AMA and the PPRC had identified this method as unfair and technically flawed. Their concern was that if physicians were not adequately compensated for their overhead costs, patient access would be impaired.

The practice cost method included in OBRA 89 separated practice costs from physician work, and attempted to maintain the total practice cost revenue of a physician specialty at roughly the same as it had been under CPR. Practice cost relative values were, therefore, based on the average proportion of a specialty's overall revenues devoted to practice expenses as a percentage of the average Medicare payment under CPR. For example, if practice costs on average account for 45% of general surgeons' gross revenue, for a service that is provided only by general surgeons and for which the average Medicare approved amount under CPR was $1000, the practice cost component of the new payment schedule would be about $450. The actual calculation is a bit more complicated with other factors coming into play. However, the example illustrates the basic idea.

The PLI relative values were also determined in the same fashion; they were based on the average proportion of a specialty's overall revenues that is devoted to PLI costs as a percentage of the average Medicare approved amount under CPR. For instance, if the PLI cost percentage in the above example was 5%, the PLI component of the new payment schedule would have been approximately $50. Although a number of concerns about this method have surfaced during the last 6 years, two factors account for the wide support it received when OBRA 89 was drafted. First, it was considered more equitable than the Harvard study's method; and second, no other alternatives would have been ready for 1992 implementation. In 2000, CMS implemented resource-based PLI relatives. The methodology used is described in Chapter 6.

In response to these concerns, Congress adopted legislation in 1994 that required the development of resource-based practice expenses, with full implementation in 1998. Since that time, however, new legislation signed by President Clinton in August 1997 revised the implementation timeline. The Balanced Budget Act of 1997 called for the CMS to collect additional data for use in developing the new practice expenses. Proposed values were published in May 1998, with a 60-day period for public comment. CMS received over 14,000 comments on its proposed rule and issued its Final Rule on November 2, 1998. CMS began implementation of the new practice expense values on January 1, 1999. The resource-based practice expense relative values will be fully implemented on January 1, 2002. Chapter 5 describes these activities.

Geographic Adjustments

Opinions varied on the degree to which the RBRVS should be geographically adjusted under the new system. Many physicians, especially those in rural areas, believed that Medicare should pay the same amount for a service regardless of where it was provided. Others believed that payments in a resource-based system should reflect geographic differences in physicians' resource costs, ie, differences in office rents, wages of nonphysician office staff, PLI costs, and cost of living.

The AMA's policy position represented one compromise on this issue, and the OBRA 89 method represented another. The AMA had stated that payments should be adjusted to reflect only differences in physicians' practice costs and PLI costs and that geographic differences in costs of living should be ignored. Geographic differences in cost of living would be reflected in the physician work component of the payment schedule.

In the payment schedule, geographic differences in all three components are determined by three geographic cost indexes. Under the OBRA 89 compromise, differences in cost of living are measured according to a geographic index of cost of living, but this index measures only one quarter of the geographic difference in cost of living. Practice cost differences are measured by a geographic index of overhead cost differences, and PLI differences by a geographic index of PLI costs.

In practice, the OBRA 89 compromise means that, if practice costs in a particular state are 10% higher than the national average, PLI costs are 12% higher, and costs of living are 8% higher, then the practice cost component of the payment will be increased by 10% above the national average payment and the PLI component will be increased by 12%, but the physician work component will be only 2% higher than the national average, because the cost-of-living index only reflects one quarter of the difference. The OBRA 89 provision substantially reduced the degree of geographic variation in payments. Whereas under CPR, payments in one community could be three or four times greater than payments in another community for the same service, the RBRVS payment system reduced this variation to within 10% to 15% of the national average for most services.

Balance Billing Limits

Retaining the right to charge patients the difference between the Medicare approved amount and the physician's full fee for the service has been a cornerstone of AMA policy since the inception of the Medicare program. Under physician DRGs or HMOs, balance billing would not have been permitted given the nature of these payment approaches. Many physicians also feared that this right would be lost if an RBRVS-based payment schedule was adopted. The PPRC's decision not to recommend mandatory assignment and the absence of such a provision from all three legislative proposals was, therefore, a major victory for organized medicine.

In the late 1980s under CPR, balance billing was limited by MAACs, which were different for each physician because they were based on each physician's customary charges in the second quarter of 1984. The OBRA 89 eliminated MAACs over a 3-year transition period that began in 1991 and replaced them with "limiting charges." The major difference between limiting charges and MAACs is that limiting charges are a specified percentage above the Medicare approved amount (including the patient's 20% coinsurance), whereas MAACs were based on what physicians charged in a base period.

Since January 1, 1993, the limiting charge for a given service in a given Medicare payment locality has been 15% above the Medicare approved amount for the service. It is the same for every physician who provides that service.

In addition, effective January 1, 1995, CMS has statutory authority to prohibit physicians and suppliers from billing Medicare patients, as well as supplemental insurers, above the limiting charge and to require that any excess charges be refunded or credited to the patient.

The OBRA 89 also retained the Participating Physician Program under the new Medicare payment system. "Participating" physicians are those who agree to accept assignment for all services that they provide to patients enrolled in the Medicare program. To give physicians an incentive to sign such an agreement, the full Medicare payment schedule amount for "nonparticipating" physicians is only 95% of the full payment schedule for participating physicians. Because the limiting charge is, in turn, based on the payment schedule for nonparticipating physicians, the effective limiting charge is 9.25% above the full Medicare payment schedule (ie, 115% x 95% = 109.25%).

In 1999, 85% of physicians elected to participate. The percentage of allowed charges for which physicians accepted assignment also has increased from 85% in 1991 to 96% in 1996. These percentages indicate that although almost one fifth of practicing physicians have retained the right to balance bill their patients, many nonparticipating physicians accept the Medicare approved amount as payment in full for most of the services they provide to Medicare patients. Balance bills as a percentage of Medicare payments also declined over the past few years. On average, balance billing represented 23% of Medicare payments in 1993, but only 15% in 1996.

Payment Updates and the Medicare Volume Performance Standard

"A relative value scale can produce any level of payment for a given specialty or service; it all depends on the conversion factor."

James S. Todd, MD[1]

During the development of the OBRA 89 payment system provisions, much of the process for updating payments over time was widely debated. The problems caused by the historical charge patterns that developed under CPR, the government's previous attempts to control Medicare's rising costs, and the PPRC's expenditure target proposal had combined to generate substantial interest in this aspect of the new payment system. In addition, physicians were skeptical that a Congress intent on reducing the federal budget deficit would all too willingly use the new payment schedule's dollar conversion factor to achieve budget savings.

The OBRA 89 provisions that were ultimately adopted authorized Congress to annually update the conversion factor based on the percentage increase in the Medicare Economic Index (MEI), a comparison of the MVPS with the actual increase in spending, and other factors. The MVPS is set annually, by either Congress or a statutory default formula, to reflect the expected growth rate in Medicare spending for physicians' services. It is supposed to encompass all the factors that contribute to this growth, including changes in payment levels, the size and age composition of the Medicare population, technology, utilization patterns, and access to care. The concept behind the conversion factor updating process is that establishing a link between payment updates and increases in the volume of services provided to Medicare patients gives physicians an incentive to decrease unnecessary and inappropriate services. Enacting the MVPS instead of expenditure targets allowed the AMA and other physician organizations to relax that link.

The Balanced Budget Act of 1997, however, replaced the MVPS with a new sustainable growth rate (SGR) system to control Medicare expenditure growth. The SGR does not rely on historical patterns of growth in volume and intensity of physician services, as did the MVPS; rather, it uses projected growth in real gross domestic product per capita. Conversion factor updates and the sustainable growth rate are described in greater detail in Chapter 10.

Budget Neutrality Adjustment

The OBRA 89 mandated that revisions to relative values resulting from changes in medical practice, coding, new data, or the addition of new services may not cause Part B expenditures to differ by more than $20 million from the spending level that would have occurred without these adjustments. Every year since 1993, CMS has projected net expenditure increases exceeding this limitation and, to limit the increase in Medicare expenditures, has made budget neutrality adjustments to the payment schedule.

CMS has applied different types of "budget neutrality" adjustments. For the 1993 through 1995 payment schedules, CMS uniformly reduced all relative value units (RVUs) across all services; in 1996, it adjusted the conversion factors. For 1997, CMS made two separate adjustments: one to the physician work RVUs and another to the conversion factors. For 1998 it also made separate adjustments, including a –0.7% adjustment for increased work RVUs for global surgical services and –0.1% applied as a behavioral offset. The latter adjustment reflects CMS's belief that the volume and intensity of physician services will increase in response to payment schedule reductions, thus lessening their impact on overall Medicare expenditures.

Annually rescaling the RVUs created an administrative burden for physician practices and third-party payers in setting compensation levels, greatly impairing the usefulness of the RBRVS to these groups. In addition, the rescaling also masks any real changes in relative values due to changes in medical practice and refinements to the RBRVS. In 1999, CMS eliminated its separate adjustment to the work RVU and instead applied budget neutrality adjustments directly to the conversion factor. Chapter 10 explains these policies in detail.

The Transition to the New System

The OBRA 89 established a 5-year transition to the new system, which began on January 1, 1992. The transition was consistent with the AMA's desire to postpone implementation until Phase II of the Harvard RBRVS study was completed, and then to proceed incrementally to avoid precipitous changes in payments and potential disruptions in patient care. In addition, the OBRA 89 transition method was intended to accelerate payment increases, principally for visits and consultations, while providing a slower transition for payment reductions.

Much of the change to the new payment levels occurred in the first year of the transition period. The first step in determining the 1992 payment levels was to adjust the CPR prevailing charges, thereby eliminating specialty differentials. The adjustment was essentially a weighted average that accounted for the frequency of each payment amount. In other words, if six different specialties in an area provided a service and six Medicare prevailing charge levels existed under CPR, the averaging process would reflect the frequency of the service provided by physicians in each specialty. The averaging process also reflected the CPR customary charges of physicians who charged less than the prevailing charge. As a result, it was possible for an adjusted prevailing charge to be somewhat less than the average prevailing charge. The CMS referred to this average charge as the "historical payment basis" for a service.

Eliminating specialty differentials placed no limit on the degree to which payments could change in 1992 due to this adjustment. For visit services formerly provided by both internists and family practitioners, for which the internists received higher payments, the adjustment created a double increase for the family practitioners: one due to the adjustment and one due to the transition to the RBRVS. For the internists, the adjustment would mean payments might be decreased and then increased in the process of calculating the 1992 payment, although the internist would only see the net effect. Medicare payments are now the same for all physicians who provide a service in a locality regardless of their specialty.

Many Medicare carriers did not recognize specialty differentials under CPR, however, and maintained only one prevailing charge level for each service. In addition, because many services are only provided by physicians in one specialty, only one prevailing charge level existed in the area. Where there was only one CPR prevailing charge, the historical payment basis may have been closer to the 1991 prevailing charge for the service, although the presence of customary charges below the prevailing charge, in general, would still have reduced the historical basis below the prevailing charge level.

In calculating the conversion factor for 1992, CMS determined that the historical payment basis for each service should be reduced by 5.5%. This reduction was intended to compensate for the fact that payments for visits were increasing faster than payments for procedures and other services were decreasing, thus increasing expenditures over what they otherwise would have been. Finally, the historical payment basis was increased by the payment update for 1992 of 1.9%. This 1.9% update was also applied to the conversion factor for the RBRVS-based payment schedule. After the 5.5% reduction and the 1.9% increase were applied, the historical payment basis was referred to as the adjusted historical payment basis (AHPB).

The next step was the actual transition to the payment schedule. In this step, the statute required that services for which the AHPB was neither 15% higher nor 15% lower than the RBRVS payment schedule be paid entirely on the basis of the new payment schedule. Services for which the schedule represented a change of more than 15% were increased or decreased from the AHPB by 15% of the full payment schedule amount in 1992. As Figure 1 illustrates, this process was intended to accelerate the change for payment increases because such increases were based on 15% of a dollar figure larger than the AHPB and payment decreases were based on 15% of a dollar amount smaller than the AHPB.

During 1993–1995, payments for services that did not move entirely to their RBRVS amounts in 1992 were incrementally increased or decreased using a blend of the 1992 transition approved amount and the RBRVS, with the proportion of the blend that is based on the full payment schedule increased each year. The annual payment update also is applied. Since 1996, payments for all services have been based entirely on the RBRVS payment schedule. The transition is described in greater detail in Chapter 10.

Standardization

The final major component of the RBRVS payment system is the process of standardization. The move to a nationally standardized payment schedule based on an RBRVS, with some variation due to geographic differences in practice costs, was a major change in Medicare's payment system. The twofold, threefold, and fourfold differences in payments across geographic areas have been eliminated. Differences by specialty in payments for the same service within a geographic area also have been eliminated.

Standardization of Medicare payment policies across local Medicare carriers also was initiated under the RBRVS payment system. Until 1992, each Medicare carrier had broad latitude to establish its own policies, including issues such as which services were included in the payment for a surgical procedure, local codes in addition to the national coding

OBRA 89 Transition Asymmetry

Percent Change in years 1 and 5

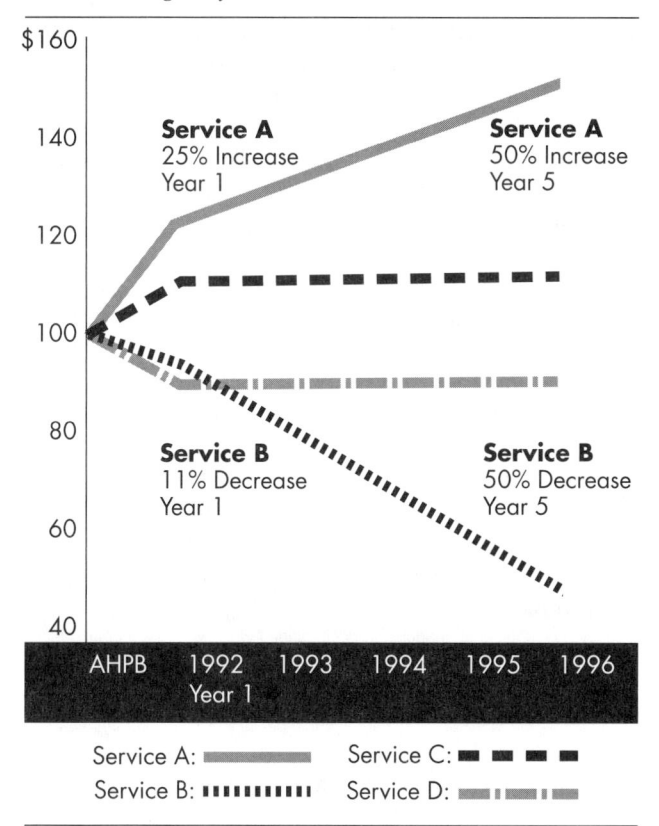

[Figure 1 graph showing:
- Service A: 25% Increase Year 1, 50% Increase Year 5
- Service B: 11% Decrease Year 1, 50% Decrease Year 5
- X-axis: AHPB Year 1, 1992, 1993, 1994, 1995, 1996
- Y-axis: $40 to $160
- Legend: Service A, Service B, Service C, Service D]

Figure 1

system, and policies for comparing Medicare payments to payments for privately insured patients.

One of the RBRVS payment system's most significant provisions substantially eliminated variation in national Medicare payment policies. Although the law did not spell out the details, it required CMS to adopt a uniform coding system for Medicare and a uniform global surgical policy and to standardize its approaches to payment for nonphysician providers, drugs and supplies, and other facets of Part B of Medicare. Chapter 11 describes all of these policies in detail.

Changes in Law and Regulations

In addition to defining these key components of the new Medicare payment system, OBRA 89 required CMS and PPRC to conduct a number of studies on issues related to the new physician payment system and make recommendations on these issues to Congress. One of these requirements directed the secretary of Health and Human Services (HHS) to publish a Model Fee Schedule (MFS) in September 1990.

The MFS, published in the Federal Register on September 4, 1990, provided an added step in CMS's normal regulatory process, giving physicians and their organizations an opportunity to review and comment on CMS's proposals for implementing the new payment system prior to a formal proposed rule. The MFS provided a detailed explanation of the new system; identified the options that CMS was considering on issues such as coding and site-of-service differentials in payment; and provided preliminary estimates of payment schedule amounts and geographic adjustments. In November 1990, Congress enacted the Omnibus Budget Reconciliation Act of 1990 (OBRA 90, PL 101-508), which changed some Medicare payment policies related to physician payment under the Medicare RBRVS. The three most significant changes:

- sharply curtailed payments for interpreting electrocardiograms (ECGs);
- reduced payments for assistants-at-surgery from 20% to 16% of the global payment for the surgery; and
- extended payment reductions for "new" physicians from their first 2 years of providing Medicare services to their first 4 years.

The legislation's ECG provision eliminated payment for interpreting ECGs whenever the ECG was provided as part of or in conjunction with a visit or consultation. Payment for these services, however, as well as for "new" physicians, was restored in 1994 under provisions of Omnibus Budget Reconciliation Act of 1993 (OBRA 93).

The *Notice of Proposed Rule Making:* 1991

On June 5, 1991, the payment reform process was almost derailed when CMS's publication of the *Notice of Proposed Rule Making (NPRM)* on Medicare physician payment in the *Federal Register* included a proposal to reduce the payment schedule's conversion factor by 16% from an otherwise budget-neutral level. The proposed reduction was clearly at odds with congressional intent as described in OBRA 89 to maintain overall Medicare spending in 1992 at the level it would have been under a continuation of CPR.

The *NPRM* prompted the AMA to initiate an extensive grassroots campaign to reverse the proposed cut before the *Final Rule* was issued. The campaign resulted in more than 100,000 comments on the *NPRM* and thousands of letters to Congress. Besides the campaign, the AMA testified before Congress and submitted detailed comments on the *NPRM,* including a legal analysis of the budget neutrality issue by the law firm of Sidley and Austin, which provided clear support for the AMA's position. As a result, 92 of the 99 members of the three congressional committees with authority over Medicare signed letters to Secretary Sullivan opposing the cuts, and 82% of the Congress indicated its support. In addition, two chairmen of the relevant subcommittees introduced legislation to prevent the reduction.

Although three factors contributed to the proposed reduction, the most offensive to physicians was CMS's "behavioral offset." Its premise was that physicians would increase the volume of their services in response to the payment reductions caused by the new payment system, and that payment levels must be reduced to compensate for this expected increase in utilization.

The AMA's comments on the *NPRM* provided a persuasive analysis opposing the proposed reduction in the conversion factor, demonstrating that the cuts clearly violated the language and intent of the law, with potentially disastrous consequences for patient access. These comments also commended CMS for its decisions to adopt the AMA's coding system as its uniform system, to allow a major role for organized medicine in updating the RBRVS, and to eliminate several CPR policies that physicians had long opposed. Details of these comments and CMS's response are discussed in the relevant chapters of this book.

The *Final Rule:* 1991

The *Final Rule* for the new Medicare physician payment system appeared in the *Federal Register* on November 25, 1991. It contained a summary of the regulation, an analysis of comments on the *NPRM* and CMS's responses, impact estimates for physicians and beneficiaries, and the regulations for the new system. It also listed the relative values for each service and geographic adjustment factors for each locality.

The *Final Rule* reflected several extremely positive changes from the *NPRM* that the AMA and other physician organizations had advocated. Most notable was the conversion factor of $30.423, which exceeded the *NPRM* conversion factor of $26.873 by 13.2%. This increase restored an estimated $10 billion to Medicare Part B over the period 1992 through 1996. The CMS also announced the payment update for 1992 of 1.9%, thus making the 1992 conversion factor $31.001.

Besides the conversion factor, the *Final Rule* contained many other substantial changes compared to the *NPRM*. For instance:

- in using a "baseline adjustment" to account for projected volume changes instead of the "behavioral offset," CMS acknowledged that volume increases result from many factors, including patient demand, rather than resulting from increases in unnecessary care;

- CMS further increased the conversion factor consistent with AMA suggestions on several technical issues;
- relative values for specific services were increased based on *NPRM* comments;
- CMS treated all relative values as "initial" for 1992 and allowed a 120-day period for public comment;
- policies on global surgical packages were substantially improved; and
- Medicare payments for drugs were limited to the average wholesale price, rather than to 85% of this price, as proposed in the *NPRM*.

Despite these changes, the AMA's House of Delegates called for substantial improvements in many important features of the payment system, including better data for the geographic indexes and eliminating discriminatory payment limits for "new" physicians and for the services of assistants-at-surgery (see Chapter 11). To help identify problems arising during implementation of the new system, the AMA established a comprehensive program to monitor changes in patient access, physician practice patterns, and errors in carrier implementation, working closely with state and county medical societies.

During 1992, the first year of implementation, the AMA worked with CMS to make the system more responsive to physician needs:

- Consistent with the AMA's March 1992 comments on the 1991 *Final Rule,* CMS enabled carriers to calculate transition amounts for about 50 new services that had dropped to full RBRVS amounts and increased about 150 technical components.
- The CMS agreed to a grace period for the old system of visit codes, allowing physicians to use these codes for the first 2 months of 1992.
- The CMS revised its definition of "new" patient for group practices to be consistent with the original intent of the CPT Editorial Panel. A "new patient" is one who has
  - not been seen by a member of the group in the same specialty in the prior 3-year period.
  - The CMS clarified several provisions of its global surgery, critical care, and other payment policies to reflect physician needs. Many of the problems identified in the first year of implementation have been resolved through either the legislative or the regulatory process, although the AMA continues to work with physicians and others in organized medicine for improvements to the Medicare RBRVS payment system.

AMA Legislative and Regulatory Activity

Several problems with Medicare's RBRVS payment system stemmed from statutory provisions of OBRA 90 and could be corrected only through legislative action. These problems included payment reductions that further reduced Medicare payments to "new" physicians and eliminating payment for interpreting ECGs.

The AMA's legislative advocacy efforts led to the introduction in 1991 and 1992 of bills that would have restored payment for ECG interpretations, repealed payment reductions for new physicians, and required CMS to use the most recent data available for compiling the geographic practice cost indexes (GPCIs). Many medical specialty societies supported these bills even though their enactment would mean slight across-the-board reductions in physician payments pursuant to budget neutrality requirements.

In August 1993, organized medicine won a substantial victory for physicians when provisions were included in OBRA 93 to restore payment for ECG interpretation and rescind payment reductions for "new" physicians. To ensure that these provisions were implemented in a budget-neutral manner, as required by OBRA 89, CMS reduced all RVUs in the 1994 payment schedule by 1.2%.

The Balanced Budget Act of 1997 gave physicians the right to contract privately with their Medicare patients for health care services, beginning in 1998. This new ability comes with a heavy price, however. Physicians who contract with one or more of their Medicare patients for Medicare covered services may not bill the program for any Medicare services for 2 years. To correct this flaw, the AMA is vigorously supporting legislative proposals that would permit Medicare beneficiaries to pursue private contracts with their physicians, without isolating physicians from the Medicare program for 2 years. In addition, the AMA has identified a number of other issues for which it will continue to work with CMS for improvement: refinement of payment policies that do not reflect resource costs, such as those for assistants-at-surgery and supplies; concurrent care policies; increased uniformity among carriers in implementing the payment system; and increased input from practicing physicians into payment policy development.

Reference

1. Todd JS. At last, a rational way to pay for physicians' services? *JAMA*. 1988;260:2439-2440.

Chapter 3
The Scope of Medicare's RBRVS Payment System

Medicare's resource-based relative value scale (RBRVS) physician payment system affects all services that were previously reimbursed according to the customary, prevailing, and reasonable (CPR) system. This means that all physicians' services are now paid according to a single cross-specialty RBRVS with payment determined by a single conversion factor. The Medicare program applies the same payment schedule to every physician's service and every physician. (The only exception is anesthesia services, whose relative value guide is discussed in Chapter 4.) The payment system also encompasses the services of radiologists, replacing a separate fee schedule for radiology that began in 1989. Chapters 4 and 5 describe the Centers for Medicare and Medicaid Services' (CMS) (formerly the Health Care Financing Administration) process for integrating the radiology fee schedule into the cross- specialty RBRVS as required by the Omnibus Budget Reconciliation Act of 1989 (OBRA 89).

With the exception of physicians' services provided to Medicare patients enrolled in a Medicare HMO, the only physicians' services not included in the revision made to the payment system are some physicians' services provided in hospitals, skilled nursing facilities, comprehensive outpatient rehabilitation facilities, and some services provided by teaching physicians.

When a physician's service is defined as being part of the general patient care activities of a hospital or nursing facility, in contrast to a service provided for the benefit of an individual patient, that service is covered under Part A. When teaching physicians act as attending physicians for their patients, their direct patient care services are paid according to the Medicare payment schedule, but other services these physicians provide may be covered differently. Under CPR, teaching physicians acting as attending physicians had separate customary charge profiles from other physicians, but these services are now all paid under the same payment schedule. The CMS significantly revised the criteria for payment for services of teaching physicians, effective July 1, 1996. These rules and the special payment rules for "provider-based" physicians' services are covered in Chapter 11.

Medicare Part B encompasses a number of services in addition to those of physicians, and Medicare's RBRVS payment system applies to many of them. They include doctors of medicine and osteopathy (MDs and DOs), optometrists, dentists, podiatrists, and chiropractors. Chapter 4 discusses assigning relative values for their services. Chapter 11 describes other features of Medicare's payment system that may be especially relevant to their practices.

In addition to the non-MD/DO practitioners identified above, Part B pays for seven categories of nonphysician practitioners' services:

- physical and occupational therapists, speech language pathologists, and audiologists;
- physician assistants;
- nurse practitioners and clinical nurse specialists in certain settings;
- certified registered nurse anesthetists;
- certified nurse midwives;
- clinical psychologists;
- clinical social workers; and
- registered dieteticians.

Each of these groups had its own coverage and payment rules under CPR, based generally on payments for services provided by physicians, and this link continues under the RBRVS-based payment system's rules. Changes in physician payment, therefore, affect payment for nonphysicians' services. Chapter 11 describes the relationship between the Medicare RBRVS and the payment rates for each of the nonphysician categories and explains the standardization of payment practices for these services.

Frequently nonphysicians provide their services "incident to" rather than independently of a physician's service. For example, "incident-to" services encompass services that nurses or physician assistants provide in a physician's office under the physician's supervision, such as an injection administered by a nurse. The CPR system did not require physicians to differentiate on a claim between services they provided directly to patients and those that nonphysician personnel provided. The services of nonphysician personnel were compensated at the physician's CPR rate. The RBRVS-based payment system's rules do not affect "incident-to" services, which will continue to be reimbursed as if they have been furnished by physicians. In 1993, CMS broadened application of the "incident-to" provision to include such services as physical exams, minor surgery, and setting simple fractures. This provision is discussed in more detail in Chapter 11. New payment rules also were developed for drugs and supplies provided on an "incident-to" basis and are covered in Chapter 11.

The Balanced Budget Act of 1997 lifted some restrictions that previously were applicable to services furnished by certain categories of nonphysician practitioners. Effective January 1, 1998, nurse practitioners, clinical nurse specialists, and physician assistants are no longer required to practice under the direct, physical supervision of an MD/DO. Nurse practitioners and clinical nurse specialists may bill and receive direct payment from Medicare. Physician assistants maintain their relationships with physicians, although they may be considered independent contractors of physicians, which previously was not allowed. Payment continues to be made through the physician assistant's employer. Additional information on these new provisions appears in Chapter 11.

The scope of the Medicare RBRVS payment system is quite comprehensive. The standardization of payment levels and diverse payment policies across different payment localities is an important, and often overlooked, aspect of the revisions made to Medicare physician payment. Chapters 4 through 8 describe the key components of this system, and Chapter 11 outlines many of the national policies enacted as part of the broad scope of the enabling legislation and regulations.

Part 2
Major Components of the RBRVS Payment System

From a practicing physician's perspective, the major components of Medicare's resource-based relative value scale (RBRVS) system are:

- the relative value scale;
- the conversion factor;
- the geographic adjustments; and
- the limits on balance billing.

Although other aspects of the payment system figured prominently in the policy making process and are important to certain groups of physicians, these four components are the key determinants of a physician's Medicare payment for a service, comprising the "bread and butter" of the payment system.

Chapters 4, 5, and 6 discuss the physician work, the practice expense and professional liability insurance (PLI) components of the RBRVS; the actual relative values for each of these components are listed in Part 5. As Figure 1 illustrates, on average, the work component comprises 55% of the total relative value for a service, the practice expense component 42%, and the PLI component 3%.

The geographic practice cost indexes are described in Chapter 7, while a list of the indexes appears in Part 5. Chapter 8 describes how the relative values, geographic adjustments, and conversion factors combine to determine the payment for a service in a locality. Part 2 concludes with Chapter 9, a description of the limits on balance billing.

Chapter 4
The Physician Work Component

Figure 1. Components of the Medicare RBRVS

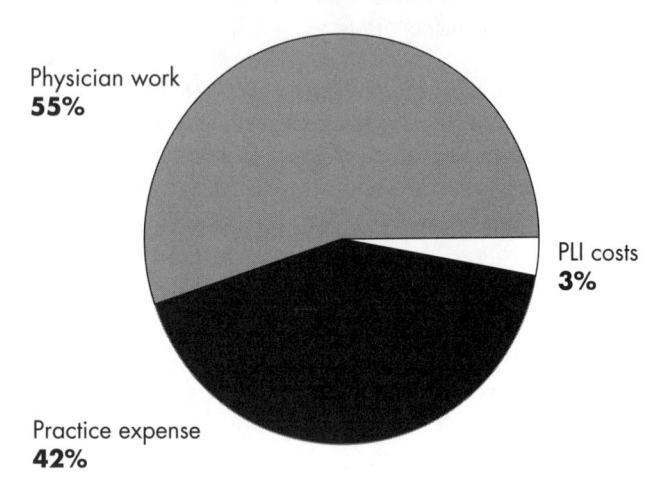

- Physician work **55%**
- PLI costs **3%**
- Practice expense **42%**

The greatest challenge in developing an RBRVS-based payment schedule was overcoming the lack of any available method or data for assigning specific values to physicians' work. The Harvard RBRVS study, therefore, played a critical role in the evolution of Medicare's payment system. Although the study contained several weaknesses, critical reviews of the data and methods concluded that it provided a reasonably valid basis for assigning relative values to the physician work component of the payment schedule. The physician work component now accounts for an average of 55% of the total relative value for a service. (See Figure 1.) The Harvard University School of Public Health, under a cooperative agreement with the Centers for Medicare and Medicaid Services (CMS) (formerly the Health Care Financing Administration), conducted the study that led to the initial relative work values, which appeared in the November 1991 *Final Rule*. The core of Harvard's landmark study was a nationwide survey of physicians to determine the work involved in each of about 800 services. About 4300 relative value estimates of the nearly 6000 services included in the 1992 Medicare relative value scale (RVS) were based directly on findings from the Harvard RBRVS study. Besides the Harvard study, the 1992 Medicare RVS also relied on findings from CMS's "refinement process," which it developed in response to public comments on the 1992 values. This refinement process also has contributed to updating the payment schedule since 1993.

Finally, values for new and revised procedures in *Physicians' Current Procedural Terminology (CPT)* are also contained in the updated relative value scales for each year. To develop recommendations for CMS regarding relative values to be assigned to these new and revised codes, the AMA and the national medical specialty societies established the AMA/Specialty Society RVS Update Process.

This chapter describes the three major sources of the physician work component relative values:

- the Harvard RBRVS study;
- The 1992 RVS refinement process; and
- the AMA/Specialty Society RVS Update Process.

The sources of relative values for anesthesiology services are discussed separately at the end of the chapter.

The Harvard RBRVS Study

Phase I of the Harvard RBRVS study, completed in September 1988, provided relative value estimates for services provided by 18 medical and surgical specialties:

- allergy and immunology,
- anesthesiology,
- dermatology,
- family practice,
- general surgery,
- internal medicine,
- obstetrics and gynecology,
- ophthalmology,
- oral and maxillofacial surgery,
- orthopedic surgery,
- otolaryngology,
- pathology,
- pediatrics,
- psychiatry,
- radiology,
- rheumatology,
- thoracic and cardiovascular surgery, and
- urology.

Phase II, completed in December 1990, expanded the RBRVS to 15 additional specialties:

- cardiology,
- emergency medicine,
- gastroenterology,
- hematology,
- infectious disease,
- nephrology,
- neurology,
- neurosurgery,
- nuclear medicine,
- oncology,
- osteopathic medicine,
- physical medicine and rehabilitation,
- plastic surgery,
- pulmonary medicine, and
- radiation oncology.

Phase II also reviewed four Phase I specialties (dermatology, ophthalmology, pathology, and psychiatry); expanded the study to include additional services provided by internists, general surgeons, and orthopedic surgeons; and included methodological refinements. Phase III, completed in August 1992, was primarily intended to revise problematic estimates from the earlier phases and expand the RBRVS to the remaining coded services. In particular, Phase III focused on a then newly developed method for assigning relative value estimates to services closely related to those included in the Harvard study's national survey of physicians, but that were not actually surveyed by the researchers.[1]

Phase IV, completed in July 1993, included research and policy recommendations regarding development of vignettes for services provided by two limited-license professions (optometry and podiatry) and one nonphysician profession (clinical psychology) and establishing work values for some psychology services; developing reference services for each major specialty; developing relative work values for services furnished on a "by-report" basis; and developing data to determine payment policies for multiple and bilateral procedures.[2]

Physician Work Defined

Before work on the RBRVS surveys could begin, the researchers needed to define physician work. The Harvard RBRVS study initially conceptualized work as the time a physician spends providing a service and the intensity with which the time is spent. To better define the non–time-related elements of work, the researchers interviewed physicians, including members of the study's Technical Consulting Groups, or TCGs. The TCGs were small groups of physicians in each studied specialty who were nominated by national medical specialty societies in a process coordinated by the AMA. As a result of these interviews, the Harvard study defined the elements of physician work as:

- time required to perform the service;
- technical skill and physical effort;
- mental effort and judgment; and
- psychological stress associated with the physician's concern about iatrogenic risk to the patient.

This definition often caused confusion because some physicians thought that work relative value units (RVUs) are determined only by the time required to perform a service. Work RVUs are based on direct estimates of physician work, however; no separate measures of time are used.

The Harvard study further divided physician work into the work involved before, during, and after a service.

The work involved in actually providing a service or performing a procedure is termed "intraservice work." For office visits, the intraservice period is defined as patient encounter time; for hospital visits, it is the time spent on the patient's floor; and for surgical procedures, it is the period from the initial incision to the closure of the incision (ie, "skin-to-skin" time).

Work prior to and following provision of a service, such as surgical preparation time, writing or reviewing records, or discussion with other physicians, is referred to as "preservice and postservice work." When preservice, intra-service, and postservice work are combined, the result is referred to as the "total work" involved in a service. For surgical procedures, the total work period is the same as the global surgical period, including recovery room time, normal postoperative hospital care, and office visits after discharge, as well as preoperative and intraoperative work.

Although the Harvard study defined physician work according to these distinct components, it did not measure work in this manner. Earlier attempts to separately measure time and intensity had produced unsatisfactory results. Instead, the study directly measured the work involved in a service. The RBRVS study's definition of physician work is important because data from this study are the major basis for the physician work component of the Medicare payment schedule. A service on the schedule with more physician work RVUs than another means that the former service involves more time, skill, effort, judgment, and stress than the latter. Efforts to refine and update the RBRVS have employed the same definition of work as the Harvard study.

Having defined and separated work into its component parts, the researchers then ensured that all surveyed physicians had the same basic service in mind when rating the work for value. The coding system used in the RBRVS is the AMA's CPT coding system. To allow physicians to rate the work of a service, the TCGs for each specialty developed "vignettes" for each coded service included in the survey of that specialty. In many cases, the vignette came directly from CPT, as in the following description (as described in CPT 1987) for CPT code 63017, a service surveyed for orthopedic surgery:

"Laminectomy for decompression of spinal cord and/or cauda equina, more than two segments; lumbar."

In other cases, particularly for visits and consultations, the TCGs designed vignettes to be representative of an average patient for the particular service being rated by that specialty. For these services, the development of a vignette ensured that each surveyed physician had the same basic service in mind. For example, the neurology vignette for CPT code 99160 (this code was replaced by CPT code 99291 in CPT 1992) reads:

"Initial hour of critical care in the ICU (intensive care unit) for a 65-year-old male who presents with a fever and status epilepticus."

The National Survey
Once the TCGs agreed on the descriptions, Harvard launched its national survey of physician work. In Phase I, researchers completed nearly 2000 telephone interviews with physicians in 18 specialties. In Phase II, they completed about 1900 interviews with physicians in 15 additional specialties.

To obtain work ratings for each of the vignettes, the study used a technique known as "magnitude estimation." Surveyed physicians were asked to use a particular service as a standard and to rate the intraservice work of about 25 other services relative to that standard.

The standard in each specialty was assigned an intraservice work value of 100. For a vignette that involved twice as much intraservice work as the standard, physicians were instructed to assign an intraservice work value of 200. Physicians would assign a value of 50 to a vignette that involved half as much intraservice work as the standard. Using this magnitude estimation method, physicians in each specialty assigned intraservice work relative values to all the vignettes on the survey for their specialty.

The Cross-Specialty Process
Harvard researchers used the national survey to develop a relative value scale for each specialty included in the study. The second step in constructing the RBRVS linked all of these specialty-specific scales onto a single scale.

The researchers organized cross-specialty panels to complete the second step. Panels consisted of about 10 physicians, each from a different specialty. The panel members, selected from the TCGs, considered potential specialty-to-specialty links, such as a single service that physicians in two or more different specialties were likely to provide. For example, the panelists determined that the following service had the same value in several different specialties:

"Decompression of carpal tunnel in a 48-year-old female, unilateral, ambulatory surgery unit."

The panels also considered pairs of different services that are typically performed by physicians in different specialties but appeared to involve equal amounts of work. The following services, for example, served as a link between two specialties:

In nephrology, "Insertion of a double-lumen femoral vein cannula for hemodialysis"; and, in general surgery, "Excisional breast biopsy of a 2-centimeter lesion."

The panels identified at least several specialty-to-specialty links for each of the studied specialties. Researchers then statistically analyzed the work ratings of the links obtained from the national survey for each specialty. This process linked all the specialty-specific scales to a common cross-specialty scale, while preserving, to the extent possible, the within specialty relationships of one service to another.

The cross-specialty process may have determined, for example, that two unilateral surgical procedures performed by different specialties, rated 80 and 120 in their respective specialty surveys, represented equal work. As a result, both might have been valued at 100 on the common scale. Assuming the magnitude estimation surveys for both services had rated the procedures as requiring 50% more work when done bilaterally, one would have been rated at 120, the other at 180 on their respective specialty scales. On the common scale, however, both bilateral procedures would be assigned a value of 150, preserving the values at 50% more than the unilateral procedures.

Preservice and Postservice Work

The RBRVS study employed several different methods to assign relative values to the preservice and postservice work involved in the surveyed services, depending on the type of service. Survey respondents rated both the intraservice work and the total work for visits and consultations in Phase II, for example, the difference being preservice and postservice work. For invasive procedures, surgeons were surveyed about the preservice and postservice time of specific components of procedures. For instance, general surgeons were surveyed about the time and work involved in a "hospital visit, 3 days post uncomplicated cholecystectomy with common bile duct exploration." Researchers then derived an "intensity per unit of time" factor from the survey data and used it to estimate preservice and postservice work from data on preservice and postservice time.

Assigning RVUs to Nonsurveyed Services

The researchers surveyed physicians about the work involved in 800 services and extrapolated work values for the remaining services. The extrapolation method grouped services into "families." For example, all coded services involving coronary artery bypass surgery became a family, as did all new patient office visits. The researchers theorized that the differences in average charges for services within a family would approximate the differences in physician work. Thus, if a nonsurveyed service in a family had a 20% higher average charge than the surveyed service, then the physician work involved in the former should be 20% higher than the latter. In practice, however, the extrapolation method often produced RVUs that seemed incongruous or paradoxical.

In Phase III of the study, the researchers developed a new extrapolation method using small groups of physicians. These groups established relationships between the surveyed and nonsurveyed services and assigned RVUs to them. The small-group process was also used to extend the RBRVS beyond the families of the surveyed services.

Phase IV, released in summer 1993, used the same small-group process to estimate work values for 227 by-report services. A review process was developed for 162 of these services, which previously had been studied in Phase III. Members of the TCG and assessment panels from Phase III were reassembled and panelists reevaluated the existing work estimates. Researchers used a single survey of the assessment panels for each specialty for the review, which followed a two-step process: ranking the services by total and intraservice work, then reviewing these values in the context of the specialty's reference services and suggesting changes where necessary. These assessments were compared with the original estimates of intraservice and total-service work from Phase III. Work value recommendations were made for 145 of the procedures, and these showed a high level of agreement with Phase III values. For services that were not previously studied, panelists rated the work of each service using magnitude estimation with multiple reference services. A total of 34 by-report services for oral and maxillofacial surgery, the major specialty studied, were reviewed.

Reviews of the RBRVS Study

After the final report of Phase I was released in September 1988, the AMA conducted an in-depth evaluation of the study's methods and results and also contracted with the Consolidated Consulting Group, Inc, for an independent evaluation. The Physician Payment Review Commission (PPRC) also evaluated the Phase I results, as did CMS, which had provided the principal funding for the study.

These evaluations identified many flaws in the study, such as the inaccurate measurement of practice costs, but the reviewers' conclusions about the core of the study—measuring physicians' intraservice work—were very positive. The Consolidated Consulting Group report on the study concluded:

"The RBRVS study's major effort—the measurement of physicians' intraservice work (ie, the work needed to perform specific services and procedures)—was successful. The RBRVS researchers . . . obtained generally accurate, reliable and consistent rankings of relative work from each of 18 specialties for about 22 representative services. These separate specialty-specific rankings were also successfully linked into a common scale. These results show that it is feasible to develop a work scale built on physicians' views about their work."

As a result of these reviews, the legislation that created the new Medicare payment system did not reflect two components of the RBRVS study: the study's method of assigning practice cost RVUs and its specialty training cost component. For the other components, the AMA and PPRC assessments recommended specific areas that needed refinement and correction.

Many of the national medical specialty societies also evaluated the study's data and results for their specialty's services. As a result, several societies requested that the Harvard researchers conduct a partial or complete restudy of their specialty's services. Some specialties turned to groups other than Harvard to reevaluate their services. For example, a group of specialty societies representing cardiovascular and thoracic surgeons jointly contracted with the consulting firm of Abt Associates for a separate study for their specialty. Finally, many of the specialty societies and individual physicians, as well as the AMA, commented on the work RVUs published in the *Notice of Proposed Rulemaking* (*NPRM*) and the November 1991 *Final Rule*.

The 1992 RVS Refinement Process

The 1992 Medicare RVS included RVUs for about 6000 CPT-coded services. Of these, about 1900 appeared for the first time in the 1991 *Final Rule*. Because there had been no opportunity for public review and comment on the RVUs for services that were excluded from the model fee schedule or the *NPRM*, all of the work RVUs in the 1991 *Final Rule* were published as "initial" RVUs.

In addition, the study was not completed in time for the January 1 implementation of the new system, although results for many of the services included in Phase III of the study had already been provided to CMS. Therefore, CMS established a process involving its carrier medical directors (CMDs) to assign work RVUs to about 800 services for which data were not available from the Harvard study. The CMS also received comments on about 1000 proposed work RVUs included in the *NPRM* and used CMDs to review these RVUs prior to publishing the final 1992 RVS.

In the 1991 *Final Rule*, CMS was careful to state that the CMD process was not intended to be a short-term revision of the Harvard RBRVS. Instead, CMS used the process to assign RVUs to low-volume services, new services, and others that Harvard did not provide, and to refine some unreasonable estimates. For example, four-graft coronary artery bypass graft RVUs were adjusted to be greater than three-graft surgery.

The CMS provided a 120-day period for public comment on the RVUs published in this first RBRVS *Final Rule*. During the comment period, CMS received about 7500 comments on the RVUs assigned to about 1000 services. Some specialty societies requested that CMS provide guidelines on how to prepare the comments, emphasizing the need for clinical arguments to support the comments.

In responding to the comments, CMS indicated that it considered principally those comments that followed its guidelines, rather than general comments regarding payment reductions. The CMS also expanded its CMD process and developed an RVS refinement process, which involved 24 review panels, each with 13 members. Panel members included 33 CMDs and 127 physicians nominated by 42 specialty societies. The multidisciplinary panels included physicians from the specialty or specialties that most frequently provide the service, physicians in related specialties, primary care physicians, and CMDs.

The objective of the review process was to allow four different panels to review each of the services. The panels' ratings of physician work were statistically analyzed to assess the consistency of ratings across the four groups.

The panels reviewed the work RVUs assigned to 791 codes. The final results from Phase III were used as one source of relevant data. The CMS retained the 1992 value for about half of these codes in the 1993 Medicare RVS. The refinement process resulted in higher values for about 360 codes and lower values for 35 codes. Notable among the code groups increased by the refinement process were:

- hernia repair;
- home visits;
- obstetrical care;
- electroencephalogram (EEG) and EEG monitoring;
- nursing facility care;
- coronary artery bypass graft surgery; and
- removal of larynx.

The CMS also reviewed 120 codes published in the 1992 *Final Notice* as interim values and subject to comment in 1993. A multispecialty panel of physicians reviewed 42 of these codes and made final RVU determinations by comparing the interim values to "reference services" whose work RVUs had not been challenged in the comment process.

1992 RVU Refinement of Evaluation and Management Codes

Work RVUs were reviewed by the CMS for the CPT evaluation and management codes for visit and consultation services, which had been introduced in *CPT 1992*. Conflicting comments on the values were made by various specialty societies. Some specialties argued that the values for the lower levels of service should have been increased to reflect higher intensity of service. Others argued that the higher levels of service failed to adequately reflect the greater intensity of providing these services. Still others argued for a more linear progression between levels 4 and 5 of each code group. In the 1992 *Final Notice,* CMS reported that the physician panel it convened on this issue could not reach a consensus. However, using data from Phase III, it increased mid- to upper-level visits to reflect a more linear progression of work and reduced some lower levels. This process also reduced the values of the follow-up inpatient consultation codes.

Work RVUs for Medicare Noncovered Services

For the 1995 RVS, as in previous years, CMS convened multispecialty panels of physicians to assist in the refinement process. The agency established final values for a number of carrier-priced and Medicare noncovered services for which it previously had published proposed values. The CMS relied strongly on the AMA/Specialty Society RVS Update Committee (RUC)'s recommendations in establishing proposed and final values, as it has each year when developing the payment schedule.

Completion of the Medicare RBRVS

In the 1994 *Final Rule,* CMS stated that with assignment of work RVUs for the 1995 RVS, it considered the RBRVS payment schedule to be "essentially" complete. Work relative value units were assigned to hundreds of codes that had been previously carrier-priced, for many commonly furnished services that were not covered by Medicare but paid by other payers, and for all pediatric services.

A mechanism to update the RBRVS on an ongoing basis was included as part of the Omnibus Budget Reconciliation Act of 1989 (OBRA 89). The statute requires that CMS conduct a comprehensive review of work relative values every 5 years. As part of this review process, all work RVUs on the 1995 RVS were open for public comment. In the November 1999 *Final Rule,* CMS again opened the 2000 RVS for public comment for 120 days. The 5-year review process and CMS's decisions are summarized later in this chapter.

The AMA/Specialty Society RVS Update Process[3]

Besides refinements to correct errors in the initial RVUs, the Medicare RVS also must be updated to reflect changes in practice and technology. The AMA updates the CPT coding system annually under an agreement with CMS to reflect such changes. The AMA maintains the coding system through the CPT Editorial Panel. Annual updates to the physician work relative values are based on recommendations from a committee involving the American Medical Association (AMA) and national medical specialty societies. The AMA/Specialty RVS Update Committee (RUC) was formed in 1991 to make recommendations to CMS on the relative values assigned to new or revised codes in *Current Procedural Terminology* (CPT).

The core of the RVS Update Process is the RUC. During its first year, the RUC established procedures for specialty societies to reconcile their different viewpoints and agree on relative value recommendations. The RUC has now completed 10 cycles of recommendations for updating the physician work component of the RBRVS, demonstrating its commitment to developing objective measures of physician work for new and revised CPT codes. The RUC has recently embarked on establishing recommendations on direct practice expense inputs for new and revised codes.

The AMA believes that updating and maintaining the Medicare RVS is a clinical and scientific activity that must remain in the hands of the medical profession and regards the RUC as the principal vehicle for refining the work and practice expense components of the RBRVS. From the AMA's perspective, the RUC provides a vital opportunity for the medical profession to continue to shape its own payment environment. For this reason, the AMA has strongly advocated that Medicare adopt the RUC's recommendations.

Structure and Process

The RUC represents the entire medical profession, with 23 of its 29 members appointed by major national specialty societies including those recognized by the American Board of Medical Specialties, those with a large percentage of physicians in patient care, and those that account for high percentages of Medicare expenditures. Three seats rotate on a two-year basis, with two reserved for internal medicine subspecialty and one for any other specialty. The RUC chair, the co-chair of the HCPAC (an advisory committee representing non-MD/DO health professionals), the chair of the Practice Expense Advisory Committee (PEAC) and representatives of the American Medical Association, American Osteopathic Association, and CPT Editorial Panel hold the remaining five seats.

The major source of specialty input for the updating process is the RUC's *Advisory Committee,* which is open to all 102 specialty societies in the AMA House of Delegates. Specialty societies that are not in the House of Delegates also may be invited to participate in developing relative values for coding changes of particular relevance to their members. Advisory Committee members designate an *RVS Committee* for their specialty, which is responsible for generating relative value recommendations using a survey method developed by the RUC. Advisors attend the RUC meeting and present their societies' recommendations, which the RUC evaluates. Specialties represented on both the RUC and the Advisory Committee are required to appoint different physicians to each committee to distinguish the role of advocate from that of evaluator.

The RUC refers procedural and methodological issues to the *Research Subcommittee,* which is composed of about one-third the members of the full RUC. This subcommittee's principal responsibility is to develop and refine the RUC's methods and processes.

The RUC also established the *Practice Expense Subcommittee* to examine the many issues relating to the development of practice expense relative values. This subcommittee also is composed of one-third of the members of the full RUC.

Most recently, the RUC formed the *Practice Expense Advisory Committee* to review and suggest changes in the CPEP data which was used to create practice expense relative values.

The *Administrative Subcommittee* also includes one-third of the RUC members and is primarily charged with the maintenance of the committee's procedural issues. This subcommittee also formulated the RUC's plans and processes for the second, five-year review of the RBRVS, which began in early 2000.

In 1992, the AMA recommended that a *Health Care Professionals Advisory Committee (HCPAC)* be established to allow for participation of limited license practitioners and allied health professionals in both the RUC and CPT processes. All of these professionals use CPT to report the services they provide independently to Medicare patients, and they are paid for these services based on the RBRVS physician payment schedule. Organizations representing physician assistants, nurses, occupational and physical therapists, optometrists, podiatrists, psychologists, registered dietitians, social workers, chiropractors, audiologists, and speech pathologists have been invited to nominate representatives to the CPT and RUC HCPACs. The CPT HCPAC fosters participation in and solicits comments from these professional organizations in coding changes affecting their members, while the RUC HCPAC allows those organizations to participate in developing relative values for new and revised codes within their scope of practice.

To further facilitate the decision-making process on issues of concern to both MDs/DOs and non-MDs/DOs, *CPT and RUC HCPAC Review Boards* were also formed. The review boards bring MDs/DOs and non-MDs/DOs together to discuss coding issues and relative value proposals. The RUC HCPAC Review Board comprises all 11 members of the current RUC HCPAC and three RUC members. For codes used by both MDs/DOs and non-MDs/DOs, the HCPAC Review Board acts much like an RUC facilitation committee. For codes used only by non-MDs/DOs, the RUC HCPAC Review Board replaces the RUC as the body responsible for developing recommendations for CMS.

Facilitation Committees are established as needed during the RUC meetings to resolve differences of opinion about relative value recommendations before they are submitted to CMS.

The RUC closely coordinates its annual cycle for developing recommendations with the CPT Editorial Panel's schedule for annual code revisions and with CMS's annual updates to the Medicare payment schedule.

The RUC process for developing relative value recommendations is as follows:

Step 1   The CPT Editorial Panel transmits its new and revised codes to the RUC staff, which then prepares a "Level of Interest" form. The form summarizes the Panel's coding actions.

Step 2   Members of the RUC Advisory Committee review the summary and indicate their societies' level of interest in developing a relative value recommendation. The societies have several options. They can:

(A) Survey their members to obtain data on the amount of work involved in a service and develop recommendations based on the survey results.

(B) Comment in writing on recommendations developed by other societies.

(C) Decide, in the case of revised codes, that the coding change requires no action because it does not significantly alter the nature of the service.

(D) Take no action because the codes are not used by physicians in their specialty.

Step 3   AMA staff develop survey instruments for the specialty societies. The specialty societies are required to survey at least 30 practicing physicians. The RUC survey instrument asks physicians to use a list of 15 to 25 services as reference points that have been selected by the specialty RVS committee.

Physicians receiving the survey are asked to evaluate the work involved in the new or revised code relative to the reference points. The survey data may be augmented by analysis of Medicare claims data and information from other studies of the procedure, such as the Harvard RBRVS study.

Step 4   The specialty RVS committees conduct the surveys, review the results, and prepare their recommendations to the RUC. When two or more societies are involved in developing recommendations, the RUC encourages them to coordinate their survey procedures and develop a consensus recommendation. The written recommendations are disseminated to the RUC before the meeting.

Step 5 The specialty advisors present the recommendations at the RUC meeting. The Advisory Committee members' presentations are followed by a thorough question-and-answer period during which the advisors must defend every aspect of their proposal(s).

Step 6 The RUC may decide to adopt a specialty society's recommendation, refer it back to the specialty society, or modify it before submitting it to CMS. Final recommendations to CMS must be adopted by a two-thirds majority of the RUC members. Recommendations that require additional evaluation by the RUC are referred to a Facilitation Committee.

Step 7 The RUC's recommendations are forwarded to CMS in May of each year. CMS convenes a meeting of selected medical directors to review the RUC's recommendations.

Step 8 The Medicare Physician Fee Schedule, which includes CMS's review of the RUC recommendations, is published late fall. The new values are considered "interim" for 1 year and are open for public comment. After 1 year, the values are considered final.

Updating Work Relative Values

Each year the RUC submits recommendations to CMS for physician work relative values based on CPT coding changes to be included in the Medicare payment schedule. The RUC has submitted more than 3000 relative value recommendations for new and revised codes for the 1993-2002 RBRVS updates. In addition, the RUC submitted more than 300 recommendations to CMS for carrier-priced or noncovered services, including preventive medicine services. Each year CMS has relied heavily upon these recommendations when establishing interim values for new and revised CPT codes. Key recommendations for each annual cycle are briefly summarized below.

The RUC submitted its first recommendations to CMS in July 1992 based on 1993 CPT coding changes to be included in the 1993 Medicare payment schedule. The recommendations addressed physician work relative values for new and revised codes spanning the entire range of physician services, including orthopedic trauma care; a new section of CPT for hospital observation care; critical care; cardiology; urology; and coronary artery bypass surgery.

The RUC's second set of recommendations, included in the 1994 Medicare RVS, again encompassed coding changes for a wide range of physician services. These recommendations included physician work values for new primary care codes for prolonged physician services and care plan oversight; the initial recommendations for pediatric services, including new codes for neonatal intensive care; pediatric surgery; hospital observation care; general surgery; skull-based surgery; and magnetic resonance angiography.

In the November 1993 *Final Rule,* CMS stated that it would defer establishing relative values for pediatric services, transplant services, and other carrier-priced and noncovered services until the RUC evaluated these codes and developed recommendations. During 1994 much of the RUC's work was devoted to developing recommendations for these codes. In May 1994, relative value recommendations were submitted for these services, including preventive medicine, newborn care, transplant surgery, and pediatric neurosurgery codes.

The third cycle of RUC recommendations for the 1995 Medicare RVS included values for orthopedic, esophageal, rectal, liver, bile duct, and endocrine surgery; neurology; and monthly end-stage renal disease. In addition, the RUC HCPAC Review Board developed its first set of work relative values, covering services for physical medicine and rehabilitation.

As previously discussed, OBRA 89 mandated that CMS conduct a comprehensive review of the RBRVS relative values on a 5-year rolling basis. As part of this 5-year review, the RUC submitted work RVU recommendations for over 1000 individual codes in September 1995. RUC activities related to this comprehensive review are detailed in the following section.

As a result of the 5-year review, the RUC submitted relatively fewer recommendations for the 1996 RVS. The RUC's relative value recommendations were reflected in the 1996 RVS for new CPT codes for trauma care and for new and revised codes for spinal procedures. Very few CPT coding changes were submitted for the RUC's consideration for 1997. Extensive work RVU changes were implemented for the 1997 RVS, however, as a result of the 5-year review. These changes are described in the "Five-Year Review" section.

The RUC submitted its sixth year of work relative value recommendations for new and revised CPT codes in May 1997. The submission included recommendations on over 200 CPT codes, including home care visits, observation same-day discharge services, various laparoscopic procedures, percutaneous abscess drainage procedures, and PET myocardial perfusion imaging. The RUC also submitted recommendations for new CPT codes proposed by the American Academy of Pediatrics. The new codes better describe services provided to children, including conscious sedation, pediatric cardiac catheterization, and attendance at delivery.

In addition, the RUC HCPAC Review Board developed recommendations in several areas, including paring, cutting, and trimming of nails; and occupational and physical therapy evaluation services.

The RUC submitted work relative values for new and revised CPT codes in May of 1998, completing its seventh year of recommendations. The RUC and the national medical specialty societies reviewed over 298 coding changes for CPT 1999 and submitted over 100 recommendations to CMS. The remainder of the codes reviewed were editorial revisions or deletions. The recommendations included additions and revisions to the following services: inpatient and outpatient psychotherapy, hallex rigidus correction with cheilectomy, breast reconstruction, and radiologic examination of the knee. In addition, the RUC HCPAC Review Board also developed one recommendation for manual manipulative therapy techniques for CPT 1999.

In May 1999, the RUC submitted its eighth year of work relative value recommendations to CMS. This year also marked the first submission of direct practice expense inputs (clinical staff, supplies, and equipment) to CMS for use in developing practice expense relative values for new and revised CPT codes. There were more than 300 coding changes for CPT 2000, however, most were considered editorial in nature or reflected laboratory services included on the Medicare Clinical Lab Payment Schedule. The RUC submitted recommendations for more than 100 new and revised CPT codes, including: critical care, deep brain stimulation, spine injection procedures, integumentary system repair, and laparoscopic urological procedures.

The RUC forwarded recommendations on 224 codes in May 2000 in its ninth submission of annual new and revised code recommendations. The major issues reviewed in this cycle included: GI endoscopy procedures; MRI procedures; anesthesia services; stereotactic breast biopsy; and endovascular graft for abdominal aortic aneurism. The RUC also reviewed public comments and submitted recommendations on nearly 900 codes as part of the second 5-year review of the RBRVS. This project is discussed in more detail in the next section.

In May 2001, the RUC submitted its 10th year of work relative value recommendations to CMS. The RUC reviewed 314 codes, including many codes describing anesthesia services, hand surgery, pediatric surgery, and urological procedures.

Five-Year Review

In addition to annual updates reflecting changes in CPT, Section 1848(C)2(B) of the Omnibus Budget Reconciliation Act of 1990 requires CMS to comprehensively review all relative values at least every 5 years and make any needed adjustments. In November 1993, CMS began preparation for this project by inviting organized medicine to develop a proposal to participate in the review process.

The RUC sought a significant role in this comprehensive review of physician work relative values and appointed a subcommittee on the 5-year review to develop this concept. To further expand organized medicine's participation in the 5-year review process, the AMA solicited comments from the executive vice presidents of all the national medical specialty societies. Consensus emerged about how to conduct the 5-year review and revolved around the following major points: 1) the RUC should play a key role; 2) the refinement should focus on correcting errors and accounting for changes in medical practice, not the whole RVS; and 3) the methods should build upon the current RUC methodology for valuing codes. In March 1994, the AMA submitted a detailed plan to CMS identifying medicine's preferred approach to dealing with organizational and conceptual issues in the 5-year review. The proposed plan incorporated much of the RUC's current methodology and built upon the cooperative approach to review and refinement the RUC and CMS had established. Further, it was consistent with the AMA's policy goal that the medical profession should have the primary responsibility for long-term maintenance and refinement of the RBRVS.

The 1994 *Final Rule* described CMS's plans for conducting the 5-year review. The agency indicated that the RUC, based on its experience in developing relative values and its ability to involve a wide range of medical specialties in the refinement process, warranted a significant role in the 5-year review.

All codes on the 1995 payment schedule were open for public comment as part of the first 5-year review. Included was the development of relative values for pediatric services. The Social Security Amendments Act of 1994 required that RVUs be developed for the full range of pediatric services, as well as determining whether significant variations existed in the work required to furnish similar services to adult and pediatric patients.

In the 1999 *Final Rule,* CMS again invited the public to comment on the work relative value for any existing CPT code. The RUC also proposed a major role in this second, 5-year review of the RBRVS. The proposal and process was very similar to the first 5-year review. CMS forwarded the public comments to the RUC in March 2000.

Scope of the 5-year Review
First 5-Year Review

The 5-year review presented an unprecedented opportunity to improve the accuracy of the physician work component of the RBRVS, as well as a significant challenge to the medical community. During the public comment period, CMS received nearly 500 letters identifying about 1100 CPT codes for review. The Carrier Medical Directors, the

American Academy of Pediatrics (AAP), and special studies conducted for three specialty societies identified additional codes for review. Following an initial review, in late February 1995, CMS referred to the RUC comments on about 3500 codes. These comments fell into the following categories: public comments on 669 codes; Carrier Medical Director comments on 387 codes; the three special studies by Abt Associates, Inc; and comments submitted by the AAP.

In approaching its task, the RUC determined that a high standard of proof would be required for all proposed changes in work values. For example, specialties were required to present a "compelling argument" in order to maintain current values for services that the comments had identified as overvalued. The RUC's methodology for evaluating codes identified by public comment was similar to that used previously for the annual updates, with some innovations designed to require compelling arguments to support requested changes. The survey was modified to require additional information regarding comparisons with the key reference services selected, as well as the extent to which the service had changed over the previous 5 years.

The RUC also established multidisciplinary work groups to help manage the large number of comments referred and to ensure objective review of potentially overvalued services. These work groups evaluated the public and Carrier Medical Director comments and developed recommendations. The full RUC treated the recommendations as consent calendars, with other RUC members and specialty society representatives extracting for discussion any work group recommendations with which they disagreed.

The RUC also considered comments on nearly 500 codes that the AAP submitted. The society believed that physician work differed depending on whether children or adults were being treated. As a result, the AAP requested that appropriate new CPT codes be added to describe different age categories of patients and that relative values be assigned. The RUC and the CPT Editorial Panel helped the AAP refine its proposal for new and revised codes, which became effective for *CPT 1997*.

Finally, the RUC considered three studies Abt Associates conducted at the request of three medical specialty societies. The RUC found that two of the studies correctly ranked ordered codes within the respective specialties, but did not reach any conclusions about the third. Following these findings, however, the specialty societies each conducted further research on individually identified codes and submitted their recommendations to the RUC.

Second 5-Year Review
CMS received only 30 public comments in response to its solicitation of misvalued codes to be reviewed in the second, 5-Year Review. However, 870 codes were identified for review as several specialties (general surgery, vascular surgery and cardiothoracic surgery) commented that nearly all of the services performed by their specialty were mis-valued. In addition, the RUC reviewed a number of codes performed by gastroenterology, obstetrics/gynecology, orthopaedic surgery, pediatric surgery, and radiology.

The process that the RUC utilized in this 5-year review was very similar to the process utilized in the first 5-Year Review. Multidisciplinary workgroups were utilized to review the large number of codes. The full RUC then reviewed and discussed the reports of these work groups.

RUC Recommendations
First 5-Year Review
In September 1995, the RUC submitted to CMS relative value recommendations for more than 1000 individual codes. These recommendations maintained values for about 60% of the codes reviewed; increased values for about one third; and decreased values for the remainder. CMS's proposed RVU changes were published in a May 1996 *Federal Register*. Overall, CMS accepted 93% of the RUC's recommendations, including 100% acceptance for several specialties. Following a public comment period, final decisions were announced in the November 22, 1996, *Federal Register*. Key results are summarized below.

- *Evaluation and Management Services*. CMS extended its review to include all 98 E/M codes that were assigned RVUs, although the RUC submitted recommendations for only a portion of these codes. The RUC asserted that the postservice work involved in E/M services had increased over the past 5 years and that the intraservice work was undervalued compared to other services on the RBRVS. CMS accepted the argument and increased work RVUs for most E/M services, including a 25% increase for *office visits* (CPT codes 99202-99215) and an average 16.6% increase for *emergency department services* (CPT codes 99281-99285). Work RVUs also were increased for *critical care, first hour* (CPT code 99291) and *office or other outpatient consultations* (CPT codes 992241-99245).
- *Anesthesia*. CMS accepted the RUC's recommendation for a 22.76% increase to the work RVUs. CMS adopted the adjustment on an interim basis and opened it to public comment since it was not part of the proposed notice. The RUC based its recommendation on results of a study conducted for the American Society of Anesthesiologists and on the expertise of the RUC Research Subcommittee. There is no defined work RVU per code for anesthesia services, which required that the adjustment be made in the aggregate on the anesthesia conversion factor.
- *Psychiatry*. CMS accepted the RUC's recommendation that the work RVUs should be increased for five psychotherapy services. The agency rejected the

CPT code descriptors, however, stating that they did not sufficiently define physician work. For Medicare reporting and payment purposes, the CPT codes were replaced with 24 temporary alphanumeric codes. These codes were time-based and differentiated between office/outpatient psychotherapy and inpatient psychotherapy; insight-oriented, behavior modifying, and/or supportive psychotherapy and interactive psychotherapy; and psychotherapy furnished with and without medical evaluation and management. The 24 temporary codes were adopted by the CPT Editorial Panel for *CPT 1998*.

Second 5-Year Review
The RUC found that several specialties presented compelling evidence that their services were indeed misvalued. As a result, the RUC submitted recommendations to CMS in October 2000 to change the work relative value for many services. These recommendations may be summarized as follows:

- increase the work relative value for 469 CPT codes,
- decrease the work relative value for 27 CPT codes,
- maintain the work relative value for 311 CPT codes, and
- refer 63 codes to the CPT Editorial Panel to consider coding changes prior to consideration of the work relative value.

The CMS published a *Proposed Rule* on June 8, 2001, and a *Final Rule* on November 1, 2001, announcing the agency's intention to accept and implement more than 95% of the RUC's recommendations on January 1, 2002. Some of the important changes are as follows:

Vascular Surgery. The American Association for Vascular Surgery and the Society for Vascular Surgery argued that vascular surgery services were historically undervalued dating back to the original Harvard studies. The RUC reviewed detailed survey data for 95 codes. The RUC recommended that 91 vascular surgical procedures be increased. CMS will implement 100% of these recommendations.

General Surgery. The American College of Surgeons and the American Society for General Surgeons submitted comments related to more than 300 services performed predominately by general surgeons. A number of rank order anomalies and historical undervalued codes were identified. The RUC recommended that 242 codes be increased, 22 be decreased, and 50 be maintained. However, CMS was convinced that further increases were warranted and will implement further changes to the general surgery relative values.

Cardiothoracic Surgery. The Society for Thoracic Surgery also commented that 89 codes describing services performed by cardiothoracic surgeons were undervalued. The RUC recommended, and CMS will implement, increases to 41 of these services. For example, the RUC was convinced that the physician work related to congenital cardiac procedures has increased over the past 5 years.

Diagnostic Mammography. The RUC reviewed data submitted by the American College of Radiology (ACR) that indicated that the increase in physician work created by the implementation of the Mammography Quality Standards Act of 1992 (MQSA). The RUC agreed that these regulations and ACR standards did require more physician time and work. CMS implemented these increases on January 1, 2002.

Routine Obstetric Care
As part of the 1994 refinement process, CMS increased work values assigned to codes for routine obstetric care in response to a joint recommendation of the American College of Obstetricians and Gynecologists (ACOG) and the American Academy of Family Physicians (AAFP). The AMA had worked with ACOG and AAFP on this recommendation and urged CMS to adopt it. The ACOG-AAFP recommendation used a "building block" approach based on existing and RUC-proposed work values for the components of the obstetrical packages. The work values for CPT code 59400 (*Routine obstetric care including antepartum care, vaginal delivery [with or without episiotomy, and/or forceps] and postpartum care*) were increased by 9% and for CPT code 59510 (*Routine obstetric care including antepartum care, cesarean delivery, and postpartum care*) by 29%.

The work values assigned to these codes equal the midrange joint recommendation. The overall RBRVS increase for these two codes (including practice expense and professional liability values and after applying the 1.3% reduction for budget neutrality) is 8% for 59400 and 27% for 59510. These increases enhanced the ability of non-Medicare RBRVS payment systems, such as state Medicaid programs, to ensure access to needed obstetrical services.

Global Surgical Services
As part of the 5-year review, the RUC recommended that the relationship between E/M services and global surgical services be evaluated and that work RVUs for the latter services be increased consistent with the 1997 RVU increases for E/M services. CMS rejected the RUC's views in its May 1996 *Proposed Rule*. The agency agreed, however, to reexamine the issue for the 1998 RVS in the November 1996 *Final Rule*.

Surgical specialty societies argued that E/M services related to a procedure were subject to the same increasing complexity as nonprocedural E/M services due to such factors as reduced inpatient lengths of stay and same-day admissions for major surgery. An additional major contributing factor is the greater utilization of home health care services, requiring the surgeon to be more involved in postservice planning and management.

Following its evaluation, CMS concluded that the work RVUs associated with global surgical services should be increased to reflect the increased evaluation and management present in the preservice and postservice portions of these services. For 1998, CMS implemented an across-the-board increase to the work RVUs for global surgical services. The change produced an average increase of 4% in services with a 10-day global period and 7% for services with a 90-day global period. To maintain budget neutrality of physician payments under the payment schedule, CMS applied a –0.7% adjustment to the conversion factor.

Future Plans

As the trend continues toward adopting the Medicare RBRVS by non-Medicare payers, including state Medicaid programs, workers' compensation plans, CHAMPUS, and state health system reform plans, it is critical that the physician work component be complete and appropriate for all patient populations.

The RUC is committed to improving and maintaining the validity of the RBRVS over time. Through the RUC, the AMA and the specialty societies have worked aggressively to identify and correct flaws and gaps in the RBRVS. In subsequent 5-year reviews, the RUC will continue to review all services considered to be inappropriately valued.

The AMA strongly supports the RUC process as the principal method to refine and maintain the Medicare RVS and believes that the RUC represents an important opportunity for the medical profession to retain professional control of the clinical practice of medicine. It will continue to support the RUC in its efforts to secure CMS adoption of its relative value recommendations.

References and Notes

1. *A National Survey of Resource-Based Relative Value Scales for Physician Services: Phase III.* Revised. Boston, Mass: Department of Health Policy and Management, Harvard School of Public Health, and Department of Psychology, Harvard University; August 30, 1992.

   Braun P, guest ed. The Resource-Based Relative Value Scale: its further development and reform of physician payment. *Med Care.* 1992;30.

2. *A National Study of Resource-Based Relative Value Scales for Physician Services: MFS Refinement.* Boston, Mass: Department of Health Policy and Management, Harvard School of Public Health, and Department of Psychology, Harvard University; July 30, 1993.

3. *The American Medical Association/Specialty Society RVS Update Process.* Chicago, Ill: American Medical Association; 2001.

Chapter 5
The Practice Expense Component

Beginning in January 1999, Medicare began a transition to resource-based practice expense relative values which establish practice expense payment for each CPT code that differ based on the site of service. Procedures which can be performed in a physicians office as well as in a hospital now have two practice expense relative values; facility and non-facility practice expense relative values. The non-facility setting includes physician offices, freestanding imaging centers, and independent pathology labs. Facility settings include all other settings, such as hospitals, ambulatory surgery centers, skilled nursing facilities, and partial hospitals. In 2002 the resource-based practice expenses will be fully transitioned and the practice expense component of the RBRVS will be resource-based. This chapter describes the method that the Centers for Medicare and Medicaid Services (CMS) (formerly the Health Care Financing Administration) used to assign practice expense in the 1991 *Final Rule* as well as the history and methodology used to develop the new resource-based practice expense relative values.

Data Used to Assign Charge Based Practice Expense RVUs

Most of the practice expense data that the CMS used to assign RVUs in the 1991 *Final Rule* were from the AMA's Socioeconomic Monitoring System 1989 Core Survey, which reflects the responses of a nationally representative sample of 4000 physicians in 34 specialties. Because the Medicare payment schedule applies to several non-MD/DO practitioner groups, CMS also used data supplied by the American Association of Oral and Maxillofacial Surgeons, the American Optometric Association, the American Podiatric Medical Association, and the American Chiropractic Association. Data for clinics and other group practice arrangements were supplied by the Medical Group Management Association. When no other data were available, CMS used averages representing all physicians.

The OBRA 89 Method

The fundamental approach used in developing the Medicare resource-based relative value scale (RBRVS) measured the average resource costs involved in providing each physician service. The basis for the work component RVUs therefore measured the average work involved in a service by surveying randomly selected samples of practicing physicians.

The OBRA 89 approach to determining the practice expense component is similar to the work component because it relies, in part, on data from the AMA's national survey of physicians' average practice costs. However, physicians generally measure practice costs as a total sum, not service by service. Surveys of practicing physicians regarding their

Table 1. Physician Practice Expense Ratios—1989
As a percentage of mean total revenue

AMA Specialty	CMS Specialty	Mean Expenses Net PLI	Mean PLI Expenses
All physicians		41.0%	4.8%
General/family practice	Family practice	52.2	3.9
	General practice	52.2	3.9
Internal medicine		46.4	2.8
General internal medicine	Internal medicine	46.4	2.8
Cardiovascular disease	Cardiovascular disease	36.1	2.7
Other	Allergy	40.5	2.6
	Gastroenterology	40.5	2.6
	Geriatrics	40.5	2.6
	Nephrology	40.5	2.6
	Pulmonary disease	40.5	2.6
Surgery		31.8	7.4
General surgery	General surgery	31.8	7.4
Otolaryngology	Otology, laryngology, rhinology	45.2	4.9
Orthopedic surgery	Orthopedic surgery	45.2	7.4
Ophthalmology	Ophthalmology	44.4	2.3
	Ophthalmology, otology, laryngology	44.4	2.3
Urological surgery	Urology	39.9	3.9
Other	Hand surgery	38.9	7.6
	Neurological surgery	38.9	7.6
	Peripheral vascular disease or surgery	38.9	7.6
	Plastic surgery	38.9	7.6
	Proctology	38.9	7.6
	Thoracic surgery	38.9	7.6
Pediatrics	Pediatrics	49.3	3.1
Obstetrics/gynecology	Gynecology	38.8	8.8
	Obstetrics	38.8	8.8
	Obstetrics-gynecology	38.8	8.8
Radiology*	Diagnostic x-ray (groups)[1]	50.5	3.3
	Global for the radiology specialties below	37.2	3.0
	Radiation therapy (professional component)	22.9	3.3
	Radiology (professional component)	22.9	3.3

AMA Specialty	CMS Specialty	Mean Expenses Net PLI	Mean PLI Expenses
	Roentgenology, radiology (professional component)	22.9%	3.3%
	Radiation therapy (technical component)	94.1	5.9
	Radiology (technical component)	94.1	5.9
	Roentgenology, radiology (technical component)	94.1	5.9
Psychiatry	Psychiatry	26.4	3.7
	Psychiatry, neurology	26.4	3.7
Anesthesiology	Anesthesiology	23.2	7.3
Pathology	Diagnostic laboratory (groups)[1]	50.5	3.3
	Pathologic anatomy, clinical	28.5	1.9
	Pathology	28.5	1.9
Other specialty			
	Dermatology	40.3	3.0
	Occupational therapy (groups)[1]	50.5	3.3
	Other medical care (groups)[1]	50.5	3.3
	Neurology	40.3	3.0
	Nuclear medicine	40.3	3.0
	Physical medicine and rehabilitation	40.3	3.0
No AMA match	Clinic or other group practice (groups)[1]	50.5	3.0
No AMA match	Oral surgery[2]	54.7	4.4
No AMA match	Optometrist[3]	52.9	0.1
No AMA match	Podiatry[4]	47.8	4.2
No AMA match	Chiropractor, licensed[5]	58.4	1.8
No AMA match	Manipulative therapy	41.0	4.8
	Miscellaneous	41.0	4.8
	Physical therapy	41.0	4.8
	Occupational therapist	41.0	4.8
	Physiotherapy	41.0	4.8

Source: *Final Rule,* p 59868.

Source: American Medical Association, 1988 1990 Socioeconomic Monitoring System Core surveys except where indicated.

[1] Source: Medical Group Management Association, 1990 Cost and Survey Production Report.

[2] Source: American Association of Oral and Maxillofacial Surgeons.

[3] Source: American Optometry Association.

[4] Source: American Podiatric Medical Association.

[5] Source: American Chiropractic Association.

[6] Source: For these remaining specialties, CMS used the practice cost percents from the AMA for all physicians.

*Note: For radiology services, the professional component percentages were based on data for radiologists with equipment expenses of $5000 or less. The technical component percentages were based on data for radiologist with equipment expenses of more than $5000.

costs of practice, therefore, provided data on the average total amount that they spend on office rents, wages of non-physician personnel, supplies, and equipment. The data did not provide the average office rent expense, for example, related to a particular service or the average nursing time required for that service.

These surveys also indicated that average practice costs vary by specialty overall and as a percentage of gross revenue. Practice costs accounted for a higher proportion of general and family physicians' revenues (52.2%) than for cardiologists' (36.1%) or neurosurgeons' (38.9%) as shown in table 1.

To distribute practice expense RVUs among the services each specialty provides, the OBRA 89 method applies the average practice cost percentage for each specialty to the 1991 average Medicare approved amount for the service. (The average approved amounts are initially expressed in dollars for this purpose and later put on the scale of RVUs, then converted back to dollars when the total RVUs for the service are multiplied by the monetary conversion factor.) For example:

- For a service that only family practitioners provide and for which the average Medicare payment in 1991 was $100, multiply the practice cost proportion (52.2%) by the $100 average approved amount. The practice expense component of the service would be assigned 52.2 (initial dollar) RVUs.
- For a service that only neurosurgeons provide and for which the average Medicare payment in 1991 was $1000, multiply the practice cost proportion (38.9%) by the $1000 average approved amount. The practice expense component of the service would be assigned 389.0 (initial dollar) RVUs.

For services provided by physicians in more than one specialty, multiply each specialty's practice cost proportion by the proportion of claims for the service that the specialty submits:

- For a service provided 70% of the time by family physicians and 30% of the time by internists and for which the average Medicare approved amount in 1991 was $100, multiply the family physicians' practice cost proportion (52.2%) by 70% and the internal medicine practice cost proportion (46.4%) by 30%. The sum of these two products becomes the practice cost proportion for the service:

$$(52.2\% \times 0.70) + (46.4\% \times 0.30) = 50.5\%$$

- This practice cost proportion is then multiplied by the $100 average approved amount:

$$(50.5\% \times 100) = 50.5$$

- The practice cost component of the service would be assigned 50.5 (initial dollar) RVUs.
- For a service that is provided 70% of the time by neurosurgeons and 30% of the time by orthopedic surgeons and for which the average Medicare approved amount in 1991 was $1000, multiply the neurosurgeons' practice cost proportion (38.9%) by 70% and the orthopedic surgeons' practice cost proportion (45.2%) by 30%. The sum of these two products becomes the practice cost proportion for the service:

$$(38.9\% \times 0.70) + (45.2\% \times 0.30) = 40.8\%$$

- This practice cost proportion is then multiplied by the $1000 average approved amount:

$$(40.8\% \times 1000) = 408$$

- The practice cost component of the service would be assigned 408 (initial dollar) RVUs.

The OBRA 89 method of assigning practice expense RVUs clearly provides a much rougher approximation of physicians' average resource costs per service than does the method of assigning work component RVUs.

Because anesthesia services are not divided into work, practice expense, and PLI cost RVUs, CMS computed the proportions of total payments for anesthesia that were comparable to these three components for other services. The portion of the anesthesiology conversion factor reflecting the work component was reduced by 42%. As for other services, to maintain a Medicare contribution comparable to the contribution under customary, prevailing, and reasonable (CPR), the portion of the conversion factor reflecting practice were not reduced.

The CMS based the 1992 practice cost on 1989 charge data "aged" to reflect 1991 payment rules because those were the most recent data available. For the 1992 payment schedule, actual 1991 charge data were used to recalculate the practice cost for some codes for which CMS had imputed values the previous year. For services with insufficient charge data and for new codes, CMS developed crosswalks to predecessor codes, where possible. Since 1993, CMS has used a similar process to establish values for such codes.

Concerns With the OBRA 89 Method

In the years immediately following implementation of the Medicare RBRVS, many organizations, especially the Physician Payment Review Commission (PPRC) and primary care specialties, expressed concern about the OBRA 89 method of calculating practice expenses. These organizations were concerned that practice expense relative values based on historical Medicare allowed charges failed to reflect the relative resource costs of providing a service. They were also concerned that statutorily designated "overvalued procedure" reductions in 1990 and 1991 lowered the practice cost RVUs to levels less than they would otherwise have been when OBRA 89 was enacted.

OBRA 93 Revisions to the Practice Expense Component

Congress adopted additional payment reductions to "overvalued" services under OBRA 93. The legislation called for reductions to the practice expense relative values for such "overvalued" procedure codes to be phased in over a 3-year period, 1994-1996. The practice expense RVUs of the affected services were reduced each year by 25% of the amount by which they exceeded the physician work RVUs but could not fall below a floor of 128% of the work RVUs. Services performed at least 75% of the time in the physician office setting were exempt from the reductions, as were services without work RVUs (eg, diagnostic tests with only a technical component). In addition, practice expense RVUs assigned to a global service were subject to the same reduction as its technical component.

Resource-Based Practice Expenses

Congress' interest in developing resource-based practice expense relative values goes back several years to 1992 when the Physician Payment Review Commission (PPRC) published a report on resource-based practice expenses. Section 121 of the Social Security Act amendments, enacted in late 1994, required development of "resource-based" practice expense relative values for implementation in 1998. It required that the new resource-based methodology consider the staff, equipment, and supplies used to provide medical and surgical services in various settings.

Developing the Methodology

To respond to the Congressional mandate, CMS contracted with Abt Associates, Inc, for a national study of physicians' practice expenses. This study was designed to have three components: use of Clinical Practice Expert Panels (CPEPs) to estimate the direct costs associated with each CPT-coded service; use of a national mail survey of 5000 practices to obtain information on practice costs and service mix; and collection of data on the price of each input, such as equipment and disposable supplies. Due to delays in the Abt study at each step in the process and Congressional concern about the validity of CMS's methodology, Congress extended the implementation deadline by 1 year to January 1999.

The CMS determined that the primary methodology for deriving resource-based practice expense values should incorporate microcosting, a cost accounting approach that identifies all direct costs associated with a particular service. This methodology was to produce a detailed database to support several analytical methods for estimating practice expense per service. Estimates for both direct and indirect practice expenses for all services under the RBRVS were to be included. Direct expenses are those for equipment, supplies, and clinical and administrative staff associated with providing a particular service to an individual patient. Indirect expenses include office rent and equipment, utilities, and staff and other costs not directly allocable to an individual service. Estimates would vary according to the site of service.

The CMS began constructing the new database in March 1995. Data were to be collected from two types of expert panels and from a detailed practicing physician survey for distribution to 5000 physician offices.

Two types of expert panels were formed:

- *Clinical Practice Expert Panels (CPEPs).* Fifteen CPEPs were formed, with membership based on nominations from medical associations. The role of the CPEPs was to produce data for Abt to use in constructing direct cost estimates. Each CPEP developed "resource profiles," a detailed list of direct cost elements associated with a service, for a selected group of reference procedures. The cost estimates were then extended to the rest of the codes in a family.
- *Clinical Practice Expert Panel Technical Expert Group (TEG).* The TEG's role was to monitor the data collection process to ensure that the data are usable by other researchers who might conduct further analyses for generating practice expense relative values. The TEG members include researchers in this area and representatives of organized medicine, including the AMA, American College of Physicians, American College of Surgeons, and American College of Radiologists. In addition, TEG meetings were attended by observers from the AMA/Specialty Society RVS Update Committee (RUC), American Hospital Association, and the PPRC.

The national mail survey was designed to collect detailed information on aggregate indirect and direct practice expenses and relate them to individual CPT codes. It also solicited information on the practice's case mix and general characteristics. The data compiled by the CPEPs and through the survey would be used by Abt to calculate indirect costs for individual services and validate direct cost estimates with review by the CPEPs. Two alternative CMS studies produced additional data to be used to allocate indirect costs across procedures. One study allocated indirect costs based on the physician time required for the service; the other set practice expense relative values so that they were the same proportion of relative value units as practice expenses are of total practice revenues within a specialty. Both studies relied on existing data, including that from the AMA's Socioeconomic Monitoring System (SMS), to determine the proportion of expenses that are direct and indirect.

The CPEPs and the national mail survey were designed to combine expert professional analysis and actual practice expense data, which could be used to develop relative values. The CPEPs were comprised of groups of physicians and other health care professionals who met to develop values for the direct cost component for each service. For each procedure on the RBRVS, the CPEPs developed lists of the practice resources required to provide the service, including the time of nonphysician clinical personnel, equipment, and supplies. The national mail survey would be used to validate the CPEP estimates, determine the proportions of practice expenses devoted to direct vs indirect expenses, and indicate how indirect costs, which include rent, furnishings, computer equipment, office supplies, and other administrative overhead costs, could be appropriately allocated across procedures. However, in April 1996, CMS announced that, due to insufficient response rates to an initial survey, it could not use the results of the survey to develop the new relative values. In September 1996, CMS announced that it had cancelled all further work on the national mail survey. At the same time, however, the CMS announced it would publish proposed practice expense RVUs in March 1997 to meet the implementation deadline of January 1, 1998.

CMS's decisions to cancel the mail survey and to proceed with plans for 1998 implementation heightened the level of concern about the process for developing resource-based practice expense relative values. In the absence of the mail survey, it was not clear where CMS would find data suitable for determining the split between indirect costs and direct costs; validating the results from the CPEP process; and allocating indirect costs among procedures. With estimates of the proportion of total costs that are direct costs ranging from 30% to 80% and the CPEP process relying on a very small number of physicians in each specialty, the lack of data on physicians' actual practice expenses made any assessment of the validity of the resource-based relative values extremely difficult.

Opposition to the Medicare Proposed Methodology

The AMA urged the Clinton administration to defer action on a Proposed Rule and to request Congress to adopt legislation extending the deadline for implementing practice expense changes. Deferment was necessary for several major reasons:

- The proposed relative values did not account for many practice expenses, including physician office staff, equipment utilization, and differences in actual practice costs of various specialties.
- A transition period and refinement process would not solve major problems with the practice expense proposal; rather, agreement must be reached on the basic methodology and the database before designing a transition and refinement process.
- Additional time was needed to allow physicians the opportunity to validate data and assumptions.
- Adopting the flawed proposed values would extend beyond the Medicare program, as some private sector payors had indicated they would implement payment cuts based on the CMS data.

In June 1997, CMS issued its proposed regulation, which included a practice expense methodology heavily dependent on the CPEP data. Instead of using actual practice expense data to verify the CPEP data, CMS used a number of assumptions and adjustments designed to improve data consistency among the expert panels. However, the AMA and some specialty societies were critical of the CMS methodology and called for a 1-year delay in implementation. During the rule's public comment period, more than 8000 comments were submitted to CMS by individual physicians, professional societies, and others. Many groups, including the AMA, argued that CMS moved too quickly and without sufficient data to implement a resource-based methodology. The AMA submitted detailed comments for improving CMS's approach, including recommendations on the following issues:

- *Direct cost data.* 1) Per-procedure cost estimates the CPEPs developed should be reviewed and errors corrected. 2) CMS's assumptions regarding use of overhead and procedure-specific equipment greatly overstate its utilization, thus significantly undervaluing equipment costs. Data on actual equipment utilization rates should be collected and used in the relative values.
- *Indirect costs.* The methodology for assigning indirect cost RVUs should recognize all staff, equipment, supplies, and expenses, not just those that can be tied to specific procedures. CMS should evaluate the relationship between the proposed relative values and physicians'

actual practice expenses and revise its methodology to account for specialty differences in the costs of operating a medical practice.

- *Multiple procedure reduction.* CMS should not apply the current multiple procedure rule for surgery to office procedures that are provided during the same encounter as a visit. Resource cost data are not available to demonstrate that physician work and practice expenses for office procedures are reduced by half when an office visit is also provided.

Legislation Revises Medicare's Proposal

Profound dissatisfaction with CMS's methodology and the proposed relative values led many physician groups, including the AMA, to work vigorously with members of Congress to enact needed legislative changes. Due to these concerns, Congress delayed the implementation of the new practice expense relative values until January 1999, and directed the General Accounting Office (GAO) to evaluate CMS's proposed methodology and data. Congress also adopted a number of provisions directed to improve the accuracy of the resource-based methodology. The provisions were included in the Balanced Budget Act of 1997. For example, it specified the data that must be used in developing the new values and required implementation over a 4-year transition period.

As a first step toward implementing a resource-based system, the law called for adjusting the practice expense values for certain services for 1998. Services whose practice expense values were proposed for reduction by CMS in the June 1997 *Proposed Rule,* and that were not performed at least 75% of the time in an office setting, were reduced to be equivalent to 110% of the work RVUs for the service. The reduction was used to increase the practice expense RVUs for office visits.

The GAO issued its report in February 1998, and its recommendations were highly consistent with AMA policy. The GAO's review of CMS's methodology found that CMS's use of the CPEPs was reasonable but that many of CMS's adjustments to the data were questionable and may have biased the cost estimates. For example, the GAO reported that "CMS capped nonphysician clinical labor time at $1^1/_2$ times the minutes used by a physician to perform a procedure. CMS has not, however, conducted tests or studies that validate these changes and thus cannot be assured that they are necessary or reasonable." The GAO recommended CMS collect additional data to validate its adjustments and assumptions and also evaluate alternative methodologies for adjusting the CPEP data.

The 1999 Resource-Based Methodology

On June 5, 1998, CMS issued a new proposal that contained two options for a practice expense methodology. The first option was referred to as the "bottom up" approach and was basically the same as the previously proposed methodology without many of the adjustments to the CPEP data. The second option was referred to as the "top-down" approach because it uses actual practice cost data developed by the AMA Socioeconomic Monitoring Survey (SMS) data, which is allocated down to individual procedures using the data collected in the CPEP process. This methodology was significantly different from previous proposals.

On November 2, 1998, CMS issued its final proposal on the practice expense relative value methodology. CMS selected the new "top-down" approach published in June 1998 with only minor changes. CMS begins it methodology by dividing practice costs into six categories: clinical labor, medical supplies, medical equipment, office expense, administrative labor, and all other expenses.

The SMS data consist of the average annual practice expense per average hours worked by physicians in a given specialty. These expense data are then multiplied by the total time spent treating Medicare patients as determined by RUC/Harvard physician time data and Medicare claims data. Each specialty cost pool is then allocated to procedures performed by that specialty using the Clinical Practice Expert Panel (CPEP) data. This process can be broken down into 6 steps.

Step 1 Specialty Practice Expenses The AMA's SMS data provide the aggregate practice expense per hour according to each specialty and cost category. This is obtained by dividing total practice expenses, as determined by the SMS survey, by total physician hours worked, also determined by the SMS survey. For those specialties not included in the SMS data, CMS crosswalked these specialties to specialties that were included in the SMS data. These data constitute the total practice expenses, which are allocated to specific codes according to the methodology discussed below in Steps 2 through 5.

Step 2 Physician Time Spent Treating Medicare Patients The frequency with which each service is performed on Medicare patients by each specialty is multiplied by the estimated physician time required to perform each service. This results in the total physician time spent treating Medicare patients according to procedure. The physician time data were taken either from the RUC surveys of new and revised codes or, for those codes that the RUC has not examined, from the original Harvard RBRVS survey. The physician time data consists of all time involved in a procedure including pre, intra, and post service time.

Step 3 Specialty Practice Expense Cost Pools A practice expense pool for each specialty and cost category is calculated by multiplying the results of step 1 by the results of Step 2. The practice expenses per hour multiplied by the total hours spent treating Medicare patients results in the total practice expenses, which will be allocated to codes according to specialty. For codes without a work relative value, CMS created a separate technical services cost pool that is not specialty specific. The costs for this technical pool were taken from specialty pools that have codes without a work RVU and allocated according to 1998 charge-based relative value units; therefore, these codes are not yet resource based.

Step 4 Allocate Practice Expense Pools to Individual Codes As Figures 2 and 3 illustrate, each specialty's cost pool is divided into six categories: clinical labor, medical supplies, medical equipment, administrative labor, office expense, and all other expenses. These six categories are further separated into two groups, which can be considered direct and indirect costs. The first group of direct costs includes clinical labor, medical supplies, and medical equipment. The second group of indirect costs includes administrative labor, office expense, and all other expenses.

The practice expense cost pools are primarily allocated to individual codes using the CPEP cost per procedure data, which establishes the relativity among codes within each specialty. Unlike previous proposed methodologies, CMS used the original CPEP data without making any adjustments; however, CMS used a different allocation method for the direct and indirect categories.

The direct cost group consisting of clinical labor, medical supplies, and medical equipment was allocated by first multiplying the CPEP costs by the Medicare frequency data for each procedure. This produces a cost per procedure and category. These CPEP cost pools are then scaled to the SMS data so that the total CPEP costs for each specialty equal the total SMS cost by specialty. Changes to the CPEP values can change the total CPEP pool and also the scaling factor resulting in the same size scaled pool but with different values assigned to individual codes. If for example, one family of codes have the CPEP inputs reduced, then the total CPEP pool is reduced, creating a larger scaling factor. Therefore, this has the effect of increasing the scaled values of the remaining codes so that the scaled pool remains the same. This results in a redistribution among codes for a specialty.

Figure 2. Overall Allocation Approach

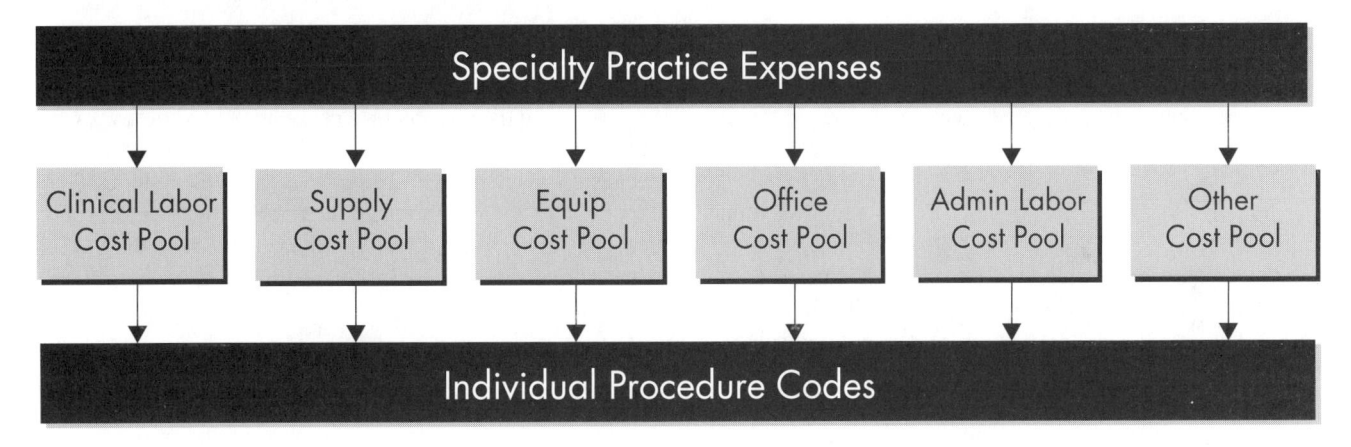

Figure 3. Cost Allocation Methodology

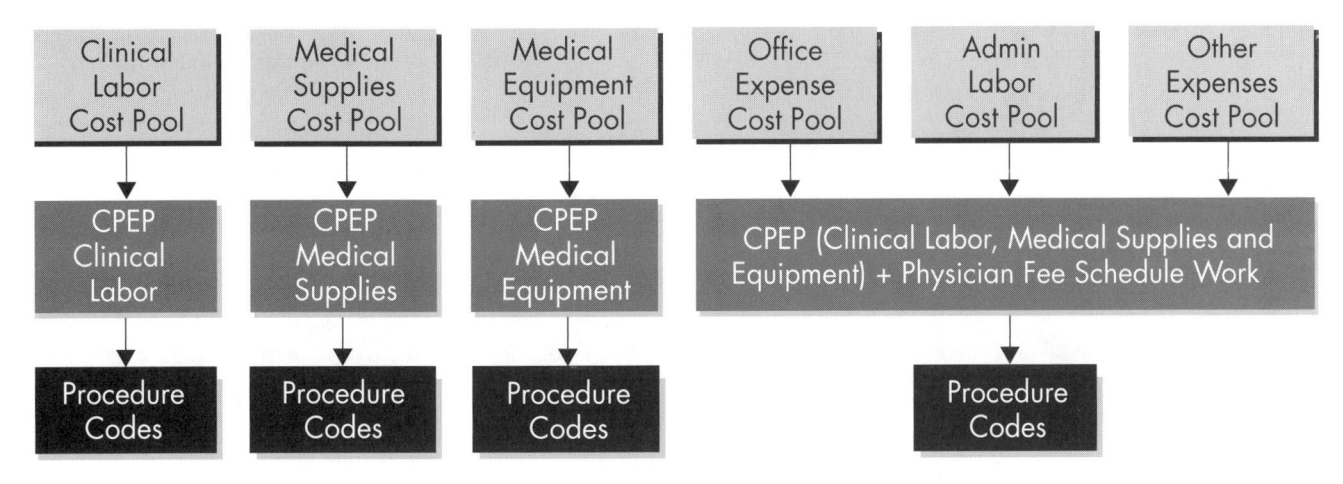

The second cost group consists of administrative labor, office expenses, and all other expenses. These costs are allocated by a combination of the direct costs calculated above and the work relative values. This methodology assumes a direct relationship between the work relative values and indirect expenses so that codes with higher work values will be assigned more indirect costs.

Step 5 Average the RVUs for Procedures Performed by More Than One Specialty For those codes performed by more than one specialty, CMS calculated a weighted average of the practice expenses based on Medicare frequency data. This weight averaging that occurs when services are provided by more than one specialty can sometimes have the effect of altering a specialty's payments when CPEP inputs are changed. When certain services have their CPEP inputs reduced, those expenses are then shifted to other services. As described above this only changes the allocation of costs but should not affect total payments for a specialty. However, when these inputs are weight averaged, a specialty can experience a decrease in costs if the specialty's costs for certain services are higher than other specialty's. The end result is sometimes a lower weighted average cost figure than the specialty's reported costs.

Step 6 Budget Neutrality Adjustment The final relative values are adjusted to match historical RVU totals to maintain budget neutrality.

During the transition period, practice expense relative value units will be a combination of the 1998 charge-based value and the new resource value. In 1999, practice expense resource values were based on 75% of the 1998 charge-based relative value and 25% on the resource-based value. In 2000 the mix will be equally weighted between the charge-based and resource-based values, and in 2001 the practice expense relative values will be 75% resource based and only 25% charged based. In 2002 the transition will be complete, with practice expense RVUs totally resource based.

SMS Data Used in CMS Methodology

The AMA's SMS specialty practice costs data plays a critical role in CMS's methodology for establishing practice expense relative values. The practice expense/hour data are based on the AMA SMS survey. The AMA has stated that these data were never collected for the purpose of developing relative values and has identified three potential problems with the use of these data for this purpose:

- The sample sizes for some specialties will be too small to permit separate calculation of expense data from SMS. Even among the larger specialties, the inherent variability of the expense data will mean that the average expense figures provided will be subject to significant sampling error.
- The response rates for the expense items tend to be low relative to other questions on the survey, leading to potential nonresponse bias.
- The SMS is a physician-level survey and physicians in group practices are asked for their share of expenses rather than the practice's expenses. Practice-level data may provide a better basis for constructing practice expense RVUs.

Although the SMS survey was not originally designed for the purpose of constructing practice expense RVUs, CMS has made it clear that it intends to use the SMS and will look for improvements during the refinement process. The AMA is already planning significant modifications to the SMS over the next few years. The AMA has also pilot tested a practice level survey and continues to explore alternative ways to collect data on physician practice expense.

Example of Practice Expense per Hour Calculation

The SMS expense per hour data were calculated according to a formula specified by CMS. This formula adjusted the SMS expense data to obtain average hourly expenses per physician in the practice. These adjustments were necessary because physicians in groups are asked for their share of expenses on SMS (rather than the total for the practice) and because only self-employed physicians are asked the SMS expense questions. The expense per hour formula is:

$$\frac{X \times nown}{(ownhrs \times nown) + (emphrs \times nemp)}$$

where: X = the respondent's share of his or her practices expenses for the previous year

$nown$ = the number of owner physicians in the respondent's practice

$nemp$ = the number of employee physicians in the respondent's practice

$ownhrs$ = an estimate of total hours+ worked in direct patient care by the respondent for the previous year

$emphrs$ = an estimate of average hours worked in direct patient care by employee physicians of the same specialty as the respondent for the previous year.

The variable $ownhrs$ is calculated as the product of the number of weeks the respondent reportedpracticing the previous

Table 2. Mean practice expenses per hour spent in patient care activities, hours and expenses adjusted for practice size (in dollars)

Specialty	# of Cases	Non-Phys Payroll Per Hour	Non-Phys Clinical Staff*	Clerical Payroll Per Hour	Office Expense Per Hour	Supplies Expense Per Hour	Equipment Expense Per Hour	Other Expense Per Hour	Total Expense Per Hour**
All Physicians	5470	27.7	12.3	15.4	19.4	7.4	3.2	11.5	69.0
General/Family Practice	587	29.7	14.8	14.9	17.7	7.9	3.1	8.8	67.1
General Internal Medicine	590	23.8	9.4	14.4	17.9	6.1	2.1	6.6	56.5
Cardiovascular Disease	140	31.0	15.8	15.2	20.7	6.2	5.9	17.8	81.6
Gastroenterology	110	25.9	8.9	17.0	18.0	3.6	2.1	12.3	61.8
Allergy/Immunology	47	61.6	36.3	25.3	31.4	16.0	4.0	15.8	128.8
Pulmonary Disease	75	19.3	6.9	12.4	15.7	2.6	1.6	6.9	46.1
Oncology w/supplies adj.	37	51.5	27.4	24.1	26.5	7.4	4.6	9.3	99.3
General Surgery	355	22.8	7.2	15.6	16.8	3.4	2.0	9.9	54.9
Otolaryngology	141	42.4	17.2	25.2	32.9	7.5	5.6	17.2	105.7
Orthopedic Surgery	289	45.1	16.6	28.5	29.7	10.3	3.8	19.1	108.0
Ophthalmology	301	50.9	25.1	25.8	34.1	10.8	8.4	21.1	125.3
Urological Surgery	156	30.9	12.4	18.5	23.2	25.5	5.3	11.3	96.2
Plastic Surgery	122	35.3	15.0	20.3	32.4	18.5	5.7	25.2	117.2
Neurological Surgery	57	34.2	8.6	25.6	28.6	1.8	1.4	16.1	82.2
Cardiac/Thoracic Surgery***	146	34.9	18.1	16.8	16.8	1.8	2.2	13.1	68.8
Pediatrics	361	25.3	12.4	12.9	18.9	10.2	1.7	8.6	64.8
Obstetrics/Gynecology	355	35.2	16.4	18.8	24.7	7.3	3.2	11.2	81.7
Radiation Oncology	46	23.2	14.0	9.2	12.1	5.4	9.7	16.4	66.8
Radiology	280	20.1	9.3	10.8	14.8	4.8	7.4	20.9	68.0
Psychiatry	487	6.8	1.7	5.1	10.5	0.4	0.4	7.2	25.3
Anesthesiology	321	15.0	11.3	3.7	5.9	0.4	0.4	5.9	27.6
Pathology w/Part A Hrs Adjustment of 1.37	119	25.2	11.2	14.0	11.9	6.8	2.0	21.0	66.9
Dermatology	137	50.9	22.5	28.4	33.4	12.6	5.4	17.2	119.4
Emergency Medicine w/adjustment for admn, other	98	18.7	3.3	15.4	2.0	0.7	0.1	11.5	33.0
Neurology	83	31.3	8.3	23.0	19.5	5.2	4.4	9.3	69.7
Phys Med/Rheumatology	101	38.6	14.9	23.7	30.7	6.5	6.2	12.2	94.2
Other Specialty	66	22.3	9.3	13.0	19.3	4.9	1.9	8.8	57.3
Vascular Surgery*** (Supplemental Data)	57	38.3	20.2	18.1	17.7	3.2	4.5	11.4	75.1
Physical and Occupational Therapy****		18.2	12.3	5.9	7.5	7.4	3.2	4.4	40.7

Source: Center for Health Policy Research, American Medical Association, 1995-1999 SMS Surveys
*Clinical staff and clerical payroll are included in total non-physician payroll.
**Total expenses exclude professional liability insurance premiums and employee physician payroll.
***CMS accepted revised data based on an oversample of Cardiothoracic surgeons and vascular using the SMS survey.
****Physical and occupational therapy based on "All Physician" for clinical staff, supplies, and equipment. It is based on salary equivalency guidelines assuming 750 square ft of office space for clerical, office and other indirect expense.

Notes:
(1) Only self-employed non-federal non-resident patient care physicians who responded to all relevant expense questions are included. Self-employed physician respondents with no practice expenses for the year are excluded.
(2) Physicians whose typical number of hours worked in patient care activities per week is missing, less than 20, or equal to 168 (3 cases) are excluded. Physicians whose number of weeks worked in the previous year is missing or less than 26 are excluded.
(3) For each respondent, total practice expense and expense components per hour are calculated as (4)/(5) below.
(4) Expenses adjusted for practice size = self-employed respondent expense * # physician owners.
(5) Hours adjusted for practice size = (respondent hours * # physician owners) + (employee physician hours (see (6) below).
(6) The typical number of hours worked in patient care activities for the employee physician(s) of a self-employed physician's practice is not known. Mean hour worked in patient care activities for employee physicians of each specialty are used as an estimate of employee physician hours.

year (*week*) and the number of hours the respondent reported spending in direct patient care activities in a typical week (*hours*). The same calculation for annual hours worked was performed for employee physicians, and the (weighted) mean of this amount was calculated for physicians of the same specialty as the respondent to obtain *emphrs*.

For solo physicians *nown* = 1 and *nemp* = 0, and the formula becomes:

$$\frac{X}{ownhrs}$$

or simply expenses divided by hours worked in direct patient care.

As an example of the expense per hour calculation for physicians in groups, suppose that a general surgeon reported that her share of the practice's office expenses was $100,000 for the previous year. Suppose she also reported that there were two owner physicians in the practice (including herself) and two employee physicians, and that she worked 50 weeks the previous year and 60 hours per week in direct patient care in a typical week. Average annual hours worked for employee physicians in general surgery were 2381.8. The necessary data for calculating office expenses per hour for this respondent are:

X	=	$100,000
nown	=	2
nemp	=	2
ownhrs	=	50 × 60 = 3000
emphrs	=	2381.8

The numerator of the expense per hour formula will be $200,000 for this physician for office expenses. This is an estimate of the *practice's* total office expenses for the previous year, assuming that physician owners share expenses equally.

The denominator of the expense per hour formula will be 10,763.8 hours for this physician. This is an estimate of total hours worked the previous year by all physicians (owners and employees) in the practice. It assumes that the average annual hours worked among all owner physicians in the practice is equal to the annual hours worked by the respondent. It also assumes that average annual hours worked among all employee physicians in the practice is equal to average annual hours worked among all employee physicians of that specialty.

Office expenses per hour for this respondent will be $18.58 ($200,000/10,763.8). These expense per hour amounts were calculated for all self-employed physicians responding to the 1994–1998 SMS surveys subject to the edits specified by CMS. The weighted mean of these expense per hour amounts was then calculated by specialty for each expense item to obtain the figures reported to CMS.

Table 2 contains the practice expense information that was provided to CMS for use in the 2002 Medicare Physician Payment System. This table contains the information on the specialties that CMS requested as well as the expense per hour information for selected crosswalked specialties.

Refinement of Resource Based Practice Expenses

The AMA is closely monitoring all phases in the development of the new relative values and continues to advocate that they be based on valid physician practice expense data. Since there is not a single universally accepted cost allocation methodology, it is especially important that CMS bases its methodology on actual practice expense data. CMS's decisions not only affect Medicare reimbursements, but since many other payment systems use the Medicare RBRVS, the change to resource-based practice expense relative values has broad implications for the entire health care system. Due to the significance of this issue, the RUC established an advisory committee to assist in refining a portion of the data used to calculate practice expense relative values.

The transition period for practice expense relative value units reflected a combination of the 1998 charge based value and the new resource value. The transition began in 1999 when practice expense resource values were based on 75% of the 1998 charge based relative value and 25% on the resource based value. In 2000 the mix was equally weighted between the charge based and resource based values and in 2001 the practice expense relative values is 75% resource based and only 25% charged based. In 2002 the transition will be complete with practice expense RVUs totally resource based.

The AMA has advocated that the practice expense relative values remain interim during the refinement process and CMS has agreed to keep the values interim during the four year transition to resource based practice expense relative values. This interim period is necessary due to the amount of refinement work that needs to occur and so physicians have an opportunity to provide CMS with new data that can be used in updating the practice expense relative values. In the November 1, 2001 *Final Rule,* CMS went further in offering to leave the practice expense values interim until refinement is complete.

The numerous issues which will be addressed in refinement can be divided into the following six categories:

- Review and refine practice expense/hour data
- Obtain and review practice expense/hour data for specialties and practitioners not included in the SMS survey

- Address anomalies, if any, in code-specific Harvard/RUC physician time data
- Address anomalies, if any, in code-specific CPEP data on clinical staff types and times, quantity and cost of medical supplies, and quantity and cost of medical equipment
- Refine, as needed, the CMS process of developing practice expense RVUs for codes that were not addressed by the CPEP process, for example, codes that were new in 1996, 1997, 1998, and 1999
- Develop practice expense RVUs for codes that will be new in 2000 and beyond

RUC Role in Refinement

The RUC has closely followed the development of resource-based practice expenses over the past several years and is committed to developing recommendations for the direct inputs associated with new and revised codes. Additionally, the RUC has begun the arduous process of reviewing the CPEP data and suggesting code specific changes in the data. The RUC will also examine other refinement issues involving the general methodology utilized to calculate practice expense RVUs.

The RUC has discussed at length its desire to provide CMS with recommendations on practice expenses for new/revised codes. The RUC has agreed that as the RUC reviews new or revised codes for the work component, the committee will also consider the direct practice expense inputs for these services. Since many aspects of the methodology for assigning indirect costs to individual codes will undergo changes during refinement, the RUC will limit its recommendations for new and revised codes to the direct inputs required to perform a service that CMS can then use to calculate practice expense RVUs. Additionally, due to possible alterations to the practice expense allocation methodology, the RUC has recommended to CMS that all new/revised codes which receive practice expense RVUs during the refinement process be considered interim and that specialties be afforded an opportunity to refine their code level cost data during the refinement process. The practice expense relative value methodology will undoubtedly undergo changes during the refinement period and the RUC is committed to providing CMS with recommendations which will produce a methodology which truly reflects the resources required to perform a service.

When CMS published the details of its current practice expense methodology in June, 1998, CMS stated that *"There is much needed improvement in the CPEP data, and the identification and correction of any CPEP errors whether in staff times, supplies, equipment, or pricing will be a major focus of our refinement process."* In response to the need to update this set of data, the RUC created a special advisory committee, the Practice Expense Advisory Committee (PEAC) to assist the RUC in refining the direct input data CMS uses to calculate practice expense relative values. The PEAC is charged to review direct expense inputs (ie, clinical time, supplies, and equipment) for individual CPT codes. The PEAC held several meetings to develop a process for reviewing the direct inputs associated with CPT codes, and is working with CMS to develop clear definitions. In September, 1999 the RUC approved the first set of direct inputs reviewed by the PEAC. These recommendations were forwarded to CMS, which then accepted a majority of the recommendations and incorporated these changes into the Medicare payment schedule for 2000. The PEAC met several times in 2000 where it continued to review the direct input data and refine its methodology for code selection and analysis.

In May 2000, the RUC submitted recommendations to CMS on direct practice expense inputs for new and revised CPT codes. The PEAC and the RUC also reviewed the Evaluation and Management codes and recommended new data be utilized to reflect clinical staff, medical supplies, and medical equipment. CMS accepted these recommendations and implemented the data on January 1, 2001. In addition, the RUC recommended, and CMS has implemented, standardized medical supply packages for nearly 600 CPT codes. These revisions to medical supplies were based on recommendations from ophthalmology, neurosurgery, and obstetrics/gynecology. The PEAC and RUC continue to refine direct practice expense inputs for individual CPT codes for future submissions to CMS.

CMS has also recently made a number of broad-based changes in the practice expense data used to calculate resource based practice expense relative value units. These are primarily "egregious errors and anomalies" that have been highlighted by specialties since the introduction of the new CMS methodology. Additionally, CMS made a number of changes in CPEP data based on specific RUC recommendations. For example, a contractor examined criteria under which CMS would use survey data to improve specialty representation in CMS's calculation of the specialty specific practice expense per hour. In 2001, CMS issued strict criteria that specialties would need to follow to submit supplemental data, and CMS has given specialties until 2003 to provide supplemental survey data.

CMS still has a number of methodological issues relating to its cost allocation methodology that need to be resolved during the refinement period. For example, codes that have no physician work values have their practice expense relative values determined by a different methodology. This methodology does not use the CPEP data, but instead uses the 1998 practice expense RVUs to allocate costs from a separate cost pool created for codes with no physician work. CMS has indicated that this is an interim measure and is currently reviewing various options. The AMA and RUC are closely monitoring CMS's progress and will continue to work with CMS to ensure that the implementation of a methodology that recognizes the actual expenses necessary to provide health care.

The work of the PEAC has contributed greatly to the refinement efforts, and 2001 was particularly successful with the PEAC refining the inputs for over 1,100 codes. CMS accepted virtually all of the PEAC recommendations. This allowed a number of specialties including dermatology, orthopaedic surgery, pathology, opthamology, and physical medicine to refine large numbers of codes that were of importance to these specialties. Also in 2001, the PEAC began using PEAC developed practice expense standards which were never before used when the data was originally collected. As a result, specialty societies were able to refine their data using standards that applied to all specialties in a uniform manner. Due to the success of the PEAC, CMS has stated that the practice expense relative values will remain interim as long as refinement is necessary. Refinement has allowed specialty societies to identify and correct errors in the original CPEP data as well as place all specialty cost data on the same scale.

Chapter 6
Professional Liability Insurance (PLI) Component

On January 1, 2000, CMS implemented resource-based professional liability insurance (PLI) relative value units. With this implementation and final transition of the resource-based practice expense relative values on January 1, 2002, components of the RBRVS will no longer be based on historical charges. This chapter explains the previous payment methodology for professional liability insurance expense and discusses the new implementation of resource-based PLI relative values.

Data Used to Assign Charge Based PLI RVUs

As explained in Chapter 5, the OBRA 89 approach to valuing the practice expense component was also utilized in creating PLI relative values. Table 1 in Chapter 5 illustrates the percentage of mean PLI expenses as a percentage of total revenue per specialty, based data from the 1988-1990 AMA Socioeconomic Monitoring System Core Survey. To distribute PLI RVUs among services, the OBRA 89 method applies the average PLI expense percentage for each specialty to the 1991 average Medicare approved amount for each service. For example:

- For a service that only family practitioners provide and for which the average Medicare payment in 1991 was $100, multiply the PLI proportion for family physicians (3.9%) by the $100 average approved amount. The PLI expense component of the service would be assigned 3.9 (initial dollar) RVUs.
- For a service that only neurosurgeons provide and for which the average Medicare payment in 1991 was $1000, multiply the PLI proportion for neurosurgeons (7.6%) by the $1000 average approved amount. The PLI expense component of the service would be assigned 76 (initial dollar) RVUs.

For services provided by physicians in more than one specialty, multiply each specialty's PLI expense proportion by the proportion of claims for the service that the specialty submits, as follows:

- For a service that is provided 70% of the time by neurosurgeons and 30% of the time by orthopedic surgeons, multiply the neurosurgeons' PLI proportion (7.6%) by 70% and the orthopedic surgeons' PLI proportion (7.4%) by 30%. The sum of these two products becomes the PLI proportion for the service:

$$(7.6\% \times 0.70) + (7.4\% \times 0.30) = 7.5\%$$

This PLI expense proportion is then multiplied by the $1000 average approved amount:

$$(7.5\% \times \$1000) = \$75$$

The PLI expense component of the service would be assigned 75 (initial dollar) RVUs.

Because anesthesia services are not divided into work, practice expense, and PLI Revues, CMS computed the proportions of total payments for anesthesia that were comparable to these three components for other services. The portion of the anesthesiology conversion factor reflecting the work component was reduced by 42%. As for other services, to maintain a Medicare contribution comparable to the contribution under customary, prevailing, and reasonable (CPR), the portion of the conversion factor reflecting PLI were not reduced.

The CMS based the 1992 PLI RVUs on 1989 charge data "aged" to reflect 1991 payment rules because those were the most recent data available. For the 1992 payment schedule, actual 1991 charge data were used to recalculate the PLI RVUs for some codes for which CMS had imputed values the previous year. For services with insufficient charge data and for new codes, CMS developed crosswalks to predecessor codes, where possible. Since 1993, CMS has used a similar process to establish values for such codes.

Creating Resource-Based PLI Relative Values

In its 1996 and 1997 Annual Reports, the Physician Payment Review Commission (PPRC) called for Congress to revise current law to allow for the development of resource-based PLI RVUs. Further, the PPRC recommended that CMS be directed "to collect data on risk groups and relative insurance premiums across insurers" that could be used in the resource-based component. The AMA generally supported the PPRC's risk-of-service approach but identified a number of issues that warrant further investigation. Additional study is needed to determine the extent to which relative premiums and classification methods differ across areas and insurers and to determine whether significant differences exist in liability premiums across physicians in a particular specialty resulting from differences in service mix. The Medicare Payment Advisory Commission (MedPAC) has also supported basing PLI RVUs not only on the physician specialty but also on the type of service. MedPAC contends that the research demonstrates that even within a specialty, the risk of malpractice claim varies according to procedure invasiveness.

The Balanced Budget Act of 1997 required the development of resource-based PLI RVUs by January 1, 2000. The CMS contracted with KPMG to provide support in developing PLI RVUs and published their review of this report, along with proposed PLI RVUs, in their July 22, 1999 *Notice of Proposed Rule-making*. CMS finalized this proposal, with relatively few changes, in the November 2, 1999 *Final Rule*. In the November 1, 2000 *Final Rule*, CMS utilized updated premium data to derive new PLI RVUs.

The CMS has computed the new resource-based PLI RVUs using actual professional liability premium data and current Medicare payment data on allowed services and charges, relative value units, and specialty payment percentages. As stated above, MedPAC had previously recommended that CMS base the new PLI RVUs on procedure-specific actual malpractice claims. CMS did not use this approach as this type of data was not available and it is not possible to correlate claims paid to a specific CPT code, when a combination of services are performed. In the Final Rule, CMS encourages MedPAC to further develop their idea, particularly as it relates to the statutory requirement to develop resource-based PLI RVUs, and submit their further analysis in comments to further physician payment schedule notices.

The steps in CMS's calculation of PLI RVUs are as follows:

1) A national average professional liability premium is calculated for each specialty using 1996-1998 data. Premiums were for a $1 million / $3 million mature claims-made-policy (a policy covering claims made rather than services provided during the policy term). CMS collected malpractice premium data for twenty specialties. For other specialties, CMS utilized premium weighted average risk factors of five selected malpractice insurers. In a few cases, CMS crosswalked one specialties risk factor to another specialty. For example, neuropsychiatry was cross-walked to psychiatry.

2) Risk factors (non-surgical and surgical) were calculated for each specialty by dividing the national average premium for each specialty by the national average premium for the specialty with the lowest average premium. For example, the thoracic surgery risk factor is 8.14 compared to psychiatry at 1.31. CMS applied the surgical risk factors to CPT codes 10000 through 69999, and the non-surgical risk factor to all others. In the November 2, 1999 and November 1, 2000 *Final Rules,* CMS acknowledged that certain codes in the "non-surgical" section of CPT may indeed be invasive and, therefore, be valued based on the surgical risk factor. CMS changed the risk factor to surgical for the cardiology catheterization, angioplasty and electrophysiology codes (92980 to 92998, 93501 to 93536, 93600 to 93612, 93618 to 93641, and 93650 to 93652). In the case of OB/GYN services, the higher obstetric premiums and risk factors were used for services that were obstetrical services, while the lower gynecology risk factor was used for all other services.

3) PLI RVUs were calculated for each CPT code. The percentage of a specific service provided by each specialty was

multiplied by the specialties' risk factor, and the product was then summed across specialties by service. This yielded a specialty-weighted PLI RVU that was then multiplied by the physician work RVU for that code to account for differences in risk-of-service. In instances where the work RVU equaled zero, CMS retained the current professional liability RVUs. CMS acknowledged that work RVUs may not be the ideal determination of risk-of-service and has requested suggestions for other indicators.

4) The calculated PLI RVUs were then rescaled for budget neutrality. The raw unadjusted resource-based PLI RVUs were multiplied by 0.0171569 to maintain budget neutrality.

As the professional liability component is only, on average, 3.2% of the total payment amount, the initial impact in the 2000 implementation to specialties were minimal. While Emergency Medicine had a 2.7% increase in total payment, all others did not increase or decrease by more than 1%.

Many of those commenting on the July 22, 1999 *Proposed Rule* argued that CMS should use more recent premium data in calculating PLI RVUs. CMS has agreed to consider these values interim until they can be verified by more recent data. In the November 1, 2000 *Final Rule,* CMS did update the PLI RVUs using 1996-1998 data, the most recent data available at this time.

The CMS plans to update the PLI data every 5 years.

As explained in the above methodology, the following is an example of how a PLI RVU will be calculated for a new CPT code:

1) The percentage of a specific service to be performed by each specialty will be assumed. This information is typically provided during the CPT and RUC Processes.

Example:

New Code X	Family Practice	20%
	Dermatology	50%
	Plastic Surgery	30%

2) This percentage is then multiplied by the specialty's risk factor

Example:

New Code X (deemed to be "surgical")
Family Practice $.20 \times 1.73 = 0.35$
Dermatology $.50 \times 1.12 = 0.56$
Plastic Surgery $.30 \times 6.57 = 1.97$

3) The products for all specialties for the procedure are then summed, yielding a specialty-weighted PLI RVU reflecting the weighted professional liability costs across all specialties for that procedure.

Example:

New Code X   2.88

4) This number will then be multiplied by the procedure's work RVU to account for differences in risk-of-service.

Example:

New Code X $2.88 \times 2.50 \text{(work rvu)} = 7.20$

5) PLI RVU from step 4 to be adjusted for budget neutrality factor used in initial implementation.

Example:

New Code X $7.20 \times 0.0171569 = .12$ PLI RVU for New Code X

The new resource-based professional liability insurance relative value units may be found in Part 5 Reference Lists.

As discussed above, CMS is now using current data to calculate the PLI relative values, which take into account specialty specific risk factors. There are three different ways that an increase in PLI expenses incurred by physicians can be reflected in Medicare payments. For example, if PLI costs increase for most specialites, these increased expenses would be reflected in the annual update to the Medical Economic Index, which is used to update the Medicare conversion factor. These increased costs would have the potential to increase the conversion factor, which would then lead to increased payments for all physicians. (See chapter 10 for an explanation of the conversion factor update.) Alternatively, if a particular specialty experiences increased PLI costs, those changes would most likely only be reflected in the relative values every 5 years when CMS updates the 3-year average of professional liability premium data. To account for geographic differences in PLI costs, CMS uses a PLI geographic adjustment based on actual PLI premium data. These geographic practice cost indexes (GPCI) adjustments are made every 3 years so a sudden increase in PLI costs in a particular region of the country may not be reflected for several years.

In calculating the resource-based PLI relative values, CMS has taken into account interspecialty and geographic variances; however, rising PLI costs for individual physicians may not be reflected in changes to the relative values or the geographic adjustments for several years. While these potential delays in reflecting increased costs may be of concern, a more significant problem is the adequacy of the Medicare conversion factor. Assuming that the relative values reflect accurate PLI data, it is the conversion factor that determines the extent that the actual PLI costs are covered by Medicare reimbursements. The decrease in the 2002 conversion factor by 5.4% only heightens the concern that Medicare payments may not cover the costs of providing care. The AMA is committed to ensuring that the data used for the conversion factor is based on accurate data.

Combining Work, Practice Expense, and PLI RVUs

The sum of the work, practice expense, and PLI RVUs for each service is the total RVUs for the service. To align the three components on a common scale, CMS converted the original Harvard scale to the same dollar scale as used for the practice expense and PLI RVUs. It then assigned a total relative value of 1.00 to established patient office visit code 99213 and rescaled all other services accordingly. The common scale comprising the total RVUs for all services relative to 99213 is the complete Medicare RBRVS. Multiplying the RVUs for all of these services by the 2002 conversion factor of $36.1992 yields the full unadjusted Medicare payment schedule. The unadjusted payment schedule is the full schedule with no geographic practice cost adjustment. It includes the 80% that Medicare pays and the 20% patient coinsurance. Part 5 lists the RVUs for each component and the unadjusted payment schedule for all of the CPT-coded services.

Chapter 7
Geographic Variation in the Payment Schedule

Support for adopting a nationally standardized payment schedule that would reduce geographic variation in Medicare payment levels developed independently of the movement for a resource-based relative value scale (RBRVS). The AMA's House of Delegates adopted policy on reducing geographic variations before setting policy on an RBRVS-based Medicare payment schedule. Even after establishing its policy on the RBRVS, the House of Delegates sought to reduce geographic inequities before implementing the RBRVS. For example, at its December 1989 meeting, the AMA adopted policy to support pegging minimum Medicare prevailing charge levels at 80% of the national average prevailing charge level.

The Omnibus Budget Reconciliation Act of 1989 (OBRA 89) provision for and implementation of geographic adjustments often has drawn as much attention to the RBRVS payment system as did the relative values. This chapter describes the geographic adjustment provision in OBRA 89, revisions made to the geographic practice cost indexes (GPCIs) in 1995 and 1997, and how and to what extent payments vary geographically under the Medicare RBRVS payment system. The chapter also explains a revised configuration of Medicare payment localities that became effective January 1, 1997. A listing of all the GPCIs may be found at the end of this publication.

The OBRA 89 Provision for Geographic Adjustment

Most health policymakers are well aware that rural communities face physician recruitment and retention problems and that people living in these communities find it difficult to obtain high-quality care. Many rural community hospitals have closed since Medicare implemented prospective pricing, emphasizing the impact that changes in government policy may have in rural areas and underscoring the health care needs of these communities.

Wide disparities in Medicare payments for the same service, with twofold to threefold differences in some cases, provoked physicians nationwide to call for a more equitable policy.[1] For many physicians, the issue was not the wide variation in earnings, but whether Medicare payment levels were sufficient to even cover their costs of practicing in rural areas. Rural communities often have a higher proportion of Medicare and Medicaid patients, providing fewer opportunities for physicians to recover costs through higher charges to private sector patients.

In response, physicians in several predominantly rural states proposed a single national payment schedule with no geographic variation in payments. This proposal did not receive widespread support, however, because it would have merely shifted the underpayment problem to urban areas. In large cities where average Medicare payments based on CPR exceeded the national average by 37%, overall shifting to a single national schedule would have reduced average payment levels by 27%.

Many other physicians believed that a policy adjusting the entire RBRVS to reflect geographic differences would be inequitable and provide insufficient relief for rural areas. Most physicians agreed that the practice expense and professional liability insurance (PLI) components of the RBRVS should be varied to reflect geographic differences, but they disagreed about whether the physician work component should be adjusted. While variation in the practice expense component would have reflected differences among localities in office rents and the wages of nonphysician office personnel in Medicare payments, variation in the work component would have reflected differences in physicians' costs of living.

Because the work component is valued according to the physician time and effort involved in a service, it may be viewed as the physician earnings component of the schedule. Earnings variations reflect costs of living and amenities. If costs of living and amenities are relatively high, then employers must pay higher wages to cover their employees' higher costs of living, but the amenities level will offset the degree to which wages must be higher. Likewise, professional workers such as lawyers, engineers, and physicians must charge higher fees to cover these higher costs, but the need for these higher fee levels is partially offset by the amenities.

Physicians who supported varying Medicare payments according to cost-of-living differences believed that higher payments were needed to offset these higher costs. Other physicians objected to variation based on cost-of-living differences, believing that the cultural, environmental, and other amenities of high-cost communities adequately compensated for their higher costs. Others objected because such variation would preserve existing payment disparities to a greater extent than variation based on overhead only.

The OBRA 89 provided for adjusting the practice expense and PLI components of the payment schedule to fully reflect geographic differences in these costs, while adjusting the physician work component to reflect only one quarter of geographic differences in costs of living.

According to this provision, each component of each service provided in a locality is adjusted for geographic cost differences. Because the proportion of relative value units (RVUs) that comprise the work, practice expense, and PLI components are different for every service, the effect of this provision varies the amount of geographic adjustment for every service. For example:

- if the work adjustment in a state is 3% below the national average, the practice expense adjustment is 10% below the national average, and the PLI adjustment is 10% below the average,
- then, in that state, a service for which practice and PLI costs represent 75% of the total RVUs will be 8.5% below the unadjusted payment schedule, and,
- in contrast, a service for which physician work RVUs represent 75% of the total RVUs will only be 5.5% below the unadjusted schedule.

Geographic Practice Cost Indexes

The OBRA 89 legislation made three geographic adjustment factors the basis for the three geographic practice cost indexes, or GPCIs (pronounced "gypsies"), developed by researchers at the Urban Institute, the Center for Health Economics Research, and JIL Systems, Inc, with funding from the Centers for Medicare and Medicaid Services (CMS) (formerly the Health Care Financing Administration). The resources involved in operating a medical practice were identified by CMS as physician work or net income; employee wages; office rents; medical equipment, supplies, and other miscellaneous expenses; and professional liability insurance. Employee wages, office rents, medical equipment, medical supplies and miscellaneous expenses are combined to comprise the practice expense GPCI. Each component within the practice expense GPCI is weighted according to its percentage of practice costs. These weights are obtained from the AMA's Socioeconomic Monitoring System Survey. The original GPCIs, in effect from 1992 through 1994, used practice cost weights from the AMA's 1987 survey.

OBRA 90 requires that the GPCIs be updated at least every 3 years. Accordingly, CMS revised the GPCIs for 1995 to 1997, 1998 to 2000, and again for 2001 to 2003. The legislation specifies that the updated GPCIs be phased in over a 2-year period, with half of the overall adjustment to occur in the first year. The data used to measure each of the three component GPCIs are more fully described in the following sections. The GPCIs for 2002 are included in the "Reference Lists" section.

Cost-of-Living GPCIs

The physician work, or cost-of-living, GPCI is not based on differences in physicians' earnings, which some researchers and CMS argue have been affected by physicians' Medicare earnings under the previous CPR payment system. The 1995 to 1997 work GPCI measures geographic differences in the earnings of all college-educated workers, based on 1990 census data. In updating the work GPCIs for 1998 to

2000 and again for 2001 to 2003, no changes were made to the data sources.

Practice Expense GPCIs

The practice expense GPCI is designed to measure geographic variation in the prices of inputs to medical practice (eg, office rent per square foot and hourly wages of staff). It does not, therefore, reflect geographic differences in the amount of space that physicians rent nor in the number of nonphysician personnel they employ. It is important to distinguish between the practice expense component of the relative value scale and the practice expense GPCI. The practice expense relative value reflects average direct and indirect expenses. The practice expense GPCI reflects only the differences in these costs across geographic areas relative to the national average.

The office rent portion of the practice expense GPCI is based on apartment rental data from the Department of Housing and Urban Development (HUD). As it did in calculating the original GPCIs, the CMS continues to use proxy data to update this index, stating that no national data for physician office rents are available. However, the CMS indicated that it would continue to search for alternative sources of commercial rental data. The employee wage portion comes from 1990 census data on wages of clerical workers, registered nurses, and health technicians. The practice expense GPCI does not reflect geographic differences in medical equipment and supply costs. The CMS has stated its belief that a national market exists for these components and that input prices do not vary specifically across geographic areas.

For 1995 to 1997, the GPCIs were updated to reflect data from the 1990 census; the cost shares attributable to employee wages, rent, and miscellaneous expenses also were updated. The same 1990 census data sources were used to update the GPCIs for 1998 to 2000 and 2001 to 2003, although updated (1996 and 2000 respectively) HUD fair market residential rent data were used.

PLI GPCI

The PLI GPCI (which Medicare regulations refer to as the "malpractice" GPCI) reflects geographic differences in premiums for a mature claims made policy providing $1 million/$3 million of coverage. Adjustments are made for mandatory patient compensation funds.

Critics of the original GPCIs were particularly dissatisfied with the CMS's calculations of the PLI GPCIs, which were based on outdated premium data drawn largely from a single nationwide carrier. Each of the subsequent updates, however, used more recent premium data, as well as data collected on 20 medical specialties and from insurers representing the majority of the market in each state. The 1995 to 1997 GPCIs were based on premium data for 1990 to 1992, while the 1998 to 2000 GPCIs are based on 1992 to 1994 data. The 2001 to 2003 PLI GPCIs are based on 1996 to 1998 data. A 3-year average was used, rather than data from the most recent single year, to achieve a more accurate indication of historic PLI premium trends.

AMA Views

The AMA continues to be concerned about CMS's use of proxies for physician resource costs in the GPCIs rather than collecting data on physicians' actual expenses.

The AMA continues to believe that the cost-of-living GPCI should be based on physician earnings or physician-comparable data, not on the earning of all professionals. The AMA also objected to CMS's assumption that a national market exists for medical equipment, supplies, and other miscellaneous expenses. Data from the AMA's SMS suggest significant geographic variations in supply costs per visit.

Variation in the GPCIs

The GPCIs allow for considerably less variation in physicians' costs of practice than under historic Medicare pre–vailing charges. Relative to a national average of "1," the 2002 practice expense GPCIs range from 1.458 (San Francisco, CA) to 0.712 (Puerto Rico), with most falling between 0.85 and 1.10. Because the cost-of-living GPCI (work) accounts for only one quarter of geographic differences, the range is even smaller, from 0.881 (Puerto Rico) to 1.094 (Manhattan, NY), with most values for this component falling between 0.97 and 1.02. The range is greatest in the PLI GPCI, from 0.275 (Puerto Rico) to 2.738 (Detroit, MI).

Because of this narrow range of variation, most Medicare payments under the fully transitioned RBRVS payment system are within 10% of the national average, rather than the twofold and threefold differences in payment common under CPR. For many areas where physicians' payments were only 60% to 70% of the national average under CPR, payments increased to 80% to 90% of the national average under the payment schedule. Conversely, in areas where Medicare's payments under CPR were twice the national average, payments declined to only 15% to 20% above the national average.

This pattern means that the GPCIs do not necessarily indicate the impact of the payment schedule on Medicare payments in an area. In fact, the opposite may be true: many areas with the lowest GPCIs experienced the highest payment increases and many areas with the highest GPCIs experienced the most severe payment reductions.

Impact of the Revised GPCIs

The three GPCI components can be combined into a composite GPCI or geographic adjustment factor (GAF) by weighting each by the share of Medicare payments accounted for by the work, practice cost, and PLI components. The GAF indicates how Medicare payments in a locality differ from the national average (with the national average cost being 1.00).

Changes in the GPCIs do not affect total Medicare physician payments, but redistribute payments among localities. The overall redistributive effects of the revisions to the GPCIs for 1995 to 1997, as compared to the 1992 GPCIs, was modest. A CMS analysis indicated that 75% of localities experienced GPCI changes of about 3% or less. An AMA analysis, comparing the GAFs for 1994 and 1996, showed that revisions in the practice cost GPCIs caused a variance of over 2% in the GAFs for about 60 localities. Revisions to the PLI GPCIs led to GAF changes of over 2% in 52 localities.

The impact of the GPCI revisions for 1998 to 2000 was even less pronounced than for the previous update, as the only data changes made were to the indexes for office rent and PLI. Seventy-six of the 89 localities experience payment changes of less than 1% for the average service over the 2-year transition period, while payment changes in 58 localities will be less than 0.5%. The largest gain for an area is 2.4% and the largest loss is 2.2% for the average service. Several localities experienced PLI GPCI changes of about 30%, reflecting the volatility in PLI premiums that occurs from year to year. Because the weight of the PLI GPCI is about 5% of the total GPCI, a 30% change in the PLI GPCI causes only a 1.5% change in payments. Two thirds of the localities, however, experience PLI GPCI changes of less than 10%.

The impacts are also minimal in 2001 to 2003 as CMS again only updated the indexes for office rent and PLI. Only 14 of the 89 fee schedule areas changed by at least 2%. Sixteen areas will change from 1% to 1.9%. The remaining 59 areas are estimated to experience payment changes of less than 1% under the revised GPCIs.

Evaluating the GPCIs

Because the geographic adjustments to the payment schedule and the resulting payment changes are such a critical part of Medicare's RBRVS payment system, the GPCIs continue to be the focus of considerable debate and critical review. Physicians in places such as Puerto Rico, Texas, New York, and Florida have argued that the GPCIs do not capture important dimensions of their practice costs, making the resulting adjustments too low.

The most serious charge leveled against the GPCIs, however, is that they fail to measure what they purport to measure. Physicians in a number of states argue that the GPCIs have no place in the RBRVS payment system because they do not accurately measure the geographic cost differences physicians face. Others feel that payments across geographic areas should be the same.

To assess how well the GPCIs measure differences in physicians' practice costs, the AMA's Center for Health Policy Research compared data reported by physicians in its SMS surveys for 1991 and 1992 with the original GPCIs.[2]

The study found generally positive results:

- Although there is room for improvement, the GPCIs do, in fact, measure a significant amount of the geographic difference in physicians' practice costs.
- The GPCIs measure variation in office expenses and personnel costs quite well, despite concerns about the representativeness and/or age of the data used to construct these GPCIs.
- Adjusting payments based on the GPCIs reflects physicians' practice costs more accurately than a single national payment schedule.

There are measurable geographic differences in the costs of supplies that should be reflected in the practice cost GPCI.

The study concluded that using the GPCIs in the RBRVS payment system was appropriate but that improving the data sources as part of the updating process is critical, particularly the data used to construct the PLI GPCI. (The PLI GPCI was not highly correlated with physicians' reported PLI expenses.) The study recommended that with the collection of new data, the magnitude of changes in geographic cost differences over time should be determined to aid in assessing how frequently the GPCIs should be updated.

Medicare Payment Localities

Medicare payment localities are geographic areas defined by the CMS for use in establishing payment amounts for physician services. Localities may be entire states, counties, or groups of counties. There were 240 localities prior to 1992, largely reflecting historic circumstances of the CPR payment system. The number dropped to 210 with RBRVS implementation, as a number of states with multiple localities converted to single payment areas. The CMS implemented a more systematic approach to defining payment localities in 1997. The new policy achieved a number of goals, including administrative simplicity, reducing urban/rural payment differences among adjacent areas, and stabilizing payment updates resulting from periodic GPCI revisions.

The new policy increased the number of statewide payment localities to 34 from 22 and further reduced the overall number of localities to 89. To define the new payment localities, the CMS compared the GAF of a locality to the average GAF of lower-cost localities in the state in an iterative process.

If the difference exceeded 5%, the locality remained a distinct payment area. Otherwise, it was combined with other payment areas or the state converted to a single locality. The 5% threshold automatically eliminated subcounty areas in all but three states, aggregating them into statewide or residual state localities. The subcounty approach, however, could not be applied in Pennsylvania, Massachusetts, and Missouri, where a major redesign to payment localities was required.

In addition to the new methodology for defining payment localities, the CMS indicated that it would continue to consider physician requests for conversion to statewide localities. The CMS has emphasized that such requests must demonstrate support for the change from both physicians whose payments would increase as well as those who would experience payment losses.

Payment Impacts
The GPCIs for the revised localities were calculated to be budget neutral within each state; ie, overall physician payment within a state would be the same as under the existing localities. The impact on payment, as a result, was small. Forty-three percent of localities experienced increases in payments, 33% experienced decreases, and 24% experienced no change. Urban areas experienced an average decrease in payments of 0.14%, while rural area payments on average increased by 1%. Specialty impacts, reflecting the disproportionate concentration of specialists in urban areas, also were slight. Average payment gains of 0.3% were projected for family and general practice physicians, while average payment decreases of 0.1% to 0.2% were projected for most medical and surgical specialty physicians.

The new localities were phased in over a 2-year period, from 1997 to 1998, in those states where at least one locality experienced payment reductions of more than 4%. Only Pennsylvania and Missouri contained localities that exceeded the threshold and, thus, were the only states affected by the transition. All localities within these states were subject to the 2-year phase-in. Localities receiving payment cuts were assigned 1997 GPCIs whose values limited the loss to 4%. Similarly, localities whose payment levels rose received only a portion of the increase in 1997.

Payment changes for all localities became fully effective in 1998.

AMA Views
The AMA, in general, supported the approach taken by CMS to redefine Medicare payment localities. The approach succeeds, in the AMA's view, in simplifying payment areas and reducing payment differences among adjacent and urban/rural geographic areas, while maintaining accuracy in tracking input prices among areas. The AMA believes, however, that the 5% threshold was too high, due to its effect on some small urban areas (eg, San Antonio, TX). Policy adopted by the AMA in December 1996 called for CMS to retain as distinct Medicare localities those cities where inclusion in a statewide locality would not allow for appropriate recognition of the higher costs associated with practice in these areas.

The AMA also urged CMS to consider locality revisions based on future GPCI changes. Such changes may be particularly important for those areas where a temporary economic downturn may have depressed their GPCIs and led to inclusion in a statewide locality.

Bonus Payments for Health Professional Shortage Areas
In addition to the geographic adjustment provision for all services, there are special payment provisions for physician services when provided in designated Health Professional Shortage Areas (HPSAs). The HPSAs are rural and inner-city areas, defined by the Public Health Service (PHS) as having a shortage of health care personnel. To help attract and retain physicians in HPSAs, Congress adopted a Medicare bonus payment program, effective in 1989. The program initially provided an incentive payment of 5% for all services furnished by physicians in rural HPSAs. In 1991, the bonus was increased to 10% and extended to services furnished by physicians in both urban and rural HPSAs.

The PHS identifies three separate types of HPSAs, each corresponding to shortages of three different categories of health personnel—primary medical care professionals, dental professionals, and mental health professionals. Separate sets of criteria are used to designate each type of HPSA. Only geographic areas with shortages of primary care physicians (defined as general or family practice, general internal medicine, pediatrics, and obstetrics and gynecology) are eligible for the Medicare bonus payments. Three criteria must be met for a geographic area to be designated as an HPSA with a shortage of primary care medical professionals:

- It must be a rational delivery area for primary medical care services.
- There must be at least 3500 people per full-time-equivalent primary care physician, or at least 3000 people per full-time equivalent primary care physician in areas with "unusually high needs for primary care services" or "insufficient capacity of existing primary care providers."
- Primary care physicians in contiguous areas must be overutilized, excessively distant, or inaccessible.

Although the ratio of primary care physicians to population is a criterion used to designate areas to receive the bonus payments, such payments are not restricted to primary care physicians nor to primary care services. They apply to any Medicare covered service provided in a designated HPSA regardless of physician specialty.

Carriers make quarterly bonus payments to physicians in addition to the allowed amount under the payment schedule. To receive the bonus payment, the claim form must indicate that the service was provided in an HPSA. Listings and maps of HPSA designations appear in Medicare carrier bulletins.

References and Notes

1. For example, the PPRC reported in its 1988 Annual Report that, while the average prevailing charge in 1987 for a family practitioner for a comprehensive office visit was $64, 5% of these visits occurred in localities where the prevailing charge was less than $30, 5% in localities where the prevailing charge was more than $111—a more than threefold difference. Likewise, the average prevailing charge for a coronary artery bypass was $4385, but 5% of charges were less than $3092 and 5% were higher than $5919—a nearly twofold difference.
2. Gillis KD, Willke RJ, Reynolds RA. Assessing the validity of the geographic practice cost indices. *Inquiry.* Fall 1993;30:265-280.

Chapter 8
The Medicare Payment Schedule

The Medicare payment schedule's impact on a physician's Medicare payments is primarily a function of three key factors:

- the resource-based relative value scale (RBRVS);
- the geographic practice cost indexes (GPCIs); and
- the monetary conversion factor.

This chapter briefly describes how these elements combine to form the payment schedule.

The enabling legislation and regulations, as well as Medicare carrier correspondence and forms, refer to the Medicare physician payment schedule as a "fee schedule." From the AMA's perspective, the distinction between a payment schedule and a fee schedule is extremely important: a fee is what physicians establish as the fair price for the services they provide; a payment is what Medicare approves as the reimbursement level for the service. All references to the "full Medicare payment schedule" include the 80% that Medicare pays and the 20% patient coinsurance. Likewise, transition "approved amounts" also include the patient coinsurance.

The Formula for Calculating the Payment Schedule

As discussed in Chapter 7, the Omnibus Budget Reconciliation Act of 1989 (OBRA 89) geographic adjustment provision requires all three components of the relative value for a service—physician work relative value units (RVUs), practice expense RVUs, and professional liability insurance (PLI) RVUs—to be adjusted by the corresponding GPCI for the locality. In effect, this provision increases the number of components in the payment schedule from three to six:

- physician work RVUs;
- physician work GPCI;
- practice expense RVUs;
- practice expense GPCI;
- PLI RVUs; and
- PLI GPCI.

The formula for calculating payment schedule amounts entails adjusting RVUs, which correspond to services, by the GPCIs, which correspond to payment localities.

The general formula for calculating Medicare payment amounts for 2002 is expressed as:

Total RVU = (work RVU[1] × work GPCI[2])
+ (practice expense RVU[3] × practice expense GPCI[2])
+ (malpractice RVU[1] × malpractice GPCI[2])
= Total RVU

Payment = Total RVU × Conversion Factor

1 The 2002 physician work practice expenses, and malpractice RVUs may be found in Part 5 of this guide (Reference Lists).

2 The GPCIs for calendar year 2002 follow the Part 5 Reference List.

3 The conversion factor for calendar year 2002 is $36.1992.

Example = Payment for CPT code 99213, *Office/outpatient visit*, provided in a nonfacility (eg, in the physician's office) in Chicago, Illinois. The payment is calculated as follows:

Total RVU = $0.67^1 \times 1.028^2 = 0.689$
+ $0.69^1 \times 1.092^2 = 0.753$
+ $0.03^1 \times 1.797^2 = 0.054$
= 1.42 RVUs for CPT code 99213 in the Chicago locality

Payment = $1.496 \times 36.1992^3 = \$54.15$

Table 3 illustrates this calculation for four services in the Chicago locality using the current 2002 conversion factor. The first procedure is provided in a nonfacility and the subsequent procedures are in the facility.

Table 3. Calculation of Locally Adjusted Payment Schedule

Service CPT Codes	Work RVUs	Work GPCIs	PE RVUs	PE GPCI	PLI RVUs	PLI GPCI	Total RVUs	Conversion Factor	Local Payment Schedule
99213	0.67	1.028	0.69	1.092	0.03	1.797	1.496	$36.1992	$54.15
27130	20.12	1.028	17.18	1.092	2.82	1.797	44.512	$36.1992	$1,611.30
33533	30.00	1.028	17.24	1.092	3.24	1.797	55.488	$36.1992	$2,008.62
71010-26	0.18	1.028	0.06	1.092	0.01	1.797	0.269	$36.1992	$9.74

Worksheets for Determining the Impact of the Medicare Payment System on Individual Physician Practices

With the Centers for Medicare and Medicaid Services' November 2001 publication of the *Final Rule* on the Medicare physician payment schedule, physicians are able to determine the impact that the Medicare physician payment schedule will have on their practices. The worksheet provided here will allow physicians to estimate their practice revenue under this payment system. In using the worksheet, the following factors and limitations should be closely noted:

- The mix and volume of, and assignment rate for, the services and procedures provided to Medicare patients, and the geographic location for the physician practice, are major factors determining the impact of the payment systems.
- The practice expense RVUs for 2002 as listed in the Part 5 Reference List are the transitioned amount (for further discussion please see Chapter 5).
- The phrase "Medicare approved amount" used throughout the worksheets includes 80% of the approved amount paid by Medicare and the 20% copayment collected by the patient.

Instructions for Appendix A:

The worksheet will enable physicians to calculate 2001 payment amounts for frequently provided procedures and services.

Step 1 Make as many copies of "Appendix A" as needed for your personal use.

Step 2 Identify the most frequent services and procedures that you provide to Medicare patients by entering each CPT code (include a modifier if appropriate) and short descriptor in columns A and B, respectively.

Step 3 Using the List of Relative Units in Part 5 of the *Physicians' Guide,* find the relative value units (RVUs) for the work, practice expense, and professional liability insurance (PLI) components of the Medicare physician payment schedule and enter each RVU in Column C. In selecting the practice expense relative values, make certain to select the appropriate site of service.

Step 4 Using the List of Geographic Practice Cost Indexes for Each Medicare Locality, from Part 5 of the *Physicians' Guide,* find the work, practice expense, and PLI GPCIs for your payment locality. For each of the three RVUs that you recorded in column C, enter the three corresponding GPCIs.

Step 5 In column C, calculate the geographically adjusted RVU for the work, practice expense, and PLI components by multiplying each RVU by each GPCI.

Step 6 In the last box of column C, calculate the total geographically adjusted RVU by summing the three geographically adjusted RVUs.

Step 7 Multiply the total geographically adjusted RVU in column C by the conversion factor, $36.1992, in column D to arrive at the full Medicare payment schedule amount and enter in column E.

Step 8 Repeat steps 3 through 7 to calculate full Medicare physician schedule amounts for each service and procedure that you provide most frequently to Medicare amounts.

Appendix A

Calculating 2002 full Medicare payment schedule amounts for most frequently provided procedures

Column A CPT Code	Column B Short Descriptor	RVU Components	Column C RVU × GPCI =	Geographic Adjusted RVU	Column D Conversion Factor	Column E Full Payment Schedule Amount
		Work	×	=		
		PE	×	=		
		PLI	×	=		
		Total Adjusted RVU	=		× $36.1992	
		Work	×	=		
		PE	×	=		
		PLI	×	=		
		Total Adjusted RVU	=		× $36.1992	
		Work	×	=		
		PE	×	=		
		PLI	×	=		
		Total Adjusted RVU	=		× $36.1992	
		Work	×	=		
		PE	×	=		
		PLI	×	=		
		Total Adjusted RVU	=		× $36.1992	
		Work	×	=		
		PE	×	=		
		PLI	×	=		
		Total Adjusted RVU	=		× $36.1992	

Instructions for Appendix B: "Nonparticipating" Physicians

The worksheet will enable physicians to calculate 2002 payment amounts for frequently provided procedures and services.

Step 1 Make as many copies of "Appendix B" as needed for your personal use.

Step 2 Identify the most frequent services and procedures that you provide to Medicare patients by entering each CPT code (include a modifier if appropriate).

Step 3 Using the List of Relative Units in Part 5 of the *Physicians' Guide,* find the relative value units (RVUs) for the work, practice expense, and professional liability insurance (PLI) components of the Medicare physician payment schedule and enter each RVU in Column B. In selecting the practice expense relative values, make certain to select the appropriate site of service.

Step 4 Using the List of Geographic Practice Cost Indexes for Each Medicare Locality, from Part 5 of the *Physicians' Guide,* find the work, practice expense, and PLI GPCIs for your payment locality. For each of the three RVUs that you recorded in column B, enter the three corresponding GPCIs.

Step 5 In column B, calculate the geographically adjusted RVU for the work, practice expense, and PLI components by multiplying each RVU by each GPCI.

Step 6 In the last box of column B, calculate the total geographically adjusted RVU by summing the three geographically adjusted RVUs.

Step 7 Multiply the total geographically adjusted RVU in column B by the conversion factor, $36.1992, in column C to arrive at the full Medicare payment schedule amount and enter in column D.

Step 8 Multiply the full Medicare payment schedule amount by 1.0925 to arrive at the nonparticipating amount. This adjustment corresponds to the Medicare approved amount for nonparticipating physicians of 95% of payment rated for participating physicians. Medicare then allows nonparticipating physicians to charge Medicare patients 15% more than the Medicare approved amount for nonparticiapting physicians. This results in payments 9.25% greater than participating physician payments.

Step 9 Repeat steps 3 through 8 to calculate full Medicare physician schedule amounts for each service and procedure that you provide most frequently to Medicare patients.

Appendix B

Calculating 2001 "nonparticipating" Medicare payments schedule amounts for most frequently provided procedures

Column A **CPT Code**	*Column B* **RVU Components**	**RVU × GPCI =**	**Geographic Adjusted RVU**	*Column C* **Conversion Factor**	*Column D* **Full Payment Schedule Amount**	*Column E* **Nonparticipating Amount**
	Work	×	=			
	PE	×	=			
	PLI	×	=			
	Total Adjusted RVU =			× $36.1992		× 1.0925 =
	Work	×	=			
	PE	×	=			
	PLI	×	=			
	Total Adjusted RVU =			× $36.1992		× 1.0925 =
	Work	×	=			
	PE	×	=			
	PLI	×	=			
	Total Adjusted RVU =			× $36.1992		× 1.0925 =
	Work	×	=			
	PE	×	=			
	PLI	×	=			
	Total Adjusted RVU =			× $36.1992		× 1.0925 =
	Work	×	=			
	PE	×	=			
	PLI	×	=			
	Total Adjusted RVU =			× $36.1992		× 1.0925 =

Chapter 9
Balance Billing Under the Payment Schedule

Two features of the Medicare program are designed to control the amount of money that patients pay out of pocket for Medicare-covered services: the Physician Participation (PAR) Program and the limiting charges. The purpose of the PAR Program is to encourage physicians to accept Medicare assignment for all claims, which means they accept the Medicare approved amount as payment in full (including the 80% that Medicare pays and the 20% coinsurance). Limiting charges restrict the amount that physicians who do not accept Medicare assignment may charge above the amount that Medicare approves.

The AMA has a long history of vigorously opposing any government policy that restricts physicians' ability to establish their own fees for the services they provide. The AMA believes that fees are a matter for discussion between patients and physicians, not a matter for government intervention. The AMA encourages physicians to accept assignment or accept no fee for their indigent patients, and to consider patients' ability to pay when making fee decisions.

To facilitate assignment acceptance for low-income patients, a number of state and county medical societies have initiated voluntary assignment programs. Laws in several states limit the amounts physicians may bill patients to either the Medicare-approved amount or a percentage amount above the approved amount.

As Chapter 2 outlined, AMA opposed both the PAR Program and the earlier limits on balance billing, called maximum allowable actual charges (MAACs), which had been in place under the customary, prevailing, and reasonable (CPR) system for several years before Congress enacted the Omnibus Budget Reconciliation Act of 1989 (OBRA 89). Although the AMA continued its strong opposition during the drafting of the legislation, Chapter 2 explained why retaining the PAR Program and MAAC-type limits under the Medicare RBRVS payment system was unavoidable, with the larger battle being the one against mandated assignment. This chapter describes the PAR Program and the limiting charges.

The PAR Program

Under Medicare law, Medicare patients must pay a $100 annual deductible for Part B services and a 20% copayment on claims for Part B services that are submitted after meeting the deductible. Throughout this book, discussion of Medicare approved amounts and Medicare payment schedule amounts refers to 100% of the Medicare amount, for which the Medicare program pays 80% and patients 20%. The difference between the physician's actual charge and the Medicare allowed amount is known as "balance billing."

Most beneficiaries have Medicare supplemental insurance, such as that provided by an employer, or "Medigap," policies to cover the costs of the deductible and coinsurance; some of these policies also cover balance billing. Medicare beneficiaries who also qualify for state Medicaid programs have their deductibles and coinsurance covered by Medicaid; assignment is mandatory for these beneficiaries.

When a physician accepts Medicare assignment, the patient is still responsible for the 20% coinsurance. Assignment acceptance limits the patient's out-of-pocket financial responsibility to this 20% coinsurance, however, and precludes the physician from charging more than the Medicare approved amount.

The PAR Program was established in 1984 to provide incentives for physicians to accept Medicare assignment. A "participating" physician, or PAR physician, agrees to accept assignment for all services provided to Medicare patients. Physicians are invited to become PAR physicians in a "Medicare Participating Physician/Supplier Agreement" (formerly referred to as the "Dear Doctor" letter) from their Medicare carrier each fall. Physicians must sign the PAR agreement and return it to the carrier by a given date. Failure to respond results in a continuation of the physician's current status. The agreement binds physicians to accept assignment for all Medicare claims during the calendar year in which the agreement is effective.

Medicare provides the following incentives for physicians to participate:

- The full payment schedule for "nonparticipating" (non-PAR) physicians is set at 95% of the full payment schedule for PAR physicians. Non-PAR approved amounts are 95% of PAR amounts for the same service.
- A directory of PAR physicians is provided to senior citizens groups and, upon request, to individual beneficiaries.
- Carriers assist PAR physicians with simplified billing procedures for Medigap coverage.
- PAR claims are processed more quickly than non-PAR claims.

The major incentive to participate in the PAR program is the payment differential. In 1997, 80% of MDs and DOs were participating. Physician participation rates vary considerably by specialty and practice location. The highest participation rates are among surgical subspecialists, including vascular surgeons (93.3%) and hematologists/ oncologists (90.4%), and lowest among general practice physicians (66.3%). Participation rates also vary widely across states. By 1999, the physician participation rate increased to approximately 85%.

According to the Physician Payment Review Commission (PPRC) in its 1997 Annual Report to Congress, 96% of Medicare charges in 1996 were submitted on an assignment basis. In 1991, 85% of physicians' allowed charges were accepted on assignment. Physician balance bills in 1996 accounted, on average, for less than 15% of Medicare payments. These percentages represent a continuing trend since the mid-1980s of increased participation and reduced balance billing.

Limiting Charges

When established in 1986, MAACs were based on a complicated formula involving an individual physician's charges in the second quarter of 1984. As a result, the variation between physicians' MAACs was as wide as their individual fees for the services they provided. The change from MAACs to limiting charges, therefore, produced an effect similar to the geographic practice cost indexes (GPCIs) because it eliminated much of the variation in payments (or, in this case, variation in charges) for the same service.

The resource-based relative value scale (RBRVS) payment schedule compressed balance billing limits relative to their wide range under CPR. Since 1993, the limiting charge has been 115% of the Medicare approved amount for non-PAR physicians. Physicians whose MAACs were considerably higher than prevailing charges under CPR now have limiting charges that exceed the payment schedule amounts by a much lower percentage. Physicians whose MAACs were only 10% more than their prevailing charges generally experienced a slight increase in payments for visit services and services for which Medicare payments were not reduced under the Medicare RBRVS payment system.

Limiting charge information is provided in the annual "Medicare Participating Physician/Supplier Agreement," which the Medicare carrier sends to each physician. The letter must also include payment information on the PAR-approved amount, the non-PAR amount, and the limiting charge for all services paid under the RBRVS payment schedule.

The limiting charge provision has applied to drugs and biologicals provided "incident to" a physician's service since January 1, 1994. In addition, the limiting charge provisions apply to all nonparticipating providers and suppliers for services on the payment schedule. Prior to 1994, only services provided by nonparticipating physicians were subject to limiting charges.

In addition to controlling patient out-of-pocket payments, the limiting charges provide an additional incentive for physicians to participate. Medicare payment schedule amounts and transition approved amounts for non-PAR physicians are 95% of payment rates for PAR physicians. Therefore, the 15% limiting charge translates into only 9.25% above the PAR approved amount for a service.

When considering whether to participate, physicians must determine whether their total revenues from balance billing would exceed their revenues as PAR physicians, particularly in light of collection costs, bad debts, and claims for which they do accept assignment. The 95% payment rate is not based on whether physicians accept assignment on the claim, but whether they are PAR physicians; when non-PAR physicians accept assignment for their low-income or other patients, they still receive only 95% of the amount PAR physicians receive for the same service. A non-PAR physician would need to collect the full limiting charge amount roughly 35% of the time they provided the service for the revenues from the service to equal those of PAR physicians. In addition to payment considerations, other factors support the decision to participate.

Assignment acceptance, for either a PAR or a non-PAR physician, also means that the Medicare carrier pays the physician the 80% Medicare payment. For unassigned claims, even though the physician is required to submit the claim to Medicare, the program pays the patient, and the physician must then collect the entire amount for the service from the patient. Because PAR physicians receive 80% of their Medicare amounts directly from Medicare, they only need to collect the 20% coinsurance from patients. For assigned claims, non-PAR physicians receive 80% of the Medicare approved amount directly from Medicare, but must bill patients for the 20% coinsurance.

Monitoring Compliance

The Centers for Medicare and Medicaid Services (CMS) (formerly the Health Care Financing Administration HCFA) received greater statutory authority to monitor compliance with Medicare balance billing limits through provisions contained in the Social Security Act Amendments of 1994. The legislation clarifies that nonparticipating physicians and suppliers may not bill patients more than the limiting charge and that patients, as well as supplemental insurers, are not liable for payment of any amount that exceeds the limiting charge. If billed charges exceed the limiting charge, carriers are required to notify the physician or other provider of the violation within 30 days. A refund or credit for the excess charges must be made to the patient within 30 days of carrier notification. Sanctions may be imposed for "knowingly and willfully" billing or collecting fees that exceed the limiting charge.

In addition, when an unassigned claim is submitted with charges that exceed the limiting charge, the law requires that limiting charge information be included on the Explanation of Medicare Benefits (EOMB), indicating the beneficiary's right to a refund if an excess charge has been collected.

Information reflecting these changes appears on the EOMB and the Limiting Charge Exception Report (LCER).

To monitor physicians' and other providers' compliance with the limiting charges, carriers are required to screen all unassigned claims. Physicians and other providers who fail to make adjustments for overcharges as outlined in the LCER are subject to sanctions that can include fines and suspension from the Medicare program for up to 5 years. Finally, the law requires the secretary of Health and Human Services (HHS) to report to Congress annually concerning the extent of limiting charge violations and the services involved.

Under CMS's Comprehensive Limiting Charge Compliance Program (CLCCP),which took effect in mid-1992, carriers issue notifications to physicians when a violation of the limiting charge has occurred. Carriers send LCERs to those physicians and other Medicare providers whose unassigned claims include charges that exceed the limiting charge by $1.

Part 3
The RBRVS Payment System in Operation

Part 3 addresses the operational details of Medicare's physician payment system. Chapter 10 explains the conversion factor and the sustainable growth rate for updating physician payment. Chapter 11 describes all of the key features in the standardization of Medicare's payment system, including the policies on global surgical packages; visit coding; payments for assistants-at-surgery; nonphysicians; drugs, services, and supplies provided "incident to" a physician's service; and other issues.

Chapter 10
Updating the Payment Schedule

The Medicare resource-based relative value scale (RBRVS) payment system was phased in during 1992-1996, with 1996 the first year that physician payments were fully based on the new payment schedule. The Omnibus Budget Reconciliation Act of 1989 (OBRA 89) and subsequent legislation have provided a process to annually update the RBRVS payment system. Key features are the methods for determining annual updates to the conversion factor and periodic updates to the relative value units (RVUs) and geographic practice cost indexes (GPCIs). This chapter explains each of these processes.

Conversion Factor Updates

Since 1992, Medicare conversion factor updates have been based on three factors:

1) the Medicare Economic Index (MEI);

2) an expenditure target "performance adjustment"; and

3) miscellaneous adjustments including those for "budget neutrality."

The first of these factors, the MEI, has been used since 1976 as a proxy for inflation in the cost of operating a medical practice. The largest single determinant of changes in the MEI is the change in hourly earnings in the general economy, which is the proxy for physicians' own time in the index. The index also includes measures of changes in:

- nonphysician compensation, including fringe benefits;
- office expenses;
- medical materials and supplies;
- professional liability insurance;
- medical equipment expenses; and
- other professional expenses.

The MEI has increased by an average of just over 2% in recent years. An MEI of 2.6% was used in determining the 2002 CF update.

The other major factor in determining conversion factor updates since 1992, the "performance adjustment," is based on a comparison of actual and target expenditures under an expenditure target system. The method of determining this factor has changed over time. Initially, the performance adjustment was based on the Medicare Volume Performance Standard (MVPS). This formula, which had been altered under the Omnibus Budget Reconciliation Act of 1993 (OBRA 93), was projected to produce substantial long-term payment cuts.

In 1997 Congress enacted key changes to the conversion factor update process as part of the Balanced Budget Act (BBA), replacing the MVPS with the Sustainable Growth Rate (SGR) system for determining updates. This system was also seriously flawed, however, and further revisions that were advocated by AMA were adopted as part of the Balanced Budget Refinement Act of 1999 (BBRA). These changes to the expenditure target system are described in greater detail in the remainder of this section.

The MVPS and conversion factor updates prior to 1998

Under the MVPS system, a target rate of fee-for-service Medicare physician spending growth was calculated each year. This target rate of growth was compared to actual spending growth for the year to determine the conversion factor update two years hence. If actual spending growth exceeded the target in a given year, for example, physicians would be penalized with a below-inflation (MEI) update two years later. If actual spending growth was below the target, then an above-inflation update would be awarded. The two-year lag was specified to allow for delays in claims processing.

This formula-driven approach to updating the conversion factor was not automatic, however. OBRA 89 gave Congress the authority to set its own conversion factor updates and spending targets. As part of its deliberations, Congress was required to consider the recommendations submitted by the Centers for Medicare and Medicaid Services (CMS) (formerly the Health Care Financing Administration) and the Physician Payment Review Commission (PPRC). If Congress failed to act on these recommendations, however, annual updates were set by the default (MVPS) formula, which had also been established under OBRA 89.

The default MVPS target rate of spending growth was based on the following factors:

- changes in Medicare payment levels,
- changes in the size and age composition of the Medicare population,
- the 5-year historical average growth in the volume and intensity of physician services, and
- changes in expenditures resulting from law and regulation.

The target was then reduced by a legislatively determined number of percentage points known as the *performance standard factor*. The performance standard factor was initially just 0.5 percentage points, but was increased to 4.0 percentage points by OBRA 93 starting in 1995.

With the modifications to the MVPS formula specified in OBRA 93, Medicare payments were projected to decline steadily over time. Payments were virtually guaranteed to fall over the long term given the structure of the MVPS system, which essentially set the target rate of spending growth at the expected rate of spending growth minus 4 percentage points. The PPRC projected that the default formula would generate annual conversion factor cuts of 2% or more indefinitely.

Separate MVPS targets for surgical and nonsurgical services were also established under OBRA 89, allowing separate conversion factors for each service category. A third service category, for primary care services, was implemented in 1994 under provisions of OBRA 93. By 1997, the separate targets and updates under the MVPS system resulted in a surgical conversion factor that was 9% higher than that for primary care, and 14% higher than that for nonsurgical services. As the conversion factors diverged, interest grew among various groups to eliminate multiple MVPSs and return to a single conversion factor.

The AMA consistently opposed multiple conversion factors and multiple MVPSs because they undermined the intent of the RBRVS payment schedule that relative payments should reflect relative resource costs across all procedures. In 1995 the AMA called for Congress to establish a single conversion factor with a transition period "as close to three years as possible." The AMA emphasized in discussions with CMS, congressional staff, and national medical specialty societies that such an approach would help to offset losses by physicians in surgical specialties.

The Sustainable Growth Rate System, 1998-1999

The Balanced Budget Act of 1997 established a single conversion factor for all physician services which was set at $36.69 for 1998. For anesthesia services, the 1998 conversion factor was set at 46% of this amount, or $16.8762.

The legislation also replaced the MVPS system with the Sustainable Growth Rate expenditure target system. In some ways the systems are similar. Under SGR, a target rate of spending growth is calculated each year with a similar set of factors. The SGR target is determined by changes in:

- fees for physician services (in practice, primarily the MEI);
- Medicare fee-for-service enrollment;
- real (inflation-adjusted) per capita Gross Domestic Product (GDP); and
- spending due to law and regulation.

A major change with the SGR is that real per capita GDP is used in place of the historical average volume growth in the target. A second major change is that the SGR system is cumulative. The target growth rate is applied to the allowed amount of spending for the prior year to determine the (dollar amount of) allowed spending for the following year. Running totals of actual and allowed spending, beginning April 1, 1997, are kept, and the performance adjustment is based on the difference between cumulative allowed and actual spending (rather than the difference between the target and actual growth rate for the second preceding year).

Although the SGR was projected by the Congressional Budget Office to reduce physician payments even more than

MVPS, the system offered the opportunity for improved payment levels if volume growth stayed low enough. Volume growth has in fact been low enough since the inception of SGR to generate positive conversion factor updates, despite the fact that the first two targets set under SGR were artificially low. The SGR targets for fiscal years 1998 and 1999 were set at 1.5% and –0.3%, respectively (see Table 4), but physician spending growth was within these limits.

For the calendar year 1999 conversion factor update (the first to be determined by the SGR system), the MEI was 2.3% and the "performance adjustment" was 0%, yielding a conversion factor update (before scaling and budget-neutrality adjustments) of 2.3%. For calendar year 2000, the MEI was 2.4% and the "performance adjustment" a positive 3%, yielding an update of 5.4%.

The SGR system as specified in the BBA had many faults though. Updates, of course, are made on a calendar year basis, but the SGR target rates of growth were set on a federal fiscal year basis (beginning October 1 and ending September 30) and allowed and actual spending were tracked on a year ending March 31 basis. CMS acknowledged in a November 2, 1998 final rule that this mismatch in time periods rendered conversion factor updates under the BBA SGR formula unstable. Updates could alternate between periods at the maximum of inflation (MEI) plus 3 percentage points, and periods at the minimum of inflation minus 7 percentage points (limits that were also imposed as part of BBA).

A second major flaw in the original SGR system regarded the correction of projection errors. Under the original SGR, CMS set a target rate of growth each fall for the coming fiscal year. This target rate of growth was based on projections of the components of the target for that year, including real per capita GDP growth and changes in fee-for-service enrollment. CMS stated in an October 31, 1997 notice that errors in projecting changes in GDP and enrollment would be corrected in subsequent years. However, in a November 2, 1998 notice, CMS stated it did not have the authority to correct these projection errors given the legislative language of the BBA.

The immediate impact of this decision for physicians was substantial. Growth in the US economy for fiscal years 1998 and 1999 was much stronger than projected by CMS. As shown in Table 4, CMS projected only 1.1% and 1.3% growth in real per capita GDP for 1998 and 1999, respectively, whereas actual growth for both years was over 3%. Fee-for-service enrollment was projected to decline by 4.3% in fiscal year 1999, but enrollment actually fell by just 1.1%. Combined, these errors reduced allowed physician spending by over 7% in just 2 years.

The AMA developed legislation to correct these problems and vigorously advocated for its implementation. The Medicare Payment Advisory Commission (MedPAC) also made several recommendations to revise the SGR in its March 1999 report to Congress, including:

- placing all elements of the SGR on a calendar year basis, and reducing the time lag between measurement of spending and the update;
- requiring CMS to correct errors in the projection of each year's SGR with actual data;
- requiring CMS to publish an estimate of the conversion factor update each year in the spring prior to the update;
- including an allowance in the SGR target for cost increases due to improvements in medical capabilities and advancements in scientific technology; and
- making an adjustment to the SGR target for changes in the composition of the fee-for-service population over time.

The AMA strongly supported these recommendations. AMA also supported other changes that would further reduce volatility in updates including using a 5-year average for GDP growth in the target and narrowing the update limits.

The Sustainable Growth Rate System—BBRA

Many of the corrections advocated by AMA and recommended by MedPAC were enacted by Congress as part of the Balanced Budget Refinement Act of 1999 (BBRA). Changes included moving to a calendar year system, correcting projection errors, and requiring a report in the spring of each year from CMS on the coming year's likely conversion factor update and SGR target. The legislation also mandated a study of the impacts of technological change and shifts in site of service on physician service utilization.

These changes had a positive impact on funding for Medicare physician services in 2001. In particular, the legislation required that CMS correct its fiscal year 2000 target that had been issued prior to passage of BBRA. This target was used to set allowed spending for the period of transition to the new calendar year SGR (the period April 1, 1999 to December 31, 1999). The target, initially estimated at just 2.1% was revised to 6.9%, increasing allowed spending for this period by nearly 5%. The correction of this error was a major factor behind the 4.5% conversion factor update for 2001 which included a 3% "performance adjustment"—the maximum bonus allowed by law.

The positive performance adjustments in 2000 and 2001 were the result of strong economic growth in 2000 (which increased target spending) combined with what appeared to be little or no growth in the utilization of Medicare physician services (which restrained actual spending). These positive trends were reversed in 2001, with a severe slowdown in the US economy, and an increase in utilization growth. In their final rule on the Medicare physician

Table 4. SGR Targets for 1998-2001 – Allowed Growth in Medicare Physician Spending:

	FY98*	FY99*	FY00*	FY00*	CY00**	CY01**
Fees (inflation)	2.3%	2.1%	2.1%	2.1%	2.1%	1.9%
Fee-for-service enrollment	–2.4%	–4.3%	–1.6%	0.5%	1.0%	3.0%
Real per-capita GDP growth	1.1%	1.3%	1.8%	3.6%	3.2%	0.7%
Law and regulation	0.6%	0.7%	–0.2%	0.6%	0.8%	0.4%
Total	1.5%	–0.3%	2.1%	6.9%	7.3%	6.1%

*Targets calculated prior to BBRA.
**Targets calculated post-BBRA and subject to correction for projection error.
Note: The FY00 target is listed twice because it was first calculated prior to BBRA, but then was revised due to BBRA to correct the projection errors in the original estimate.

payment schedule for 2002, CMS projected that actual spending would exceed target spending by a wide margin in 2001, resulting in a significant pay cut under the SGR in 2002. In addition, CMS discovered it had failed to include many new codes beginning in 1998 in its measurement of actual spending. Correcting this error further reduced their published 2002 update to –5.4%, which includes a –7% "performance adjustment"—the maximum penalty allowed by law.

The payment updates for 2001 and 2002 illustrate the strong link between economic growth and Medicare payments that exists under the current SGR system. They also illustrate the instability of Medicare physician payments that remains even with the refinements of BBRA. During the BBRA debate in the summer of 1999, the AMA advocated for further changes to the SGR system to reduce volatility, including using a 5-year average for GDP growth in the target and narrowing the update limits. These proposals were not incorporated in BBRA.

Under the SGR, Medicare physician payment updates over the long term will depend primarily on how close actual growth in the utilization of Medicare physician services is to the targeted rate of real per-capita GDP growth. A rough idea of future changes to the Medicare conversion factor can be obtained given assumptions about utilization growth and growth in the economy. In particular, each percentage point that actual utilization growth exceeds the target of real per-capita GDP growth translates into a one percentage point annual cut in real Medicare physician payments. For example, if utilization growth averages 4.5% and GDP growth averages 1.5% then inflation-adjusted Medicare physician pay will fall by an average of 3% per year—*indefinitely*.

Given the short term instability and long-term uncertainty of Medicare pay under SGR, the AMA continues to advocate for changes in this payment update formula.

Updating the Relative Values

The relative values for new and revised procedures also must be regularly updated to reflect changes in medical practice and technology. The AMA's CPT coding system, through the work of the AMA CPT Editorial Panel, reflects such changes as it revises and develops new CPT codes. The AMA and the national medical specialty societies established the AMA/Specialty Society RVS Update Committee (RUC) to make annual recommendations to the CMS on the work RVUs assigned to new and revised CPT codes. A primary objective of this process is that new RVUs, developed by the medical profession, will be available for use with new or revised CPT codes in the same year that these codes are introduced. The CMS has used the RUC's recommendations as the principal basis for the work RVUs assigned to new and revised codes for each year's updated payment schedules since 1993. Since 1999, the RUC has submitted recommendations for refining and updating the practice expense relative values. The AMA regards the RUC as the principal vehicle for refining the work and practice expense components and strongly advocates Medicare adoption of the RUC's recommendations.

The RUC worked with CMS to complete the RBRVS and to ensure that it is appropriate for all patient populations. A rigorously updated and validated RBRVS is of critical importance as the trend toward adoption of the Medicare RBRVS by non-Medicare payers continues. The RUC played a major role in the 5-year review processes of the RBRVS and is committed to improving and maintaining the validity of the RBRVS over time. Chapter 4 includes a detailed description of the RUC and the update process, including results from the past 5-year review processes.

This process does not, however, constitute the exclusive means for CMS to receive advice and recommendations on new and revised RVUs, as interim values are subject to a public notice and comment period. In addition, CMS relies on carrier medical directors (CMDs) to review recommended RVUs for new and revised services, as well as on practicing physicians appointed by national medical specialty societies to serve on multispecialty physician panels.

Budget neutrality. The OBRA 89 specified that changes in RVUs resulting from changes in medical practice, coding, new data, or addition of new services could not cause Part B expenditures to differ by more than $20 million from the spending level that would occur in the absence of these adjustments. Each year since 1993, CMS has projected net expenditure increases exceeding the $20 million limitation as the result of RVU refinements and the addition of new codes.

To limit the increase in Medicare expenditures as mandated by the statute, CMS has applied various adjustments to the payment schedule to ensure budget neutrality. For the 1993-1995 payment schedules, CMS achieved budget neutrality by uniformly reducing all RVUs across all services. The RVUs were reduced by 2.8% in 1993; 1.3% in 1994; and 1.1% in 1995. For the 1996 payment schedule, however, CMS applied a budget neutrality adjustment to the conversion factors rather than across RVUs.

The AMA strongly objected to using the RVUs as a mechanism to preserve budget neutrality. Such annual budget neutrality adjustments cause confusion among the many non-Medicare payers, as well as physician practices, that adopt the RBRVS payment system. Rather than adjusting the conversion factors, however, the AMA has favored developing a separate budget neutrality factor to simplify private payer use of the RBRVS.

CMS applied two separate budget neutrality adjustments for the 1997 payment schedule. First, to adjust for changes in payments resulting from the 5-year review of the RBRVS, CMS reduced the RVUs for physician work by 8.3% through a budget neutrality adjuster applied to the work RVUs. A separate budget neutrality adjustment was made through a reduction to the conversion factors of 1.5%. This adjustment was due to new payment policies and changes in RVUs from CPT coding changes (0.6%), as well as anticipated changes in the behavioral offset (0.9%). Budget neutrality for 1998 was achieved by reducing the conversion factor by 0.8%.

In 1999, CMS eliminated the separate 8.3% reduction in work RVUs and now applies this budget neutrality adjustments directly to the conversion factor. To ensure that the adjustment only applied to the work relative values, CMS then increased the practice expense and malpractice RVUs. In addition, CMS adjusted the practice expense and malpractice relative values to ensure that the percentages of fee schedule allowed charges for work, practice expense, and malpractice premiums equal the new percentages represented in the revised Medicare Economic Index (MEI). The changes due to the MEI weights resulted in changes to the conversion factor and the practice expense and malpractice relative values. Work now increased from 54.2 percent of the total to 54.5 percent, the practice expense portion increased from 41.0 percent to 42.3 percent, and the malpractice portion decreased from 4.8 percent to 3.2 percent. To maintain stable work RVUs as a result of these adjustments, CMS changed the practice expense and malpractice RVUs which are then offset by an adjustment to the conversion factor.

In 2000, the conversion factor is a result of the changes in the MEI weights, the elimination of the separate work adjuster, the SGR update, and the behavioral offset. This last adjustment reflects CMS's belief that the volume and intensity of physician services will increase in response to payment schedule changes, thus increasing overall Medicare expenditures.

1999 Conversion factor		$34.7315
2000 Update		5.47%
Other 1999 factors		
Budget Neutrality (Pulse Oximetry Bundle)	.07%	
Behavioral offset	–0.127%	
Net effect of 2000 factors		5.42%
2000 Conversion factor		$36.6137

The adjusted conversion factor in 2001 was computed as follows:

2000 Conversion Factor	$36.6137
2001 Update	1.05163
2001 Legistative Adjustment	0.99800
Volume and Intensity Adjustment	0.99800
Other Factors	0.99700
2001 Conversion Factor	$38.2581

The adjusted conversion factor in 2002 was computed as follows:

2001 Conversion Factor	$38.2581
2002 Update	0.9523
Budget-Neutrality Adjustment: 5-Year Review	0.9954
Behavior Offset	0.9982
2002 Conversion Factor	$36.1992

Updating the GPCIs

OBRA 90 requires that the GPCIs be updated at least every 3 years. As a result, they were revised for 1995 to 1997, 1998 to 2000, and for 2001 to 2003. The revisions were phased in over a 2- year period, with half the overall adjustment in each year. The resulting changes in payments are distributed among localities and do not affect total Medicare payments. Medicare payment localities were substantially revised for 1997 to achieve several CMS goals, including administrative simplification, reduced urban/rural payment differences and reduced payment differences among adjacent areas, and stabilization of payment updates resulting from the periodic GPCI revisions. As a result, the number of payment areas dropped from 240 to 89. GPCIs for the revised localities were developed and became fully effective in 1997 for all payment areas except those in Missouri and Pennsylvania. Changes to the GPCIs in these states exceeded a specified threshold and, thus, were transitioned in 1988 and 1999.

Chapter 11
Standardizing Medicare Part B: RBRVS Payment Rules and Policies

The resource-based relative value scale (RBRVS) payment system required the development of national payment policies and their uniform implementation by the Medicare carriers. As Chapter 2 described, under customary, prevailing, and reasonable payment (CPR) each Medicare carrier established its own policies, including issues such as which services were included in the payment for a surgical procedure. As with the elimination of specialty differentials and customary charges, there was no transition period for standardizing carrier payment policies under the RBRVS payment system. Standardization of payment policies became effective January 1, 1992. This revised edition of the Guide reflects CMS's clarifications and new policies issued since implementation, as well as new policies published in the November 2000 *Final Rule* and effective for services provided January 1, 2001.

One of the most significant standardization provisions included in the Omnibus Budget Reconciliation Act of 1989 (OBRA 89) was the requirement that CMS adopt a uniform coding system for Medicare. In the June 1991 *Notice of Proposed Rulemaking (NPRM),* CMS stated that the AMA's Current Procedural Terminology (CPT) would serve as that uniform system. CPT 2001 includes nearly 8000 codes to describe physicians' services, including codes for evaluation and management (E/M) that became effective January 1, 1992. These codes are used to describe visit and consultation services and were developed for use under Medicare's RBRVS-based payment system. They are described briefly in this chapter.

The CPT is maintained and updated annually by the AMA's CPT Editorial Panel. To ensure that CPT appropriately reflects the services provided by the broader spectrum of physician specialties, the CPT Advisory Committee assists the Editorial Panel in reviewing proposals for changes in codes and new codes. The Advisory Committee includes representatives from more than 100 specialty societies, as well as 11 representatives on the AMA CPT Health Care Professionals Advisory Committee (HCPAC).

In addition to the five-digit CPT codes, CMS recognizes other alphanumeric codes for some nonphysician services and supplier services, such as ambulances. Together, the CPT codes and the alphanumeric codes comprise the Health Care Common Procedural Coding System, or HCPCS.

As Chapter 3 outlined, besides coding, CMS established a multitude of national policies as part of the revisions to the payment system, including uniform national policies on payment for:

- global surgical packages;
- assistants-at-surgery;
- "incident-to" services;
- supplies and drugs;

- technical component–only services;
- iagnostic tests;
- nonphysicians' services; and
- several other aspects of Medicare Part B.

In reviewing this chapter, it is important for physicians to understand that the carriers are required to implement these policies in a uniform manner nationally. Carriers do not have an option to develop a different policy for their local area.

Defining a Global Surgical Package: Major Surgical Procedures

A global surgical package for major surgical procedures refers to a payment policy of bundling payment for the various services associated with an operation into a single payment covering the operation and these other services, such as postoperative hospital visits. It is common practice among surgeons to bill for such global surgical packages, which generally include the immediate preoperative care, the operation itself, and the normal, uncomplicated follow-up care. Under the CPR payment system, Medicare carriers were allowed a wide latitude in establishing a global package, resulting in global surgery policies that varied from carrier to carrier and from service to service. (For a more detailed discussion of CPR, refer to Chapter 1.) For example, about half of the carriers included preoperative care in their global surgery packages. In addition, carrier policies for the number of days included in postoperative care differed widely, from 0 to 270 days after surgery.

Revising Medicare's physician payment system required a nationally standardized definition of what constitutes the preoperative and postoperative time periods, as well as the specific services included in these periods. In the 1991 *Final Rule,* CMS identified specific services included in the global surgical package when provided by the physician who performs the surgery: preoperative visits the day before the surgery; intraoperative services that are normally a usual and necessary part of a surgical procedure; services provided by the surgeon within 90 days of the surgery that do not require a return trip to the operating room and follow-up visits provided during this time by the surgeon that are related to recovery from the surgery; and postsurgical pain management.

Each component of CMS's global surgical policy—evaluation or consultation, preoperative visits by the surgeon, intraoperative services, and postoperative period—is discussed below in further detail. Following the summary of the global surgery package is a discussion on using six coding modifiers (-24, -25, -57, -58, -78, and -79) the CPT

Editorial Panel established in 1992 and 1993 and CMS adopted for payment purposes. These modifiers identify a service or procedure furnished during the global period that is not a usual part of the global surgical package and for which separate payment may be made. Also covered in this chapter in the section on "Modifiers" are definitions for multiple surgery (-51) and for providers furnishing less than the full global package (-54, -55, -56). Physician work relative value units (RVUs) for surgical services were generally based on the Harvard RBRVS study, which included:

- preoperative visits on the day before surgery or the day of surgery;
- the hospital admission workup;
- the primary operation;
- immediate postoperative care, including dictating operative notes, talking with the family and other physicians;
- writing orders;
- evaluating the patient in the recovery room;
- postoperative follow-up on the day of surgery; and
- postoperative hospital and office visits.

Initial Evaluation or Consultation by the Surgeon

The surgeon's initial evaluation or consultation is considered a separate service from the surgery and is paid as a distinct service, even if the decision, based on the evaluation, is not to perform the surgery. Previously, some carriers bundled the initial evaluation or consultation into the global surgery payment if it occurred within the week prior to the surgery and, in some cases, even within 24 hours of surgery. If the decision to perform a major surgery (surgical procedures with a 90-day global period) is made on the day of or the day prior to the surgery, separate payment is allowed for the visit at which the decision is made if adequate documentation is submitted with the claim demonstrating that the decision for surgery was made during a specific visit. Modifier -57 (Decision for surgery) is used to indicate that an evaluation and management (E/M) service resulted in the initial decision to perform the surgery.

Preoperative Visits by the Surgeon

In the 1991 *Final Rule,* CMS adopted a preoperative period that includes any visits by the surgeon, in or out of the hospital, for 1 day prior to the surgery. It is important to note that CMS emphasized that preoperative billings are carefully monitored as part of carrier postpayment medical necessity review and a longer preoperative period may be adopted later.

Intraoperative Services

All intraoperative services that are normally included as a necessary part of a surgical procedure are included in the global package.

Complications Following Surgery

If a patient develops complications following surgery that require additional medical or surgical services but do not require a return trip to the operating room (for example, a stitch pop), Medicare will include these services in the approved amount for the global surgery, with no separate payment made. However, if the complications require the patient's return to the operating room for any reason for care determined to be medically necessary, these services are paid separately from the global surgery amount. Modifier -78 is reported in this instance.

CMS defines "operating room" as a:

"place of service specifically equipped and staffed for the sole purpose of performing procedures. The term 'operating room' includes a cardiac catheterization suite, a laser suite, and an endoscopy suite. It does not include a patient room, a minor treatment room, a recovery room or an intensive care unit (unless the patient's condition was so critical there would be insufficient time for transportation to an operating room)."

Separate payment is allowed for treatment for complications requiring expertise beyond that of the surgeon. Full payment will be made to the physician who provides such treatment. In addition, separate payment is allowed for the following tests when performed during the global period of a major surgery: visual field (92081-92083), fundus photography (92250), and fluorescein angiography (92235).

Postoperative Services by the Surgeon

The global surgery package includes a standard postoperative period of 90 days when no separate payment is made for the surgeon's visits or services. Postoperative services specifically identified by CMS as part of the global package are:

- dressing changes;
- local incisional care;
- removal of operative packs; removal of cutaneous sutures, staples, lines, wires, tubes, drains, casts, and splints;
- insertion, irrigation, and removal of urinary catheters;
- routine peripheral intravenous lines and nasogastric and rectal tubes; and
- change and removal of tracheostomy tubes.

Exceptions to the postoperative period when separate payment is allowed include the surgeon's E/M services that are unrelated to the diagnosis for which the surgery was performed. These services are paid separately by appending modifier -24 to the appropriate level of E/M service and submitting appropriate documentation.

Services provided by the surgeon for treating the underlying condition and for a subsequent course of treatment that is not part of the normal recovery from the surgery are also paid separately. The CMS provides an example of a urologist who performs surgery for prostate cancer and subsequently administers chemotherapy services. The chemotherapy services would not be part of the global surgery package. When reporting these circumstances, modifier -79 should be included.

Full payment for the procedure (not just the intraoperative services) is allowed for situations when distinctly separate but related procedures are performed during the global period of another surgery (eg, reconstructive and burn surgery) in which the patient is admitted to the hospital for treatment, discharged, and then readmitted for further treatment. When the decision is made prospectively or at the time of the first surgery to perform a second procedure (ie, to stage a procedure), modifier -58 (Staged or related procedure or service by the same physician during the postoperative period) should be reported.

When postoperative care following surgery is provided by a nonsurgeon for an underlying condition or medical complication, it is reported and will be considered as concurrent care and should be reported using the appropriate E/M code. The nonsurgeon should not append modifier -55 when reporting such services.

To determine if a procedure is part of a global package, refer to the List of Relative Value Units in Part 5. The column headed "Global Period" indicates the appropriate global period (eg, 090) or one of the following alpha codes:

MMM = A service furnished in uncomplicated maternity cases including antepartum care, delivery, and postpartum care. The usual global surgical concept does not apply.

XXX = Global concept does not apply.

YYY = Global period is to be set by the carrier (eg, unlisted surgery code).

ZZZ = The code is part of another service and falls within the global period for the other service.

Postoperative Pain Management

Payment for physician services related to patient-controlled analgesia is included in the surgeon's global payment. Pain management by continuous epidural is paid by reporting CPT code 62319 on the first day of service. This code includes the catheter and injection of the anesthetic substance. Payment will be allowed for CPT code 01996 for daily management of the epidural drug administration after the day on which the catheter was introduced. Payment is not allowed for both 01966 and 62279 on the same day. The global surgical payment will be reduced if postpayment audits indicate that a surgeon's patients routinely receive pain management services from an anesthesiologist.

Duration of the Global Surgical Period
The preoperative period for major surgeries is the day immediately prior to the day of surgery, and the postoperative period is 90 days immediately following the day of surgery. Services provided on the day of surgery but prior to the surgery are considered preoperative, while services furnished on the same day but after the surgery are considered postoperative.

Rebundling of CPT-4 Codes
The CMS implemented the first phase of a new correct coding initiative (CCI) January 1, 1996, with the stated goal to reduce program expenditures by detecting inappropriate coding on Medicare claims and denying payment for them. Code edits detect "unbundling" or reporting a CPT code for each component of a service rather than a single, comprehensive code for all services provided.

The coding matrix enables carriers to identify "unbundled" codes billed with a more comprehensive procedure code and "mutually exclusive" coding combinations. According to CMS, this "correct coding initiative" improves the carriers' ability to detect inappropriate billing code combinations, such as a comprehensive code with component code combinations and coding combinations that would not be performed at the same time. The bundling initiative seeks to eliminate carrier-specific interpretations of CMS's bundling policy.

The AMA and a number of medical specialty societies expressed concerns to CMS that the proposed coding edits contained many errors and that implementation should be delayed until revisions were made. In response to these requests, CMS removed some edits and adopted other edit changes. CMS moved forward with the project, however, due to strong pressure from members of Congress to adopt more restrictive coding practices similar to coding rules that have been implemented by the private sector.

In response to widespread criticism about the coding edits, the AMA formed the Correct Coding Policy Committee (CCPC) to establish a process that would allow organized medicine to formally provide input to CMS on proposed code edits. The CCPC works with specialty societies to evaluate proposed code edits and submits recommendations to CMS for revisions to improve appropriateness of the edits. In response to CCPC recommendations, CMS has dropped or revised many proposed edits. The AMA believes that such a process is essential to preserve the AMA's leadership in maintaining the CPT coding system and determining what constitutes correct or incorrect coding.

Minor Surgery and Nonincisional Procedures (Endoscopies)

In 1992, a major revision was made in Medicare payment policy for endoscopic procedures and other minor surgeries for which global packages have generally not been established. No payment will be made for a visit on the same day a minor surgical or endoscopic procedure is performed, unless a separate, identifiable service is also provided. The CMS provides the following example:

"Payment for a visit would be allowed in addition to payment for suturing a scalp wound if, in addition, a full neurological exam is made for a patient with head trauma. If the physician only identified the need for sutures and confirmed allergy and immunization status, billing for a visit would not be appropriate."

Payment for the visit will be made by including modifier -25 when a separate, identifiable E/M service is provided. The carrier may contact those who bill extensively for visits on the same day as a minor surgery or endoscopy to request documentation for their billings.

There is no postoperative period for endoscopies performed through an existing body orifice. Endoscopic surgical procedures that require an incision for insertion of a scope will be covered under the appropriate major or minor surgical policy.

Minor surgeries will include a postoperative period of either 0 or 10 days. For procedures with a 10-day global period, the global fee includes all postoperative services related to recovery from the surgery. Payment for unrelated E/M services provided during this time is allowed when billed with modifier -24. To determine the global period for a minor surgery, refer to the "Global Period" column included in the "List of Relative Value Units" in Part 5.

Multiple Endoscopic Procedures
Special rules apply to multiple endoscopic procedures and to some dermatologic procedures. In the case of multiple endoscopic procedures, the full value of the higher valued endoscopy will be recognized, plus the difference between the next highest endoscopy and the base endoscopy. The CMS provides the following example:

"In the course of performing a fiberoptic colonoscopy (CPT code 45378), a physician performs a biopsy on a lesion (code 45380) and removes a polyp (code 45385) from a different part of the colon. The physician bills for codes 45380 and 45385. The value of code 45380 and code 45385 both have the value of the diagnostic colonoscopy (45378) built in. Rather than recognizing 100 percent for the highest

valued procedure (45385) and 50 percent for the next (45380), the carrier pays the full value of the higher valued endoscopy (45385) plus the difference between the next highest endoscopy (45380) and the base endoscopy (45378)."

In situations when two series of endoscopies are performed, the special endoscopy rules are applied to each series, followed by the multiple surgery rules of 100% and 50%. In the case of two unrelated endoscopic procedures (eg, 46606 and 43217), the usual multiple surgery rules apply. When two related endoscopies and a third unrelated endoscopy (eg, 43215, 43217, and 45305) are performed in the same operative session, the special endoscopic rules apply only to the related endoscopies. To determine payment for the unrelated endoscopy, the multiple surgery rules are applied. The total payment for the related endoscopies are considered one service and the unrelated endoscopy as another service.

For some dermatology services the CPT descriptors contain language, such as "additional lesion," to indicate that multiple surgical procedures have been performed (for example, 11201, 17001, and 17002). The multiple procedures rules do not apply because the RVUs for these codes have been adjusted to reflect the multiple nature of the procedure. These services are paid according to the unit. A 50% reduction in value for the second procedure applies to dermatologic codes in the following series: 11400, 11600, 17260, 17270, 17280. If dermatologic procedures are billed with other procedures, the multiple surgery rules apply.

Payment to Assistants-at-Surgery

By law, payment for services of assistants-at-surgery is the lower of the actual charge or 16% of the payment schedule amount for the global surgical service. (Prior to 1991, the law limited payment for assistant-at-surgery services to 20% of the prevailing charge for the surgical service.) In addition, the law provides that payment for services of assistants-at-surgery may be made only when the most recent national Medicare claims data indicate that a procedure has used assistants at surgery in at least 5% of cases based on a national average percentage. To determine when payment for an assistant-at-surgery is not allowed, refer to the List of Relative Value Units in Part 5 under the "Payment Policy Indicators" column. The notation "A" indicates that CMS does not allow payment for a surgical assistant; "A+" indicates that payment is allowed when documentation is provided to establish that a surgical assistant was medically necessary.

In its comments to CMS on the 1991 *Final Rule,* the AMA opposed the arbitrary limits set by Congress for authorizing services of an assistant-at-surgery and cautioned that quality considerations may demand using an assistant even when the data indicate that an assistant is rarely required.

CPT Modifiers

Modifiers to the CPT procedure codes are used to describe special circumstances under which the basic service was provided. With implementation of the Medicare RBRVS, the use of modifiers was standardized to establish national payment policies. The following sections describe reporting of the CPT modifiers and Medicare payment policies. Individual Medicare carriers may still use local modifiers, but only for purposes other than payment, for example, to identify claims exempt from certain utilization or medical review screening. Refer to CPT 2002 for additional details on modifiers and their proper use.

Unrelated E/M Service by the Same Physician During a Postoperative Period (Modifier -24)

This modifier indicates that an E/M service was provided by the surgeon during the postoperative period for reasons unrelated to the original procedure. It is added to the appropriate level of E/M service, or the separate five-digit modifier 09924 may be used.

This modifier is primarily intended for use by the surgeon. In most circumstances, subsequent hospital care (99231- 99233) provided by the surgeon during the same hospitalization as the surgery will be considered by the carrier to be related to the surgery. Separate payment for such visits will not be made, even if reported with modifier -24, unless documentation is submitted demonstrating that the care is unrelated to the surgery. Two exceptions to this policy are for treatment provided for immunotherapy management furnished by the transplant surgeon and critical care for a burn or trauma patient. Modifier -24 should be reported in these situations and appropriate documentation submitted with the claim.

When a visit is provided in the outpatient setting, an ICD-9- CM code indicating why the encounter is unrelated to the surgery may be sufficient documentation if it is clear the service is unrelated. If the ICD-9-CM code does not make this clear, a brief narrative explanation is required. Carriers will review all claims submitted with the -24 modifier.

Significant, Separately Identifiable E/M Service by the Same Physician on the Same Day of the Procedure or Other Service (Modifier -25)

This modifier was revised to indicate that on the day a procedure or service was performed the patient's condition required a significant, separately identifiable E/M service "above and beyond" the other service provided or beyond the usual preoperative and postoperative care associated with the procedure that was performed.

For example, the revised modifier -25 can be used with the preventive medicine codes. When a significant problem is encountered while performing a preventive medicine E/M service, requiring additional work to perform the key components of the E/M service, the appropriate office outpatient code also should be reported for that service with the modifier -25 appended. Modifier -25 allows separate payment for these visits without requiring documentation with the claim form.

This policy applies only to minor surgeries and endoscopies for which a global period of 0 to 10 days applies. (The global period is included in the List of Relative Value Units in Part 5 of this book.) For example, if a gastroenterologist examines an established patient on Monday and schedules the patient for an endoscopy on Tuesday, only the endoscopy can be billed for the Tuesday encounter, because that was the sole purpose of the encounter. If the global period concept does not apply to the minor surgery or endoscopy, separate payment is made for the services and visit on the same day.

Multiple Procedures (Modifier -51)

The definition of this modifier was changed for CPT 1999 to indicate: "When multiple procedures, other than Evaluation and Management Services, are performed at the same session by the same provider, the primary procedure or service may be reported as listed. The additional procedure(s) or services(s) may be identified by appending the modifier '-51' to the additional procedure or service code(s) . . . Note: This modifier should not be appended to designated "add-on" codes (eg, 22612, 22614)."

Medicare payment policy is based on the lesser of the actual charge or 100% of the payment schedule for the procedure with the highest payment, while payment for the second through fifth surgical procedures is based on the lesser of the actual charge or 50% of the payment schedule. Surgical procedures beyond the fifth are priced by carriers on a "by-report" basis. The payment adjustment rules do not apply if two or more surgeons of different specialties (eg, multiple trauma cases) each perform distinctly different surgeries on the same patient on the same day. The CMS has clarified that payment adjustment rules for multiple surgery, cosurgery, and team surgery do not apply to trauma surgery situations when multiple physicians from different specialties provide different surgical procedures. Modifier -51 is used only if one of the same surgeons individually performs multiple surgeries.

Under CMS's previous policy, carriers based payment for the second procedure on the lesser of the actual charge or 50% of the payment schedule amount; the third, fourth, and fifth procedures were each based on 25%; any subsequent procedures were paid on a by-report basis.

Discontinued Procedure (Modifier -53)

This modifier is used to indicate that the physician elected to terminate a surgical or diagnostic procedure. In 1999, the CPT definition for this modifier was editorially revised to clarify its intent for outpatient physician reporting of this circumstance. The 2002 CPT definition states "due to extenuating circumstances or those that threaten the well being of the patient, it may be necessary to indicate that a surgical or diagnostic procedure was started but discontinued.

Note: This modifier is not used to report the elective cancellation of a procedure prior to the patient's anesthesia induction and/or surgical preparation in the operating suite. For outpatient hospital/ambulatory surgery center (ASC) reporting of a previously scheduled procedure/service that is partially reduced or cancelled as a result of extenuating circumstances or those that threaten the well being of the patient prior to or after administration of anesthesia, see modifiers -73 and -74."

Distinct Procedural Service (Modifier -59)

CPT 2002 provides the following definition: "Under certain circumstances, the physician may need to indicate that a procedure or service was distinct or independent from other services performed on the same day. Modifier '-59' is used to identify procedures/services that are not normally reported together but are appropriate under the circumstances. This may represent a different session or patient encounter, different procedure or surgery, different site or organ system, separate incision/excision, separate lesion, or separate injury (or area of injury in extensive injuries) not ordinarily encountered or performed on the same day by the same physician. However, when another already established modifier is appropriate it should be used rather than modifier '-59.'"

Bilateral Surgery (Modifier -50)

The bilateral modifier is used to indicate cases in which a procedure normally performed on only one side of the body was performed on both sides of the body. The CPT descriptors for some procedures specify that the procedure is bilateral. In such cases, the bilateral modifier is not used for increased payment. The Harvard research described above for multiple surgical procedures found similar results for the physician work required for bilateral procedures. Medicare has maintained the policy of approving 150% of the global amount when the bilateral modifier is used. If additional procedures are performed on the same day as the bilateral surgery, they should be reported with modifier -51. The multiple surgery rules apply, with the highest valued procedure paid at 100% and the second through fifth procedures paid at 50%. All others beyond the fifth are paid on a by-report basis.

When identical procedures are performed by two different physicians on opposite sides of the body or when bilateral procedures requiring two surgical teams working during the same surgical session are performed, the following rules apply:

- The surgery is considered cosurgery (see modifier -62) if CPT designates the procedure as bilateral (eg, 27395). The CMS payment rules allow 125% of the procedure's payment amount divided equally between the two surgeons.
- If CPT does not designate the procedure as bilateral, CMS payment rules first calculate 150% of the payment amount for the procedure. Then the cosurgery rule is applied: split 125% of that amount between the two surgeons.

Decision for Surgery (Modifier -57)

This modifier is used to indicate that an E/M service resulted in the initial decision to perform the surgery. It may be identified by adding the modifier -57 to the appropriate level of E/M service, or the separate five-digit modifier 09957 may be used. Use of modifier -57 is limited to operations with 90-day global periods. Modifier -57 allows separate payment for the visit at which the decision to perform the surgery was made, if adequate documentation is submitted demonstrating that the decision for surgery was made during a specific visit.

Staged or Related Procedure or Service by the Same Physician During the Postoperative Period (Modifier -58)

This modifier is used to indicate that the physician performed a procedure or provided a service during the postoperative period that was (a) planned prospectively at the time of the initial procedure (ie, "staged"); (b) more extensive than the original procedure; or (c) for therapy following a diagnostic surgical procedure. These circumstances may be reported by adding modifier -58 to the staged or related procedure, or the separate five-digit modifier 09958 may be used. This modifier is not used to report the treatment of a problem that requires a return to the operating room. If a diagnostic biopsy precedes the major surgery performed on the same day or in the postoperative period of the biopsy, modifier -58 should be reported with the major surgical procedure code, for which full payment is allowed (eg, mastectomy within 10 days of a needle biopsy). Additionally, if a less extensive procedure fails and a more extensive procedure is required, the second procedure should be reported with modifier -58. If the less extensive procedure and the more extensive procedure are performed as staged procedures, the second procedure should be reported with modifier -58.

Return Trip to the Operating Room for a Related Procedure During a Postoperative Period (Modifier -78)

This modifier is used to indicate that a subsequent procedure related to the initial procedure was performed during the postoperative period of the initial procedure. This modifier should be reported when complications arising from the surgery require use of the operating room. Report this modifier by adding -78 to the related procedure or by using the separate five-digit modifier 09978.

Payment for reoperations is made only for the intraoperative services. No additional payment is made for preoperative and postoperative care because CMS considers these services to be part of the original global surgery package. The approved amount will be set at the value of the intraoperative service the surgeon performed when an appropriate CPT code exists, for example, 32120 (Thoracotomy, major; for postoperative complications). However, if no CPT code exists to describe the specific reoperation, the appropriate "Unlisted Procedures" code from the surgery section of CPT would be used. Payment in these cases is based on up to 50% of the value of the intraoperative service that was originally provided.

Unrelated Procedure by the Same Physician During a Postoperative Period (Modifier -79)

This modifier is used to indicate that the operating surgeon performed a procedure on a surgical patient during the postoperative period for problems unrelated to the original surgical procedure. Separate payment for the unrelated procedure is allowed under these circumstances and is reported by appending modifier -79 to the procedure code or by using the separate five-digit modifier 09979. Modifier -79 is used to report, for example, an appendectomy performed during the global period of a mastectomy by the same surgeon.

Unusual Services or Reduced Services (Modifiers -22, -52, -60)

Carriers continue to have authority to increase payment for unusual circumstances (-22 or -60) or decrease payment for reduced services (-52), based on review of medical records and other documentation. Modifier -22 may be reported when services provided is greater than that usually required for the listed procedure. Documentation of the unusual circumstances must accompany the claim (eg, a copy of the operative report and a separate statement written by the physician explaining the unusual amount of work required).

Providers Furnishing Less Than the Global Package (Modifiers -54, -55, and -56)

When more than one physician provides services that are part of a global surgery package, the following modifiers are used to designate the scope of services:

Modifier -54—surgical care only

Modifier -55—postoperative management only

Modifier -56—preoperative management only (CMS does not recognize this modifier for payment purposes; reported for information purposes only)

Questions arise about apportioning payment for global surgery packages in which more than one physician provides services. Examples include surgery by an itinerant surgeon with follow-up care provided by a local physician; cataract surgery by an ophthalmologist with follow-up care provided by an optometrist; and follow-up care provided by a cardiologist for cardiovascular surgery performed by a thoracic surgeon.

Under the CPR payment system, total payment for all parts of a surgical service furnished by several physicians could not exceed the amount paid if only one physician had provided all the services in the global package—although it appears this policy was not uniformly implemented by carriers. This policy was adopted in the 1991 *Final Rule*.

The AMA objected to this policy, because inequities result when an internist or other physician provides the preoperative or postoperative care. The Harvard RBRVS study surveyed only preoperative and postoperative care when provided by the surgeon who furnished the intraoperative care, which the AMA believes is not an appropriate basis for determining payment when another physician, who must be familiar with the patient, furnishes some of the services.

Consistent with the AMA's objections, CMS revised its payment rules. This modified policy allows a physician who assumes postsurgical responsibility for a patient during the hospital stay to report subsequent hospital visits in addition to the postsurgery portion of the global fee. Physicians assuming postsurgical responsibility should report appropriate subsequent hospital care codes for the inpatient hospital care and the surgical code with modifier -55 for the postdischarge care. The surgeon reports the appropriate surgery code with the -54 modifier.

The surgeon's payment, which includes preoperative, intraoperative, and postoperative hospital services, is based on the preoperative and intraoperative portions of the global payment. Where more than one physician bills for postoperative care, however, the postoperative percentage of the global payment is apportioned according to the number of days each physician was responsible for the patient's care.

When postoperative recovery care is split between several physicians, they must agree on the transfer of care. The agreement may be a letter or an annotation in the discharge summary, hospital record, or ambulatory surgical center (ASC) record. The physician assuming the patient's care reports the appropriate procedure code with the -55 modifier but may not report any services included in the global period until at least one service has been provided. If the surgeon relinquishes care at the time of discharge, only the date of surgery needs to be indicated when billing with modifier -54. However, if the surgeon provides care after the patient is discharged, it is also necessary to show date of surgery, date of discharge, and date on which postoperative care was relinquished to another physician.

When a physician other than the surgeon provides occasional postoperative services during the global period, separate payment is allowed. These services should be reported with the appropriate E/M codes. Physicians should code for services provided and take particular care in using correct ICD-9-CM codes. Payment is not included in the global fee as long as these services are occasional and unusual and do not reflect a pattern of postoperative care. However, separate payment is not allowed if the physician is the covering physician (eg, locum tenens) or part of the same group as the surgeon who performed the procedure and provided most of the postoperative care included in the global package.

Physicians Who Assist at Surgery (Modifiers -80, -81, -82)

Current law requires the approved amount for assistant surgeons to be set at the lower of the actual charge or 16% of the global surgical approved amount. In addition, the law requires that payment for services of assistant surgeons be made only when the most recent national Medicare claims data indicate that a procedure has used assistants in at least 5% of cases based on a national average percentage. To determine if services are subject to this payment restriction, refer to the List of Relative Value Units in Part 5 under the "Payment Policy Indicator" column. Full payment for the assistant surgeon's services may be made for some procedures if documentation is provided establishing medical necessity. These procedures are indicated by an "A+" in the "Payment Policy Indicator" column. (Also see modifiers -50, -62, -81.)

Cosurgeons and a Surgical Team (Modifiers -62, -66)

Cosurgery or team surgery may be required because of the complexity of the procedure(s), the patient's condition, or both. The additional surgeon(s) is not acting as an assistant at surgery in these circumstances. The definition of this modifier was changed for CPT 1999 to indicate: "When two surgeons work together as primary surgeons performing distinct part(s) of a single reportable procedure, each surgeon should report his/her distinct operative work by adding the modifier '-62' to the procedure code. If additional procedure(s) (including add-on procedure[s]) are performed during the same surgical session, separate code(s) may be reported with the modifier '-62' added as long as both surgeons continue to work together as primary surgeons. Note: If a cosurgeon acts as an assistant in the performance of additional procedure(s) during the same surgical session, those services may be reported using separate procedure codes(s) with the modifier '-80' or modifier '-81' added as appropriate." Payment is based on 125% of the global amount, which is divided equally between the two surgeons. Documentation to establish medical necessity for both surgeons is required for some services. To determine if this requirement applies, refer to the "List of Relative Value Units" in Part 5.

Team surgery involves a single procedure (reported as a single procedure code) that requires more than two surgeons of different specialties and is reported by each surgeon (with the same procedure code) with modifier -66. Payment amounts are determined by carrier medical directors (CMDs) on an individual basis. To determine if CMS requires documentation to establish medical necessity for team surgeons, refer to the List of Relative Value Units.

Multiple Modifiers

To standardize use of multiple modifiers, the payment rules limit payment adjustment to a maximum of two modifiers. Claims for which additional modifiers may apply are priced manually by the carriers.

Modifiers Not Affecting Payment Levels

Carriers may continue to use CPT numeric and HCPCS alphanumeric modifiers and carrier unique local modifiers (HCPCS level 3 modifiers beginning with the letters W through Z) that do not affect payment amounts. The local modifiers may be used for administrative purposes, such as utilization review, but cannot be used to increase or decrease payment levels.

Travel

Payment for travel in unusual circumstances will be allowed using CPT code 99082, "unusual travel," but is subject to carrier review of documentation to support the nature of the travel. Payment for this code is primarily intended to compensate physicians, in particular pathologists, radiologists, and anesthesiologists, who routinely travel to rural hospitals where these specialties are not available on a routine basis. The CMS provides an example of "unusual travel" as travel of more than 100 miles one way.

Telephone Management

Separate payment is not made for telephone consultations. The CMS considers this service to be bundled into the RVUs for the appropriate E/M code. The AMA is working to achieve CMS adoption of a proposal to allow payment for such services when they cannot be reasonably considered part of a specific E/M service.

Payment for "New" Physicians

Prior to 1994, legislative requirements imposed lower payment schedule amounts on "new physicians," defined as those in their first through fourth years of submitting Medicare claims. Effective January 1, 1994, provisions contained in OBRA 93 repealed these payment reductions. As a result, payments to "new physicians" and other health care providers under the RBRVS payment system are no longer subject to these percentage reductions.

Payment for Provider-Based and Teaching Physicians

Medicare payment regulations distinguish between the *direct* patient care services of hospital-based physicians and services related to *general* patient care. The latter category of services are payable to the facility as Part A services through the hospital prospective pricing system or on a reasonable cost basis.

Payment for direct patient care services is covered under Medicare Part B. Such payment may be made to the teaching hospital when it elects to be paid for physicians' direct medical and surgical services on a reasonable cost basis; otherwise, payment is made directly to the teaching physician who provided the services. The CMS defines direct patient care as follows:

- the service is personally furnished by the physician;
- the service contributes directly to an individual patient's diagnosis or treatment; and
- the service is ordinarily provided by a physician.

In the December 8, 1995, *Final Rule*, CMS described new payment rules for teaching physicians when services are provided by an intern or resident working under the supervision of the teaching physician. The regulations were developed with input from the AMA, national medical specialty societies, Association of American Medical Colleges, and Medical Group Management Association.

Prior to implementing the new rules, CMS required the attending physician to establish a professional relationship with the patient in order to bill for services provided by a resident or intern under the attending physician's supervision. The requirement and criteria defining such a relationship were eliminated in recognition of the fact that groups of physicians may share the teaching and supervision duties of residents who provide care to individual patients. The new rules acknowledge that payable services provided by teaching physicians occur in a variety of circumstances not limited to the inpatient setting. Finally, in defining appropriate supervision of residents, the new rules give the teaching physician greater flexibility to determine when "physical presence" is required.

The new policy clarifies that the teaching physician must be present only for the "key portion" of time during which a resident performs a procedure. During a surgical or other complex procedure, the teaching physician must be present during all critical portions of the procedure and be immediately available during the entire service. The rules allow payment for supervision of two concurrent major surgical procedures if the surgeon is physically present for the key portions of each procedure (ie, the key portions cannot take place at the same time) and another surgeon is standing by to assist in the first procedure. Only one surgeon can bill for each procedure concurrently. To receive payment for supervision of evaluation and management services, the teaching physician must be physically present during that portion of the visit that determines the level of service billed. Presence of the teaching physician must be documented in the patient's medical record.

The CMS also recognized that requiring the teaching physician's physical presence is inherently incompatible with the nature of some residency training programs and acknowledged that, under certain circumstances, payment may be appropriate even though the teaching physician is not present to supervise the resident or intern. For family practice and other residency training programs that meet specified criteria, CMS established a limited exception to the physical presence requirement. Payment will be allowed for low- to mid-level E/M services (CPT codes 99201-99203 and 99211-99213) furnished by a resident without the presence of a teaching physician if specified criteria are met. Included among the criteria is a requirement that the teaching physician supervise no more than four residents at any given time and be immediately available to those residents. Other criteria set requirements for the entities in which the services are furnished, establish minimum training requirements for residents who provide services, and identify the range of services that residents must provide.

The CMS indicated that the residency training programs most likely to meet the exception criteria are family practice and some programs in general internal medicine, geriatrics, and pediatrics. In the 1996 *Final Rule,* CMS clarified that obstetric and gynecologic residency programs or others focusing on women's health care would qualify for the exception if all other criteria are met.

The CMS also established an exception to the payment rules for services provided by residents in psychiatric programs. Under this exception, the physical presence requirement is satisfied if the teaching physician observes services furnished to the patient by the resident (psychiatric as well as E/M services) through a one-way mirror or video equipment and meets with the patient following the visit.

Changes made in the carrier instructions (May 30, 1996) clarified that it is appropriate to bill for qualified services performed by a teaching physician when in the presence or with the assistance of a medical student. Language in the 1996 *Final Rule* seemed to indicate that such services would be considered noncovered by the Medicare program. For additional information on how the new policy affects teaching physicians in particular specialties, physicians may want to contact their local carrier and request a copy of CMS's implementation guidelines developed for Medicare carriers.

Professional/Technical Component Services

Professional and technical component modifiers were established for some services to distinguish the portion of a service furnished by a physician. The professional component includes the physician work and associated overhead and professional liability insurance (PLI) costs involved in three types of services:

- diagnostic tests that involve a physician's interpretation, such as cardiac stress tests and electroencephalograms;
- diagnostic and therapeutic radiology services; and
- physician pathology services.

The technical component of a service includes the cost of equipment, supplies, technician salaries, etc. The global charge refers to both components when billed together. For services furnished to hospital outpatients or inpatients, the physician may bill only for the professional component, because the statute requires that payment for nonphysician services provided to hospital patients be paid only to the hospital. This requirement applies even if the service for a hospital patient is performed in a physician's office.

Radiology Services

Prior to the introduction of the Medicare payment schedule in January 1992, payment for radiology services was based on a separate radiology fee schedule. Although this fee schedule had separate values for professional component only, technical component only, and global services, these relative values were not divided into work, practice expense, and PLI components. The professional component services on the radiology fee schedule were divided into these components and linked to the overall RBRVS payment schedule. Practice expense and PLI RVUs are calculated as for other services. The RVUs for technical component–only radiology services are based on values for such services from the radiology fee schedule. The CMS has indicated that it will consider developing new rules for reporting global radiology services by radiology groups under contract to a hospital.

The physician payment schedule established standardized payment practices for three types of radiological procedures that were subject to carrier variations under the old fee schedule for radiologist services:

- interventional radiological procedures;
- radiation therapy services; and
- low-osmolar contrast media (LOCM).

Interventional radiological procedures. Separate payments are made, at the full approved amounts, for both the radiological portion (the supervision and interpretation code) of an interpretative radiologic service and for the primary medical-surgical service. Additional services associated with the procedure will be payable at reduced amounts: 50% of the otherwise payable approved amount for up to five additional procedures. Any additional procedures are payable by report.

Special payment rules apply to surgical intervention procedures for vascular studies: 100% to the first major family of vessels; 50% to the second through fifth; additional procedures are paid by report.

Radiation therapy services. The RVUs for the technical component of radiology services are generally based on the estimated average allowance for each technical component service based on the radiologist fee schedule. However, after analyzing the costs of free-standing radiation oncology centers, CMS indicated in the 1991 *Final Rule* that it had increased the RVUs to cover the costs of these centers. The RVUs for the technical component codes were therefore increased by 14.2%.

LOCM. In April 1989 carrier payment policies for LOCM (also known as nonionic contrast material) were frozen, and CMS undertook a study to determine if the high additional cost of using LOCM justified the benefits. Effective January 1, 1992, separate payment was made for LOCM for all intrathecal procedures and for intra-arterial and intravenous radiological procedures when it is used for nonhospital patients with the following specified characteristics:

- a history of previous adverse reaction to contrast material, with the exception of a sensation of heat, flushing, or a single episode of nausea or vomiting;

- a history of asthma or allergy;
- significant cardiac dysfunction, including recent or imminent cardiac decompensation, severe arrhythmia, unstable angina pectoris, recent myocardial infarction, and pulmonary hypertension;
- generalized severe debilitation; or
- sickle cell disease.

The separate payment for LOCM is based on the lower of the drug's estimated actual acquisition cost or its published wholesale price, adjusted by an 8% reduction. The 8% reduction is applied because the technical component RVUs for these procedures take into account the use of high-osmolar contrast media, which average about 8% of the cost of LOCM.

Portable X-ray

With the elimination of specialty differentials, the payment policy for portable x-ray service suppliers was changed to make the technical, professional, and transportation components payable according to the physician payment schedule.

Recognizing the additional costs portable x-ray suppliers incur in setting up equipment and positioning patients, a level 2 HCPCS code (Q0092) and national RVUs were established to reflect a per procedure equipment setup fee. The setup fee was calculated using carrier locality weights and, for 1998, was set at 0.31 RVU with no geographic adjustment. Carriers are instructed to continue pricing transportation costs locally.

Medicare allows separate payment for transporting equipment furnished by approved suppliers of portable x-ray services, which is used to perform x-rays and diagnostic mammograms. These services are billed by reporting HCPCS code R0070. The Balanced Budget Act of 1997 reinstated payment for transporting ECG equipment for services furnished after December 31, 1997, and before January 1, 1999. These services are billed by reporting HCPCS code R0076 with CPT codes 93000 (a 12-lead ECG with interpretation and report) or 93005 (a 12-lead ECG, tracing only, without interpretation and report).

Diagnostic Tests

Under the RBRVS payment schedule, CMS established criteria to identify which services are considered diagnostic tests and include a technical component and a method to determine the technical component relative value. Diagnostic tests are defined by the following two criteria:

- The service is diagnostic rather than therapeutic in nature.
- The physician's professional service is separable from the technical component of the test, meaning the professional diagnostic service is not so integrally related to performing the test as to make separation a practical impossibility.

The professional component RVU is the physician work RVU plus practice expense and PLI RVUs based on 1991 average allowed charges. The relative value for the technical component is based on the difference between the 1991 average approved amount for the global service and the 1991 average approved amount for the professional component. This formula will apply whenever a substantial volume of service is billed for either global or professional component services, and at least a 21% difference exists between the global and professional component average approved amounts. An alternate formula for services not meeting these criteria is based on the actual charge data for the component with the most charge data and an assumption that the technical component is 21% of the global services value.

For those services that do not have a professional component, RVUs are based on the 1991 average approved amount for the service itself. Diagnostic tests without a professional component are subject to the practice expense and PLI geographic practice cost index only.

Coverage Conditions for Diagnostic Tests

Medicare payment policy for diagnostic tests, including radiologic procedures, covers such tests only when ordered by the physician responsible for a patient's treatment and when that physician will use the test results in managing the patient's specific medical problems. Coverage also is allowed when ordered by a physician who is consulting for another physician. Nonphysicians, such as PAs, NPs, nurse specialists, nurse midwives, and clinical psychologists, also would be able to order these services if it is within their scope of practice.

It is recognized that a patient may have several treating physicians in various circumstances. CMS defined specific situations in which physicians will be recognized as the "treating physician":

- an "on-call" physician with responsibility for a patient's care during a period when the patient's physician is unavailable;
- a patient's primary care physician who refers the patient to a specialist;
- a specialist who is managing only one aspect of a patient's care; and
- different members of a group practice who treat a patient at different times.

CMS allows two exceptions to the above requirements:

- x-rays ordered by a physician to be used by a chiropractor to demonstrate subluxation of the spine for a patient receiving manual manipulation treatments; and
- diagnostic mammograms ordered by a physician based on the findings of a screening mammogram even though the physician does not treat the patient.

New requirements became effective January 1, 1998, for physician supervision of diagnostic x-ray and other diagnostic tests. The new rules apply only to the technical component of diagnostic procedures that are paid under the Medicare RBRVS payment schedule. (They do not apply to diagnostic procedures furnished to hospital patients nor to diagnostic laboratory tests.) All such diagnostic tests would require one of the three levels of appropriate physician supervision that CMS adopted: "general," "direct," or "personal."

Diagnostic procedures, such as magnetic resonance imaging, procedures in which contrast materials are used, and certain x-rays, would require general or direct supervision. Cardiovascular stress tests, cardiac catheterization, and radiological supervision and interpretation procedures either would require general supervision or must be performed personally by the physician. The List of Relative Value Units in Part 5 includes an indicator denoting the required level of physician supervision, as assigned by CMS, for all relevant CPT codes.

The statute exempts several diagnostic tests that would otherwise meet CMS's physician supervision requirements. These exceptions are diagnostic mammography procedures; diagnostic tests personally furnished by a qualified audiologist; diagnostic psychological testing services personally furnished by a clinical psychologist or a qualified independent psychologist; and diagnostic tests personally performed by some physical therapists, as specified by regulations.

The Balanced Budget Act of 1997 also removed the restriction on the areas and settings in which nurse practitioners (NPs), clinical nurse specialists (CNSs), and physician assistants may be paid under the physician payment schedule for services if furnished by a physician. CMS will modify the exceptions for diagnostic x-ray and other diagnostic tests to specify that no physician supervision of NPs and CNSs is required for diagnostic tests performed by NPs and CNSs when they are authorized by the State to perform these tests. CMS also changed regulations to state that diagnostic tests that a PA is legally authorized to perform under state law require only a general level of physician supervision of the PA.

Purchased Diagnostic Tests

In accordance with legislative requirements, CMS eliminated the physician markup for diagnostic tests performed by an outside supplier and purchased by a physician. When billing for a purchased diagnostic test, the physician must identify the supplier and the supplier's provider number and the amount the supplier charged the billing physician. Patients may be charged only the applicable deductible and coinsurance amounts. The CMS applies these provisions to the technical component for all physician pathology services purchased from another laboratory.

In the 1995 *Final Rule,* CMS announced that it would no longer allow separate payment by the carriers for transporting diagnostic equipment, except under specified circumstances. The rule, which applies CMS's policy for travel expenses to transportation of diagnostic equipment, holds that any costs for travel associated with providing a particular service are included in the practice expense RVUs for that service. The CMS will allow separate payment only for the transportation of equipment used to perform x-rays and diagnostic mammograms furnished by approved suppliers of portable x-ray services. These services are reported by HCPCS level 2 code R0070 or R0075 and are paid at the carrier's discretion. Effective January 1, 1996, payment for transportation of electrocardiographic equipment will be bundled into payment for the ECG service. Other transportation services may be billed on a "by report" basis with CPT code 99082 (Unusual travel).

Pathology Services

Physician pathology services were placed on the payment schedule effective January 1, 1992. These services are usually provided in a hospital or independent laboratory. The professional component of these services includes study of the specimen and interpretation of test results, while technician preparation of the material constitutes the technical component. When a physician performs these services in a hospital, only the professional component may be billed by the physician; the technical component costs are included in the hospital's payment. Effective January 1, 2001, hospitals may only bill for the technical component of pathology services furnished to its inpatients. When physician pathology services are performed in a physician's office or in an independent laboratory, a global billing is submitted.

In the 1991 *Final Rule,* CMS established a technical component for pathology services when furnished through a laboratory that is independent of a hospital and separate from a physician's office. This technical component is set at 15% of the 1991 adjusted historical charge for the professional component. (This adjustment was based on a Congressional assumption that the technical component for pathology services provided in an independent laboratory is approximately 15% of the professional component.) In addition, a hospital laboratory furnishing surgical pathology services to nonhospital patients is acting as an independent laboratory and is paid similarly for the technical component services.

In the 1992 *Final Notice,* in response to recommendations from the College of American Pathologists, CMS increased the payment for the technical component of physician pathology services to 30% of the professional component of these services. The payment increase was based on cost data for the technical component of anatomic pathology services furnished by hospital laboratories.

The GPCIs are used to adjust the technical component RVUs in the same way as described above for radiology and diagnostic tests. Division of the technical component RVUs into practice cost and PLI portions is based on historical practice cost data for pathologists.

Clinical Consultation Services

Clinical consultations (codes 80500 and 80502) are professional component services only. Criteria for payment are that the service:

- is requested by the patient's attending physician;
- relates to a test result outside the clinically significant normal or expected range in view of the condition of the patient;
- results in a written narrative report included in the patient's medical record; and
- requires the exercise of medical judgment by the consultant physician.

A standing order is no longer accepted by Medicare carriers as a substitute for an individual request by the patient's attending physician. CMS eliminated the standing order policy effective January 1, 1998, to address concerns that Medicare may be allowing payment for medically unnecessary services.

Clinical Laboratory Services

Medicare Part B pays for clinical laboratory diagnostic tests performed in independent clinical laboratories, hospital outpatient departments, and physician offices. Payment is made according to a laboratory payment schedule established by the local Medicare carrier for each test or procedure. Each payment schedule is set at 60% of the prevailing charge level in each area but payments are capped by a "national limitation amount." Effective January 1, 1998, this national limit became 74% of the median of all the payment schedules established for each test for each kind of laboratory setting.

Payment is made at 100% of the payment schedule amount, with no deductible or coinsurance required. The laboratory must accept assignment for the services performed (unless the services are rendered in a rural health clinic). Physicians must accept assignment for tests performed by the laboratory in their offices but are not required to accept assignment for other Medicare covered services furnished, even if the other services are billed together with the laboratory services.

Physicians are prohibited from billing Medicare or Medicare patients for laboratory services with any kind of a markup. Laboratories participating in the Medicare program must meet additional requirements, including disclosure of ownership and quality standards as provided by the Clinical Laboratory Improvement Act.

Clinical Laboratory Interpretation Services

The 1991 *Final Rule* created a new category of pathology service, clinical laboratory interpretation services. The CMS has identified a number of clinical laboratory codes for which a separate payment under the payment schedule can be made. These codes are found in the "Pathology and Laboratory" section of the List of Relative Value Units.

The codes are payable under the payment schedule if they are furnished to a patient by a hospital pathologist or independent laboratory. Payment criteria for these codes are as follows:

- The attending physician requests the interpretation service. (A hospital's standing order policy also fulfills this requirement.)
- The service results in a written report.
- The service requires the medical judgment of the pathologist.

Modifier -26, professional component, should be included with the clinical laboratory code.

Payment for Supplies, Services, and Drugs Furnished Incident to a Physician's Service

Separate payment is made for services that are incidental to a physician's service and for supplies for specified services when provided in the office setting.

Supplies

Office medical supplies are generally considered by CMS to be practice expenses, and payment is included in the practice expense portion of the service or procedure for which they were provided. Such supplies are considered "incident to" the physician's service. For example, surgical dressings are considered "incident to" when they are furnished during an office visit to treat a patient's accidental cut or scrape.

Separate payment is allowed for surgical dressings furnished to treat a wound that is the result of a surgical procedure performed by the physician, or after debridement of the wound. The CMS has clarified that primary surgical dressings are covered as long as they are medically necessary.

CMS also allows separate payment for supplies used to treat fractures or dislocations; separate payment is allowed for splints, casts, and other devices if provided in the physician's office. These supplies are separately payable under the reasonable charge payment methodology.

Beginning in 2001, the casting supplies were removed from the practice expenses for all HCPCS codes, including the CPT codes for fracture management and for casts and splints. For settings in which CPT codes are used to pay for services that include the provision for a cast or splint, new temporary codes are being established to pay physicians and other practitioners for the supplies used in creating casts. The work and practice expenses involved in the creation of the cast or splint should continue to be coded using the appropriate CPT code. The use of the new temporary codes will replace less specific coding for the casting and splinting supplies. For additional information on these temporary codes, including payment information, please see Appendix C in the back of this book.

Durable Medical Equipment

Durable medical equipment (DME) refers to such items as wheelchairs, crutches, and other equipment that is used repeatedly, as well as to such items as surgical dressings and urologic supplies. The DME is covered under Medicare Part B when furnished to a patient for use in the home, if it is considered reasonable and medically necessary. Medicare payment for inexpensive and other routinely purchased DME is made according to a payment schedule, effective January 1993, which is based solely on CMS's estimate of the national cost for purchasing the item. Prior to 1994, physicians and other suppliers submitted claims for DME to the local Medicare Part B carrier. In response to Congressional concerns about fraud and abuse and to streamline administrative operations, however, the CMS consolidated DME claims processing from local Medicare carriers into four DME regional carriers (DMERC).

Under the revised DMERC policies, physicians and suppliers who sell or rent DME, prosthetics, orthotics, and other supplies (DMEPOS) must obtain a separate Medicare "supplier" identification number and submit claims to the appropriate DMERC. Jurisdiction for DMERC claims submission is based on the beneficiary's permanent address.

The AMA opposed this policy because its requirements add significantly to the administrative burden on physician practices. The AMA believes that low-cost supplies should be exempt from DME regulatory requirements. In response, CMS removed some of these supplies from the DME payment schedule.

Incident-to Services

Medicare covers services that are provided "incident to" a physician's service by a nonphysician employee and pays for them under the payment schedule as if the physician performed the services. Coverage of incident-to services applies to part- and full-time nonphysician employees, such as nurses, psychologists, technicians, and therapists, and to licensed nonphysician practitioners. Services provided by leased employees also may be billed under the incident-to provision, effective October 1, 1996. Leased employees must work under a written agreement with the supervising physician or group practice.

Incident-to services must be provided in the physician's office under the direct personal supervision of the physician, although such supervision does not require the presence of the physician in the same room with the physician assistant or other nonphysician employee (unless otherwise provided by state law). The CMS has indicated that to satisfy the direct supervision requirements, the physician must be immediately available to provide the nonphysician employee with assistance and directions if needed. Furthermore, CMS guidelines state that patient contact is not required of the physician on each occasion that a nonphysician employee provides a service. According to CMS, the requirement would be met if the physician initiates the course of treatment and provides subsequent services that reflect his or her active participation in managing the patient's treatment.

The CMS broadened the application of the incident-to payment provision in 1993 to include services "ordinarily performed by the physician," such as physical exams, minor surgery, setting casts or simple fractures, and reading x-rays. Prior to adopting this policy, CMS defined reimbursable incident-to services very narrowly, for example, administering injections, taking blood pressures and temperatures, and changing dressings.

The Balanced Budget Act of 1997 included changes to Medicare requirements for payment for services furnished by nurse practitioners, clinical nurse specialists, and physician assistants. Effective January 1, 1998, these practitioners no longer are required to work under the direct, personal supervision of an MD or DO. In addition, nurse practitioners and clinical nurse specialists may receive payment for services directly from Medicare at 85% of the physician payment schedule. Physicians may want to evaluate current employment arrangements with these practitioners in response to the new requirements. CMS has indicated that it will issue revised rules in the near future regarding the new provisions relative to requirements for services provided on an incident-to basis.

Further discussion of the changes made to payment for services of nonphysician practitioners under the Balanced Budget Act appears at "Payment for Nonphysicians."

Drugs

Drugs provided on an outpatient basis are covered under Part B as incident to a physician's service. Payment for drugs is limited to those that cannot be self-administered, generally drugs that must be administered by injection.

Prior to January 1, 1998, payment for drugs and biologicals not paid on a cost or prospective payment basis was based on the lower of the billed charge or the average wholesale price (AWP). The median of the average national wholesale generic prices was used for drugs with multiple sources. Effective January 1, 1998, Medicare payment for such drugs is the lower of the actual charge or 95% of the AWP. Physician fees for drugs provided on an incident-to basis are subject to limiting charge restrictions.

Injections. In general, if the physician provides a subcutaneous, intramuscular, intravenous, or intra-arterial injection (CPT codes 90782, 90783, 90784, 90788) in conjunction with a visit, no additional payment is made for administering the injection. Separate payment is made for the drug injected, but CMS considers the resource costs of administering the drug (including nondrug supplies) to be bundled into the payment for the visit. The CMS allows payment, however, for administering the injection when only noncovered services are furnished on the same day. Separate payment, however, is allowed for joint injections (CPT codes 20600, 20605, 20610) when reported with modifier -25.

Insulin is generally not covered because it can be self-administered. It can be covered, however, if it is administered in an emergency situation.

Vaccinations. Vaccinations and inoculations are covered if they are directly related to treatment of an injury or to direct exposure to a disease (for example, antirabies or tetanus); if furnished as preventive immunizations (for example, smallpox or polio), they are not covered. There are a number of exceptions to this limitation, however:

Blood clotting factors for hemophilia are covered even when self-administered; supplies related to the administration of blood clotting factors are also covered.

Pneumococcal pneumonia and influenza vaccines are covered for all patients. Hepatitis B vaccine is covered for patients at risk of contracting hepatitis B.

Immunosuppressive therapy drugs are covered when administered to an organ transplant recipient within 36 months after the date of the transplant. (The "date of transplant" is defined by CMS as the date of discharge from the hospital.) Drugs not directly related to rejection control, such as antibiotics that can be self-administered, are not covered.

Osteoporosis drugs and their administration, under certain conditions, are covered even if they may be self-administered. The drug must be injectable and used for treatment of a bone fracture related to postmenopausal osteoporosis.

Oral cancer drugs are covered, effective January 1, 1994, even when self-administered, if they contain anticancer chemotherapeutic agents having the same active ingredients and are used for the same indications as anticancer drugs that are covered when administered intravenously. Four drugs currently meet the above requirements: cyclophosphamide tablets, etoposide capsules, methotrexate tablets, and melphalan tablets. Medicare allows individual carrier approval for "off-label" uses of oral anticancer drugs in an anticancer chemotherapy regimen if the carrier determines that their use is generally considered medically acceptable. To reduce regional variations among carriers, OBRA 93 established specific criteria for medical acceptability of off-label uses: supported by at least one of the three major drug compendia; not listed as "not indicated" in any of the three compendia; or supported by clinical research that appears in peer-reviewed medical literature.

Chemotherapy management. Separate payment is allowed for cancer chemotherapy injections (CPT codes 96400-96450) in addition to the visit furnished on the same day as the injection. Separate payment is allowed for chemotherapy administration by both push and infusion techniques on the same day. The CMS's previous policy allowed payment for only one method of chemotherapy administration on a given day.

The CMS has clarified its payment policy for chemotherapy administration in the office setting on a day in which there is no direct contact between the patient and the physician. The physician work associated with chemotherapy administration, including review of lab results, adjusting medication dosages, and discussing patient care issues with the nursing staff, should be reported with CPT code 99211. These services are covered as incident-to services, which are more fully described under "Incident-to Services" in this section.

Separate payment for hydration therapy infusion (CPT codes 90780 and 90781) and the administration of other drugs such as antiemetics and corticosteroids is not made when provided at the same time as chemotherapy infusion (CPT codes 96410, 96412, and 96414). Separate payment for the drugs will continue to be made, however. Separate payment also will be made when hydration therapy or the infusion of a nonchemotherapy drug is provided on the same day but sequentially to the chemotherapy infusion, rather than at the same time.

Antigens. As a result of changes made in OBRA 93, antigen services are paid under the physician payment schedule, effective for services furnished on or after January 1, 1995. At the same time, CMS announced that it would delete the level 2 HCPCS J codes for antigen services and no longer recognize the complete service codes (CPT codes 95120-95134). Physicians may bill only CPT codes 95144-95149, 95165, and 95170 representing the antigen extract itself and the physician's professional service in creating the extract.

Payment for Nonphysicians

In addition to incident-to services, the Medicare program provides separate coverage and payment for limited license practitioners and seven categories of nonphysician practitioners. As discussed below, the payment rules governing these services vary considerably according to such factors as site of service, medical supervision, and other circumstances.

Limited License Practitioners

The physician payment schedule applies to optometrists, chiropractors, dentists, oral and maxillofacial surgeons, and podiatrists when they furnish the specific services for which long-standing provisions of the Medicare law consider them to be physicians.

All carriers have implemented nationally standardized payment practices for nonphysician practitioners by using CPT codes for these services, where applicable; in all other instances, the appropriate HCPCS code is maintained. Payment amounts for each nonphysician category will be calculated by carriers. The CMS uses the specialty designation of these nonphysician practitioners to collect and analyze data on the services they provide.

Approved amounts for nonphysicians' services under the payment schedule are tied to approved amounts for physicians' services in the locality. That is, the payment schedule for nonphysicians' services is implemented in the same manner as the payment schedule for physicians' services. In the section that follows, therefore, the term "payment schedule" refers to the full Medicare payment schedule amount for a particular physician's service in the locality.

Chiropractors

CPT codes for chiropractic manipulative treatment (CPT codes 98940-98943) were introduced for CPT 1997. In assigning work RVUs to these services, CMS accepted the recommendation of the AMA/Specialty Society RVS Update Committee (RUC) HCPAC Review Board that the codes represented services and work essentially parallel to those of the osteopathic manipulation codes (CPT codes 98925-98929). Thus, the same RVUs were assigned to chiropractic manipulative treatment as for osteopathic manipulative treatment. CPT code 98943 is not recognized for payment by Medicare.

Effective, January 1, 2000, Medicare will no longer require an x-ray to show a subluxation of the spine for coverage of treatment. Medicare will pay for a chiropractic manual manipulation of the spine to correct a subluxation if the subluxation has resulted in a neuromusculoskeletal condition for which manipulation is appropriate treatment.

Physical/Occupational Therapists, Speech-Language Pathologists, and Audiologists

The CPT codes for physical medicine services were substantially revised for CPT 1995 and work RVU recommendations were developed according to the RUC process. The 1995 work RVUs established for these codes represent the first time that work RVUs for physical medicine services have been based on the work associated with furnishing the service. Previously, work RVUs for the physical medicine codes were based on historic charges. The CMS indicated in the 1995 *Final Rule,* however, that CPT codes 97545 and 97546 will continue to be carrier priced until better definitions for these services are developed.

The full range of CPT codes 97010 through 97770 may be reported by occupational and physical therapists in independent practice if the service is within the scope of practice. Payment for these services is made according to the Medicare payment schedule. Physical and occupational therapy services must be furnished as part of a written treatment plan that the physician or therapist caring for the patient establishes and the provider of the services must be qualified within the state's scope-of-practice laws.

A new CPT code was established for CPT 1999 to describe Manual Therapy Techniques, including mobilization and manipulation. It is expected that the primary users of this new code 97140 will be physical and occupational therapists as it is a better way to describe the spectrum of services they provide. This new code was developed after two years of discussion of the Manual Therapy Techniques Workgroup who recommended distinct coding nomenclature for osteopathic manipulative treatment(OMT), chiropractic manipulative treatment(CMT) and manual therapy techniques performed by physical therapists and occupational therapists. This new code replaces five codes (97122, 97250, 97260, 97261, 97265).

Effective January 1, 1999, all outpatient physical therapy services including outpatient speech—language pathology were to be subject to an annual cap of $1500 per Medicare beneficiary according to the Federal Register published November 2, 1998. The cap would apply to all outpatient therapy with the exception of therapy provided in hospital outpatient departments. The Balanced Budget Refinement Act placed a moratorium on Medicare Part B outpatient therapy caps.

Physician Assistants

The Balanced Budget Act of 1997 eliminated the Medicare requirement that Physician Assistants(PAs) practice under the direct, physical supervision of an MD/DO. The provision allows states to determine the required level of supervision; most states call for the physician to be accessible to the PA by electronic communication.

PAs can maintain their relationships with physicians, but they can also be considered independent contractors of physicians, which previously was not allowed. Payment would continue to be made through the PA's employer, which could be a physician or medical group. Payment would be the lower of 85% of the Medicare RBRVS or the actual charge. Medicare payment would be the same regardless of practice location. Previously, payment varied according to practice setting or whether performed in a rural Health Professional Shortage Area.

Nurse Practitioners and Clinical Nurse Specialists

The Balanced Budget Act of 1997 also allows nurse practitioners (NPs) and clinical nurse specialists (CNSs) to practice without the direct, physical supervision of an MD/DO and, further, allows these practitioners to receive direct Medicare payment. Medicare payment continues to be the lesser of 85% of the Medicare RBRVS or the actual charge and does not vary by practice setting. However, as outlined in the November 2, 1998 *Federal Register,* beginning January 1, 1999 both NPs and CNSs have to meet newly expanded certification requirements to be able to bill Medicare for their services. "A Nurse Practitioner must now meet the following qualifications: 1) Possess a master's degree in nursing; 2) Be a registered professional nurse who is authorized by the state in which the services are furnished to practice as a NP in accordance with state law, and; 3) Be certified as a nurse practitioner by the American Nurses Credentialing Center or other recognized national certifying bodies that have established standards for nurse practitioners." "Clinical Nurse Specialists must also meet similar qualifications to bill for Medicare Part B coverage of his or her services including: 1) Be a registered nurse who is currently licensed to practice in the state where he or she practices and be authorized to perform the services of a clinical nurse specialist in accordance with state law; 2) Have a master's degree in a defined clinical area of nursing from an accredited educational institution; and 3) Be certified as a clinical nurse specialist by the American Nurses Credentialing Center." The new rules in the November 2, 1998 *Federal Register* also outlined the policy for NPs and CNS in states with no regulations on their collaboration with a physician(s) as such that " NPs and CNSs must document their scope of practice and indicate the relationships that they have with physicians to deal with issues outside their scope of practice."

Certified Registered Nurse Anesthetists

The same RVS is used to determine payment for both physician anesthesia services and certified registered nurse anesthetist (CRNA) services. The conversion factor for a nonmedically directed CRNA will be limited to the anesthesia CF applicable in that locality. All services must be furnished on an assignment basis. Beginning in 1998,

Medicare will pay on a uniform basis for the provision of anesthesia services, whether performed by a physician alone or with a team.

Nurse Midwives

Effective January 1, 1994, payment may be made for services provided by a nurse midwife as authorized by state law, including obstetric and gynecologic services, if otherwise covered when provided by a physician. Nurse midwives are paid the lower of the actual charge or 65% of the physician payment schedule amount. Services must be provided on an assignment basis.

Clinical Psychologists

Medicare payment for diagnostic and therapeutic services provided by clinical psychologists was linked to the Medicare RBRVS payment schedule, effective January 1, 1997. Payment for such services is at 100% of the Medicare RBRVS. Previously, Medicare paid only for psychological testing services under the RBRVS payment schedule and paid for therapeutic services according to locality-based payment schedules determined by Medicare carriers. Diagnostic services provided by practitioners who do not meet the requirements for a clinical psychologist continue to be paid on a reasonable charge basis.

As part of the 5-year review of the Medicare RBRVS, CMS developed 24 temporary HCPCS Level II codes for reporting psychotherapy services. These codes differentiate by type of psychotherapy service provided, as well as the setting in which the service is furnished. They also allow psychotherapy services to be reported with and without medical evaluation and management services.

Only psychiatrists may perform and bill those codes that include medical evaluation and management. Clinical psychologists are not licensed to provide such services to Medicare patients and, therefore, may report only those codes involving nonmedical evaluation services. Clinical psychologist services, other than diagnostic services, furnished outside of the hospital inpatient setting are subject to the mental health services limitation (payment is limited to 62.5% of the payment schedule). All services must be provided on an assignment basis. Diagnostic tests performed by an independently practicing psychologist (who is not a clinical psychologist) are paid as are other diagnostic tests, if ordered by a physician.

Effective with *CPT 1998,* new CPT codes for psychotherapy (90801-90899) and psychological diagnostic testing services (96100-96117) replaced the HCPCS codes. The temporary HCPCS codes were crosswalked to the new CPT codes, as were the RVUs. Recently, five organizations, the American Academy of Child and Adolescent Psychiatry (AACAP), American Nurses Association, American Psychiatric Association (APA), American Psychological Association(ApA) and the National Association of Social Workers (NASW), conducted a survey of these 24 psychotherapy codes and work RVUs were submitted by the RUC in May 1998. CMS accepted the recommendations after applying a uniform 6.7% reduction across all of the codes to attain budget neutrality.

Clinical Social Workers

The distinction that applies to clinical psychologists regarding diagnostic and therapeutic services is also applicable to clinical social workers (CSWs). Payment for CSW therapeutic services will be limited to 75% of the clinical psychologist payment schedule amount, while payment for diagnostic services will be according to the physician payment schedule.

Registered Dietitians

Section 105 of the Medicare, Medicaid, and SCHIP Benefits Improvement and Protection Act of 2000 created a benefit for medical nutrition therapy (MNT) for certain Medicare patients who have diabetes or a renal disease. This benefit was implemented on January 1, 2002. Medicare Part B will pay for MNT services furnished by a registered dietitian or nutrition professional when the beneficiary is referred for the service by the beneficiary's "treating physician." The *treating physician* is defined to mean the primary care physician or specialist coordinating care for the beneficiary with diabetes or renal disease. The statute specifies that the Medicare payment for MNT services must equal 80% of the lesser of the actual charge for the services or 85% of the amount determined under the physician payment schedule for the same services if furnished by a physician. The MNT services should be reported using CPT codes 97802-97804. CMS also clarified that medical nutrition therapy cannot be provided incident to a physician's service unless the physician also meets the qualifications to bill Medicare as a registered dietitian or nutrition professional.

E/M Codes and Other Coding Issues Under the Physician Payment Schedule

Background

In 1989, the AMA's CPT Editorial Panel began revising the CPT coding system for visits and consultations. The Panel developed new codes for visits and consultations in order to improve the coding uniformity for these services and to improve the codes' appropriateness for use in an RBRVS-based payment schedule. On a parallel track, CMS was required by law to establish a uniform procedure coding system for physician services, including visits and consultations, as part of the standardization of Medicare policies. There was considerable geographic variation in the use of CPT visit codes prior to 1992.

The CPT Editorial Panel developed new codes for office visits, hospital visits, and consultations, taking into account recommendations of the panel's Ad Hoc Committee on Visits and Levels of Service, a special AMA/Physician Payment Review Commission Consensus Panel, and research from Phases I, II, and III of the Harvard study. Issues that the panel considered included the appropriateness of using time in visit coding, the number of levels of service, the need for different codes for different sites of service, and the need for different codes for new and established patients.

The AMA and CMS conducted a two-part pilot test in January 1991. As the first phase, specialty societies developed clinical descriptions of typical patient visits; physicians from five specialties were then asked to select codes for the case studies. Discussions of the new codes' strengths and weaknesses followed. In the second phase, a field test conducted in California, Kentucky, New York, and South Carolina, physicians actually used the new codes in their clinical practices. Pilot test results indicated the proposed codes could be used reliably by practicing physicians.

Based on the pilot study results, the panel refined the proposed codes and implemented them in 1992. The CMS accepted the proposed visit codes as developed by the CPT Editorial Panel. The new codes have enabled physicians to select the proper CPT code more easily and help to assure that physicians receive the correct payment for the E/M services they provide. The 1992 CPT codes for evaluation and management services adopted for use under the RBRVS payment system differ fundamentally from the previous version in the way they define and categorize codes. The familiar levels of service were replaced by a more precise method of assigning codes based primarily on extent of history and examination, and the complexity of medical decision making involved in diagnosing and treating a patient's problem(s). Four contributory components, usually less important, are counseling, coordination of care, nature of presenting illness, and time taken to perform the service.

Including typical time is intended to assist physicians in selecting the most appropriate level of E/M services. It represents physician face-to-face time for office and outpatient visits and unit/floor time for hospital visits. Consistent with the CPT approach to these codes, CMS emphasized in the 1991 *Final Rule* that time is an ancillary factor and is included to help physicians select the appropriate code. In most instances, it does not matter how much time a visit takes, provided the medical record documents the major components needed to qualify a visit for a particular code.

The E/M codes are divided into categories, such as location of service, and subcategories, such as new or established patient. The *CPT 1998* contains visit codes in several categories, including "Prolonged services," "Care plan oversight," and "Critical care" codes. Clinical examples and coding guidelines are included as an appendix in *CPT 1998*

to illustrate proper reporting of the revised visit codes. In addition, *CPT Assistant,* a quarterly newsletter published by the AMA Department of Coding and Nomenclature, provides in-depth discussion of proper usage of these and other CPT codes.

Refinements to the E/M Codes

The work RVUs for the E/M codes were revised by CMS for 1993 as a result of comments received from several specialty societies. The comments reflected widely differing views among specialty societies about the intensity of work involved in providing E/M services. The CMS determined that, based on comments received and data from Phase III of the Harvard study, the RVUs for visits should increase in a linear fashion so that the work per unit of time is the same for every code within a given class regardless of the duration of the visit. As a result, work RVUs were increased for the mid- to upper-level codes and slightly decreased for other E/M services.

CMS reevaluated the work RVUs for all 98 E/M services as part of the 5-year review of the RBRVS. The agency agreed with the RUC's argument that these services were undervalued in relationship to other services and that the preservice and postservice work involved had increased over time. As a result, work RVUs were increased in varying amounts for many of these services, including a 25% increase for office visits (CPT codes 99202-99215), an average 16.6% increase for emergency department services (CPT codes 99281-99285), and smaller increases for critical care, first hour (CPT code 99291), and office or other outpatient consultations (CPT codes 992241-99245).

Significant revisions were made to the CPT codes for 1998 for observation same-day discharge (99234-99236), nursing facility discharge (99315-99316), home care visits (99341-99350), and care plan oversight, including the addition of new codes. Work RVUs for many of the codes subsequently were changed. Coding changes and work RVUs for these codes are described more fully in the following section.

Reporting the E/M Codes

CMS reporting and payment guidelines differ in some respects from the CPT codes for certain E/M services. Coding changes and Medicare payment policies effective for 2000 are described below.

Physician care plan oversight services. Physician care plan oversight services were first recognized for Medicare payment in 1995, although on a more limited basis than described in CPT. For 1997, CMS eliminated for Medicare payment purposes the CPT definition of the care plan oversight code (99375) and replaced it with three temporary HCPCS codes (G0064-G0066) to eliminate confusion that the agency believed had arisen among physicians about proper reporting. The temporary codes specified the type of facility that provided care to the patient: home health agency, hospice, and nursing facility. Medicare allowed payment, however, only for physician oversight services provided to home health and hospice patients.

The CPT codes for care plan oversight services, as revised for *CPT 1998,* retain the changes that CMS adopted in the 1997 HCPCS codes. The CPT Editorial Panel, however, adopted six codes for care plan oversight services (99374-99380), two for each facility, that differentiate between the amount of physician time spent: 15 to 29 minutes and 30 minutes or more. Although new work RVUs were assigned to each code for 1998, Medicare recognizes for payment only CPT codes 99375 (home health care supervision, 30 minutes or more) and 99378 (hospice care supervision, 30 minutes or more).

For CPT 2001, the care plan oversight codes were revised to reflect the range of settings in which the services are applicable and to clarify that the time the physicians spends communicating with non-health professionals should also be included. CMS has stated that existing policy that this communication is included in the payment for evaluation and management services. CMS has, therefore, established new codes, G0181 and G0182, to describe the care plan oversight codes that they will now cover. The AMA objects to this action and will work with specialty societies and CMS to resolve this issue.

Home services. CPT 1998 includes new codes for new patient home visits (99344 and 99345) and established patient home visits (99350). The home visit codes for new patients will allow physicians to report comprehensive history and examination with medical decision making of moderate and high complexity. The new code for established patient home visits allows the physician to report services for those patients presenting with problems of moderate to high severity.

Prolonged physician services. Effective January 1, 1994, CMS adopted for payment a series of codes developed for *CPT 1994* to report prolonged physician services.

Prolonged physician service with direct (face-to-face) patient contact (CPT codes 99354-99357) is used when a physician provides prolonged services that involve direct (face-to-face) patient contact beyond the usual service, in the outpatient (99354 and 99355) and inpatient (99356 and 99357) settings. These codes provide incentives for physicians to furnish care in the most appropriate setting and reduce the incidence of more costly emergency department visits and hospital admissions. For guidance in selecting the appropriate prolonged service code, refer to the clinical examples in *CPT 1998*.

In addition, CMS developed the following criteria to determine when payment will be allowed for these codes.

- The physician must furnish and bill one of the following CPT codes for the patient on the same day:

    To bill CPT code 99354: 99201-99205, 99212-99215, 99241-99245.

    To bill CPT code 99355: 99354 and one of the E/M codes required for 99354 to be used.

    To bill CPT code 99356: 99221-99223, 99231-99233, 99251-99255, 99261-99263, 99301-99303, 99311-99313.

- To bill CPT code 99357: 99356 and one of the E/M codes required for 99356 to be used.

The time counted toward payment for prolonged E/M services includes only direct face-to-face contact between the physician and the patient (even if the service is not continuous).

The medical record must document the content of the E/M service that was billed and duration and content of prolonged services personally furnished by the physician after the typical time of the E/M service was exceeded by 30 minutes.

The CMS further specified that time counted toward the use of the prolonged services codes does not include "time that a patient spends occupying an examination or treatment room while there is no direct physician-patient contact" nor does it include time spent with a nonphysician practitioner for "incident-to" services.

The CPT codes 99354 and 99355 are considered primary care services for purposes of the payment schedule update, while CPT codes 99356 and 99357 are updated as nonsurgical services. The CMS did not assign RVUs to the codes for prolonged physician services without direct face-to-face patient contact (CPT codes 99358 and 99359).

Other Issues for Reporting the E/M Codes

Since implementation of the Medicare RBRVS, CMS has issued a number of clarifications and policy changes concerning reporting of the E/M codes under specific circumstances. These reporting and coding issues are described below.

Revised definition of "new patient" for selecting appropriate visit codes by group practices.

In 1992, CMS revised its definition of "new patient" for group practices to be consistent with the original intent of the CPT Editorial Panel in developing the visit codes. "New patients" are those who have not been seen by a member of the group in the same specialty during the prior 3-year period.

Annual routine (asymptomatic) exam in conjunction with a visit.

The CMS revised Medicare payment policy for the routine physical exam when performed at the same time as a medically necessary covered E/M service. Although Medicare does not cover routine physical exams, physicians generally were able to bill their patients at their regular fees for these services prior to May 1992.

In a May 29, 1992, memorandum issued to carriers, CMS stated that physicians could not divide the visit or consultation into covered and noncovered portions. Accordingly, if a symptom or medical condition was followed up during the annual exam, the physician was to report the visit with the appropriate level of E/M code. The visit was considered a covered E/M service, and the limiting charge applied. The physician could not separately bill the patient for the *noncovered E/M services*. Variation in carrier interpretation of the CMS guidelines allowed some physicians to report a higher level code appropriate for the overall encounter, while others were limited to reporting codes appropriate for the *covered services only*.

Revised CMS policy, for services rendered on or after October 30, 1993, allows physicians to bill the patient for noncovered visit services provided as part of routine physical examinations. The Preventive Medicine Services codes (99381-99379) should be reported for these services. The physician may continue to bill patients for noncovered *procedures,* such as routine chest x-ray.

Payment for the covered visit services is the lesser of the physician's actual charge or the Medicare approved amount, if the physician accepts assignment. If assignment is not accepted, Medicare bases its payment on the lesser of the physician's actual charge or 95% of the allowed amount. The physician, in addition to collecting the coinsurance, may bill up to his or her limiting charge. The physician's charge to the patient for the noncovered portion of the E/M service is the difference between the physician's *usual fee* for a routine physical exam and his/her *usual fee* (not the Medicare allowed amount) for the covered visit.

The CMS's rationale for the revised policy is that the covered visit services are considered to be provided in lieu of a part of the routine physical exam that is of equal value to the visit. Because the basis of noncoverage is a specific statutory exclusion rather than medical necessity, there is no statutory authority to preclude physicians from billing the patient for the noncovered portion of the E/M service. Therefore, the physician is not required to notify the patient in advance that the physical exam is a noncovered service.

Preoperative medical clearance by the primary care physician. Effective June 28, 1993, a primary care or specialist physician who performs a preoperative consultation or a postoperative evaluation for a new or established patient at the request of the surgeon may bill the appropriate consultation code. The CMS's previous policy required the physician (if he/she had seen the patient within the previous 3 years) to report either an established patient office code or the appropriate subsequent hospital care code. All criteria for use of the consultation codes as identified in CPT 1998 must be met. The CMS has identified the following CPT requirements as the most relevant for reporting a preoperative consultation:

- The surgeon must request the opinion or advice of the physician regarding the evaluation and/or management of a specific problem.
- The surgeon's request for a consultation and the need for consultation must be documented in the patient's medical record.
- The consultant's opinion and any services ordered or performed must be documented in the patient's medical record and must be communicated to the surgeon.
- The physician must have provided all of the services necessary to meet the CPT description of the level of service billed.

The patient's medical record should support these criteria. The CMS provides these guidelines:

In an inpatient setting, the request may be documented as part of a plan written in the requesting surgeon's progress note, an order in a hospital record, or a specific written request for the consultation.

In an office or other outpatient setting, the request may be documented by specific written request for the consultation from the requesting surgeon, or the physician's records may reference the request.

The medical record should identify the specific problem that was the reason for the consultation; describe the extent of history, physical, and decision making that supports the level of consultation code billed; and include the consultant's findings and recommendations to the requesting surgeon.

Postoperative consultations by nonsurgeons. A physician who performs a postoperative evaluation for a new or established patient at the request of the surgeon may bill the appropriate consultation code. However, if the physician had already provided the preoperative consultation, the same physician may not also bill for a postoperative consultation code. The same criteria as described above for using the consultation codes must be met for a postoperative consultation.

The CMS provides the following example:

". . . if the surgeon requests the opinion or advice of a physician regarding a specific problem that has arisen following the surgery and also requests that the physician assume responsibility for the management of that problem during the postoperative period, the physician may bill the initial encounter with the appropriate consultation code and subsequent encounters with the appropriate subsequent hospital care codes. This example applies whether the patient is new or established to the physician."

However, if the surgeon only refers the patient for the management of a specific condition during the postoperative period—and does not request specific advice from the physician—a consultation may not be billed. The CMS considers these services as concurrent care. The services should be reported with the appropriate level of visit codes, not a consultation code.

In *CPT 2000,* a number of changes have been made to the consultation notes to clarify any misinterpretation of the intent and use of the outpatient and inpatient consultation codes (99241-99255). The revisions clarify the following issues:

- A physician consultant may initiate diagnostic and/or therapeutic services at the same or subsequent visit;
- The written or verbal request for a consult may be made by a physician or other appropriate source and documented in the patient's medical record;
- The consultant's opinion and any services that were ordered or performed must also be documented in the patient's medical record and communicated by written report to the requesting physician or other appropriate source;
- In the hospital setting, the consulting physician should use the appropriate inpatient hospital consultation code for the initial encounter and then subsequent hospital care codes (not follow-up consultation codes). In the office setting, the appropriate established patient code should be used.

Critical care. In 1992, CMS issued a revised and reduced list of services bundled into critical care codes 99291 and 99292. These codes are 36000, 36410, 36415, 36600, 71010, 71020, 91055, 92953, 93561, 93562, 94656, 94657, 94760, 94761, and 94762. Separate payment will be made when services other than these are reported with the provision of critical care.

The critical care codes 99291 and 99292 should be reported when critical care is provided to a patient upon admission to the emergency department. If critical care is required upon admission to the emergency department, CMS has indicated that the physician should report only the appropriate critical care code. Payment will not be made for emergency department services reported for the same encounter as critical care when provided by the same physician. However, if the physician provided emergency department services to a patient and later the same day provided critical care to the patient, each encounter should be reported and separate payment would be made. Similarly, if the physician provides a hospital visit to a patient who later that same day requires critical care, the physician should report both encounters and separate payment would be made. The CMS has specified that documentation must be submitted when E/M services are reported on the same day as critical care.

Critical care services provided during the global period for a seriously injured or burned patient are not considered to be related to a surgical procedure and may be paid separately. The CMS has indicated that preoperative and postoperative critical care may be paid separately from the global payment if (1) the patient requires the physician's constant attendance, and (2) the critical care is unrelated to the specific anatomic injury or the general surgical procedure performed. To report preoperative critical care, the appropriate critical care code and modifier -25, as well as supporting documentation, must be submitted. To report postoperative critical care, the appropriate critical care code and modifier -24, as well as supporting documentation, must be submitted.

In 2000, several important revisions were made to the critical care codes to clarify long-standing misinterpretations among Medicare Carriers. These revisions included: 1) the elimination of the word "unstable"; 2) expansion of the definition of critical care to include care provided after the initial intervention; 3) replacing the term "constant attendance" to "constant attention"; 4) inclusion of language that critical care services include treatment and prevention of further deterioration; 5) inclusion of language making the determination of time for these codes consistent with CPT instructions for hospital inpatient E/M codes; and 6) inclusion of family discussion time as part of the intra- service work, which is consistent with the definition of work for E/M services in a hospital setting. In CPT 2001, CPT clarified that critical care services are those where "there is a high probrobility of imminent or life threatening deterioration in the patient's condition." The Panel also further clarified examples of vital organ system failure. For further detail on the new nomenclature for the critical care services, refer to *CPT 2001.* The RUC reviewed these changes and determined that the revisions were for clarification only and did not change the physician work required to perform the service. Unfortunately, CMS did not agree with the RUC and decreased the work relative values for both 99291 and 99292 by 10%. The AMA, RUC, and several specialty societies objected to these decreases and argued that CMS should revert back to the 1999 work RVUs. In the November 1, 2000 *Final Rule,* CMS announced that it will restore the work relative values for critical care as a result of the further clarification in CPT.

Emergency department services. The emergency department visit codes (99281-99285) should be reported whenever physicians, regardless of whether they are "assigned" to the emergency department, provide services to a patient registered in the emergency department. The emergency department codes may not be used for services provided in a physician's office, even though the services are for an emergency. The critical care codes (99291 and 99292) may be reported for these circumstances. In addition, CMS issued the following guidelines for reporting emergency department services provided to the same patient by a primary care physician and an emergency department physician:

"If a primary care physician advises his/her own patient to go to an emergency department of a hospital for care and subsequently is asked by the emergency department physician to come to the hospital to evaluate the patient and to advise the emergency department physician as to whether the patient should be admitted to the hospital or be sent home, the physicians should report the services as follows:

a) *If the patient is admitted to the hospital by the primary care physician, then that physician should report only the appropriate level of the initial hospital care codes (99221-99223) because all E/M services provided by that physician in conjunction with that admission are considered part of the initial hospital care when performed on the same date as the admission. The emergency department physician should report the appropriate level of the emergency department codes.*

b) *If the emergency department physician sends the patient home, based on the advice of the primary care physician, then he/she should report the appropriate level of the emergency department codes. The primary care physician also should report the appropriate level of the emergency department codes. It would be inappropriate to report the consultation codes because the primary care physician is responsible for the overall management of the patient."*

Observation Care Services. Observation Care Services codes (99217 – 99220, and 99234 – 99236) should be reported when evaluation and management services are provide to patients designated/admitted as "observation status" in a hospital. It is not necessary that the patient be located in an observation area designated by the hospital. In the *November 1, 2000 Final Rule,* CMS announced very specific policies for the reporting these services. These policies are outlined below:

- When a patient is admitted to an observation status for less than 8 hours on the same date, CPT codes for *Initial Observation Care* (99218 through 99220) should be used by the physician and no discharge code should be reported.
- When a patient is admitted to an observation status for more than 8 hours, on the same calendar date, then CPT codes for *Observation or Inpatient Care Services, Including Admission and Discharge Services* (99234 through 99236) should be reported.
- When a patient is admitted for observation care and then discharged on a different calendar date, the physician should use CPT codes for *Initial Observation Care* (99218 through 99220) and the CPT code for *Observation Discharge* (99217).

The physician must satisfy the document requirements for both admission to and discharge from inpatient or outpatient care to bill the codes 99234, 99235, and 99236. The length of time for observation care or treatment status also must be documented.

Psychotherapy. Separate payment is not allowed for E/M services provided on the same day by the same physician as individual psychotherapy. This policy applies to E/M services whether provided in the hospital or at other sites (eg, office and nursing home). The AMA has protested this policy to CMS, pointing out that it conflicts with current CPT instructions. These instructions recognize medical psychotherapy as a therapeutic procedure that is distinct from those services reported with the E/M codes.

Ventilator management on the same day as an E/M service. Ventilator management codes (CPT codes 94656, 94657, 94660, and 94662) continue to be separately payable services under the payment schedule. However, when these codes are billed with an E/M service for the same patient on the same day, CMS will consider the ventilator management services bundled and will pay only the E/M code.

Pulse oximetry. CMS will bundle payment for pulse oximetry services (CPT codes 94760 and 94761) when provided on the same date as other services. CMS implemented this policy on January 1, 2001 because as technology has progressed, been simplified, and reduced in cost, pulse oximetry is considered a routine minor part of a procedure or visit.

Anesthesia services provided by nonanesthesiologists. Payment for standby surgical team.

The CMS considers services furnished by the standby surgical team to be hospital services and paid by the hospital; consequently, physicians are precluded from billing the patient for these services.

Allergen immunotherapy. The CMS clarified that it will not allow payment for an office visit provided on the same day as allergen immunotherapy (CPT codes 95115, 95117, 95144-95199) unless separate identifiable services are performed. This policy is consistent with CPT coding language: "Office visit codes may be used in addition to allergen immunotherapy, if and only if, other identifiable services are provided at that time."

E&M Documentation Guidelines

In June of 2000, the Centers for Medicare and Medicaid Services (CMS), then the Health Care Financing Administration, issued draft Evaluation and Management Documentation Guidelines. These guidelines were revised in December 2000. They focused on correct documentation of E&M encounters with Medicare beneficiaries and offered an alternative approach through clinical examples. CMS contracted with Aspen Systems Corporation to develop clinical examples which were intended to illustrate acceptable E&M documentation practices, provide guidance for clinical practitioners, and to promote consistent medical review of E&M claims by Medicare Carriers. The clinical examples were to illustrate the guidelines for various levels of physical examination and medical decision making. Aspen developed clinical examples for 16 medical specialties from identification-stripped medical records obtained from Medicare Carriers throughout the country. In May 2001, Aspen introduced the examples and their methods to organized medicine to begin an in depth review by physicians and Carrier Medical Directors.

At the time of the introduction, specialty societies had many questions regarding how the clinical examples would be used in practice, the availability of Carrier feedback to the specialties, coordination between Carriers and specialty societies, and next steps. Also, the possibility that the clinical examples were based on medical records that were "downcoded" was raised as a serious concern. Since medical records were not available for some specialties, the issue was raised of the ability to develop sufficient clinical examples for all E&M services for all specialties. The participating specialty societies and Carriers were given a short time frame (60 days) to review a large volume of clinical examples.

On June 26, 2001, the AMA hosted a specialty society meeting designed to collect broad specialty society reaction to the CMS/Aspen clinical examples. This meeting resulted in a specialty sign-on letter to Thomas Scully, Administrator of CMS. The letter attempted to capitalize on the Bush Administration's efforts to reduce the regulatory burden on physicians and called on CMS to re-examine the need for documentation guidelines and their commitment to the development of clinical examples. The letter made the point that it would be more appropriate for organized medicine to develop its own examples that accurately reflect appropriate levels of patient care, rather than use those suggested by the CMS contractor.

On July 19, 2001, the Department of Health and Human Services (HHS) responded to medicine's concerns indicating that HHS was willing to address the E&M documentation burden. CMS stopped all work on the Aspen project and the 2000 Documentation Guidelines. (Carriers will continue to use either the 1995 or the 1997 Documentation Guidelines.) The announcement was a direct response to advocacy efforts by the AMA and the specialty societies and represents a significant concession to the physician community. In follow-up statements, CMS indicated that they believed that E&M coding should also be reviewed and it was their belief that physicians may be having problems with the E&M descriptors and CPT coding guidelines.

The AMA, through the CPT Editorial Panel, is responsible for maintaining CPT codes and thus, the preferred approach would be to address ambiguities with the code descriptors and coding guidelines through the established CPT Panel process. The Panel opted to form an E&M Workgroup to address CMS's concerns. Initial discussions were held with CMS on the proposed scope and composition of the Workgroup. The Federal Advisory Committee Act (FACA) has prevented CMS from organizing its own task force, and the Workgroup provides a viable approach to resolve CMS's coding concerns. CMS is supportive of the Workgroup and will participate in its deliberations. In November 2001, at the CPT Annual Advisory Committee and Editorial Panel Meeting, the issue of a Panel E&M Workgroup was discussed. Advisors from the specialty societies were given the Workgroup's prospective goals and work parameters developed through detailed discussions with CMS. Following the Advisors' discussion, the Panel voted unanimously to form a Workgroup that would report back to the Panel in November 2002 through the normal Advisory Committee process.

The Panel E&M Workgroup will include representatives from several specialties, Physician Payment Advisor Council (PPAC), a Carrier Medical Director, the Blue Cross Blue Shield Association, and the AMA Board Ad Hoc Task Force on E&M Documentation Guidelines. The Workgroup's charge is to enhance the functionality and utility of CPT Evaluation and Management (E&M) codes by recommending changes in code descriptors, codes selection criteria, and/or code levels to improve understanding among physicians. E&M codes must reflect current clinical practice and continue to describe physician work, while reducing the need for documentation guidelines and ensuring that any remaining documentation guidelines are oriented toward facilitating patient care. To assist in their examination of E&M coding, the Workgroup will collect data through physician surveys and oral and written testimony, and will perform analyses of existing and alternative coding structures.

New Legislative Initiatives to Detect Fraud and Abuse

Under provisions of the Health Insurance Portability and Accountability Act of 1996, the secretary of HHS and the attorney general are required to jointly establish a national health care fraud and abuse control program to coordinate federal, state, and local law enforcement to combat fraud related to health plans. The creation of a Health Care Fraud and Abuse Control Account also was called for, whereby the assessment of civil money penalties and fines from court cases would be transferred into the Federal Hospital Insurance Trust Fund.

The law also authorizes CMS to contract with private entities to carry out certain review activities previously performed by local Medicare carriers. These private contractors which may include carriers will conduct medical and utilization review and fraud review, and determine when Medicare is the secondary payer. The legislation requires that they adopt the commercial standards and claims processing software technology currently used by private insurers. CMS is expected to begin phasing in the new authority later this year.

Congressional members' continuing concerns about health fraud and abuse are reflected in the Balanced Budget Act of 1997. The new law extends to 10 years or makes permanent Medicare and Medicaid program exclusion requirements for individuals convicted of a felony related to health care fraud and other specified offenses. Provisions are designed to identify beneficiaries and to report suspected Medicare fraud and abuse. These include requirements that the Explanation of Medicare Benefits (EOMB) form contain the toll-free telephone number for reporting complaints of suspected fraudulent activity; and that Medicare carriers and intermediaries give beneficiaries itemized bills for Medicare services within 30 days upon request. Other provisions target durable medical equipment (DME) suppliers and home health agencies.

AMA Views

The AMA has consistently opposed the establishment of a fraud and abuse control account funded by fines and penalties collected from convictions for health care offenses. Such an account constitutes a bounty system, and provides inappropriate incentives for objective implementation of the fraud and abuse program. The AMA will closely monitor government enforcement activities to ensure fairness.

The AMA also is concerned that CMS's current approach to waste, fraud, and abuse mixes two issues that should be separated: correct coding policy and fraud and abuse in Medicare claims. It is believed that only 1% to 2% of physicians are involved in filing fraudulent claims. Bad editing procedures, however, punish all physicians (and their Medicare patients) by denying payment and refusing coverage for medically necessary services. The AMA and CMS have worked cooperatively on CMS's Correct Coding Initiative (CCI). The CCI, implemented by CMS in January 1996, is aimed at detecting and denying payment for inappropriate coding on Medicare claims.

The AMA believes that the problem of health care fraud is serious. At the same time, physicians cannot be expected to fulfill their obligations without standards to guide them. Therefore, the AMA has called for public and private payers and fraud enforcement agencies to work with the medical profession to clearly define the conduct that constitutes fraud and abuse. To assist the medical profession and the public understand fraudulent health practices, the AMA is working to develop informational materials for use by state medical associations and other members of the Federation.

Payment Policy Changes due to Legislation

The Balanced Budget Act of 1997 expanded the Medicare benefits package to include coverage for some preventive medicine services. Effective January 1, 1998, Medicare covers an annual mammography screening for all women beneficiaries more than 39 years of age; colorectal cancer screening tests for beneficiaries 50 years of age and older; and screening pelvic examinations (including a clinical breast exam) for women beneficiaries. Frequency limits and coverage conditions for the new benefits are described below.

The Medicare, Medicaid, and SCHIP Benefits Improvement and Protection Act of 2000 (BIPA) was enacted on December 21, 2000, and provides for revisions to policies applicable to the physician payment schedule. This legislation created Medicare coverage changes for several services including: enhancements to screening mammography, pelvic examinations, colonoscopy, and telehealth; new coverage for screening for glaucoma; new coverage for medical nutrition therapy performed by registered dietitians and nutrition professionals.

Screening Mammography

Mammography screening is a covered benefit for all women beneficiaries more than 39 years of age. The Balanced Budget Act waived the Part B deductible. The statute defines "screening mammography" (CPT code 76092) as a radiologic procedure furnished to a woman who does not have signs or symptoms of breast disease, for the purpose of early detection of breast cancer. It includes a physician's interpretation of the results of the procedure.

Previously, the screening mammography benefit varied according to a woman's age and level of risk for developing breast cancer. Coverage for women 40 to 49 years of age was provided annually or twice per year for beneficiaries considered to be at high risk; coverage for women 50 to 64 years of age was annually; and coverage every 2 years for women over 64 years of age.

For medical purposes, the definition of "diagnostic" mammography was expanded beginning in January 1996 to include as candidates for this procedure "asymptomatic men or women who have a personal history of breast cancer or a personal history of biopsy-proven disease." The definition of "biopsy-proven disease" includes both benign and malignant neoplasms.

On January 1, 2002, payment for screening mammography will no longer be established by statute. Instead, it will be based on the RBRVS and the physician payment schedule. BIPA also required CMS to pay for new digital technologies for both screening and diagnostic mammography beginning January 1, 2002.

Colorectal Cancer Screening

Colorectal cancer screening is covered for Medicare patients 50 years of age and older. The statute specified coverage for screening fecal occult blood tests, screening flexible sigmoidoscopy, and screening colonoscopy. Flexibility in the statute allowed CMS to expand the new benefit to include coverage for screening barium enema examinations.

The statute specified frequency limitations for Medicare coverage according to type of test. Fecal occult blood tests are covered annually and only if ordered in writing by the patient's attending physician.

Screening flexible sigmoidoscopy examinations are covered once every 48 months. Screening colonoscopy examinations are covered once every 24 months for patients at high risk of developing colorectal cancer. The statute defines "high-risk" patients as those with a family history of such disease, prior experience of cancer or precursor neoplastic polyps, a history of chronic digestive disease condition (including inflammatory bowel disease, Crohn's disease, or ulcerative colitis), the presence of any appropriate recognized gene markers for colorectal cancer, or other predisposing factors. Medicare requires that an MD or DO perform screening flexible sigmoidoscopies and screening colonoscopies.

Screening barium enema examinations may be covered as an alternative to a flexible sigmoidoscopy once every 48 months for Medicare patients who are not at high risk for developing colorectal cancer. For high-risk patients, screening barium enemas may be covered once every 24 months as an alternative to a screening colonoscopy. (Current policy allows payment for diagnostic barium enemas that are performed to evaluate a patient's specific complaint or to monitor an existing medical condition for patients with a history of colon cancer.) Screening barium enema exams are covered only if ordered in writing by the patient's attending physician.

The BIPA also added coverage of screening colonoscopies once every 10 years for individuals not at high risk for colorectal cancer. However, in the case of an individual who is not at high risk for colorectal cancer but who has had a screening flexible sigmoidoscopy within the last 4 years, the statute provides that payment may be made for a screening colonoscopy only after at least 47 months have passed following the month in which the last screening flexible sigmoidoscopy was performed. In addition, the statute provides that, in the case of an individual who is not at high risk for colorectal cancer but who does have a screening colonoscopy performed on or after July 1, 2001, payment may be made for a screening flexible sigmoidoscopy only after at least 119 months have passed following the month in which the last screening colonoscopy was performed.

Reporting and Payment

CMS developed new HCPCS codes for use in reporting the new services. The agency also developed relative values for the new codes, which are listed in the List of Relative Value Units in Part 5.

Payment for screening fecal occult blood tests is at the same rate as diagnostic fecal occult blood tests (CPT code 82270) and is made under the clinical laboratory fee schedule.

Screening flexible sigmoidoscopies (HCPCS code G0104) are paid at rates consistent with payment for similar or related services under the physician payment schedule but may not exceed the rates for a diagnostic flexible sigmoidoscopy (CPT code 45330). If during the course of the screening flexible sigmoidoscopy a lesion or growth is detected that results in a biopsy or removal of the growth, the physician should bill for a flexible sigmoidoscopy with biopsy or removal rather than use the new HCPCS code.

Payment for screening colonoscopy will be made under HCPCS code G0121 colorectal screening; colonoscopy for an individual not meeting critical for high risk. Payment for screening colonoscopies (HCPCS code G0105) is consistent with that for similar or related services under the payment schedule but may not exceed that for a diagnostic colonoscopy (CPT code 45378). If during the course of the screening colonoscopy a lesion or growth is detected that results in a biopsy or removal of the growth, the physician should bill for a colonoscopy with biopsy or removal rather than codes G0105 or G0121.

HCPCS codes G0106 (Colorectal cancer screening; alternative to G0104, screening sigmoidoscopy, barium enema) and G0120 (Colorectal cancer screening; alternative to G0105, screening colonoscopy, barium enema) should be used to report the barium enema when it is substituted for either the sigmoidoscopy or the colonoscopy, as indicated by the code nomenclature. The RVUs for these procedures are the same as for the diagnostic barium enema procedure (CPT code 74280). Physicians should use HCPCS codes G1021 (Colorectal cancer screening; colonoscopy on individual not meeting criteria for high risk [noncovered]) and G1022 (Colorectal cancer screening; barium enema [noncovered]) when the high-risk criteria are not met, or a barium enema is performed but not as a substitute for either a sigmoidoscopy or colonoscopy.

Pelvic Examination

The Balanced Budget Act provided for Medicare coverage of screening pelvic examinations (including a clinical breast examination) for all women beneficiaries, subject to certain frequency and other limitations. The statute waived the Part B deductible requirement.

Under the statute, the examination should include at least seven of the 11 elements listed for such an exam, as specified in the *Documentation Guidelines for Evaluation and Management Services*. Effective July 1, 2001, BIPA amended the coverage of pelvic examinations to provide that a woman qualifies for coverage of a screening pelvic examination (including a clinical breast examination) once every 2 years (rather than once every 3 years as provided by the BBA of 1997). However, it would allow annual pelvic exams for certain women of childbearing age and for women at high risk for cervical or vaginal cancer.

Annual screening pelvic examinations would be covered if one of the following conditions is met:

- The woman is of childbearing age and has had an examination indicating the presence of cervical or vaginal cancer or other abnormality during any of the preceding 3 years.
- The woman is considered by her physician or other practitioner to be at high risk of developing cervical or vaginal cancer.

Based on recommendations made by the National Cancer Institute and the Centers for Disease Control and Prevention, the Medicare program adopted the following as high-risk factors for cervical cancer:

- early onset of sexual activity (less than 16 years of age);
- multiple sexual partners (five or more in a lifetime);
- history of a sexually transmitted disease (including the human immunodeficiency virus [HIV]; and
- absence of three negative Pap smears or any Pap smears within the previous 7 years.

Prenatal exposure to diethylstilbestrol is considered the high-risk factor for development of vaginal cancer. Based on recommendations from the American College of Gynecologists and Obstetricians and other groups, a woman of childbearing age is considered to be a premenopausal woman and is considered by her physician or other practitioner to be of childbearing age, based on her medical history or other findings.

Medicare coverage requirements of the Balanced Budget Act specify that screening pelvic examinations must be performed by an MD or DO, or by a certified nurse midwife, physician assistant, nurse practitioner, or clinical nurse specialist who is authorized by state law to perform the examination.

Screening for Glaucoma

Section 102 of the BIPA provides for Medicare coverage under Part B for screening for glaucoma for individuals with diabetes, a family history of glaucoma, or others determined to be at "high risk" for glaucoma, effective for services furnished on or after January 1, 2002. Payment will be allowed for one glaucoma screening examination per year. Payment for glaucoma screening will be bundled if provided on the same date as an E&M service, or when it is provided as part of any ophthalmology service. When glaucoma screening is the only service provided, or when it is provided as part of an otherwise noncovered service (for example, preventive services visit), physicians should report either G0117 (when performed directly by optometrist or ophthalmologist) or G0118 (when performed under the supervision of an optometrist or ophthalmologist).

Medical Nutrition Therapy

Section 105 of the Medicare, Medicaid, and SCHIP Benefits Improvement and Protection Act of 2000 created a benefit for medical nutrition therapy (MNT) for certain Medicare patients who have diabetes or a renal disease. This benefit was implemented on January 1, 2002. Medicare Part B will pay for MNT services furnished by a registered dietitian or nutrition professional when the beneficiary is referred for the service by the beneficiary's "treating physician." The treating physician is defined to mean the primary care physician or specialist coordinating care for the beneficiary with diabetes or renal disease. The statute specifies that the Medicare payment for MNT services must equal 80% of the lesser of the actual charge for the services or 85% of the amount determined under the physician payment schedule for the same services if furnished by a physician. The MNT services should be reported using CPT codes 97802-97804. CMS also clarified that medical nutrition therapy cannot be provided incident to a physician's service unless the physician also meets the qualifications to bill Medicare as a registered dietitian or nutrition professional.

Other Payment Policy Changes Adopted Under the RBRVS

Described below are payment policies CMS has adopted since implementation of the payment schedule.

Evaluation of psychiatric records and reports (90825) and family counseling services (90887). The CMS bundled payment for these services into the payment for other psychiatric services and redistributed the RVUs for CPT codes 90825 and 90887 across other psychiatric codes. The CMS stated its belief that CPT codes 90825 and 90887 describe activities that are generally performed as part of the prework and postwork of other psychiatric services.

X-rays and ECGs taken in the emergency department. The CMS's policy generally allows separate payment for only one interpretation, by either the radiologist/cardiologist or emergency department physician, of an ECG or x-ray furnished to an emergency department patient. Payment for a second interpretation may be allowed in unusual circumstances, such as a "questionable finding," for which the physician performing the initial procedure believes another physician's expertise is needed. Previously, some Medicare carriers paid separately for an interpretation provided by the emergency department physician and a second interpretation by a hospital's radiologist or cardiologist.

Payment will be made for the interpretation that is used to diagnose and treat the patient. The criteria for reporting the applicable CPT code must be fully met, including written documentation of the interpretation that is prepared for the patient's medical record. Payment is allowed for a verbal interpretation furnished by the radiologist/cardiologist that is conveyed to the treating physician and that is later prepared as a written report. In this circumstance, the emergency department physician should not bill for the interpretation. In addition, interpretations furnished via teleradiology are payable interpretations when used to diagnose and treat the patient.

Finally, CMS encourages hospitals to work with their medical staffs to establish guidelines for the billing of x-ray and ECG interpretations for emergency department patients, which will avoid multiple claims submission.

End-stage renal disease. *Hospital inpatient dialysis on the same date as an E/M service.* Payment for subsequent hospital visits (CPT codes 99231-99233) and follow-up inpatient consultations (CPT codes 99261-99263) is bundled into the inpatient dialysis code (CPT codes 90935-90947), but separate payment is allowed for an initial hospital visit (CPT codes 99221-99223), initial inpatient consultation (CPT codes 99251-99255), and hospital discharge services (CPT code 99238) on the same date as inpatient dialysis. The RVUs for E/M codes performed on the same day as dialysis were redistributed into the RVUs for each of the four dialysis codes.

Payment for end-stage renal disease–related services. These services were made payable under the payment schedule in 1995. In assigning relative values to these codes, CMS accepted the RUC's overall approach of using different office visit codes as "building blocks" for the monthly capitation payment (MCP). In the 1995 *Final Rule*, CMS defined the MCP as a "comprehensive monthly payment that covers all physician services associated with the continuing medical management of a maintenance dialysis patient" and specified the services included in and excluded from the MCP. The RVUs assigned to these services were slightly increased for 1996, and CMS reclassified the service category from nonsurgical to primary care.

Therapeutic apheresis. Although payment is made for the physician work component of therapeutic apheresis in the hospital and nonhospital settings, CMS will not pay for both therapeutic apheresis and certain E/M codes on the same date. Separate payment is made for an initial hospital visit, initial consultations, and hospital discharge services. Separate payment is not allowed for established patient office visits, subsequent hospital care, or follow-up inpatient consultations when furnished on the same date as therapeutic apheresis. Separate payment for services provided to establish the required vascular access will be allowed, if performed by the physician.

The policy was implemented in a budget-neutral manner by bundling the payment for the specified E/M codes performed on the same date as therapeutic apheresis into the payment for the therapeutic apheresis service.

AMA Advocacy Efforts

In describing Medicare's payment rules, this chapter indicated several areas where positive changes were made by CMS to proposed and existing policies as a result of advocacy efforts by the AMA and other physicians' organizations. For example:

- Policies on global surgical packages were substantially improved in 1992 by eliminating the proposed global payments for endoscopic procedures, reducing the global period for minor surgeries from 30 to 10 days, and shortening the preoperative period.
- Payments for drugs are limited to the average wholesale price, rather than 85% of this price, as proposed in the June 5, 1991, NPRM.
- Policy for the annual routine exam in conjunction with a visit was revised to allow physicians to bill patients for noncovered E/M services.
- Policy for preoperative medical clearance by the primary care physician for a new or established patient was revised to allow billing of the appropriate consultation code.
- Policy for physician care plan oversight services was broadened from the June 24, 1994, Proposed Rule to include payment for these services when provided to hospice patients; during the month of hospital discharge; and during the global period of another service.
- The multiple surgery rule was revised to base payment for the third through fifth procedures on 50% of the payment schedule.

In addition, physicians realized significant victories in payment policy changes, which restored payment for interpreting ECGs and eliminated payment reductions for physicians in their first through fourth years of providing services to Medicare patients.

Despite these changes, however, the AMA and much of organized medicine remain strongly opposed to several of CMS's current Medicare policies. Because several of these inequitable regulations were required by law, the AMA's House of Delegates has called for changes in legislation aimed at:

- elimination of the unfounded payment limits for the services of assistants-at-surgery; and
- elimination of the discriminatory 50% copayment for mental health services.

As a result, the AMA will continue working to secure these and other changes in the Medicare statutes. The AMA is working on a number of payment policy issues to make the payment system more responsive to physician needs, including refinement of payment policies that do not reflect resource costs (eg, payment for supplies); increased uniformity among carriers in implementing CMS policies; and better input from practicing physicians into development of payment policies.

The CMS established a formal role for physician involvement with Medicare carrier medical policy in late 1992. Carrier Advisory Committees (CACs) now serve as advisory bodies to each carrier. The Practicing Physician Advisory Council frequently consults with the CACs in establishing its agenda. The Council's recommendations are submitted to CMS for its consideration.

The CACs are composed of physicians (as defined by Medicare statute) who are appointed by state medical associations and state specialty societies. This representation includes a member from each of 30 specialties identified by CMS, the state medical association, the national medical specialty association, and five limited license practitioners. The CMD and a physician selected by the CAC serve as cochairs. The CAC's role is to encourage communication between physicians and the carrier by enabling physicians to participate in developing local medical review policy and to identify and pursue needed improvements in Medicare carrier administration.

Part 4
The RBRVS Payment System in Your Practice

Chapter 12
Practice Management Under the RBRVS: Implications for Physicians

Bringing All the Changes Together

The Medicare resource-based relative value scale (RBRVS) payment system implemented fundamental changes in the way Medicare pays for physician services. The first year of RBRVS implementation, in particular, required substantial adjustments for the many physicians accustomed to Medicare's customary, prevailing, and reasonable (CPR) payment system. Although the complete transition to payments based fully on the RBRVS payment schedule occurred in 1996, the Medicare RBRVS payment system continues to evolve. For example, the relative value units (RVUs) assigned to the physician work component are adjusted each year in response to Current Procedural Terminology (CPT) coding changes; and the original geographic practice cost indexes have been updated in 1995 to 1997, 1998 to 2000, and for 2001 to 2003. In addition, CMS is implementing a new resource-based methodology for assigning practice expense RVUs which will be fully implemented in 2002. Professional liability insurance (PLI) relative values became resource based in 2000 and were updated with new data in 2001.

This chapter briefly describes the fundamental elements of the RBRVS and suggests elements for consideration in an audit of basic practice management techniques. In addition, it reviews those aspects of the Medicare program that may significantly affect physician practices, including the PAR program, Medicare requirements related to electronic data interchange, and recently adopted provisions related to private contracting with Medicare patients.

Physician Payment Under the RBRVS

The impact of the Medicare RBRVS payment system on a physician's practice is determined, in large part, by the volume of services the practice provides to Medicare patients, the mix of visit and procedural services it provides, and the geographic location of the practice. The four basic elements of the Medicare RBRVS that most greatly influence physician practices are:

- payment based on a national standard RBRVS payment schedule;
- payment adjustments for geographic differences in resource costs;
- balance billing limited to 115% of the Medicare allowed amount; and
- standardization of Medicare carrier payment policies.

The RBRVS. The RBRVS pays for physicians' services according to a national standard payment schedule that is based on physicians' resource costs. As discussed in detail in Chapter 8, the major effect of the RBRVS is redistribution of payments among specialties by narrowing the gap between payments for visits and procedures. In general, the RBRVS has resulted in increased payments for visits, consultations, and other evaluation and management (E/M) services, and decreased payments for surgery, imaging, anesthesiology, and other procedural services.

Geographic payment variations. Payment based on a national standard payment schedule has narrowed considerably the wide range of geographic variation in payments that existed under customary, prevailing, and reasonable (CPR). Payments in localities where practice costs are relatively high are greater than payments in lower-cost localities. Because there is less variation in costs than there was in Medicare prevailing charges, areas with low prevailing charges relative to the national average generally have experienced increased payments under the RBRVS; areas with very high prevailing charges relative to the national average generally have experienced decreased payments. These geographic payment variations are described in detail in Chapter 7.

Limiting charges. Limiting charges apply to all nonparticipating physician payments and, generally, are more restrictive than those imposed prior to RBRVS implementation. The limiting charge since 1993 has been 15% more than the Medicare-approved amount (including the 80% that Medicare pays and patients' 20% coinsurance) for nonparticipating physicians. Nonparticipating physician payments are set at 95% of participating physician amounts.

For a detailed discussion of limiting charges, refer to Chapter 9.

Medicare payment based on a national standard RBRVS payment schedule required that all carriers uniformly implement Medicare's payment rules. The shift to standardized payment policies across Medicare carriers resulted in payments that are more predictable and consistent than under CPR.

Global surgical packages. The global surgery policy under the RBRVS resulted in major payment adjustments for some surgeons. For example, standardized policy under the RBRVS includes a postoperative period of 90 days. For those surgeons accustomed to a postoperative period of 30 days or less, this longer postoperative period meant a decline in billing volume for follow-up visits. When other than normal surgical care is provided during this time, however, physicians may appropriately bill and receive separate payment for these services. Careful use of the appropriate CPT modifiers to indicate these services, as outlined in Chapter 11, will help avoid unnecessary claims denials. In addition, the global surgery policy specifically allows surgeons to bill for related services provided beyond the 90-day postoperative period.

Medicare RBRVS payment policy for minor surgeries and endoscopies eliminates payment for a visit on the same day, unless a separate E/M service is also provided during the visit. Properly using modifier -25 in this circumstance will help ensure that the claim is paid appropriately.

Evaluation and management (E/M) codes. Major changes to the CPT codes for E/M services were adopted for 1992, the first year of Medicare RBRVS implementation. For information on proper coding of these and other services, physicians should obtain the 2001 edition of the AMA's *Physicians' Current Procedural Terminology.*

The Practice Management Audit

Physicians may want to consider conducting an audit of office management practices to ensure that they are reflective of current RBRVS policies, as well as other Medicare requirements. The audit could be conducted by designated office staff or an outside consulting firm. Physician payment seminars sponsored by medical societies, carriers, and practice management consulting firms are tools available to medical practices as an alternative to outside consultants.

The volume of Medicare services provided by the practice should determine how much time and expense to invest in an audit. If a practice treats a large number of Medicare patients, or if a previous financial analysis indicated that the RBRVS payment system significantly affects practice revenues, retaining a consultant may be a useful investment.

Office Management Practices

The practice management audit might include an evaluation of office management practices to ensure efficient operations. This evaluation should ensure that systems are in place to implement all aspects of the RBRVS payment system, as well as other Medicare requirements as discussed in the following sections.

Educating office staff is important in adapting office management practices to changes in the RBRVS payment system. For example, appropriate staff should be knowledgeable about CPT coding changes, RVU revisions, and new Medicare payment policies, particularly for those services provided most frequently by the practice. Proficiency in using the new documentation guidelines for E/M services is also important for most practices. Numerous workshops and seminars are available for billing and other office staff, as well as physicians, through medical societies, hospitals, carriers, and practice management firms.

Medical practices should formalize their payment and collection procedures and communicate these policies to patients. Practices with a large Medicare patient base may want to collect payment when services are provided as a way to accelerate cash flow. This policy should be conveyed to patients during their initial visit. Information about patients' insurance plans should also be obtained at that time. The physician is required to file all Medicare claims for the patient, even if they are unassigned. Medicare prohibits any charge to the patient for this service. Statutes also prohibit Medicare carriers from imposing any fees on physicians related to claims filing, appeals, assigning unique provider identifier numbers, or for responding to inquiries on the status of pending claims.

Incomplete Claims

As part of efforts to streamline claims processing, CMS has developed a new policy to reduce the number of claims that enter into the formal appeals process. Whereas previously carriers denied incomplete or invalid claims, which would start the appeals process, they must now return such claims to physicians as "unprocessable." Incomplete claims lack required information (eg, no provider number), while invalid claims contain complete and necessary information that is somehow illogical or incorrect. The claims are returned by the carrier with notification for correction and resubmission. No "initial determination" is made. Carriers must provide an explanation of errors and allow correction or resubmission of the claim.

Medigap and Other Supplemental Benefits

Billing procedures are simplified when Medicare patients assign their Medigap payments to a participating physician. When the participating physician submits a claim to the Medicare carrier for a patient with non–employment-related Medigap coverage, the carrier automatically sends the claim to the Medigap insurer for payment of all coinsurance and deductible amounts due under the Medigap policy. The Medigap insurer must make payment directly to the physician.

Physicians and other providers are required to obtain information from their Medicare patients about coverage by other health benefit plans and to include this information on the claim form. It is important to maintain records of your patients' health care coverage that may be primary to Medicare, because carriers may search their records dating from January 1, 1983, to recover payments for which they believe Medicare may be the secondary payer. Supplemental claims are forwarded automatically to the private insurer if the insurer contracts with the Medicare carrier to send Medicare claim information electronically. Otherwise, the patient must file the supplemental claim.

In instances when another insurer is primary to Medicare but pays only part of the doctor's bill, Medicare makes a supplemental payment. Total payment to the physician, however, may not exceed the 20% copayment or deductible on assigned claims. The physician should refund any excess payment to the supplemental insurer.

When assignment is not accepted, physicians may bill the supplemental insurer up to their limiting charge for the service. The Social Security Act Amendments of 1994 provide that supplemental insurers, as well as Medicare beneficiaries, are not liable for payment of any amount in excess of the limiting charge. Effective for services provided on or after January 1, 1995, nonparticipating physicians and suppliers may not bill supplemental insurers in excess of the limiting charge. Physicians and suppliers who collect payments from a Medicare beneficiary or supplemental insurer that exceed the limiting charge are required to refund the excess amount. Previously, many interpreted the statute to mean that billing and accepting payment from the supplemental insurer up to the private payer's allowed amount was an acceptable billing practice, even though this amount may have exceeded the physician's limiting charge for the service.

Electronic Data Interchange

To help reduce the administrative costs of our health care system, the AMA supports the development of a uniform claim form and voluntarily expanding electronic claims processing by public and private health insurers. Electronic claims can be processed at a lower cost and with greater accuracy than paper claims due to reduced administrative time and paperwork. In addition, electronic claims processing can accelerate cash flow through faster claims payment and can quickly verify receipt of transmitted claims. Cost savings associated with processing electronically filed claims and the goal of a nationwide electronic health care information network have led CMS to adopt incentives for the Medicare program that may encourage physicians to file claims electronically. Such incentives include faster payment for claims submitted electronically; free billing and remittance software; on-line access to claims status and eligibility data for participating physicians; and access for participating physicians to toll-free telephone numbers for electronic claims submission. In addition, CMS has extended to all physicians, not just those who file claims electronically, the option of electronic fund transfers rather than payment by checks.

In addition, the growing interest in electronic claims processing led CMS to adopt standardized formats for the electronic submission of claims. Finally, provisions contained in the Health Insurance Portability and Accountability Act of 1996 (HIPAA) are likely to accelerate the use of electronic data interchange. The legislation requires adoption of standards for administrative and financial electronic health care transactions, including unique identifiers for all physicians and other health care providers, as well as for health plans, employers, and individuals. These new systems are described below.

Standardized Electronic Formats

Under new CMS requirements that became effective in July 1996, Medicare claims submitted electronically must be in one of two standard formats: the X12 837 format or the National Standard Format. Proprietary formats no longer will be accepted by Medicare carriers. One advantage of the X12 837 is the corresponding standards developed by the American National Standard Institute (ANSI) for related transactions, such as eligibility and claims status inquiries.

Administrative Simplification

HIPAA calls for the adoption of standards for the following electronic health care transactions:

- health claims or equivalent encounter information;
- health claims attachments;
- enrollment and disenrollment in a health plan;
- eligibility for a health plan;
- health care payment and remittance advice;
- health plan premium payments;
- first report of injury;
- health claims status;
- referral certification and authorization; and
- coordination of benefits

Payers and clearinghouses will be required to accept the standard health care transactions from any physician or other provider who desires to use a standard electronic transaction. The timetable outlined in the Act originally required the secretary of Health and Human Services (HHS) to adopt most standards no later than February 1998. The timelines have been delayed with a compliance date of October 16, 2002. Health plans and clearinghouses will be required to comply with the new requirements. The statute, however, places no mandate on physicians to submit claims electronically.

National Provider Identifier

HIPAA also calls for development of a new identification system for all health care providers that will also replace the current CMS identifier, the Unique Physician Identification Number (UPIN). The new system will assign a unique national provider identifier (NPI) to all physicians and other providers including those that treat Medicare patients and could serve both as a unique identifier and as a billing number. Physicians will keep the assigned NPI throughout their careers, even if they change specialties or relocate their practice.

The CMS has indicated that it may provide NPI directories, similar to the current UPIN directories, to physicians and other health care providers.

The NPI will be linked to an electronic database maintained by the Department of Health and Human Services (HHS) that includes such information as name, practice address, specialty, type of practice, education, licensing, and credentials of the physician or provider. The NPI system is part of an intergovernmental effort that is intended to allow the identification of the same provider across federal programs. To encourage use of a nationally uniform identification system across all payers, HHS plans to make the NPI available to other insurers for use in their claims processing systems.

The AMA has expressed its concerns about the need to protect physicians' confidentiality, as well as the accuracy of baseline information, under NPI implementation. The AMA has offered its assistance to HHS on verification of physician source data for the NPI through the AMA Physician Masterfile, similar to previous efforts to determine accuracy of physician data for assignment of the current UPIN. The AMA will continue to work with HHS on development of the new identifier system to ensure that these issues are appropriately resolved.

National Payer Identifier

Third party payers are currently identified in a variety of ways, resulting in claims payment errors and delays. A major new initiative currently under way at HHS, initiated by HIPAA and known as PAYERID, will assign a unique identifier to each payer of health care claims to standardize and simplify coordination of benefits. PAYERID will allow CMS to track beneficiary coverage by other insurers and better coordinate benefits with state Medicaid agencies, Medigap insurers, and other payers, as well as contribute to identification of appropriate payers in accordance with the Medicare Secondary Payer Program. It is anticipated that CMS will require the PAYERID on claims forms, although an implementation date has not yet been established.

Access to the electronic database containing the unique payer identifiers will be available through health care network operators, claims clearinghouses, and large payers. The AMA will work with CMS to ensure that such information is easily available to physicians who do not subscribe to a claims clearinghouse. Controls placed on the PAYERID application process and access to the database will minimize the potential for fraud and abuse.

Related AMA Activities

The AMA is a leader in promoting administrative simplification and the development of standards for health care transactions through its participation in two policymaking bodies, the National Uniform Claim Committee (NUCC) and the Workgroup for Electronic Data Interchange (WEDI). An AMA representative chairs the NUCC and is a member of the WEDI Board of Directors. With passage of the Health Insurance Portability and Accountability Act, the NUCC and WEDI have a formal consultative role regarding the standards for health care transactions selected by the secretary.

The Participation Decision

A medical practice should evaluate whether to sign a participation agreement with Medicare along with other financial considerations. The advantages and disadvantages of each decision are discussed below.

Participation

Participation may present a significant advantage to a practice's cash flow, particularly if it has a substantial volume of Medicare claims. When 80% of the Medicare approved amount is paid directly to the physician, rather than to the patient, the payment collection process may be faster and completed with fewer administrative requirements than for nonparticipating claims. When selecting a physician, many Medicare patients consider participation an important advantage because they are responsible only for the annual deductible and 20% copayment for Medicare-covered services. Participating physicians also benefit because their names are published in directories provided to senior citizen groups and because they receive participation emblems from Medicare to display in their offices.

Participating physicians must agree to accept Medicare's approved amount as payment in full for all covered services for the duration of the calendar year. The opportunity to change participation status is only offered once per year, usually during November when the carriers send the Medicare Participating Physician/Supplier Agreement (formerly referred to as the Dear Doctor letters).

Nonparticipation

Nonparticipating physicians have some advantages not available to participating physicians. They may choose to accept assignment on a claim-by-claim basis, and this freedom of choice may be an important philosophical consideration when making the participation decision. Nonparticipating physicians are allowed to bill Medicare patients for covered services above the Medicare-approved amount, which is referred to as "balance billing." Beginning in 1986, however, when maximum allowable actual charges (MAACs) were imposed, the amount a nonparticipating physician could bill a Medicare patient in excess of the approved amount was subject to limitations. In 1991, limiting charges replaced MAACs.

Since January 1993, the limiting charge has been 15% more than the Medicare-approved amount for nonparticipating physicians. Medicare payments for nonparticipating physicians are 95% of payment rates for participating physicians. As a result, the 15% limiting charge translates into only 9.25% more than the participating physician payment schedule. Medical practices should evaluate the advantage of balance billing based on their success in collecting payments and on the extra costs associated with billing patients.

As explained in Chapter 9, carriers closely monitor physician compliance with the limiting charges. Under CMS's Comprehensive Limiting Charge Compliance Program (CLCCP), when a physician bills a patient in excess of the limiting charge (by at least $1 or more), the physician is notified of the overcharges on a biweekly or case-by-case basis through a Limiting Charge Exception Report. Patients are informed of overcharges on the Explanation of Medicare Benefits (EOMB). When limiting charge violations occur, the physician must refund to the patient any payment that exceeds the charge limit. The carrier may request that physicians provide documentation verifying that they made appropriate refunds to the patient.

The Social Security Act Amendments of 1994 gave CMS statutory authority to enforce Medicare balance billing limits for nonparticipating physicians and suppliers. Effective January 1, 1995, if billed charges exceed the limiting charge, carriers are required to notify the physician or other provider of the violation within 30 days. The physician or other provider must refund or credit the excess charges to the patient within 30 days of carrier notification. Sanctions may be imposed against physicians and other providers for "knowingly and willfully" billing or collecting fees that exceed the limiting charge.

The law also requires carriers to provide limiting charge information on the EOMB form following submission of an unassigned claim with charges that exceed the limiting charge. The form must also indicate the beneficiary's right to a refund if an excess charge was collected. To monitor physicians' and other providers' compliance with the limiting charges, carriers are required to screen all unassigned claims.

The AMA has urged Congress to ensure that due process safeguards are applied in any enforcement process that is adopted. These safeguards should include the opportunity for physicians to protest a refund request in situations such as "downcoding" by the carrier that are beyond the physician's control. For further details on the participation program, refer to Chapter 9.

Copayments and Deductibles

Medicare beneficiaries are liable for a monthly Part B premium for 2002 of $54.00, an annual deductible of $100, and 20% coinsurance for most services. In most cases, the physician (or other health care provider) must collect the deductible and coinsurance from the patient or the patient's Medigap insurer.

The HHS inspector general considers it fraudulent practice to routinely waive patients' Medicare copayments and deductibles. Under the RBRVS, if the copayments and/or deductibles are routinely waived, the charge minus this portion of the payment is considered to be the physician's actual charge. Medicare continues to pay at the lower of the actual charge or the approved amount. A physician's office must be able to demonstrate that it made a good faith effort to collect from the patient. Letters and records of phone calls that the physician's office or a collection agency makes to the patient would provide appropriate documentation that a good faith effort was made to collect from the patient.

Discussing Fees With Patients

AMA policy supports disclosure by physicians, hospitals, and other health care providers of the fees charged to patients prior to providing services. Such disclosure enables patients to make informed and cost-conscious health care choices. Physicians may provide this information to patients or prospective patients on request or, in the absence of a request, by volunteering the information. Physicians may volunteer fee information in a variety of ways: by posting fees in the office waiting area, by providing information for inclusion in directories, or through discussions with patients and families.

Medical practices should establish a specific policy for discussing charges with patients to ensure that they consistently observe patient concerns. Physicians and office staff should be familiar with this policy, which should be sensitive to patients' financial and family considerations. For example, the physician should first ask patients if they would like to discuss the physician's charges before initiating such a discussion, because the patient may want a spouse or other family member to participate. Such consideration is especially important if a major surgical procedure is planned or when the physician anticipates that a service may not be a covered benefit. Prior to the discussion, the physician may want to obtain background information on the patient's insurance and have some knowledge about expected hospital expenses, if applicable.

When discussing charges, physicians also may want to explain their participation status and the concerns that influenced their decision. If possible, any discussion of payment policies with patients should take place in the business office or consultation room, rather than in the examining room.

Written information about charges and participation status may be very useful to Medicare patients. The information might be a simple list of charges for frequently provided services that could include the Medicare-approved amount, the physician's actual charge, and an explanation of the limiting charge, if applicable. Other information could include the physician's participation status and the patient's responsibility for copayments and deductibles. A summary of charges and payment policies can be printed as a brochure and made available in the physician's waiting room or posted on the wall. Patients can then take home the information to review and share with family members, and they can refer to it for later discussions with the physician. The best opportunity to review the brochure or list of charges and payment policies with new patients, however, is during the initial office visit.

Private Contracting

Physicians who wish to enter into private contracts with Medicare patients may do so without fearing that such contracts would not be considered legally binding. Provisions in the Balanced Budget Act of 1997, which became effective January 1, 1998, give physicians and their Medicare patients the freedom to privately contract to provide health care services outside the Medicare system. These private contracts have to meet specific requirements, which include that:

- Medicare does not pay for the services provided or contracted for;
- the contract is in writing and signed by the beneficiary before any item or service is provided;
- the contract is not entered into at a time when the beneficiary is facing an emergency or urgent health situation; and
- the physician signs and files an affidavit agreeing to forgo receiving any payment from Medicare (either directly, on a capitated basis, or from an organization that receives Medicare reimbursement directly or on a capitated basis) for items or services provided to any Medicare beneficiary for the following 2-year period.

In other words, the new right comes with a hefty price; physicians who privately contract with even one Medicare patient cannot participate or receive any payment from Medicare for 2 years.

In addition, the contract must state unambiguously that by signing the private contract, the beneficiary gives up all

Medicare payment for services furnished by the "opt out" physician; agrees not to bill Medicare or ask the physician to bill Medicare; is liable for all of the physician's charges, without any Medicare balance billing limits; acknowledges that Medigap or any other supplemental insurance will not pay toward the services; and acknowledges that he or she has the right to receive services from physicians for whom Medicare coverage and payment would be available. Nothing prohibits beneficiaries from seeing their physician for non–Medicare-covered services such as routine annual physical exams, cosmetic surgery, hearing aids, and eye exams.

To opt out, a physician must file an affidavit that meets the criteria specified above and which is received by the carrier at least 30 days before the first day of the next calendar quarter. The physician must renew the opt-out every two years to continue to privately contract. A physician who "knowingly and willingly" submits a claim or receives any payment from Medicare during the affidavit's two-year period will lose the rights provided under the private contract provision, and will not be eligible to receive Medicare payments for any service provided to any patient, for the remainder of the period.

Over the past few years, several bills were introduced in Congress attempting to change the private contracting rules. For example, in 1998, the Medicare Beneficiary Freedom to Contract Act, also known as the Kyl-Archer Bill was introduced. The Act would have repealed the requirement that physicians give up their Medicare reimbursement for two years if they enter into a private contract. The Act also would have made it explicit that a patient could enter into a private contract with their physicians on a case-by-case basis for any length of time, take steps to ensure that private contracting does not lead to fraud, and protected taxpayers from double payment for services rendered under private contracts. Further, in March 1999, the Medicare Preservation and Restoration Act was introduced in the U.S. House of Representatives. This Act sought to repeal the entire Medicare private contracting provision of the BBA and clarify that private contracts are prohibited under Medicare for Medicare-covered services. The supposed reasoning behind the Act was to retain Medicare's balance billing limits to guarantee beneficiaries reasonable and fair prices. Both bills have essentially died in committee.

The AMA has consistently advocated for the basic right of physicians to privately contract with their patients in appropriate circumstances. Requiring physicians to opt out of Medicare for 2 years as a condition for private contracting creates an onerous and unfair situation for both physicians and patients. The AMA is committed to pursuing appropriate legislative and legal means to permanently preserve that patient's basic right to privately contract with physicians for wanted or needed health care services, while also working to ensure that important beneficiary protections are maintained.

Using the RBRVS to Establish Physician Charges

The AMA believes that a strong fee-for-service sector is essential to patient choice and must be a central feature of the health care marketplace. To strengthen the viability of fee-for-service medicine in the current marketplace, the AMA developed a new approach to fee-for-service based on a national standard RBRVS. This approach, which is explained in Chapter 13, holds that RBRVS relative values could provide the basis for public and private physician fee and payment systems. Using RBRVS under this approach would apply only to the RBRVS relative values, not to Medicare's conversion factors, balance billing limits, geographic practice cost indexes (GPCIs), or other inappropriate Medicare payment policies.

Using a National Standard RBRVS

A national standard RBRVS for physicians and payers would rely on advance disclosure of physician and other provider fees, hospital and facility charges, and health plan payments. Under this principle, fee-for-service physicians and health plans could offer the cost predictability that is often cited as a hallmark of managed care plans. Patients could use this information to help choose a physician, use plan payment levels to help choose a plan with the best coverage, and, through such comparisons, estimate out-of-pocket costs.

A national standard RBRVS offers one method for physicians to establish their charges. Using the RBRVS, physicians can establish their fees based on a dollar conversion factor that they select.[1]

Table 5. Calculating a Conversion Factor Using the RBRVS: An Illustration

Service	RVUs/Service	Service Frequency	Frequency × RVUs	Fees	Frequency × Fees
A	9	10	90	$500	$ 5,000
B	2	15	30	$ 90	$ 1,350
C	12	10	120	$600	$ 6,000
D	1	50	50	$ 60	$ 3,000
Total			290		$15,350

Total RVUs = sum of RVUs for each service multiplied by frequency = 290.
Total fees = sum of fee per service multiplied by frequency = $15,350.
Conversion factor = total fees divided by total RVUs = $52.93.

Establishing the Conversion Factor

The methodology described below offers one alternative to physicians for establishing a conversion factor that maintains current practice revenue. Other methods could also be used. The initial calculation of a conversion factor provides the starting point for determining physician charges. Adjustments could then be made in accordance with other considerations, such as the local market for the physicians' services.

A conversion factor using RBRVS relative values can be calculated with information on the types of physician services provided, utilization, and current billed charges. In order for the conversion factor to accurately reflect the practice's charge levels, it is recommended that services representing 85% to 90% of the practice's volume be included in the calculations. As a result, determining a conversion factor for a multispecialty group practice will be more complex than for a single specialty.

A conversion factor is determined by dividing the total fees for all services provided (fee for each service multiplied by service frequency) by total RVUs (RVUs for each service multiplied by frequency). Total RVUs by CPT code can be found in Part 5, List of Relative Value Units. Table 5 illustrates how to set up the worksheet for calculating a conversion factor. Physicians may want to consider developing an electronic spreadsheet to complete the calculations.

Note

1. Establishing a conversion factor is the equivalent of setting fees for antitrust purposes, and the law requires that this be done independently by each physician or physician group.

Chapter 13
Non-Medicare Use of the RBRVS: New Survey Data

Since the adoption of Medicare's resource-based relative value scale (RBRVS) in 1992, the American Medical Association (AMA) has conducted national surveys of public and private payers to assess the effects of this payment method in non-Medicare health markets. The basis for these surveys is a persistent concern on the part of the AMA that policies implemented by the government could have consequences for non-Medicare payers. The AMA is committed to an RBRVS that will be an accurate, comprehensive standard uniformly covering all medical services nationwide. For this reason it is important to understand the extent to which the RBRVS has been adopted outside of Medicare, the different payment policies used by payers, and the use of Medicare payment policies. While many payers may claim to use the RBRVS, adjustments to payment policies, large numbers of conversion factors, and other adjustments may result in a payment system that differs from Medicare's RBRVS system.

This chapter analyzes recent data collected in fall of 2001 from 226 different public and private payers. The survey showed that 74% of respondents use the RBRVS in at least one product line. This compares with a 63% adoption rate from the 1998 survey, a 32% adoption rate from a 1993 Deloitte & Touche survey, and a 28% adoption rate from a Physician Payment Review Commission (PPRC) study for its 1995 Annual Report to Congress. This suggests that non-Medicare use of the RBRVS continues to increase and is in wide use by a variety of payers.

Survey Design

The survey instrument was structured to capture data from a variety of different payers in both public and private sectors. In addition to collecting data on the use of the RBRVS, the survey also asked questions regarding conversion factors, payment policies used with the RBRVS, product lines where the RBRVS is used, and the respondents' opinion of the RBRVS. In order to facilitate longitudinal analysis, the instrument contained some of the same questions as previous AMA surveys and the 1993 Deloitte & Touche survey.

The survey sample contained Medicaid agencies, state workers' compensation plans, Blue Cross/Blue Shield affiliated plans, health insurance companies, and a variety of managed care organizations. A letter was sent to the Medical Directors of payers in the summer of 2001 and a follow-up letter was sent in September to those plans that had not responded. The overall response rate was 20%.

Characteristics of Respondents

Respondents self-designated their primary payer type, resulting in the following self-description:

- 8%   Blue Cross/Blue Shield
- 32%   Health maintenance organization/point of service
- 12%   Preferred provider organization
- 20%   Medicaid
- 7%   Workers' compensation
- 21%   Other, which includes traditional fee-for-service, IPAs, physician hospital organizations, and TRICARE

In addition to the type of payer the respondents consider themselves, respondents can be described by the number of physicians they have under contract, and the number of beneficiaries. Responses to these two questions can be divided into ranges.

Number of physicians under contract:

- Less than or equal to 5000   63%
- 5001 to 10,000   13%
- 10,001 to 20,000   14%
- Greater than 20,000   10%

Number of beneficiaries:

- Less than or equal to 100,000   46%
- 100,001 to 500,000   32%
- 500,001 to 1,000,000   12%
- Greater than 1,000,000   10%

As Figure 4 illustrates, the data can be divided into four payer types. Blue Cross/Blue Shield plans accounted for 8% of the respondents, Medicaid accounted for 20%, managed care organizations (MCOs), which include HMOs, POS plans, and PPOs, accounted for 44%, and other non-Medicare accounted for 28%. The four types of payers will be analyzed after the responses of all respondents are examined. For purposes of this analysis, BC/BS plans were considered as a separate payer category although most of the BC/BS plans characterized themselves as primarily a PPO. The BC/BS plans tended to offer a greater number of plan types than the other managed care organizations (5 vs 3). Most of the BCBS plans offered HMO, PPO, POS and traditional fee-for-service plans. Also, the BCBS plans were larger in terms of number of enrollees and number of providers under contract (1.5 million vs .5 million). For these reasons, and also to allow for comparisons with prior year's data, we continued to include a separate payer category for BC/BS plans. Those payers that identified themselves primarily as either a PPO, HMO, or POS plan are included in one managed care organization category. The group of other non-Medicare payers includes TRICARE, workers' compensation, and other fee-for-service providers.

Figure 4. Payers

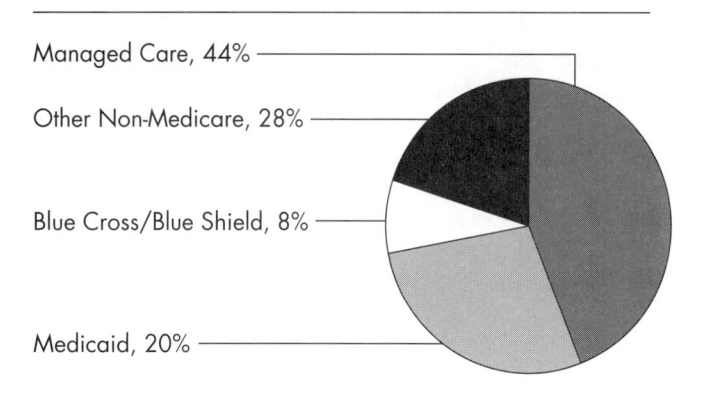

- Managed Care, 44%
- Other Non-Medicare, 28%
- Blue Cross/Blue Shield, 8%
- Medicaid, 20%

Adoption Rate, All Payers

As previously mentioned, 74% of the respondents currently use the RBRVS. Of this group using the RBRVS, 83% have adopted and fully implemented it, and 17% have decided to adopt the system and are in the process of implementation. Additionally, 7% of the survey respondents are examining the potential use of the Medicare RBRVS. This indicates that 81% of respondents are either using the RBRVS or considering its use. Alternatively, only 9% have considered, but decided not to adopt, and 10% have not considered it at all. Also of those using the RBRVS, 95% use all three components (work, practice expense, and professional liability insurance) while only 5% use either the work RVUs only or a combination of the work and PE RVUs.

Use of RBRVS by All Payers

Those respondents who indicated that they use the RBRVS were asked to identify the product lines where they have implemented the RBRVS. Historically, the RBRVS has been used primarily by traditional fee-for-service insurers, but the data show that use of RBRVS is now widespread by various types of payers. Part of this can be due to the continued dominance of fee-for-service payment mechanisms, even by managed care companies. Since respondents can use the RBRVS in more than one product line, the percentages will sum to more than 100%.

Respondents who use the RBRVS in:

- Fee-for-service   44%
- HMO   55%
- PPO   54%
- POS   47%

The data show that managed care organizations continue to use the RBRVS to a greater extent than traditional fee-for-service payers. This indicates that the RBRVS is applicable not only to fee-for-service insurers, but to a wide range of product lines. As long as a managed care plan continues to base some payments on a fee-for-service basis, it can effectively utilize the RBRVS to determine payments within a managed care framework.

We also found that for those payers that use the RBRVS in at least one product line, the RBRVS is used extensively. Seventy-nine percent of the respondents indicated that they use the RBRVS for at least 75% of the physicians that the payer has made payments to or has under contract. In fact, for 53% of the respondents who use the RBRVS, all of the physicians under contract are reimbursed with an RBRVS methodology.

Percentage of physicians under contract who are subject to the RBRVS:

Percentage of Physicians Subject to RBRVS	Percentage of Payers
■ All physicians under contract	53%
■ 75%-99% of physicians	26%
■ 50%-74% of physicians	7%
■ 1%-49% of physicians	14%

While the RBRVS establishes the relativity among procedures, it is the conversion factor that also determines the final payment amount. The AMA has been concerned that private payers would use the conversion factors and associated payment policies only to contain costs. Such an inappropriate use of the RBRVS could have negative consequences for patient access; however, the current survey shows that with the exception of Medicaid, the conversion factor amounts were generally in excess of Medicare.

- Sixty percent of survey respondents had more than one conversion factor. The distribution of the number of conversion factors is as follows:

  - Single conversion factor   41%
  - Two conversion factors   26%
  - Three or four conversion factors   16%
  - Greater than four conversion factors 17%

While Medicare switched to a single conversion factor in 1998, the survey data indicate that a majority of the respondents continue to use multiple conversion factors. Most frequently the conversion factors were arranged by surgical, nonsurgical, or primary care. Some payers also adjust the conversion factor by plan type, such as PPO and HMO, and for rural or urban practice setting.

- For all payers, the average conversion factor was $41.70, with a minimum of $10.75 and a maximum of $78.49. At the time of the survey, Medicare had a single conversion factor of $38.26.

To obtain a better understanding of how the payers varied conversion factors among specialties we asked those respondents who had multiple conversion factors to provide the conversion factors for a number of specialties. As seen in Figure 5, payers that differentiated among specialties applied the highest conversion factor to surgery and the lowest to primary care. For those payers that did not differentiate among specialties, the average conversion factor was $38.22.

Figure 5. Average Conversion Factor by Specialty

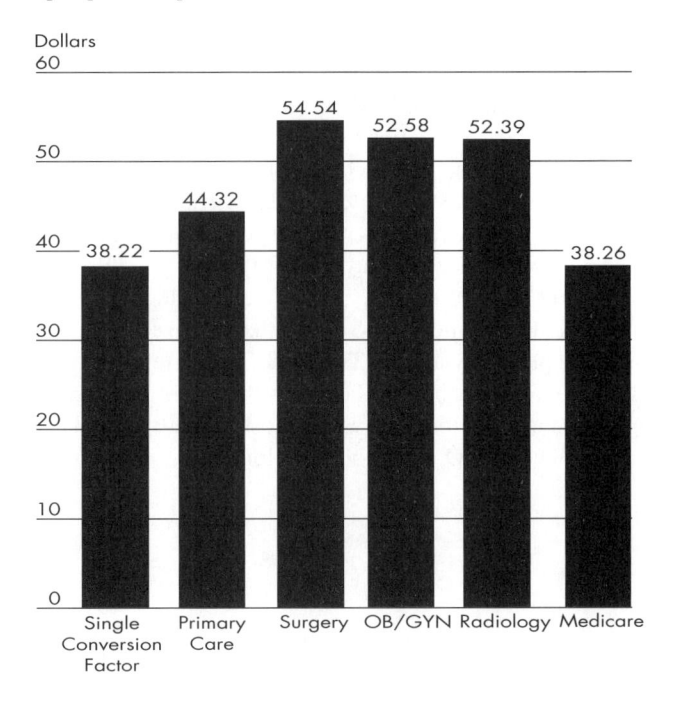

Specialty	Dollars
Single Conversion Factor	38.22
Primary Care	44.32
Surgery	54.54
OB/GYN	52.58
Radiology	52.39
Medicare	38.26

Figure 6. Average Anesthesia Conversion Factor

Anesthesia	Medicare
35.66	17.83

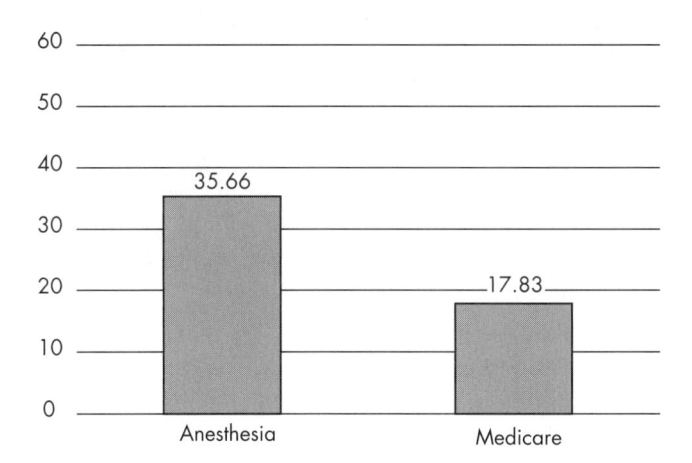

Figure 6 shows the conversion factor for anesthesia services compared to the Medicare conversion factor. Since anesthesia services are reimbursed according to a different relative value scale and methodology than other physician services, the anesthesia conversion factor is listed in a separate figure. See page 453 for a description of anesthesiology payments.

- For payers that used a single conversion factor for all physicians who receive reimbursement under the RBRVS the average conversion factor was $38.22 with a minimum of $10.75 and a maximum of $60.
- For primary care services the average conversion factor was $44.32 with a minimum of $16.37 and a maximum of $61.21.
- For surgical services the average conversion factor was $54.54 with a minimum of $22.41 and a maximum of $91.53.
- For obstetrical/gynecological services, the average conversion factor was $52.58 with a minimum of $30.23 and a maximum of $87.80.
- For radiology services the average conversion factor was $52.39 with a minimum of $11.61 and a maximum of $95.65
- For anesthesia services, the average conversion factor was $35.66 with a minimum of $8.20 and a maximum of $58.00. In 2001, the Medicare anethesia conversion factor was $17.83.

We also asked respondents the extent to which they have adopted a variety of Medicare payment policies. The acceptance of these policies is an important aspect of correctly implementing the RBRVS system. Below are the acceptance rates for respondents for 1998 and the current survey. The acceptance rates appear to be consistently high for the global surgical periods and the multiple survey reduction. The Medicare site of service differential increased in acceptance since 1998 most likely due to payers gaining a better understanding of this policy since it has been in use for several years. The site of service differential relates to differences in practice expenses between services provided in a facility such as a hospital and a non-facility such as a physician's office. CMS has structured the practice expense methodology to recognize more physician costs when services are provided in the office as compared to when services are performed in the hospital. The reasoning behind this policy is that physicians incur more expenses such as staff and supplies when they are performing services in their office as opposed to performing services in the hospital where staff and supply expenses are incurred by the hospital. The hospital then receives separate payment through Medicare Part A.

Respondents who use the RBRVS use:

	2001	1998
■ Global surgical periods	73%	74%
■ Multiple surgery reduction	85%	84%
■ Medicare site of service differentials	55%	26%
■ Geographic practice cost indexes (GPC's)	51%	45%

We also asked respondents who use the RBRVS which of the following six modifiers they accept. Thirty-five percent of the respondents indicated they accepted all six of the modifiers.

	2001	1998
■ 22—Unusual procedural services	68%	81%
■ 25—Significant, separately identifiable E/M service by the same physician on the same day of the procedure	79%	75%
■ 26—Professional component	95%	92%
■ 51—Multiple procedures	90%	89%
■ 57—Decision for surgery	48%	64%
■ 59—Distinct procedural service	50%	63%

While both groups indicate their acceptance of modifiers, the use of claims-editing software may affect the acceptance of modifiers. Seventy-seven percent of the respondents indicated that they use a commercial or internally developed claims-editing package, or a combination of commercial and internally developed systems. Therefore, if a particular claims-editing package does not recognize certain modifiers, then most likely, payers use of the software will result in certain modifiers automatically recognized or rejected. Only 23% of respondents do not use such software to process claims.

The responses to the policy questions indicate that payers continue to be likely to implement Medicare payment policies. Payers' acceptance of these policies is critical to properly implement the RBRVS system. It is not sufficient to use only the Medicare established RVUs and then not recognize modifiers or use a large number of conversion factors, or not update those conversion factors. Such a system would resemble Medicare's RBRVS in name only, since the actual implementation of the system would be quite different.

One important facet of the RBRVS methodology that non-Medicare payers should implement is the use of current CPT codes and relative values. Each year, new services are assigned relative values and existing codes receive revised relative values. Therefore, it is important that payers continually update their fee schedule so physicians and other health care providers are reimbursed according to the most recent relative values and payment policies. Eighty-nine percent of respondents indicated that they update their conversion factor at least annually. While users of RBRVS seem to accept many of the Medicare payment policies, a majority of respondents (59%) continue to use multiple conversion factors that differentiate among specialties and health plans.

One Medicare policy that may have significant implications for non-Medicare payers is the Medicare conversion factor. Although we did not specifically ask respondents if they link their conversion factor to the Medicare conversion factor, 44% of respondents who provided conversion factor data indicated that their conversion factor is based on a percentage of the Medicare conversion factor. This may be another important area where Medicare policies affect private payers and is especially relevant this year where the Medicare conversion factor will decline by 5.4%. Although we cannot determine what effect the Medicare conversion factor decrease will have on private payers determination of conversion factors, there is a potential that private payers that link their conversion factor to the Medicare conversion factor may also decrease their conversion factor by the same percentage. Therefore, a decrease in the Medicare conversion factor may have even greater repercussions than originally anticipated.

While we were primarily interested in learning the extent to which payers who use the RBRVS recognize modifiers, we also wanted to compare their responses with those of payers who do not use the RBRVS. It is important to remember that payers' acceptance of modifiers is not reliant on payers' use of the RBRVS, since the CPT modifiers can be used in a variety of payment systems. We found that, generally, payers who do not use the RBRVS are less likely to recognize the six modifiers we surveyed. Twenty-four percent of the respondents who do not use the RBRVS indicated that they recognize all six modifiers compared to 35% for those payers that use the RBRVS.

However, even for those respondents who do not use the RBRVS, we found a high rate of acceptance for some modifiers.

	2001	1998
■ 22—Unusual procedural services	68%	68%
■ 25—Significant, separately identifiable E/M service by the same physician on the same day of the procedure	68%	62%
■ 26—Professional component	90%	80%
■ 51—Multiple procedures	83%	80%
■ 57—Decision for surgery	35%	52%
■ 59—Distinct procedural service	53%	54%

Adoption of the RBRVS Among the Four Payer Types

We divided the payer types into four categories: managed care organizations, Medicaid, Blue Cross/Blue Shield (BC/BS), and other non-Medicare plans. Use of the RBRVS, conversion factors applied to the RBRVS, and payment policies associated with the RBRVS vary among these four different payer types.

As illustrated by Figure 7, the adoption rate for the RBRVS varies among the four types of payers, with a majority of all payer types. A significant number of the BC/BS plans and MCOs use the RBRVS. Additionally, 64% of Medicaid and 76% of other non-Medicare plans use the system.

The current adoption rates of RBRVS are higher than those in the 1998 survey, with the exception of the BC/BS plans. The 1998 survey respondents indicated that 63% of all respondents adopted the RBRVS compared to 74% for 2001. The individual payer groups compared to the 2001 data are as follows:

	2001	1998
BC/BS	78%	87%
MCO	86%	69%
Medicaid	64%	55%
Other	76%	44%

Figure 7. Percentage That Use the RBRVS

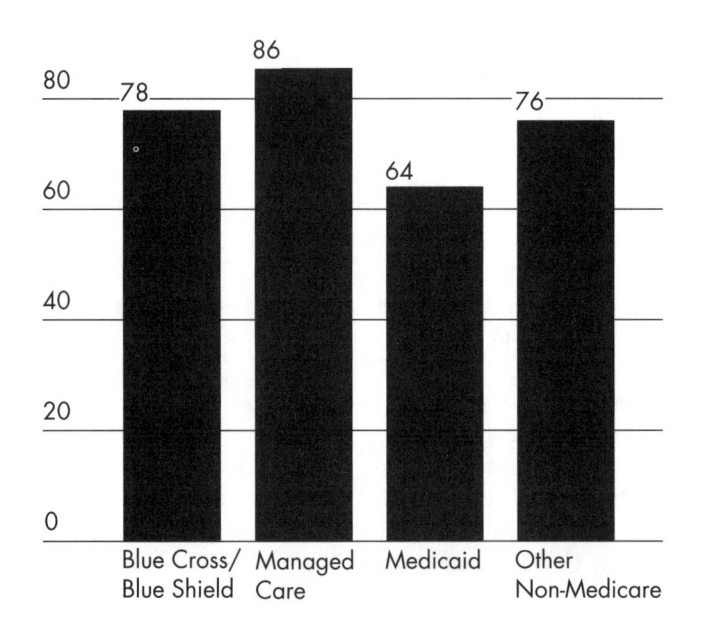

- Of the BC/BS plans using the RBRVS, 93% have adopted and fully implemented the RBRVS. Additionally, 7% are undergoing implementation.

- Of the MCOs using the RBRVS, 84% have adopted and fully implemented the RBRVS. Additionally, 16% of MCO respondents are undergoing implementation.

- Of the Medicaid plans using the RBRVS, 75% have adopted and fully implemented the RBRVS. Additionally, 25% of Medicaid respondents are undergoing implementation.

- Of the other non-Medicare plans using the RBRVS, 85% have adopted and fully implemented the RBRVS. Additionally, 15% of non-Medicare respondents are in the process of implementing the RBRVS.

These data demonstrate that most of the respondents that use the RBRVS have fully implemented the payment system.

Use of the RBRVS Among the Four Payer Types

The four payer types use the RBRVS in different ways which are related to the types of plans they offer. For example, since Medicaid agencies are public payers, it would be expected that their use of the RBRVS would involve mainly fee-for-service medicine, lower conversion factors, and, possibly, greater use of Medicare payment policies. Conversely, MCO payers would use the RBRVS mostly in PPOs and HMOs that do not use capitation exclusively, and might use unique payment policies to implement the RBRVS.

Product Line Application of RBRVS

Figure 8 illustrates the variation in product line application of the RBRVS. The four payer categories demonstrate that use of the RBRVS is widespread among the four types of product lines. The survey of BC/BS plans found that a large percentage of respondents used the RBRVS heavily in both fee-for-service medicine and managed care services. In fact, 69% of BC/BS plans' PPO products used the RBRVS as compared to fee-for-service at 64%. The other largely private sector group, the managed care group, had the highest usage rates among all four types of products. Eighty-two percent of the MCO PPO plans used the RBRVS as well as 74% of their fee-for-service plans. The Medicaid plans used the RBRVS as expected, primarily for fee-for-service (57%) and for the HMO product line (8%). As expected, this group did not use the RBRVS at all for other types of plans. The stated lack of RBRVS use in managed care by Medicaid is due to the contracting out of Medicaid managed care activities so Medicaid officials may not be aware of RBRVS usage in Medicaid Managed care products.

Conversion Factors Used

Since the conversion factor determines the dollar value of a service, this perhaps more than any other component impacts physicians and patients. Figure 9 shows the average conversion factors for each payer category for 2001. Medicare's conversion factor for 2001 is shown as a basis for comparison. BC/BS and MCO respondents had conversion factors that exceeded Medicare's, at $45.76 and $43.96. As expected,

Figure 8. Variations in Product Lines

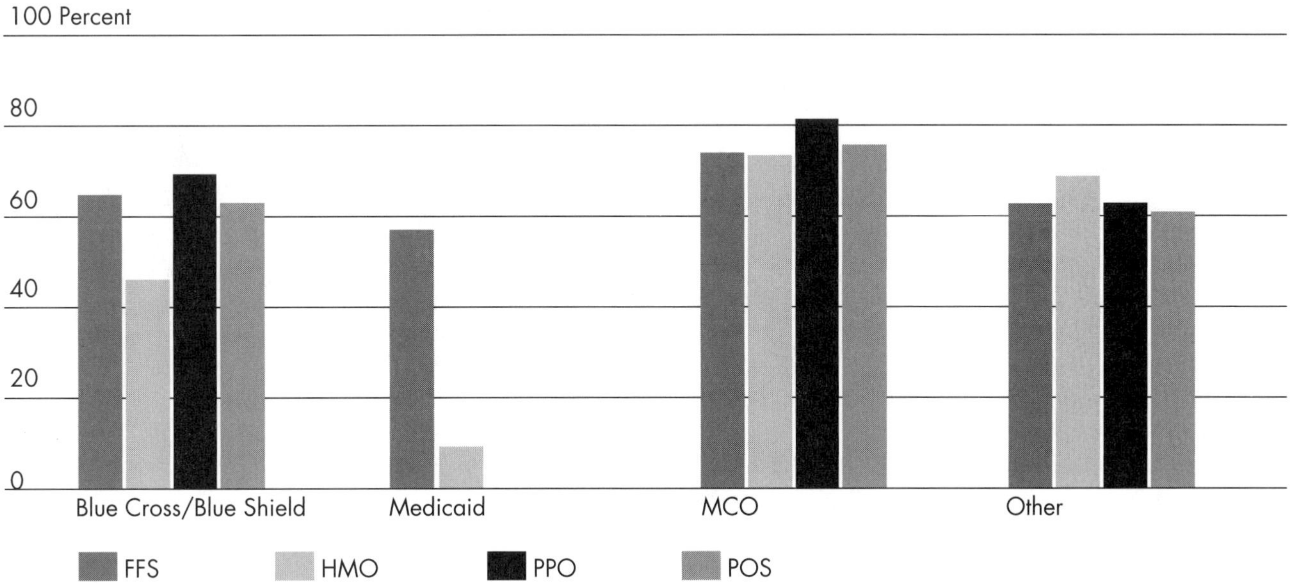

Medicaid had the lowest conversion factor at $28.23. The number of conversion factors and the division of payment among specialties or plans is another important aspect of the application of conversion factors.

Figure 9. Average Conversion Factor, 2001

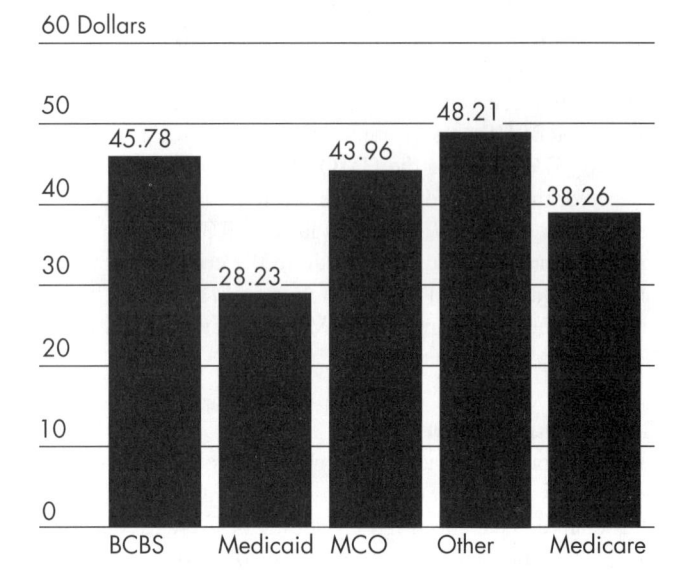

60 Dollars

- BCBS: 45.78
- Medicaid: 28.23
- MCO: 43.96
- Other: 48.21
- Medicare: 38.26

The distribution of the number of conversion factors differed among payer groups is shown below. Fifty-nine percent of the respondents had multiple conversion factors. The most common division of conversion factors was between surgical and non-surgical or primary care. Several respondents had different conversion factors for different product lines or for care inside and outside of plans. For all payer types except Medicaid that differentiated among specialties, the conversion factors for surgery exceeded the conversion factors for the other specialties. The Medicaid agencies on the other hand, established their highest conversion factor for OB/GYN services.

Number of Conversion Factors By Payer Type

	Single CF	2 or 3 CFs	4 or Greater CFs
BCBS	50%	17%	33%
MCO	40%	23%	37%
Medicaid	45%	32%	23%
Other	37%	29%	34%

Payment Policies

As shown in Figure 10, all the payer categories showed a high propensity to adopt Medicare payment policies. The most common policy adopted was the multiple surgery reduction with BC/BS and Medicaid respondents at 92%,

Figure 10. Medicare Adoption Policies

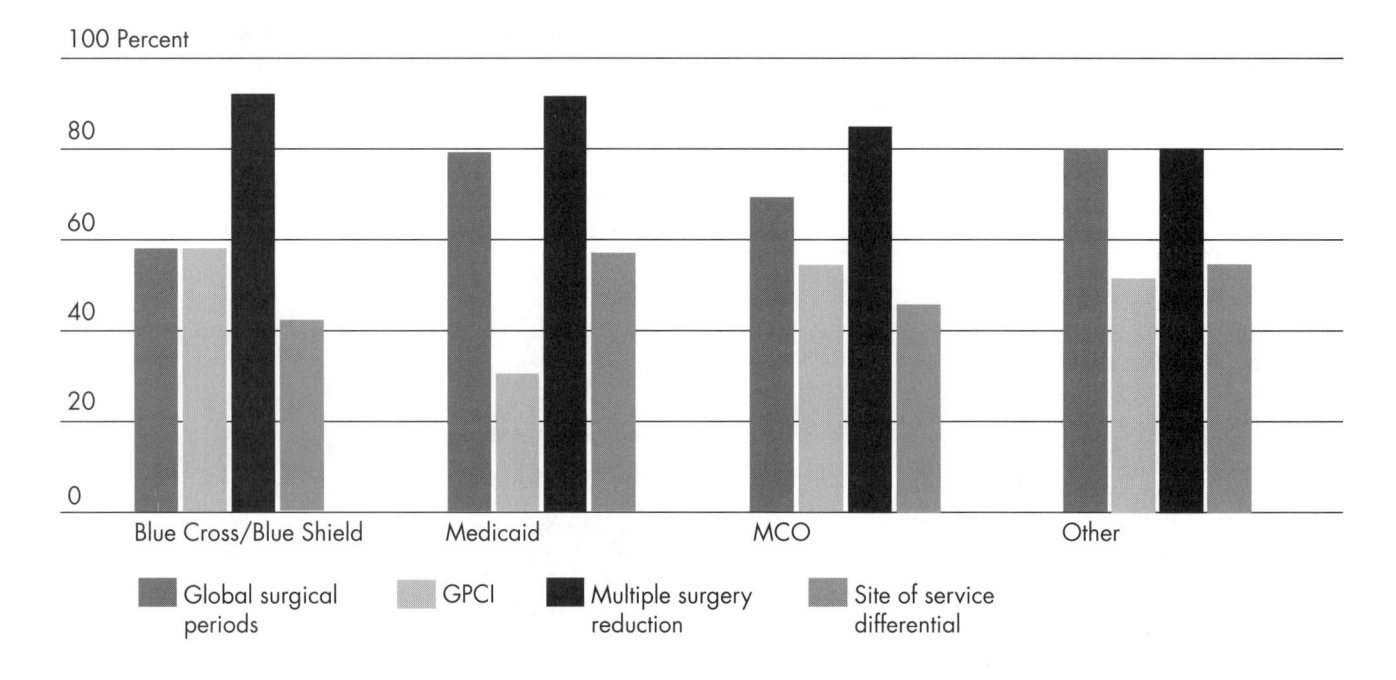

100 Percent

Categories (by group): Blue Cross/Blue Shield, Medicaid, MCO, Other

Legend: Global surgical periods, GPCI, Multiple surgery reduction, Site of service differential

MCOs at 85%, and other non-Medicare at 80%. The adoption of global surgical periods was also widespread but showed a decrease over the 1998 survey: BC/BS respondents at 58% compared to 80% in 1998 and Medicaid at 78% compared to 87% in 1998. MCOs stayed the same at 69%, and other non-Medicare at 80% compared to 26%, utilized global surgical periods.

Opinion of the RBRVS

In addition to questions on use of the RBRVS, product lines, conversion factors, and payment policies, we attempted to obtain payers' opinion of the RBRVS by asking a series of questions related to possible benefits and drawbacks of the RBRVS system. These questions were asked of all respondents, both those that use the RBRVS and those that do not. Respondents could select from five categories: strongly agree, agree, no opinion, disagree, or strongly disagree. The questions were divided into positive and negative issues that could be associated with the RBRVS.

Percent of respondents who agree or strongly agree that the RBRVS successfully addresses the following issues:

	2001	1998
■ Controls health care costs	39%	37%
■ Allows for payment based on actual resources utilized	68%	67%
■ Makes system compatible with Medicare	66%	68%
■ Makes physician payment more equitable across specialties	65%	70%
■ Rationalizes physician payment	71%	74%
■ Increase control over physician payment	54%	53%
■ Make it easy to implement and update each year	70%	69%

From this table it is apparent that at least 54% of the respondents agreed or strongly agreed that the RBRVS successfully addressed all of the aforementioned issues (except the RBRVS' ability to control costs). However, it is important to note that this data includes respondents who do not incorporate RBRVS into their payment policies. When the same responses are divided into RBRVS and non-RBRVS users, the results are quite different.

Percent of RBRVS and non-RBRVS users who agree or strongly agree that the RBRVS successfully addresses the following issues:

	RBRVS Users	Non-RBRVS Users
■ Controls health care costs	46%	21%
■ Allows for payment based on actual resources utilized	74%	46%
■ Makes system compatible with Medicare	74%	46%
■ Makes physician payment more equitable across specialties	71%	44%
■ Rationalizes physician payment	80%	38%
■ Increase control over physician payment	61%	31%
■ Makes it easy to implement and update each year	76%	50%

This table demonstrates there is a clear difference in opinion of the perceived benefits of the RBRVS system among these two groups. For example, 80% of the RBRVS users agree or strongly agree that RBRVS successfully rationalizes physician payment while only 38% of non-RBRVS users concur. According to this table, at least 61% of RBRVS users agreed that the RBRVS system successfully addressed all of the aforementioned issues (except the RBRVS' ability to control costs). The ease of implementing and updating, the ability to rationalize payment and allowing for payment to be based on actual resources used are the major perceived benefits among the RBRVS users. However, the ability to make payments more equitable across specialties and the compatibility with Medicare also ranked above 70%. The potential drawbacks of the RBRVS system were also assessed in the survey.

Percent of respondents who agree or strongly agree that the following are potential drawbacks to the RBRVS system:

	2001	1998
■ Problems with methodology	30%	26%
■ Potential to disrupt beneficiary access to physician services	17%	32%
■ Potential to disrupt physician relations	30%	12%
■ Current system better	10%	6%
■ RBRVS is too complicated	13%	10%

This table demonstrates that no more than 30% of the respondents agreed or strongly agreed with any of the potential drawbacks. The greatest drawbacks appear to be the potential to disrupt physician relations and problems associated with the methodology, both at 30%. However, only 10% of respondents agreed or strongly agreed that the current system of physician payment used by the payer is better. When comparing the responses of the users and non-users of RBRVS to these questions it was discovered that basically both groups recognized these drawbacks equally with the exception of the questions asking if the current system is better and whether the RBRVS is too complicated. However, these two potential drawbacks of the RBRVS system were expected to be greater within the non-RBRVS users responses.

Factors That Influence Adoption of RBRVS

The AMA survey asked a question regarding the factors that influence an organization's adoption of the RBRVS. This was an attempt to examine the elements that contributed to adoption or nonadoption. In essence, it is another measure of the payer's perception of the RBRVS, this time in terms of application of the RBRVS to their individual needs.

Percentage of respondents who selected the following as an influence over their adoption of the RBRVS:

	2001	1998
■ Impact and effectiveness of RBRVS under Medicare	51%	48%
■ Competitors have adopted RBRVS	44%	45%
■ Assurances that Medicare adjustments to the RBRVS will not negatively affect its accuracy/consistency	23%	37%
■ Physicians demand payment under RBRVS	35%	29%
■ Physician participation in setting values for work and practice expense	35%	28%

The factors that influence adoption can be divided into those that are internal forces to the system and those that are driven by external forces. The purpose of this division is to distinguish those that organized medicine, payers, and the government may be able to control and those that are determined by market forces. From these responses it is evident that payers are primarily concerned over the same issues of concern to the AMA. Both seek to maintain the soundness and effectiveness of the RBRVS system. This is a factor that is internal to the system but can be affected by the care and maintenance provided by the medical community and CMS. Other factors internal to the system are: physician participation in setting values for work and practice expense, and that all three components of the RBRVS are resource based. Several of these factors, such as physician participation and making all three components resource based, have already been achieved. It is interesting to note that physician participation in setting the values has increased in importance, while the assurances that Medicare adjustments will not negatively effect the accuracy of the RBRVS has declined as an influence. This could be a recognition of a greater understanding of the important role that physicians play in maintaining the RBRVS, in spite of inappropriate payment policies instituted by CMS that sometimes may affect the accuracy of the RBRVS.

Several factors listed by the respondents are outside of the RBRVS system and subject to the control of other forces such as the market. These external influences over adoption include competitors' adoption of RBRVS, physicians demand payment under the RBRVS, and the impact and effectiveness of RBRVS under Medicare. Some of these external factors, especially adoption of RBRVS by competitors, are highly ranked influences.

None of the respondents rated the factors influencing adoption very high; all but one are below 50%, and most are lower than the 1998 survey responses. This suggests that there are other factors that impact a payer's decision. Some of these may be specific to the health care market the payer serves, part of the organizational structure of the payer, or contingent on political decisions of state legislatures.

Other Uses of the RBRVS

In addition to using the RBRVS for its primary purpose as a payment mechanism for specific procedures, payers have begun to use the RBRVS for other purposes. We asked questions relating to physician practice management activities that involve utilizing the RBRVS. We found that 71% of those respondents who use the RBRVS also use the RBRVS for at least one practice management activity. As shown in Figure 11, almost all payers use the RBRVS in contract negotiations, 33% use it for developing capitation rates, 26% for individual or group physician profiles, and 15% for physician productivity benchmarks.

These results demonstrate once again the adaptability of the RBRVS to meet various needs of payers. While this survey asked payers their use of the RBRVS in these activities, individual physicians can also use the RBRVS for various practice management activities. In fact, they may find themselves at a disadvantage relative to payers if they do not. The use of individual physician and group profiles can provide a wealth of information to physicians if used in a constructive manner; however, they could also possibly be used by payers for economic credentialing. Also, if physicians are receiving data from several payers, the data may be skewed and not provide a complete picture of a physician's practice. Therefore, it often becomes necessary for physicians to compile the necessary data to so they can examine their own performance as well as their group's performance.

One common use for RVUs is to calculate the costs per RVU and make a comparison to the reimbursement. This

Figure 11. Practice Management Activities

- Individual/group physician profile: 26
- Physician productivity benchmarks: 15
- Contract negotiations: 79
- Capitation rates: 33

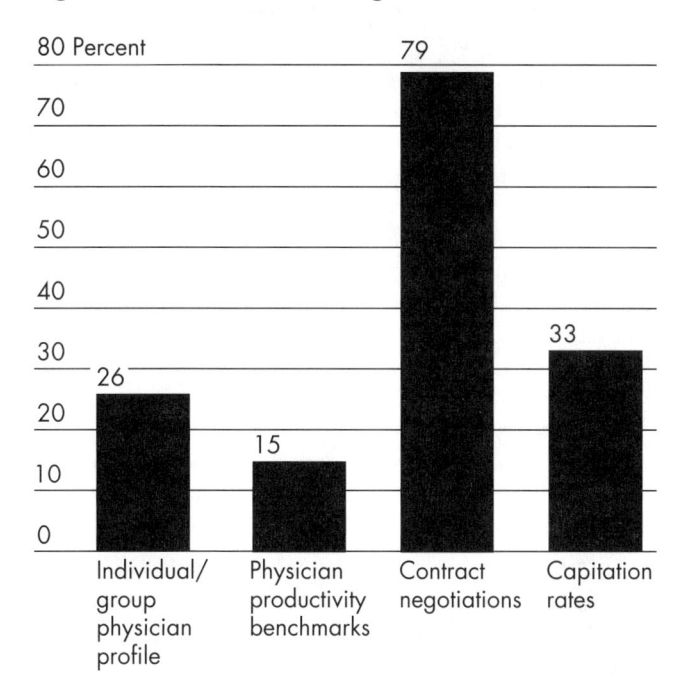

analysis can allow a physician to determine which procedures may be under reimbursed by payers. Also, RVU analysis is one method for comparing productivity among physicians in a group. For example, a group of physicians wanting to examine their collective as well as their individual physician performance would need to collect RVU data for a period of time. First, the group would compile the total work RVUs associated with individual physicians by multiplying the frequency associated with each CPT code billed during a period of time by the work RVU for each code. This would allow the physicians to examine the total work RVUs associated for each physician and for the group as a whole. Physicians could use these data as one method for beginning to assess physician performance, identify variations and causes for the variations, and possibly make adjustments to the group's remuneration policies.

Conclusion

The two recent AMA surveys and comparisons with other past surveys, such as the 1993 Deloitte & Touche and 1994 PPRC studies, reveal a continuing increase in non-Medicare use of the RBRVS. The current study also shows that all non-Medicare users of the RBRVS had a high rate of adoption of Medicare payment policies, indicating a high probability of incorporating new policies. Also shown was a willingness on the part of users to adapt the RBRVS to their own needs such as using the RBRVS in various practice management related activities. These results confirm the necessity of maintaining the RBRVS as an accurate, comprehensive standard, uniformly containing all medical services nationwide.

The RBRVS is not simply Medicare's method of physician payment. This study shows that payers are using the RBRVS in multiple product lines, including increasingly in managed care. Although the RBRVS is maintained by and for Medicare, it has evolved into a payment and data collection mechanism that is well beyond the Medicare program and fee-for-service medicine.

Part of the reason for such extensive and diverse utilization is the perception that the RBRVS is rational and equitable. This is not to say that problems do not exist or that RBRVS is viewed favorably by all parties. It is clear that those that have adopted the RBRVS have a more favorable view of the RBRVS as compared to those that have not adopted the RBRVS. The critical task is to continue cooperative efforts at maintaining the relativity and accuracy of the RBRVS system, while simultaneously expanding the breadth of health care services covered.

AMA Position on Medicare Physician Payments and Fee-for-Service

The AMA supports fee for service as one payment option for the Medicare program and a means to enhance patient choice in the health care marketplace. Although the AMA has been a leader in initiating improvements to the RBRVS, AMA policy does not endorse a specific payment mechanism, but instead, states that use of RBRVS relative values is one option that could provide the basis for both public and private physician payment systems. RBRVS relative values could provide the basis for both public and private physician payment systems independent of Medicare's conversion factor and payment policies such as balance billing limits. Using an updated and rigorously validated RBRVS, both physicians and payers could establish their fees and payments using their own, widely publicized conversion factors. Physicians could base their fees on a national standard RBRVS. They would set their fees based on a physician conversion factor they had adopted. Practice overhead costs and the market value of their services would help determine this conversion factor.

- Physicians using this method would inform patients of their dollar conversion factor before providing a service.
- Physicians who have contracts with specific health plans could negotiate for alternate conversion factors with these plans.

As a result, physicians would benefit from payment components developed with the assistance of CPT and the RUC. Finally, physicians would obtain simplified and easily understood means of disclosing fees to patients and protect their ability to establish their own fees.

Beneficiaries would receive information on conversion factors and patients, and they would benefit from cost-containing competition among physicians. They also would obtain predictability and comparability of physician charges and out-of-pocket costs. Finally, they would have a basis on which to compare coverage among third-party payers.

Payers could also make their fee-for-service payments to physicians using payment schedules based on a national standard RBRVS.

- This approach could apply to traditional insurance, benefit payment schedules, and managed care programs (eg, PPOs and IPAs) that make fee-for-service payments.
- No physician would be forced to accept a payment schedule amount as payment in full without a contract to do so.

Payers would thus avoid costly provider-specific fee profiles and payment schedules, obtain the means to standardize payment policies, benefit by eliminating automatic links between their outlays and physician charges, be protected against cost shifting, be better able to predict expenditures on physician services, and enhance their ability to negotiate payment schedules with physicians. The AMA supports the position that the RBRVS should not be implemented by private payers as a cost-containment device. Medicare could also benefit from such an approach that would allow physicians to set their own conversion factors. Under this more flexible approach, Medicare could set regional conversion factors at a level that would guarantee a certain level of access. If CMS sets the conversion factor at a reasonable level, a substantial number of physicians would choose to accept that conversion factor thus guaranteeing a predetermined level of access to care. However, other physicians would be free to establish their own conversion factor. Patients would then be able to choose among those physicians that accept the standard conversion factor or those that have established their own conversion factor.

Bibliography

Physician Payment Review Commission. *Annual Report to Congress,* Physician Payment Review Commission; 1995: 399-408.

Prince TR. *Strategic Management for Health Care Entities: Creative Frameworks for Financial and Operational Analysis.* Chicago, IL: American Hospital Publishing Inc; 1998: 434-437.

Swem RT. How and why private payers are using the RBRVS: 1993 Deloitte & Touche survey of physician payment methods. Presented at the Non-Medicare Adoption of the RBRVS Plenary Session III, May 5, 1994.

Part 5
Reference Lists

List of Relative Value Units, Payment Schedule, and Payment Policy Indicators

This list presents:

- the relative value units (RVUs) for the three components of each physician's service covered by the Medicare program;
- the unadjusted payment Medicare amount for each service (including the 80% that Medicare pays and the 20% patient coinsurance);
- the global period covered by the payment;
- applicable payment policy indicators for assistant surgeon, cosurgeon, and team surgeon; multiple and bilateral surgery;

The RVUs are listed according to either their numeric five-digit code in the AMA's CPT *(Physicians' Current Procedural Terminology, Fourth Edition)* coding system for physicians' services or their alphanumeric five-digit Health Care Common Procedural Coding System (HCPCS) code. The CPT comprises level 1 of the HCPCS that Medicare uses. Alphanumeric HCPCS codes comprise level 2 of HCPCS and appear toward the end of the list.

In this list, each CPT code is also identified by a heading, eg, Surgery: Musculoskeletal System; Pathology and Laboratory: Hematology and Coagulation, and by a brief description, eg, Revision of Knee Joint, Removal of Lung. These descriptions are included to help physicians identify the services they provide, but they do not contain sufficient information to code a service. For example, five codes (27441, 27442, 27443, 27445, and 27446) are described as "Revision of Knee Joint." Full descriptions of each of the CPT-coded services are contained in *CPT 2002,* which may be obtained by calling 800 621-8335.

Codes describing a professional component–only or technical component–only service are also accompanied by modifiers -26 (professional only) and -TC (technical component). If the physician provides both the technical and professional components of a service (which is called the "global service"), no modifier should be used.

All five-digit numeric codes, two-digit numeric modifiers, service descriptions, instructions, and/or guidelines are copyright 2001 American Medical Association (AMA). No payment schedules, fee schedules, relative value units, scales, conversion factors, or components thereof are included in CPT. The AMA is not recommending that any specific relative values, fees, payment schedules, or related listings be attached to CPT. Any relative value scales or related listings assigned to the CPT codes are not those of the AMA, and the AMA is not recommending use of these relative values.

The RVU schedule contains all coded services included in the Medicare physician payment schedule. Several categories of codes that were included in the November 1, 2000 *Federal Register* have been omitted from this list:

- many codes for services not covered by Medicare;
- deleted codes;
- codes that are covered by Medicare but not included in the physician payment schedule, and for which payment continues under the previous rules, ie, clinical diagnostic laboratory services, ambulance services; and
- bundled codes, which are services or supplies that are only payable as part of another service, ie, a telephone call from a hospital nurse regarding care of a patient is not separately payable because it is included in the payment for other services such as hospital visits.

For approximately 50 services not covered by the Medicare program, but for which payment is frequently allowed by other payers, CMS has assigned relative values. These services are included in the table and are denoted by an asterisk (§) immediately to the right of the CPT code.

For the CPT- and HCPCS-coded services included in the list of RVUs, the following information is provided:

- **Work RVUs.** RVUs for the physician work component of the service. Chapter 4 provides an explanation of the resource-based relative value scale (RBRVS) and the physician work component.
- **Practice expense RVUs.** RVUs for the practice expense component of the service are explained in Chapter 5. The 2002 practice expense RVUs are now fully resource based, and CMS assigned two different levels (nonfacility or facility) of practice expense RVUs to each code, depending on the site of service. Facility includes hospitals (inpatient, outpatient, and emergency department), ambulatory surgical centers (ASCs), and skilled nursing facilities (SNFs). Nonfacility includes all other settings.
- **PLI RVUs.** RVUs for the professional liability insurance (PLI) component of the service. The *Federal Register* refers to this component as the "malpractice" component or the "malpractice" RVUs. Chapter 6 explains the PLI component.

Where no RVUs have been assigned, "0.00" appears in each of the RVU columns. These services are priced by the carrier. Carriers will generally establish payment amounts for these services on an individual case basis after reviewing documentation, such as an operative report.

- **Medicare payment schedule.** This column is the full payment amount for a service under the Medicare RBRVS, excluding the adjustment for geographic location. It includes both the 80% that Medicare pays and the 20% patient coinsurance. The limiting charge for a service is 109.25% of the payment schedule amount. There are separate payment totals according to whether the service was provided in a facility or nonfacility.

Unadjusted payment amounts are calculated by summing the RVUs for all three components of a service and multiplying the sum by the 2002 conversion factor of $36.1992.

To calculate the full 2002 payment schedule amount for a locality, refer to Chapter 8 and to the List of Geographic Practice Cost Indexes for each Medicare Locality that appears in this section.

- **Global period.** The global period refers to the number of postoperative days of care that are included in the payment for a global surgical package, ie, an 090 in the column means that 90 days of postoperative care is included in the payment. Medicare policies on global packages are described in Chapter 11. The following alpha codes also appear in this column:

XXX = The global concept does not apply to the code.

YYY = The global period is to be set by the carrier.

ZZZ = The code is part of another service and falls within the global period for the other service.

MMM = A service furnished in uncomplicated maternity cases, including antepartum care, delivery, and postpartum care. The usual global surgical concept does not apply.

- **Payment policy indicators.** Pending CMS review of the levels of physician supervision, CMS is defering decisions regarding levels of physician supervision to the individual Medicare carriers.
- Special payment policies apply to some procedure codes for the use of cosurgeons, team surgeons, and assistants-at-surgery; site of service; supplies; and multiple and bilateral service. Assistant-at-surgery services are not payable for those codes where an **A** appears in the Payment Policies Indicator column. An **A+** indicates this payment restriction applies unless medical necessity is established.

A **C** indicates that payment for a cosurgeon is allowed, while a **C+** indicates that documentation establishing medical necessity is required before payment for the cosurgeon would be allowed.

A **T** indicates that payment for a surgical team is allowed and paid on a by-report basis. A **T+** indicates team surgeons are payable if medical necessity is established and are paid on a by-report basis.

A **M** indicates that Medicare's standard multiple surgery rule applies, which allows 100% of the global payment schedule for the highest valued procedure and 50% of the global payment schedule for the second through fifth procedures. Subsequent procedures are priced by the carrier.

A **Me** indicates that special Medicare rules apply if the procedure is billed with another endoscopy in the same family (ie, another endoscopy that has the same base procedure). Under **Me,** Medicare pays the full value of the highest valued endoscopy, plus the difference between the next highest valued procedure and the base endoscopy. For example, in the course of performing a fiberoptic colonoscopy (CPT Code 45378), a physician performs a biopsy on a lesion (code 45380) and removes a polyp (code 45385) from a different part of the colon. The physician bills for codes 45380 and 45385. The value of codes 45380 and 45385 have the value of the diagnostic colonoscopy (45378) built in. Rather than paying 100% for the highest valued procedure (45385) and 50% for the next (45380), Medicare pays the full value of the highest valued endoscopy (45385), plus the difference between the next highest endoscopy (45380) and the base endocopy procedure (45378). Assuming the following are the fee schedule amounts for these codes:

45378	Diagnostic colonoscopy	$459.37
45380	Colonoscopy with biopsy	$571.22
45385	Colonoscopy with polypectomy	$571.22

Medicare would pay the full value of 45385 ($571.22), plus the difference between 45380 and 45378 ($44.88), for a total of $616.61. If an endoscopic procedure with an **Me** is billed with the -51 modifier with other procedures that are not endoscopies, then the standard rules for multiple surgeries apply.

Medicare RBRVS: The Physicians' Guide

Relative value units

CPT Code and Modifier	Description	Work RVU	Non Facility Practice Expense RVU	Facility Practice Expense RVU	PLI RVU	Total Non Facility RVUs	Medicare Payment Non Facility	Total Facility RVUs	Medicare Payment Facility	Global Period	Payment Policy Indicators*
Surgery: Integumentary system											
10021	Fna w/o image	1.27	1.02	1.02	0.10	2.39	$86.52	2.39	$86.52	XXX	A+
10021-26	Fna w/o image	1.27	0.55	0.55	0.07	1.89	$68.42	1.89	$68.42	XXX	A+
10021-TC	Fna w/o image	0.00	0.47	0.47	0.03	0.50	$18.10	0.50	$18.10	XXX	A+
10022	Fna w/image	1.27	1.11	1.11	0.08	2.46	$89.05	2.46	$89.05	XXX	A+
10022-26	Fna w/image	1.27	0.48	0.48	0.05	1.80	$65.16	1.80	$65.16	XXX	A+
10022-TC	Fna w/image	0.00	0.63	0.63	0.03	0.66	$23.89	0.66	$23.89	XXX	A+
10040	Acne surgery	1.18	1.00	0.54	0.05	2.23	$80.72	1.77	$64.07	010	A M
10060	Drainage of skin abscess	1.17	1.51	0.70	0.08	2.76	$99.91	1.95	$70.59	010	A M
10061	Drainage of skin abscess	2.40	1.88	1.48	0.17	4.45	$161.09	4.05	$146.61	010	A M
10080	Drainage of pilonidal cyst	1.17	2.18	0.75	0.09	3.44	$124.53	2.01	$72.76	010	A M
10081	Drainage of pilonidal cyst	2.45	3.02	1.61	0.19	5.66	$204.89	4.25	$153.85	010	A M
10120	Remove foreign body	1.22	1.52	0.36	0.10	2.84	$102.81	1.68	$60.81	010	A M
10121	Remove foreign body	2.69	2.99	1.83	0.25	5.93	$214.66	4.77	$172.67	010	A M
10140	Drainage of hematoma/fluid	1.53	1.54	0.90	0.15	3.22	$116.56	2.58	$93.39	010	A M
10160	Puncture drainage of lesion	1.20	0.74	0.43	0.11	2.05	$74.21	1.74	$62.99	010	A M
10180	Complex drainage, wound	2.25	1.51	1.33	0.25	4.01	$145.16	3.83	$138.64	010	A M
11000	Debride infected skin	0.60	0.66	0.24	0.05	1.31	$47.42	0.89	$32.22	000	A M
11001	Debride infected skin add-on	0.30	0.37	0.11	0.02	0.69	$24.98	0.43	$15.57	ZZZ	A
11010	Debride skin, fx	4.20	2.53	2.10	0.45	7.18	$259.91	6.75	$244.34	010	A M
11011	Debride skin/muscle, fx	4.95	3.90	2.69	0.53	9.38	$339.55	8.17	$295.75	000	A M
11012	Debride skin/muscle/bone, fx	6.88	5.52	4.35	0.89	13.29	$481.09	12.12	$438.73	000	A M
11040	Debride skin, partial	0.50	0.55	0.22	0.05	1.10	$39.82	0.77	$27.87	000	A M
11041	Debride skin, full	0.82	0.69	0.34	0.08	1.59	$57.56	1.24	$44.89	000	A M
11042	Debride skin/tissue	1.12	1.04	0.47	0.11	2.27	$82.17	1.70	$61.54	000	A M
11043	Debride tissue/muscle	2.38	2.72	1.42	0.24	5.34	$193.30	4.04	$146.24	010	A M

Code	Description									
11044	Debride tissue/muscle/bone	3.06	3.30	1.86	0.34	6.70	$242.53	5.26	$190.41	010	M	A
11055	Trim skin lesion	0.43	0.52	0.19	0.02	0.97	$35.11	0.64	$23.17	000	M	A
11056	Trim skin lesions, 2 to 4	0.61	0.59	0.26	0.03	1.23	$44.53	0.90	$32.58	000	M	A
11057	Trim skin lesions, over 4	0.79	0.66	0.34	0.04	1.49	$53.94	1.17	$42.35	000	M	A
11100	Biopsy of skin lesion	0.81	1.49	0.38	0.04	2.34	$84.71	1.23	$44.53	000	M	A
11101	Biopsy, skin add-on	0.41	0.71	0.20	0.02	1.14	$41.27	0.63	$22.81	ZZZ		A
11200	Removal of skin tags	0.77	1.20	0.32	0.04	2.01	$72.76	1.13	$40.91	010	M	A
11201	Remove skin tags add-on	0.29	0.53	0.12	0.02	0.84	$30.41	0.43	$15.57	ZZZ		A
11300	Shave skin lesion	0.51	1.05	0.22	0.03	1.59	$57.56	0.76	$27.51	000	M	A+
11301	Shave skin lesion	0.85	1.12	0.39	0.04	2.01	$72.76	1.28	$46.33	000	M	A+
11302	Shave skin lesion	1.05	1.21	0.49	0.05	2.31	$83.62	1.59	$57.56	000	M	A+
11303	Shave skin lesion	1.24	1.36	0.55	0.06	2.66	$96.29	1.85	$66.97	000	M	A+
11305	Shave skin lesion	0.67	0.77	0.29	0.04	1.48	$53.57	1.00	$36.20	000	M	A+
11306	Shave skin lesion	0.99	1.02	0.44	0.05	2.06	$74.57	1.48	$53.57	000	M	A+
11307	Shave skin lesion	1.14	1.15	0.51	0.05	2.34	$84.71	1.70	$61.54	000	M	A+
11308	Shave skin lesion	1.41	1.29	0.62	0.07	2.77	$100.27	2.10	$76.02	000	M	A+
11310	Shave skin lesion	0.73	1.15	0.34	0.04	1.92	$69.50	1.11	$40.18	000	M	A+
11311	Shave skin lesion	1.05	1.24	0.51	0.05	2.34	$84.71	1.61	$58.28	000	M	A+
11312	Shave skin lesion	1.20	1.32	0.58	0.06	2.58	$93.39	1.84	$66.61	000	M	A+
11313	Shave skin lesion	1.62	1.63	0.74	0.09	3.34	$120.91	2.45	$88.69	000	M	A+
11400	Removal of skin lesion	0.91	1.68	0.36	0.06	2.65	$95.93	1.33	$48.14	010	M	A
11401	Removal of skin lesion	1.32	1.83	0.53	0.09	3.24	$117.29	1.94	$70.23	010	M	A
11402	Removal of skin lesion	1.61	2.61	0.98	0.12	4.34	$157.10	2.71	$98.10	010	M	A
11403	Removal of skin lesion	1.92	2.84	1.12	0.16	4.92	$178.10	3.20	$115.84	010	M	A
11404	Removal of skin lesion	2.20	3.02	1.19	0.18	5.40	$195.48	3.57	$129.23	010	M	A
11406	Removal of skin lesion	2.76	3.33	1.41	0.25	6.34	$229.50	4.42	$160.00	010	M	A
11420	Removal of skin lesion	1.06	1.52	0.44	0.08	2.66	$96.29	1.58	$57.19	010	M	A
11421	Removal of skin lesion	1.53	1.84	0.64	0.11	3.48	$125.97	2.28	$82.53	010	M	A

* **M** = multiple surgery adjustment applies
Me = multiple endoscopy rules may apply
B = bilateral surgery adjustment applies
A = assistant-at-surgery restriction

A+ = assistant-at-surgery restriction unless medical necessity established with documentation
C = cosurgeons payable
C+ = cosurgeons payable if medical necessity established with documentation

T = team surgeons permitted
T+ = team surgeons payable if medical necessity established with documentation
$ = indicates services that are not covered by Medicare.

CPT five-digit codes, two-digit numeric modifiers, and descriptions only are © 2001 American Medical Association

Medicare RBRVS: The Physicians' Guide

Relative value units

CPT Code and Modifier	Description	Work RVU	Non Facility Practice Expense RVU	Facility Practice Expense RVU	PLI RVU	Total Non Facility RVUs	Medicare Payment Non Facility	Total Facility RVUs	Medicare Payment Facility	Global Period	Payment Policy Indicators*
11422	Removal of skin lesion	1.76	2.60	1.08	0.14	4.50	$162.90	2.98	$107.87	010	M A
11423	Removal of skin lesion	2.17	3.02	1.26	0.17	5.36	$194.03	3.60	$130.32	010	M A
11424	Removal of skin lesion	2.62	3.20	1.43	0.21	6.03	$218.28	4.26	$154.21	010	M A
11426	Removal of skin lesion	3.78	3.81	1.89	0.34	7.93	$287.06	6.01	$217.56	010	M A
11440	Removal of skin lesion	1.15	2.26	0.53	0.08	3.49	$126.34	1.76	$63.71	010	M A
11441	Removal of skin lesion	1.61	2.48	0.74	0.11	4.20	$152.04	2.46	$89.05	010	M A
11442	Removal of skin lesion	1.87	2.91	1.30	0.14	4.92	$178.10	3.31	$119.82	010	M A
11443	Removal of skin lesion	2.49	3.41	1.64	0.18	6.08	$220.09	4.31	$156.02	010	M A
11444	Removal of skin lesion	3.42	3.92	2.08	0.25	7.59	$274.75	5.75	$208.15	010	M A
11446	Removal of skin lesion	4.49	4.37	2.58	0.30	9.16	$331.58	7.37	$266.79	010	M A
11450	Removal, sweat gland lesion	2.73	4.20	1.03	0.26	7.19	$260.27	4.02	$145.52	090	M A
11451	Removal, sweat gland lesion	3.95	5.23	1.33	0.39	9.57	$346.43	5.67	$205.25	090	M A+
11462	Removal, sweat gland lesion	2.51	4.32	0.98	0.23	7.06	$255.57	3.72	$134.66	090	M A+
11463	Removal, sweat gland lesion	3.95	5.67	1.67	0.40	10.02	$362.72	6.02	$217.92	090	M A+
11470	Removal, sweat gland lesion	3.25	4.97	1.26	0.30	8.52	$308.42	4.81	$174.12	090	M A
11471	Removal, sweat gland lesion	4.41	5.54	1.74	0.40	10.35	$374.66	6.55	$237.10	090	M A+
11600	Removal of skin lesion	1.41	2.48	1.08	0.09	3.98	$144.07	2.58	$93.39	010	M A
11601	Removal of skin lesion	1.93	2.52	1.36	0.12	4.57	$165.43	3.41	$123.44	010	M A
11602	Removal of skin lesion	2.09	2.66	1.40	0.13	4.88	$176.65	3.62	$131.04	010	M A
11603	Removal of skin lesion	2.35	2.93	1.49	0.16	5.44	$196.92	4.00	$144.80	010	M A
11604	Removal of skin lesion	2.58	3.27	1.56	0.18	6.03	$218.28	4.32	$156.38	010	M A
11606	Removal of skin lesion	3.43	3.88	1.85	0.28	7.59	$274.75	5.56	$201.27	010	M A
11620	Removal of skin lesion	1.34	2.47	1.09	0.09	3.90	$141.18	2.52	$91.22	010	M A
11621	Removal of skin lesion	1.97	2.56	1.41	0.12	4.65	$168.33	3.50	$126.70	010	M A
11622	Removal of skin lesion	2.34	2.87	1.60	0.15	5.36	$194.03	4.09	$148.05	010	M A
11623	Removal of skin lesion	2.93	3.30	1.86	0.20	6.43	$232.76	4.99	$180.63	010	M A
11624	Removal of skin lesion	3.43	3.72	2.08	0.25	7.40	$267.87	5.76	$208.51	010	M A

Code	Description									
11626	Removal of skin lesion	4.30	4.48	2.57	0.35	9.13	$330.50	7.22	$261.36	010	M	A
11640	Removal of skin lesion	1.53	2.51	1.29	0.10	4.14	$149.86	2.92	$105.70	010	M	A
11641	Removal of skin lesion	2.44	2.94	1.78	0.15	5.53	$200.18	4.37	$158.19	010	M	A
11642	Removal of skin lesion	2.93	3.37	2.03	0.18	6.48	$234.57	5.14	$186.06	010	M	A
11643	Removal of skin lesion	3.50	3.83	2.32	0.24	7.57	$274.03	6.06	$219.37	010	M	A
11644	Removal of skin lesion	4.55	4.81	2.95	0.33	9.69	$350.77	7.83	$283.44	010	M	A
11646	Removal of skin lesion	5.95	5.68	3.77	0.46	12.09	$437.65	10.18	$368.51	010	M	A
11719	Trim nail(s)	0.17	0.25	0.07	0.01	0.43	$15.57	0.25	$9.05	000	M	A
11720	Debride nail, 1-5	0.32	0.34	0.13	0.02	0.68	$24.62	0.47	$17.01	000	M	A
11721	Debride nail, 6 or more	0.54	0.44	0.22	0.04	1.02	$36.92	0.80	$28.96	000	M	A
11730	Removal of nail plate	1.13	0.83	0.46	0.09	2.05	$74.21	1.68	$60.81	000	M	A
11732	Remove nail plate, add-on	0.57	0.30	0.24	0.05	0.92	$33.30	0.86	$31.13	ZZZ		A
11740	Drain blood from under nail	0.37	0.81	0.14	0.03	1.21	$43.80	0.54	$19.55	000	M	A
11750	Removal of nail bed	1.86	1.75	0.78	0.16	3.77	$136.47	2.80	$101.36	010	M	A
11752	Remove nail bed/finger tip	2.67	2.20	1.77	0.33	5.20	$188.24	4.77	$172.67	010	M	A
11755	Biopsy, nail unit	1.31	1.10	0.60	0.06	2.47	$89.41	1.97	$71.31	000	M	A+
11760	Repair of nail bed	1.58	1.80	1.28	0.17	3.55	$128.51	3.03	$109.68	010	M	A
11762	Reconstruction of nail bed	2.89	2.28	1.95	0.32	5.49	$198.73	5.16	$186.79	010	M	A
11765	Excision of nail fold, toe	0.69	1.14	0.51	0.05	1.88	$68.05	1.25	$45.25	010	M	A
11770	Removal of pilonidal lesion	2.61	3.11	1.26	0.24	5.96	$215.75	4.11	$148.78	010	M	A
11771	Removal of pilonidal lesion	5.74	5.80	4.01	0.56	12.10	$438.01	10.31	$373.21	90	M	A
11772	Removal of pilonidal lesion	6.98	6.95	4.44	0.68	14.61	$528.87	12.10	$438.01	90	M	A
11900	Injection into skin lesions	0.52	0.77	0.23	0.02	1.31	$47.42	0.77	$27.87	000	M	A
11901	Added skin lesions injection	0.80	0.89	0.38	0.03	1.72	$62.26	1.21	$43.80	000	M	A
11920	Correct skin color defects	1.61	2.25	0.81	0.17	4.03	$145.88	2.59	$93.76	000	M	A+
11921	Correct skin color defects	1.93	2.78	1.02	0.21	4.92	$178.10	3.16	$114.39	000	M	A+
11922	Correct skin color defects	0.49	0.40	0.26	0.05	0.94	$34.03	0.80	$28.96	ZZZ		A+
11950	Therapy for contour defects	0.84	1.23	0.47	0.06	2.13	$77.10	1.37	$49.59	000	M	A+

* **M** = multiple surgery adjustment applies
Me = multiple endoscopy rules may apply
B = bilateral surgery adjustment applies
A = assistant-at-surgery restriction

A+ = assistant-at-surgery restriction unless medical necessity established with documentation
C = cosurgeons payable
C+ = cosurgeons payable if medical necessity established with documentation

T = team surgeons permitted
T+ = team surgeons payable if medical necessity established with documentation
§ = indicates services that are not covered by Medicare.

131 CPT five-digit codes, two-digit numeric modifiers, and descriptions only are © 2001 American Medical Association

Medicare RBRVS: The Physicians' Guide

Relative value units

CPT Code and Modifier	Description	Work RVU	Non Facility Practice Expense RVU	Facility Practice Expense RVU	PLI RVU	Total Non Facility RVUs	Medicare Payment Non Facility	Total Facility RVUs	Medicare Payment Facility	Global Period	Payment Policy Indicators*	
11951	Therapy for contour defects	1.19	1.47	0.49	0.10	2.76	$99.91	1.78	$64.43	000	M	A+
11952	Therapy for contour defects	1.69	1.65	0.64	0.17	3.51	$127.06	2.50	$90.50	000	M	A+
11954	Therapy for contour defects	1.85	2.62	0.97	0.19	4.66	$168.69	3.01	$108.96	000	M	A+
11960	Insert tissue expander(s)	9.08	NA	11.54	0.88	NA	NA	21.50	$778.28	090	M	A
11970	Replace tissue expander	7.06	NA	5.15	0.77	NA	NA	12.98	$469.87	090	M	A
11971	Remove tissue expander(s)	2.13	6.10	4.07	0.21	8.44	$305.52	6.41	$232.04	090	M	A+
11975 §	Insert contraceptive cap	1.48	1.58	0.59	0.14	3.20	$115.84	2.21	$80.00	XXX		
11976	Removal of contraceptive cap	1.78	1.72	0.69	0.17	3.67	$132.85	2.64	$95.57	000	M	A+
11977 §	Removal/reinsert contra cap	3.30	2.31	1.32	0.31	5.92	$214.30	4.93	$178.46	XXX		
11980	Implant hormone pellet(s)	1.48	1.14	0.58	0.10	2.72	$98.46	2.16	$78.19	000	M	A
11981	Insert drug implant device	1.48	1.58	0.59	0.14	3.20	$115.84	2.21	$80.00	XXX	M	A+
11982	Remove drug implant device	1.78	1.70	0.71	0.17	3.65	$132.13	2.66	$96.29	XXX	M	A+
11983	Remove/insert drug implant	3.30	2.31	1.32	0.31	5.92	$214.30	4.93	$178.46	XXX	M	A+
12001	Repair superficial wound(s)	1.70	2.13	0.44	0.13	3.96	$143.35	2.27	$82.17	010	M	A
12002	Repair superficial wound(s)	1.86	2.21	0.95	0.15	4.22	$152.76	2.96	$107.15	010	M	A
12004	Repair superficial wound(s)	2.24	2.47	1.07	0.17	4.88	$176.65	3.48	$125.97	010	M	A
12005	Repair superficial wound(s)	2.86	3.04	1.25	0.23	6.13	$221.90	4.34	$157.10	010	M	A
12006	Repair superficial wound(s)	3.67	3.59	1.59	0.31	7.57	$274.03	5.57	$201.63	010	M	A
12007	Repair superficial wound(s)	4.12	4.26	1.85	0.37	8.75	$316.74	6.34	$229.50	010	M	A C+
12011	Repair superficial wound(s)	1.76	2.30	0.45	0.14	4.20	$152.04	2.35	$85.07	010	M	A
12013	Repair superficial wound(s)	1.99	2.45	0.99	0.16	4.60	$166.52	3.14	$113.67	010	M	A
12014	Repair superficial wound(s)	2.46	2.72	1.11	0.18	5.36	$194.03	3.75	$135.75	010	M	A
12015	Repair superficial wound(s)	3.19	3.38	1.31	0.24	6.81	$246.52	4.74	$171.58	010	M	A
12016	Repair superficial wound(s)	3.93	3.89	1.58	0.32	8.14	$294.66	5.83	$211.04	010	M	A
12017	Repair superficial wound(s)	4.71	NA	1.93	0.39	NA	NA	7.03	$254.48	010	M	A+
12018	Repair superficial wound(s)	5.53	NA	2.18	0.46	NA	NA	8.17	$295.75	010	M	C+
12020	Closure of split wound	2.62	2.51	1.44	0.24	5.37	$194.39	4.30	$155.66	010	M	A

Code	Description										
12021	Closure of split wound	1.84	1.65	1.02	0.19	3.68	$133.21	3.05	$110.41	010	M	A
12031	Layer closure of wound(s)	2.15	2.21	0.81	0.15	4.51	$163.26	3.11	$112.58	010	M	A
12032	Layer closure of wound(s)	2.47	2.84	1.36	0.15	5.46	$197.65	3.98	$144.07	010	M	A
12034	Layer closure of wound(s)	2.92	3.12	1.51	0.21	6.25	$226.25	4.64	$167.96	010	M	A
12035	Layer closure of wound(s)	3.43	3.20	1.73	0.30	6.93	$250.86	5.46	$197.65	010	M	A
12036	Layer closure of wound(s)	4.05	5.33	2.50	0.41	9.79	$354.39	6.96	$251.95	010	M	A
12037	Layer closure of wound(s)	4.67	5.57	2.86	0.49	10.73	$388.42	8.02	$290.32	010	M	A+	C+
12041	Layer closure of wound(s)	2.37	2.41	0.87	0.17	4.95	$179.19	3.41	$123.44	010	M	A
12042	Layer closure of wound(s)	2.74	3.03	1.49	0.17	5.94	$215.02	4.40	$159.28	010	M	A
12044	Layer closure of wound(s)	3.14	3.22	1.67	0.24	6.60	$238.91	5.05	$182.81	010	M	A
12045	Layer closure of wound(s)	3.64	3.54	1.93	0.34	7.52	$272.22	5.91	$213.94	010	M	A
12046	Layer closure of wound(s)	4.25	6.24	2.62	0.40	10.89	$394.21	7.27	$263.17	010	M	A+
12047	Layer closure of wound(s)	4.65	7.21	2.86	0.41	12.27	$444.16	7.92	$286.70	010	M	A	C+
12051	Layer closure of wound(s)	2.47	3.11	1.49	0.16	5.74	$207.78	4.12	$149.14	010	M	A
12052	Layer closure of wound(s)	2.77	3.00	1.47	0.17	5.94	$215.02	4.41	$159.64	010	M	A
12053	Layer closure of wound(s)	3.12	3.20	1.63	0.20	6.52	$236.02	4.95	$179.19	010	M	A
12054	Layer closure of wound(s)	3.46	3.52	1.72	0.25	7.23	$261.72	5.43	$196.56	010	M	A
12055	Layer closure of wound(s)	4.43	4.49	2.27	0.35	9.27	$335.57	7.05	$255.20	010	M	A
12056	Layer closure of wound(s)	5.24	7.31	3.26	0.43	12.98	$469.87	8.93	$323.26	010	M	A+
12057	Layer closure of wound(s)	5.96	6.31	3.66	0.50	12.77	$462.26	10.12	$366.34	010	M		C+
13100	Repair of wound or lesion	3.12	3.39	1.93	0.21	6.72	$243.26	5.26	$190.41	010	M	A
13101	Repair of wound or lesion	3.92	3.59	2.39	0.22	7.73	$279.82	6.53	$236.38	010	M	A
13102	Repair wound/lesion add-on	1.24	0.75	0.60	0.10	2.09	$75.66	1.94	$70.23	ZZZ		A
13120	Repair of wound or lesion	3.30	3.48	1.95	0.23	7.01	$253.76	5.48	$198.37	010	M	A
13121	Repair of wound or lesion	4.33	3.84	2.52	0.25	8.42	$304.80	7.10	$257.01	010	M	A
13122	Repair wound/lesion add-on	1.44	0.89	0.67	0.12	2.45	$88.69	2.23	$80.72	ZZZ		A
13131	Repair of wound or lesion	3.79	3.75	2.30	0.25	7.79	$281.99	6.34	$229.50	010	M	A
13132	Repair of wound or lesion	5.95	4.57	3.38	0.32	10.84	$392.40	9.65	$349.32	010	M	A

* **M** = multiple surgery adjustment applies
Me = multiple endoscopy rules may apply
B = bilateral surgery adjustment applies
A = assistant-at-surgery restriction

A+ = assistant-at-surgery restriction unless medical necessity established with documentation
C = cosurgeons payable
C+ = cosurgeons payable if medical necessity established with documentation

T = team surgeons permitted
T+ = team surgeons payable if medical necessity established with documentation
§ = indicates services that are not covered by Medicare.

CPT five-digit codes, two-digit numeric modifiers, and descriptions only are © 2001 American Medical Association

Medicare RBRVS: The Physicians' Guide

Relative value units

CPT Code and Modifier	Description	Work RVU	Non Facility Practice Expense RVU	Facility Practice Expense RVU	PLI RVU	Total Non Facility RVUs	Medicare Payment Non Facility	Total Facility RVUs	Medicare Payment Facility	Global Period	Payment Policy Indicators*
13133	Repair wound/lesion add-on	2.19	1.23	1.08	0.17	3.59	$129.96	3.44	$124.53	ZZZ	A
13150	Repair of wound or lesion	3.81	5.19	2.75	0.29	9.29	$336.29	6.85	$247.96	010	M A
13151	Repair of wound or lesion	4.45	5.07	3.19	0.28	9.80	$354.75	7.92	$286.70	010	M A
13152	Repair of wound or lesion	6.33	5.78	4.14	0.38	12.49	$452.13	10.85	$392.76	010	M A
13153	Repair wound/lesion add-on	2.38	1.38	1.20	0.18	3.94	$142.62	3.76	$136.11	ZZZ	A
13160	Late closure of wound	10.48	NA	6.47	1.19	NA	NA	18.14	$656.65	090	M A
14000	Skin tissue rearrangement	5.89	7.58	4.83	0.46	13.93	$504.25	11.18	$404.71	090	M A
14001	Skin tissue rearrangement	8.47	8.72	6.18	0.65	17.84	$645.79	15.30	$553.85	090	M A
14020	Skin tissue rearrangement	6.59	8.05	5.56	0.50	15.14	$548.06	12.65	$457.92	090	M A
14021	Skin tissue rearrangement	10.06	9.29	7.38	0.69	20.04	$725.43	18.13	$656.29	090	M A
14040	Skin tissue rearrangement	7.87	8.19	6.27	0.53	16.59	$600.54	14.67	$531.04	090	M A
14041	Skin tissue rearrangement	11.49	9.90	8.17	0.68	22.07	$798.92	20.34	$736.29	090	M A
14060	Skin tissue rearrangement	8.50	8.64	7.13	0.59	17.73	$641.81	16.22	$587.15	090	M A
14061	Skin tissue rearrangement	12.29	10.85	9.08	0.75	23.89	$864.80	22.12	$800.73	090	M A
14300	Skin tissue rearrangement	11.76	10.11	8.68	0.88	22.75	$823.53	21.32	$771.77	090	M A
14350	Skin tissue rearrangement	9.61	NA	6.48	1.09	NA	NA	17.18	$621.90	090	M A+
15000	Skin graft	4.00	2.51	1.91	0.37	6.88	$249.05	6.28	$227.33	000	A
15001	Skin graft add-on	1.00	0.64	0.43	0.11	1.75	$63.35	1.54	$55.75	ZZZ	
15050	Skin pinch graft	4.30	4.98	4.12	0.46	9.74	$352.58	8.88	$321.45	090	M A
15100	Skin split graft	9.05	6.27	6.26	0.94	16.26	$588.60	16.25	$588.24	090	M A
15101	Skin split graft add-on	1.72	1.40	0.76	0.18	3.30	$119.46	2.66	$96.29	ZZZ	A
15120	Skin split graft	9.83	8.62	6.97	0.87	19.32	$699.37	17.67	$639.64	090	M A
15121	Skin split graft add-on	2.67	1.83	1.23	0.27	4.77	$172.67	4.17	$150.95	ZZZ	A C+
15200	Skin full graft	8.03	9.90	5.64	0.73	18.66	$675.48	14.40	$521.27	090	M A
15201	Skin full graft add-on	1.32	1.00	0.68	0.14	2.46	$89.05	2.14	$77.47	ZZZ	A+
15220	Skin full graft	7.87	9.38	6.47	0.68	17.93	$649.05	15.02	$543.71	090	M A
15221	Skin full graft add-on	1.19	0.92	0.60	0.12	2.23	$80.72	1.91	$69.14	ZZZ	A

Code	Description										
15240	Skin full graft	9.04	9.01	7.27	0.77	18.82	$681.27	17.08	$618.28	090	M	A
15241	Skin full graft add-on	1.86	1.47	0.95	0.17	3.50	$126.70	2.98	$107.87	ZZZ	M	A
15260	Skin full graft	10.06	9.01	7.74	0.63	19.70	$713.12	18.43	$667.15	090	M	A
15261	Skin full graft add-on	2.23	1.59	1.16	0.17	3.99	$144.43	3.56	$128.87	ZZZ	M	A
15342	Cultured skin graft, 25 cm	1.00	2.18	1.04	0.09	3.27	$118.37	2.13	$77.10	010	M	A
15343	Culture skn graft addl 25 cm	0.25	0.42	0.10	0.02	0.69	$24.98	0.37	$13.39	ZZZ	M	A
15350	Skin homograft	4.00	7.78	4.23	0.42	12.20	$441.63	8.65	$313.12	090	M	A
15351	Skin homograft add-on	1.00	0.85	0.42	0.11	1.96	$70.95	1.53	$55.38	ZZZ	M	A
15400	Skin heterograft	4.00	4.89	4.89	0.40	9.29	$336.29	9.29	$336.29	090	M	A
15401	Skin heterograft add-on	1.00	1.59	0.47	0.11	2.70	$97.74	1.58	$57.19	ZZZ	M	A
15570	Form skin pedicle flap	9.21	7.80	6.37	0.96	17.97	$650.50	16.54	$598.73	090	M	A
15572	Form skin pedicle flap	9.27	8.08	6.34	0.93	18.28	$661.72	16.54	$598.73	090	M	A
15574	Form skin pedicle flap	9.88	8.61	7.14	0.92	19.41	$702.63	17.94	$649.41	090	M	A
15576	Form skin pedicle flap	8.69	8.89	6.55	0.72	18.30	$662.45	15.96	$577.74	090	M	A
15600	Skin graft	1.91	6.66	2.51	0.19	8.76	$317.10	4.61	$166.88	090	M	A+
15610	Skin graft	2.42	5.90	2.67	0.25	8.57	$310.23	5.34	$193.30	090	M	A+
15620	Skin graft	2.94	7.04	3.54	0.28	10.26	$371.40	6.76	$244.71	090	M	A
15630	Skin graft	3.27	6.09	3.83	0.28	9.64	$348.96	7.38	$267.15	090	M	A
15650	Transfer skin pedicle flap	3.97	5.69	3.99	0.36	10.02	$362.72	8.32	$301.18	090	M	A+
15732	Muscle-skin graft, head/neck	17.84	NA	11.63	1.50	NA	NA	30.97	$1,121.09	090	M	C+
15734	Muscle-skin graft, trunk	17.79	NA	11.49	1.91	NA	NA	31.19	$1,129.05	090	M	C+
15736	Muscle-skin graft, arm	16.27	NA	11.14	1.78	NA	NA	29.19	$1,056.65	090	M	A	C+
15738	Muscle-skin graft, leg	17.92	NA	11.47	1.95	NA	NA	31.34	$1,134.48	090	M	C+
15740	Island pedicle flap graft	10.25	8.74	7.20	0.62	19.61	$709.87	18.07	$654.12	090	M	A
15750	Neurovascular pedicle graft	11.41	NA	8.45	1.12	NA	NA	20.98	$759.46	090	M	
15756	Free muscle flap, microvasc	35.23	NA	22.50	3.11	NA	NA	60.84	$2,202.36	090	M	C
15757	Free skin flap, microvasc	35.23	NA	22.54	3.37	NA	NA	61.14	$2,213.22	090	M	C
15758	Free fascial flap, microvasc	35.10	NA	22.75	3.52	NA	NA	61.37	$2,221.54	090	M	C

* M = multiple surgery adjustment applies
Me = multiple endoscopy rules may apply
B = bilateral surgery adjustment applies
A = assistant-at-surgery restriction

A+ = assistant-at-surgery restriction unless medical necessity established with documentation
C = cosurgeons payable
C+ = cosurgeons payable if medical necessity established with documentation

T = team surgeons permitted
T+ = team surgeons payable if medical necessity established with documentation
$ = indicates services that are not covered by Medicare.

135 CPT five-digit codes, two-digit numeric modifiers, and descriptions only are © 2001 American Medical Association

Medicare RBRVS: The Physicians' Guide

Relative value units

CPT Code and Modifier	Description	Work RVU	Non Facility Practice Expense RVU	Facility Practice Expense RVU	PLI RVU	Total Non Facility RVUs	Medicare Payment Non Facility	Total Facility RVUs	Medicare Payment Facility	Global Period	Payment Policy Indicators*		
15760	Composite skin graft	8.74	9.27	6.93	0.72	18.73	$678.01	16.39	$593.30	090	M		A
15770	Derma-fat-fascia graft	7.52	NA	6.14	0.78	NA	NA	14.44	$522.72	090	M		C+
15775	Hair transplant punch grafts	3.96	3.12	1.60	0.43	7.51	$271.86	5.99	$216.83	000	M		A+
15776	Hair transplant punch grafts	5.54	3.97	2.97	0.60	10.11	$365.97	9.11	$329.77	000	M		A+
15780	Abrasion treatment of skin	7.29	6.41	6.13	0.41	14.11	$510.77	13.83	$500.63	090	M		A+
15781	Abrasion treatment of skin	4.85	5.17	4.83	0.27	10.29	$372.49	9.95	$360.18	090	M		A
15782	Abrasion treatment of skin	4.32	4.37	4.09	0.21	8.90	$322.17	8.62	$312.04	090	M		A+
15783	Abrasion treatment of skin	4.29	5.02	3.51	0.26	9.57	$346.43	8.06	$291.77	090	M		A+
15786	Abrasion, lesion, single	2.03	1.73	1.29	0.11	3.87	$140.09	3.43	$124.16	010	M		A
15787	Abrasion, lesions, add-on	0.33	0.39	0.18	0.02	0.74	$26.79	0.53	$19.19	ZZZ			A
15788	Chemical peel, face, epiderm	2.09	3.15	1.07	0.11	5.35	$193.67	3.27	$118.37	090	M		A
15789	Chemical peel, face, dermal	4.92	5.65	3.32	0.27	10.84	$392.40	8.51	$308.06	090	M		A
15792	Chemical peel, nonfacial	1.86	2.87	1.63	0.10	4.83	$174.84	3.59	$129.96	090	M		A+
15793	Chemical peel, nonfacial	3.74	NA	3.81	0.17	NA	NA	7.72	$279.46	090	M		A+
15810	Salabrasion	4.74	4.04	4.04	0.42	9.20	$333.03	9.20	$333.03	090	M		A+
15811	Salabrasion	5.39	5.85	5.06	0.52	11.76	$425.70	10.97	$397.11	090	M		A+
15819	Plastic surgery, neck	9.38	NA	6.24	0.77	NA	NA	16.39	$593.30	090	M		A+
15820	Revision of lower eyelid	5.15	10.34	7.13	0.30	15.79	$571.59	12.58	$455.39	090	M	B	A+
15821	Revision of lower eyelid	5.72	11.87	7.34	0.31	17.90	$647.97	13.37	$483.98	090	M	B	A+
15822	Revision of upper eyelid	4.45	10.58	6.58	0.22	15.25	$552.04	11.25	$407.24	090	M	B	A
15823	Revision of upper eyelid	7.05	11.38	7.60	0.32	18.75	$678.74	14.97	$541.90	090	M	B	A
15824	Removal of forehead wrinkles	0.00	0.00	0.00	0.00	0.00	$0.00	0.00	$0.00	000	M	B	A+
15825	Removal of neck wrinkles	0.00	0.00	0.00	0.00	0.00	$0.00	0.00	$0.00	000	M	B	A+
15826	Removal of brow wrinkles	0.00	0.00	0.00	0.00	0.00	$0.00	0.00	$0.00	000	M	B	A+
15828	Removal of face wrinkles	0.00	0.00	0.00	0.00	0.00	$0.00	0.00	$0.00	000	M	B	A+
15829	Removal of skin wrinkles	0.00	0.00	0.00	0.00	0.00	$0.00	0.00	$0.00	000	M	B	A+
15831	Excise excessive skin tissue	12.40	NA	8.14	1.30	NA	NA	21.84	$790.59	090	M		C+

Code	Description								
15832	Excise excessive skin tissue	11.59	NA	8.04	1.21	NA	20.84	$754.39	090	M	C+
15833	Excise excessive skin tissue	10.64	NA	7.34	1.17	NA	19.15	$693.21	090	M	A+
15834	Excise excessive skin tissue	10.85	NA	7.59	1.18	NA	19.62	$710.23	090	M	A+
15835	Excise excessive skin tissue	11.67	NA	7.94	1.13	NA	20.74	$750.77	090	M	A+
15836	Excise excessive skin tissue	9.34	NA	6.51	0.95	NA	16.80	$608.15	090	M	A+
15837	Excise excessive skin tissue	8.43	7.30	6.38	0.78	$597.65	15.59	$564.35	090	M	A+
15838	Excise excessive skin tissue	7.13	NA	5.70	0.58	NA	13.41	$485.43	090	M	A+
15839	Excise excessive skin tissue	9.38	7.64	5.97	0.88	$647.97	16.23	$587.51	090	M	A+
15840	Graft for face nerve palsy	13.26	NA	10.10	1.15	NA	24.51	$887.24	090	M	A
15841	Graft for face nerve palsy	23.26	NA	14.68	2.65	NA	40.59	$1,469.33	090	M	C+
15842	Flap for face nerve palsy	37.96	NA	22.81	3.99	NA	64.76	$2,344.26	090	M	C+
15845	Skin and muscle repair, face	12.57	NA	8.81	0.80	NA	22.18	$802.90	090	M	
15850 §	Removal of sutures	0.78	1.43	0.31	0.04	$81.45	1.13	$40.91	XXX		
15851	Removal of sutures	0.86	1.64	0.35	0.05	$92.31	1.26	$45.61	000	M	A
15852	Dressing change, not for burn	0.86	1.93	0.36	0.07	$103.53	1.29	$46.70	000	M	A
15860	Test for blood flow in graft	1.95	1.35	0.84	0.13	$124.16	2.92	$105.70	000	M	A+
15876	Suction assisted lipectomy	0.00	0.00	0.00	0.00	$0.00	0.00	$0.00	000	M	A+
15877	Suction assisted lipectomy	0.00	0.00	0.00	0.00	$0.00	0.00	$0.00	000	M	A+
15878	Suction assisted lipectomy	0.00	0.00	0.00	0.00	$0.00	0.00	$0.00	000	M	A+
15879	Suction assisted lipectomy	0.00	0.00	0.00	0.00	$0.00	0.00	$0.00	000	M	A+
15920	Removal of tail bone ulcer	7.95	NA	5.90	0.83	NA	14.68	$531.40	090	M	A+
15922	Removal of tail bone ulcer	9.90	NA	7.78	1.06	NA	18.74	$678.37	090	M	C+
15931	Remove sacrum pressure sore	9.24	NA	5.89	0.95	NA	16.08	$582.08	090	M	A
15933	Remove sacrum pressure sore	10.85	NA	8.32	1.14	NA	20.31	$735.21	090	M	A+
15934	Remove sacrum pressure sore	12.69	NA	8.48	1.35	NA	22.52	$815.21	090	M	A
15935	Remove sacrum pressure sore	14.57	NA	10.12	1.56	NA	26.25	$950.23	090	M	C+
15936	Remove sacrum pressure sore	12.38	NA	8.81	1.32	NA	22.51	$814.84	090	M	A
15937	Remove sacrum pressure sore	14.21	NA	10.75	1.51	NA	26.47	$958.19	090	M	C+

* **M** = multiple surgery adjustment applies
Me = multiple endoscopy rules may apply
B = bilateral surgery adjustment applies
A = assistant-at-surgery restriction

A+ = assistant-at-surgery restriction unless medical necessity established with documentation
C = cosurgeons payable
C+ = cosurgeons payable if medical necessity established with documentation

T = team surgeons permitted
T+ = team surgeons payable if medical necessity established with documentation
§ = indicates services that are not covered by Medicare.

137 CPT five-digit codes, two-digit numeric modifiers, and descriptions only are © 2001 American Medical Association

Medicare RBRVS: The Physicians' Guide

Relative value units

CPT Code and Modifier	Description	Work RVU	Non Facility Practice Expense RVU	Facility Practice Expense RVU	PLI RVU	Total Non Facility RVUs	Medicare Payment Non Facility	Total Facility RVUs	Medicare Payment Facility	Global Period	Payment Policy Indicators*		
15940	Remove hip pressure sore	9.34	NA	6.17	0.98	NA	NA	16.49	$596.92	090	M	A	
15941	Remove hip pressure sore	11.43	NA	10.44	1.23	NA	NA	23.10	$836.20	090	M	A+	
15944	Remove hip pressure sore	11.46	NA	8.77	1.21	NA	NA	21.44	$776.11	090	M	A+	
15945	Remove hip pressure sore	12.69	NA	9.73	1.38	NA	NA	23.80	$861.54	090	M	A+	
15946	Remove hip pressure sore	21.57	NA	14.65	2.32	NA	NA	38.54	$1,395.12	090	M	C+	
15950	Remove thigh pressure sore	7.54	NA	5.43	0.80	NA	NA	13.77	$498.46	090	M	A	
15951	Remove thigh pressure sore	10.72	NA	8.07	1.14	NA	NA	19.93	$721.45	090	M	A+	C+
15952	Remove thigh pressure sore	11.39	NA	7.86	1.19	NA	NA	20.44	$739.91	090	M	A	C+
15953	Remove thigh pressure sore	12.63	NA	9.24	1.38	NA	NA	23.25	$841.63	090	M	A	C+
15956	Remove thigh pressure sore	15.52	NA	10.71	1.64	NA	NA	27.87	$1,008.87	090	M	A	C+
15958	Remove thigh pressure sore	15.48	NA	11.20	1.66	NA	NA	28.34	$1,025.89	090	M	A	C+
15999	Removal of pressure sore	0.00	0.00	0.00	0.00	0.00	$0.00	0.00	$0.00	YYY	M	A+	C+ T+
16000	Initial treatment of burn(s)	0.89	1.09	0.27	0.06	2.04	$73.85	1.22	$44.16	000	M	A	
16010	Treatment of burn(s)	0.87	1.21	0.37	0.07	2.15	$77.83	1.31	$47.42	000	M	A	
16015	Treatment of burn(s)	2.35	2.01	1.03	0.22	4.58	$165.79	3.60	$130.32	000	M	A	
16020	Treatment of burn(s)	0.80	1.20	0.27	0.06	2.06	$74.57	1.13	$40.91	000	M	A	
16025	Treatment of burn(s)	1.85	1.94	0.69	0.16	3.95	$142.99	2.70	$97.74	000	M	A	
16030	Treatment of burn(s)	2.08	3.36	0.97	0.18	5.62	$203.44	3.23	$116.92	000	M	A	
16035	Incision of burn scab, initi	3.75	NA	1.56	0.36	NA	NA	5.67	$205.25	090	M	A	
16036	Incise burn scab, addl incis	1.50	NA	0.62	0.11	NA	NA	2.23	$80.72	ZZZ		A	
17000	Detroy benign/premal lesion	0.60	1.10	0.28	0.03	1.73	$62.62	0.91	$32.94	010	M	A	
17003	Destroy lesions, 2-14	0.15	0.24	0.07	0.01	0.40	$14.48	0.23	$8.33	ZZZ		A	
17004	Destroy lesions, 15 or more	2.79	2.56	1.30	0.12	5.47	$198.01	4.21	$152.40	010	M	A	
17106	Destruction of skin lesions	4.59	4.88	2.88	0.28	9.75	$352.94	7.75	$280.54	090	M	A	
17107	Destruction of skin lesions	9.16	6.92	5.28	0.53	16.61	$601.27	14.97	$541.90	090	M	A	
17108	Destruction of skin lesions	13.20	8.87	7.26	0.89	22.96	$831.13	21.35	$772.85	090	M	A+	
17110	Destruct lesion, 1-14	0.65	1.11	0.26	0.04	1.80	$65.16	0.95	$34.39	010	M	A	

Code	Description										
17111	Destruct lesion, 15 or more	0.92	1.13	0.41	0.04	2.09	$75.66	1.37	$49.59	010	M	A
17250	Chemical cautery, tissue	0.50	0.76	0.21	0.04	1.30	$47.06	0.75	$27.15	000	M	A
17260	Destruction of skin lesions	0.91	1.37	0.39	0.04	2.32	$83.98	1.34	$48.51	010	M	A
17261	Destruction of skin lesions	1.17	1.48	0.56	0.05	2.70	$97.74	1.78	$64.43	010	M	A
17262	Destruction of skin lesions	1.58	1.69	0.76	0.07	3.34	$120.91	2.41	$87.24	010	M	A
17263	Destruction of skin lesions	1.79	1.80	0.83	0.08	3.67	$132.85	2.70	$97.74	010	M	A
17264	Destruction of skin lesions	1.94	1.87	0.87	0.08	3.89	$140.81	2.89	$104.62	010	M	A
17266	Destruction of skin lesions	2.34	2.08	1.05	0.11	4.53	$163.98	3.50	$126.70	010	M	A
17270	Destruction of skin lesions	1.32	1.57	0.60	0.06	2.95	$106.79	1.98	$71.67	010	M	A
17271	Destruction of skin lesions	1.49	1.65	0.72	0.06	3.20	$115.84	2.27	$82.17	010	M	A
17272	Destruction of skin lesions	1.77	1.79	0.86	0.07	3.63	$131.40	2.70	$97.74	010	M	A
17273	Destruction of skin lesions	2.05	1.93	0.97	0.09	4.07	$147.33	3.11	$112.58	010	M	A
17274	Destruction of skin lesions	2.59	2.21	1.20	0.11	4.91	$177.74	3.90	$141.18	010	M	A
17276	Destruction of skin lesions	3.20	2.52	1.84	0.15	5.87	$212.49	5.19	$187.87	010	M	A
17280	Destruction of skin lesions	1.17	1.41	0.54	0.05	2.63	$95.20	1.76	$63.71	010	M	A
17281	Destruction of skin lesions	1.72	1.77	0.83	0.07	3.56	$128.87	2.62	$94.84	010	M	A
17282	Destruction of skin lesions	2.04	1.93	0.99	0.09	4.06	$146.97	3.12	$112.94	010	M	A
17283	Destruction of skin lesions	2.64	2.23	1.24	0.11	4.98	$180.27	3.99	$144.43	010	M	A
17284	Destruction of skin lesions	3.21	2.52	1.51	0.14	5.87	$212.49	4.86	$175.93	010	M	A
17286	Destruction of skin lesions	4.44	3.23	2.52	0.22	7.89	$285.61	7.18	$259.91	010	M	A
17304	Chemosurgery of skin lesion	7.60	7.76	3.74	0.31	15.67	$567.24	11.65	$421.72	000		A
17305	2nd stage chemosurgery	2.85	3.60	1.40	0.12	6.57	$237.83	4.37	$158.19	000		A
17306	3rd stage chemosurgery	2.85	3.64	1.41	0.12	6.61	$239.28	4.38	$158.55	000		A
17307	Followup skin lesion therapy	2.85	3.62	1.43	0.12	6.59	$238.55	4.40	$159.28	000		A
17310	Extensive skin chemosurgery	0.95	1.54	0.48	0.05	2.54	$91.95	1.48	$53.57	000		A
17340	Cryotherapy of skin	0.76	0.39	0.27	0.04	1.19	$43.08	1.07	$38.73	010	M	A
17360	Skin peel therapy	1.43	1.46	0.73	0.06	2.95	$106.79	2.22	$80.36	010	M	A
17380	Hair removal by electrolysis	0.00	0.00	0.00	0.00	0.00	$0.00	0.00	$0.00	000	M	A+

* **M** = multiple surgery adjustment applies
   Me = multiple endoscopy rules may apply
   B = bilateral surgery adjustment applies
   A = assistant-at-surgery restriction

A+ = assistant-at-surgery restriction unless medical necessity established with documentation
C = cosurgeons payable
C+ = cosurgeons payable if medical necessity established with documentation

T = team surgeons permitted
T+ = team surgeons payable if medical necessity established with documentation
S = indicates services that are not covered by Medicare.

139 CPT five-digit codes, two-digit numeric modifiers, and descriptions only are © 2001 American Medical Association

Medicare RBRVS: The Physicians' Guide

Relative value units

CPT Code and Modifier	Description	Work RVU	Non Facility Practice Expense RVU	Facility Practice Expense RVU	PLI RVU	Total Non Facility RVUs	Medicare Payment Non Facility	Total Facility RVUs	Medicare Payment Facility	Global Period	Payment Policy Indicators*
17999	Skin tissue procedure	0.00	0.00	0.00	0.00	0.00	$0.00	0.00	$0.00	YYY	M			T+
19000	Drainage of breast lesion	0.84	1.27	0.30	0.07	2.18	$78.91	1.21	$43.80	000	M	B	A	C+
19001	Drain breast lesion add-on	0.42	0.86	0.15	0.03	1.31	$47.42	0.60	$21.72	ZZZ	M	B	A	
19020	Incision of breast lesion	3.57	7.13	3.51	0.35	11.05	$400.00	7.43	$268.96	090	M	B	A	
19030	Injection for breast x-ray	1.53	3.70	0.54	0.07	5.30	$191.86	2.14	$77.47	000	M	B	A	
19100	Bx breast percut w/o image	1.27	1.50	0.45	0.10	2.87	$103.89	1.82	$65.88	000	M	B	A	
19101	Biopsy of breast, open	3.18	5.27	1.97	0.20	8.65	$313.12	5.35	$193.67	010	M	B	A	
19102	Bx breast percut w/image	2.00	5.13	0.71	0.13	7.26	$262.81	2.84	$102.81	000	M	B	A	
19103	Bx breast percut w/device	3.70	12.73	1.31	0.16	16.59	$600.54	5.17	$187.15	000	M	B	A	
19110	Nipple exploration	4.30	9.79	4.56	0.44	14.53	$525.97	9.30	$336.65	090	M	B	A	
19112	Excise breast duct fistula	3.67	10.91	3.19	0.38	14.96	$541.54	7.24	$262.08	090	M	B	A+	
19120	Removal of breast lesion	5.56	5.18	3.20	0.56	11.30	$409.05	9.32	$337.38	090	M	B	A	
19125	Excision, breast lesion	6.06	5.36	3.36	0.61	12.03	$435.48	10.03	$363.08	090	M	B	A	C+
19126	Excision, addl breast lesion	2.93	NA	1.06	0.30	NA	NA	4.29	$155.29	ZZZ			A	C+
19140	Removal of breast tissue	5.14	10.26	3.79	0.52	15.92	$576.29	9.45	$342.08	090	M	B	A	
19160	Removal of breast tissue	5.99	NA	4.62	0.61	NA	NA	11.22	$406.16	090	M	B	A+	
19162	Remove breast tissue, nodes	13.53	NA	8.07	1.38	NA	NA	22.98	$831.86	090	M	B		C+
19180	Removal of breast	8.80	NA	6.08	0.88	NA	NA	15.76	$570.50	090	M	B		C+
19182	Removal of breast	7.73	NA	5.06	0.79	NA	NA	13.58	$491.59	090	M	B		C+
19200	Removal of breast	15.49	NA	9.33	1.51	NA	NA	26.33	$953.12	090	M	B		C+
19220	Removal of breast	15.72	NA	9.52	1.56	NA	NA	26.80	$970.14	090	M	B		C+
19240	Removal of breast	16.00	NA	8.94	1.62	NA	NA	26.56	$961.45	090	M	B		C+
19260	Removal of chest wall lesion	15.44	NA	9.12	1.64	NA	NA	26.20	$948.42	090	M			C+
19271	Revision of chest wall	18.90	NA	11.13	2.27	NA	NA	32.30	$1,169.23	090	M			C+
19272	Extensive chest wall surgery	21.55	NA	12.36	2.54	NA	NA	36.45	$1,319.46	090	M			C+
19290	Place needle wire, breast	1.27	2.95	0.45	0.06	4.28	$154.93	1.78	$64.43	000	M	B	A	
19291	Place needle wire, breast	0.63	1.74	0.22	0.03	2.40	$86.88	0.88	$31.86	ZZZ			A+	

Code	Description											
19295	Place breast clip, percut	0.00	2.83	2.83	0.01	2.84	$102.81	2.84	$102.81	ZZZ	M	B	A+
19316	Suspension of breast	10.69	NA	8.00	1.15	NA	NA	19.84	$718.19	090	M	B	A	C+
19318	Reduction of large breast	15.62	NA	10.64	1.69	NA	NA	27.95	$1,011.77	090	M	B	A	C+
19324	Enlarge breast	5.85	NA	4.41	0.63	NA	NA	10.89	$394.21	090	M	B	A+	
19325	Enlarge breast with implant	8.45	NA	7.00	0.90	NA	NA	16.35	$591.86	090	M	B	A+	
19328	Removal of breast implant	5.68	NA	4.73	0.61	NA	NA	11.02	$398.92	090	M	B	A	
19330	Removal of implant material	7.59	NA	5.41	0.81	NA	NA	13.81	$499.91	090	M	B	A	
19340	Immediate breast prosthesis	6.33	NA	3.30	0.68	NA	NA	10.31	$373.21	ZZZ	M	B	A	C+
19342	Delayed breast prosthesis	11.20	NA	8.15	1.21	NA	NA	20.56	$744.26	090	M	B	A+	C+
19350	Breast reconstruction	8.92	14.55	7.09	0.95	24.42	$883.98	16.96	$613.94	090	M	B	A	
19355	Correct inverted nipple(s)	7.57	12.42	5.93	0.80	20.79	$752.58	14.30	$517.65	090	M	B	A+	
19357	Breast reconstruction	18.16	NA	14.40	1.96	NA	NA	34.52	$1,249.60	090	M	B	A	C+
19361	Breast reconstruction	19.26	NA	12.45	2.08	NA	NA	33.79	$1,223.17	090	M	B	A	C+
19364	Breast reconstruction	41.00	NA	25.45	3.91	NA	NA	70.36	$2,546.98	090	M	B	A	C+
19366	Breast reconstruction	21.28	NA	12.02	2.27	NA	NA	35.57	$1,287.61	090	M	B	A	C+
19367	Breast reconstruction	25.73	NA	15.77	2.78	NA	NA	44.28	$1,602.90	090	M	B	A	C+
19368	Breast reconstruction	32.42	NA	19.04	3.51	NA	NA	54.97	$1,989.87	090	M	B	A	C+
19369	Breast reconstruction	29.82	NA	18.29	3.24	NA	NA	51.35	$1,858.83	090	M	B	A	C+
19370	Surgery of breast capsule	8.05	NA	6.39	0.86	NA	NA	15.30	$553.85	090	M	B	A	
19371	Removal of breast capsule	9.35	NA	7.46	1.01	NA	NA	17.82	$645.07	090	M	B	A	
19380	Revise breast reconstruction	9.14	NA	7.35	0.98	NA	NA	17.47	$632.40	090	M	B	A	
19396	Design custom breast implant	2.17	7.08	0.87	0.23	9.48	$343.17	3.27	$118.37	000	M	B	A+	
19499	Breast surgery procedure	0.00	0.00	0.00	0.00	0.00	$0.00	0.00	$0.00	YYY	M	B	A+	C+	T+

Surgery: Musculoskeletal system

Code	Description											
20000	Incision of abscess	2.12	2.23	1.20	0.17	4.52	$163.62	3.49	$126.34	010	M	B	A
20005	Incision of deep abscess	3.42	3.07	2.22	0.34	6.83	$247.24	5.98	$216.47	010	M	B	A
20100	Explore wound, neck	10.08	6.49	4.12	0.99	17.56	$635.66	15.19	$549.87	010	M	B	
20101	Explore wound, chest	3.22	3.03	1.64	0.24	6.49	$234.93	5.10	$184.62	010	M	B	A

*M = multiple surgery adjustment applies
Me = multiple endoscopy rules may apply
B = bilateral surgery adjustment applies
A = assistant-at-surgery restriction

A+ = assistant-at-surgery restriction unless medical necessity established with documentation
C = cosurgeons payable
C+ = cosurgeons payable if medical necessity established with documentation

T = team surgeons permitted
T+ = team surgeons payable if medical necessity established with documentation
§ = indicates services that are not covered by Medicare.

141 CPT five-digit codes, two-digit numeric modifiers, and descriptions only are © 2001 American Medical Association

Medicare RBRVS: The Physicians' Guide

Relative value units

CPT Code and Modifier	Description	Work RVU	Non Facility Practice Expense RVU	Facility Practice Expense RVU	PLI RVU	Total Non Facility RVUs	Medicare Payment Non Facility	Total Facility RVUs	Medicare Payment Facility	Global Period	Payment Policy Indicators*		
20102	Explore wound, abdomen	3.94	3.43	1.85	0.35	7.72	$279.46	6.14	$222.26	010	M		A
20103	Explore wound, extremity	5.30	4.41	3.01	0.57	10.28	$372.13	8.88	$321.45	010	M		A+
20150	Excise epiphyseal bar	13.69	NA	9.72	0.96	NA	NA	24.37	$882.17	090	M	B	C+
20200	Muscle biopsy	1.46	1.72	0.62	0.17	3.35	$121.27	2.25	$81.45	000	M		A
20205	Deep muscle biopsy	2.35	4.04	0.98	0.23	6.62	$239.64	3.56	$128.87	000	M		A
20206	Needle biopsy, muscle	0.99	3.27	0.36	0.06	4.32	$156.38	1.41	$51.04	000	M		A
20220	Bone biopsy, trocar/needle	1.27	4.96	2.98	0.06	6.29	$227.69	4.31	$156.02	000	M		A
20225	Bone biopsy, trocar/needle	1.87	4.47	3.06	0.11	6.45	$233.48	5.04	$182.44	000	M		A
20240	Bone biopsy, excisional	3.23	NA	4.15	0.33	NA	NA	7.71	$279.10	010	M		A
20245	Bone biopsy, excisional	7.78	NA	6.91	0.44	NA	NA	15.13	$547.69	010	M		A
20250	Open bone biopsy	5.03	NA	4.37	0.50	NA	NA	9.90	$358.37	010	M		A
20251	Open bone biopsy	5.56	NA	4.86	0.79	NA	NA	11.21	$405.79	010	M		A
20500	Injection of sinus tract	1.23	5.34	3.91	0.10	6.67	$241.45	5.24	$189.68	010	M		A
20501	Inject sinus tract for x-ray	0.76	3.32	0.27	0.03	4.11	$148.78	1.06	$38.37	000	M		A
20520	Removal of foreign body	1.85	5.62	3.62	0.17	7.64	$276.56	5.64	$204.16	010	M		A
20525	Removal of foreign body	3.50	7.26	4.40	0.40	11.16	$403.98	8.30	$300.45	010	M		A
20526	Ther injection carpal tunnel	0.86	0.78	0.39	0.06	1.70	$61.54	1.31	$47.42	000	M		A
20550	Inject tendon/ligament/cyst	0.86	0.85	0.28	0.06	1.77	$64.07	1.20	$43.44	000	M		A
20551	Inject tendon origin/insert	0.86	0.78	0.39	0.06	1.70	$61.54	1.31	$47.42	000	M		A
20552	Inject trigger point, 1 or 2	0.86	0.78	0.39	0.06	1.70	$61.54	1.31	$47.42	000	M		A
20553	Inject trigger points, > 3	0.86	0.78	0.39	0.06	1.70	$61.54	1.31	$47.42	000	M		A
20600	Drain/inject, joint/bursa	0.66	0.67	0.37	0.06	1.39	$50.32	1.09	$39.46	000	M	B	A
20605	Drain/inject, joint/bursa	0.68	0.78	0.38	0.06	1.52	$55.02	1.12	$40.54	000	M	B	A
20610	Drain/inject, joint/bursa	0.79	0.96	0.44	0.08	1.83	$66.24	1.31	$47.42	000	M	B	A
20615	Treatment of bone cyst	2.28	4.89	2.52	0.19	7.36	$266.43	4.99	$180.63	010	M		A
20650	Insert and remove bone pin	2.23	5.06	3.19	0.28	7.57	$274.03	5.70	$206.34	010	M		A	C+
20660	Apply, remove fixation device	2.51	NA	1.49	0.48	NA	NA	4.48	$162.17	000	M		A

Code	Description									
20661	Application of head brace	4.89	NA	6.74	0.92	NA	12.55	$454.30	090	M		A	
20662	Application of pelvis brace	6.07	NA	5.12	0.81	NA	12.00	$434.39	090	M		A+	
20663	Application of thigh brace	5.43	NA	4.94	0.77	NA	11.14	$403.26	090	M		A+	
20664	Halo brace application	8.06	NA	8.55	1.49	NA	18.10	$655.21	090	M		A	
20665	Removal of fixation device	1.31	2.33	1.25	0.17	3.81	2.73	$98.82	010	M		A+	
20670	Removal of support implant	1.74	5.73	3.42	0.23	7.70	5.39	$195.11	010	M		A	
20680	Removal of support implant	3.35	5.04	5.04	0.46	8.85	8.85	$320.36	090	M		A+	
20690	Apply bone fixation device	3.52	NA	1.91	0.47	NA	5.90	$213.58	090	M		A	
20692	Apply bone fixation device	6.41	NA	3.57	0.60	NA	10.58	$382.99	090	M			C+
20693	Adjust bone fixation device	5.86	NA	12.98	0.85	NA	19.69	$712.76	090	M		A	
20694	Remove bone fixation device	4.16	8.96	6.30	0.57	13.69	11.03	$399.28	090	M		A	
20802	Replantation, arm, complete	41.15	NA	28.95	5.81	NA	75.91	$2,747.88	090	M	B		C+
20805	Replant, forearm, complete	50.00	NA	38.72	3.95	NA	92.67	$3,354.58	090	M	B		C+
20808	Replantation hand, complete	61.65	NA	56.41	6.49	NA	124.55	$4,508.61	090	M	B		C+
20816	Replantation digit, complete	30.94	NA	49.50	3.01	NA	83.45	$3,020.82	090	M			C+
20822	Replantation digit, complete	25.59	NA	45.97	3.07	NA	74.63	$2,701.55	090	M			C+
20824	Replantation thumb, complete	30.94	NA	49.10	3.48	NA	83.52	$3,023.36	090	M	B		C+
20827	Replantation thumb, complete	26.41	NA	45.65	3.21	NA	75.27	$2,724.71	090	M	B		C+
20838	Replantation foot, complete	41.41	NA	25.82	5.85	NA	73.08	$2,645.44	090	M	B		C+
20900	Removal of bone for graft	5.58	5.97	5.97	0.77	12.32	12.32	$445.97	090	M			C+
20902	Removal of bone for graft	7.55	NA	8.91	1.06	NA	17.52	$634.21	090	M			C+
20910	Remove cartilage for graft	5.34	9.09	6.94	0.50	14.93	12.78	$462.63	090	M		A+	
20912	Remove cartilage for graft	6.35	NA	7.68	0.55	NA	14.58	$527.78	090	M		A+	
20920	Removal of fascia for graft	5.31	NA	5.44	0.54	NA	11.29	$408.69	090	M		A	
20922	Removal of fascia for graft	6.61	8.50	6.28	0.88	15.99	13.77	$498.46	090	M			C+
20924	Removal of tendon for graft	6.48	NA	7.03	0.82	NA	14.33	$518.73	090	M			C+
20926	Removal of tissue for graft	5.53	NA	6.54	0.73	NA	12.80	$463.35	090	M		A	
20931	Spinal bone allograft	1.81	NA	0.98	0.34	NA	3.13	$113.30	ZZZ		B	A	C+

*M = multiple surgery adjustment applies
Me = multiple endoscopy rules may apply
B = bilateral surgery adjustment applies
A = assistant-at-surgery restriction

A+ = assistant-at-surgery restriction unless medical necessity established with documentation
C = cosurgeons payable
C+ = cosurgeons payable if medical necessity established with documentation

T = team surgeons permitted
T+ = team surgeons payable if medical necessity established with documentation
S = indicates services that are not covered by Medicare.

143 CPT five-digit codes, two-digit numeric modifiers, and descriptions only are © 2001 American Medical Association

Medicare RBRVS: The Physicians' Guide

Relative value units

CPT Code and Modifier	Description	Work RVU	Non Facility Practice Expense RVU	Facility Practice Expense RVU	PLI RVU	Total Non Facility RVUs	Medicare Payment Non Facility	Total Facility RVUs	Medicare Payment Facility	Global Period	Payment Policy Indicators*			
20937	Spinal bone autograft	2.79	NA	1.54	0.43	NA	NA	4.76	$172.31	ZZZ	M	B		C+
20938	Spinal bone autograft	3.02	NA	1.64	0.52	NA	NA	5.18	$187.51	ZZZ	M	B		C+
20950	Fluid pressure, muscle	1.26	NA	2.15	0.16	NA	NA	3.57	$129.23	000	M		A+	
20955	Fibula bone graft, microvasc	39.21	NA	30.52	4.35	NA	NA	74.08	$2,681.64	090	M			C+
20956	Iliac bone graft, microvasc	39.27	NA	28.18	5.77	NA	NA	73.22	$2,650.51	090	M			C+
20957	Mt bone graft, microvasc	40.65	NA	21.71	5.74	NA	NA	68.10	$2,465.17	090	M			C+
20962	Other bone graft, microvasc	39.27	NA	28.54	5.19	NA	NA	73.00	$2,642.54	090	M			C+
20969	Bone/skin graft, microvasc	43.92	NA	33.31	4.34	NA	NA	81.57	$2,952.77	090	M			C+
20970	Bone/skin graft, iliac crest	43.06	NA	30.08	4.64	NA	NA	77.78	$2,815.57	090	M			C+
20972	Bone/skin graft, metatarsal	42.99	NA	18.23	6.07	NA	NA	67.29	$2,435.84	090	M			
20973	Bone/skin graft, great toe	45.76	NA	30.52	4.65	NA	NA	80.93	$2,929.60	090	M			C+
20974	Electrical bone stimulation	0.62	0.47	0.34	0.09	1.18	$42.72	1.05	$38.01	000	M		A	
20975	Electrical bone stimulation	2.60	NA	1.42	0.42	NA	NA	4.44	$160.72	000	M			C+
20979	Us bone stimulation	0.62	0.58	0.25	0.04	1.24	$44.89	0.91	$32.94	000	M		A	
20999	Musculoskeletal surgery	0.00	0.00	0.00	0.00	0.00	$0.00	0.00	$0.00	YYY	M		A+	T+
21010	Incision of jaw joint	10.14	NA	7.24	0.54	NA	NA	17.92	$648.69	090	M	B	A+	
21015	Resection of facial tumor	5.29	NA	7.38	0.52	NA	NA	13.19	$477.47	090	M		A	
21025	Excision of bone, lower jaw	10.06	7.40	7.00	0.79	18.25	$660.64	17.85	$646.16	090	M		A	
21026	Excision of facial bone(s)	4.85	5.23	5.12	0.40	10.48	$379.37	10.37	$375.39	090	M		A	
21029	Contour of face bone lesion	7.71	7.18	6.73	0.74	15.63	$565.79	15.18	$549.50	090	M		A+	
21030	Removal of face bone lesion	6.46	5.47	4.94	0.60	12.53	$453.58	12.00	$434.39	090	M		A	
21031	Remove exostosis, mandible	3.24	3.39	2.19	0.28	6.91	$250.14	5.71	$206.70	090	M		A	
21032	Remove exostosis, maxilla	3.24	3.38	2.47	0.27	6.89	$249.41	5.98	$216.47	090	M		A	
21034	Removal of face bone lesion	16.17	10.59	10.59	1.37	28.13	$1,018.28	28.13	$1,018.28	090	M			C+
21040	Removal of jaw bone lesion	2.11	3.03	1.81	0.19	5.33	$192.94	4.11	$148.78	090	M		A	
21041	Removal of jaw bone lesion	6.71	5.68	4.46	0.56	12.95	$468.78	11.73	$424.62	090	M		A	
21044	Removal of jaw bone lesion	11.86	NA	8.33	0.87	NA	NA	21.06	$762.36	090	M			C+

Code	Description										
21045	Extensive jaw surgery	16.17	NA	10.63	1.20	NA	NA	28.00	$1,013.58	090	M			C+
21050	Removal of jaw joint	10.77	NA	11.93	0.84	NA	NA	23.54	$852.13	090	M	B	A+
21060	Remove jaw joint cartilage	10.23	NA	10.59	1.16	NA	NA	21.98	$795.66	090	M	B		C+
21070	Remove coronoid process	8.20	NA	6.36	0.67	NA	NA	15.23	$551.31	090	M	B	A+
21076	Prepare face/oral prosthesis	13.42	9.87	7.41	1.36	24.65	$892.31	22.19	$803.26	010	M		A+
21077	Prepare face/oral prosthesis	33.75	24.83	18.64	3.43	62.01	$2,244.71	55.82	$2,020.64	090	M	B	A+
21079	Prepare face/oral prosthesis	22.34	17.55	12.90	1.59	41.48	$1,501.54	36.83	$1,333.22	090	M		A
21080	Prepare face/oral prosthesis	25.10	19.72	14.49	2.55	47.37	$1,714.76	42.14	$1,525.43	090	M		A
21081	Prepare face/oral prosthesis	22.88	17.97	13.21	1.87	42.72	$1,546.43	37.96	$1,374.12	090	M		A+
21082	Prepare face/oral prosthesis	20.87	15.35	11.53	1.46	37.68	$1,363.99	33.86	$1,225.70	090	M		A+
21083	Prepare face/oral prosthesis	19.30	15.16	11.14	1.96	36.42	$1,318.37	32.40	$1,172.85	090	M		A+
21084	Prepare face/oral prosthesis	22.51	17.68	12.99	1.57	41.76	$1,511.68	37.07	$1,341.90	090	M		A+
21085	Prepare face/oral prosthesis	9.00	6.62	4.97	0.65	16.27	$588.96	14.62	$529.23	010	M		A+
21086	Prepare face/oral prosthesis	24.92	19.58	14.39	1.86	46.36	$1,678.19	41.17	$1,490.32	090	M	B	A+
21087	Prepare face/oral prosthesis	24.92	18.33	13.76	2.22	45.47	$1,645.98	40.90	$1,480.55	090	M		A+
21088	Prepare face/oral prosthesis	0.00	0.00	0.00	0.00	0.00	$0.00	0.00	$0.00	090	M		A+
21089	Prepare face/oral prosthesis	0.00	0.00	0.00	0.00	0.00	$0.00	0.00	$0.00	090			A
21100	Maxillofacial fixation	4.22	5.66	3.70	0.18	10.06	$364.16	8.10	$293.21	090	M		A+
21110	Interdental fixation	5.21	5.25	4.48	0.28	10.74	$388.78	9.97	$360.91	090	M		A
21116	Injection, jaw joint x-ray	0.81	7.88	0.30	0.05	8.74	$316.38	1.16	$41.99	000	M		A
21120	Reconstruction of chin	4.93	7.96	4.98	0.29	13.18	$477.11	10.20	$369.23	090	M		A	C+
21121	Reconstruction of chin	7.64	7.68	6.65	0.56	15.88	$574.84	14.85	$537.56	090	M		
21122	Reconstruction of chin	8.52	NA	7.95	0.59	NA	NA	17.06	$617.56	090	M		
21123	Reconstruction of chin	11.16	NA	7.68	1.16	NA	NA	20.00	$723.98	090	M			C+
21125	Augmentation, lower jaw bone	10.62	9.56	7.84	0.72	20.90	$756.56	19.18	$694.30	090	M		
21127	Augmentation, lower jaw bone	11.12	10.66	7.33	0.76	22.54	$815.93	19.21	$695.39	090	M			C+
21137	Reduction of forehead	9.82	NA	8.20	0.53	NA	NA	18.55	$671.50	090	M		
21138	Reduction of forehead	12.19	NA	8.82	1.47	NA	NA	22.48	$813.76	090	M			C+

* **M** = multiple surgery adjustment applies
Me = multiple endoscopy rules may apply
B = bilateral surgery adjustment applies
A = assistant-at-surgery restriction

A+ = assistant-at-surgery restriction unless medical necessity established with documentation
C = cosurgeons payable
C+ = cosurgeons payable if medical necessity established with documentation

T = team surgeons permitted
T+ = team surgeons payable if medical necessity established with documentation
$ = indicates services that are not covered by Medicare.

145 CPT five-digit codes, two-digit numeric modifiers, and descriptions only are © 2001 American Medical Association

Medicare RBRVS: The Physicians' Guide

Relative value units

CPT Code and Modifier	Description	Work RVU	Non Facility Practice Expense RVU	Facility Practice Expense RVU	PLI RVU	Total Non Facility RVUs	Medicare Payment Non Facility	Total Facility RVUs	Medicare Payment Facility	Global Period	Payment Policy Indicators*	
21139	Reduction of forehead	14.61	NA	8.23	1.02	NA	NA	23.86	$863.71	090	M	C+
21141	Reconstruct midface, lefort	18.10	NA	10.69	1.63	NA	NA	30.42	$1,101.18	090	M	C+
21142	Reconstruct midface, lefort	18.81	NA	13.80	1.16	NA	NA	33.77	$1,222.45	090	M	C+
21143	Reconstruct midface, lefort	19.58	NA	11.21	0.90	NA	NA	31.69	$1,147.15	090	M	C+
21145	Reconstruct midface, lefort	19.94	NA	11.69	2.09	NA	NA	33.72	$1,220.64	090	M	
21146	Reconstruct midface, lefort	20.71	NA	11.61	2.13	NA	NA	34.45	$1,247.06	090	M	
21147	Reconstruct midface, lefort	21.77	NA	12.07	1.52	NA	NA	35.36	$1,280.00	090	M	
21150	Reconstruct midface, lefort	25.24	NA	17.20	1.09	NA	NA	43.53	$1,575.75	090	M	
21151	Reconstruct midface, lefort	28.30	NA	21.35	1.98	NA	NA	51.63	$1,868.96	090	M	C+
21154	Reconstruct midface, lefort	30.52	NA	21.03	4.86	NA	NA	56.41	$2,042.00	090	M	
21155	Reconstruct midface, lefort	34.45	NA	23.20	5.48	NA	NA	63.13	$2,285.26	090	M	C+
21159	Reconstruct midface, lefort	42.38	NA	21.72	6.74	NA	NA	70.84	$2,564.35	090	M	
21160	Reconstruct midface, lefort	46.44	NA	30.39	4.39	NA	NA	81.22	$2,940.10	090	M	C+
21172	Reconstruct orbit/forehead	27.80	NA	16.39	1.91	NA	NA	46.10	$1,668.78	090	M	
21175	Reconstruct orbit/forehead	33.17	NA	19.79	5.16	NA	NA	58.12	$2,103.90	090	M	C+
21179	Reconstruct entire forehead	22.25	NA	18.94	2.48	NA	NA	43.67	$1,580.82	090	M	
21180	Reconstruct entire forehead	25.19	NA	18.33	2.15	NA	NA	45.67	$1,653.22	090	M	C+
21181	Contour cranial bone lesion	9.90	NA	8.46	0.97	NA	NA	19.33	$699.73	090	M	A+
21182	Reconstruct cranial bone	32.19	NA	21.97	2.53	NA	NA	56.69	$2,052.13	090	M	C+
21183	Reconstruct cranial bone	35.31	NA	22.93	2.75	NA	NA	60.99	$2,207.79	090	M	C+
21184	Reconstruct cranial bone	38.24	NA	19.54	4.12	NA	NA	61.90	$2,240.73	090	M	
21188	Reconstruction of midface	22.46	NA	15.86	1.85	NA	NA	40.17	$1,454.12	090	M	
21193	Reconst lwr jaw w/o graft	17.15	NA	10.77	1.53	NA	NA	29.45	$1,066.07	090	M	C+
21194	Reconst lwr jaw w/graft	19.84	NA	12.44	1.39	NA	NA	33.67	$1,218.83	090	M	
21195	Reconst lwr jaw w/o fixation	17.24	NA	12.36	1.20	NA	NA	30.80	$1,114.94	090	M	
21196	Reconst lwr jaw w/fixation	18.91	NA	12.83	1.62	NA	NA	33.36	$1,207.61	090	M	C+
21198	Reconstr lwr jaw segment	14.16	NA	12.30	1.05	NA	NA	27.51	$995.84	090	M	C+

Code	Description									
21199	Reconstr lwr jaw w/advance	16.00	NA	10.85	NA	NA	28.11	$1,017.56	090	M		C+
21206	Reconstruct upper jaw bone	14.10	NA	9.39	1.26	NA	24.50	$886.88	090	M		C+
21208	Augmentation of facial bones	10.23	8.95	8.62	1.01	$727.60	19.77	$715.66	090	M		A+
21209	Reduction of facial bones	6.72	8.05	6.54	0.92	$556.38	13.86	$501.72	090	M		
21210	Face bone graft	10.23	8.82	8.28	0.60	$721.45	19.39	$701.90	090	M		A
21215	Lower jaw bone graft	10.77	8.95	7.48	0.88	$751.50	19.29	$698.28	090	M		A	C+
21230	Rib cartilage graft	10.77	NA	10.85	1.04	NA	22.58	$817.38	090	M		A+
21235	Ear cartilage graft	6.72	11.90	8.36	0.96	$692.85	15.60	$564.71	090	M		A
21240	Reconstruction of jaw joint	14.05	NA	11.79	0.52	NA	26.99	$977.02	090	M	B		C+
21242	Reconstruction of jaw joint	12.95	NA	10.85	1.15	NA	25.20	$912.22	090	M	B		C+
21243	Reconstruction of jaw joint	20.79	NA	13.97	1.40	NA	36.61	$1,325.25	090	M	B		C+
21244	Reconstruction of lower jaw	11.86	NA	9.56	1.85	NA	22.37	$809.78	090	M			C+
21245	Reconstruction of jaw	11.86	24.85	10.25	0.95	$1,360.73	22.99	$832.22	090	M		
21246	Reconstruction of jaw	12.47	10.20	10.20	0.88	$864.44	23.88	$864.44	090	M		
21247	Reconstruct lower jaw bone	22.63	NA	20.17	1.21	NA	45.01	$1,629.33	090	M			C+
21248	Reconstruction of jaw	11.48	8.91	7.86	2.21	$774.66	20.35	$736.65	090	M		A
21249	Reconstruction of jaw	17.52	11.44	10.35	1.01	$1,098.65	29.26	$1,059.19	090	M		A+
21255	Reconstruct lower jaw bone	16.72	NA	13.16	1.39	NA	31.01	$1,122.54	090	M			C+
21256	Reconstruction of orbit	16.19	NA	13.87	1.13	NA	31.10	$1,125.80	090	M			C+
21260	Revise eye sockets	16.52	NA	13.54	1.04	NA	31.31	$1,133.40	090	M			C+
21261	Revise eye sockets	31.49	NA	20.04	1.25	NA	53.73	$1,944.98	090	M			C+
21263	Revise eye sockets	28.42	NA	15.09	2.20	NA	45.67	$1,653.22	090	M			C+
21267	Revise eye sockets	18.90	NA	14.75	2.16	NA	35.00	$1,266.97	090	M			C+
21268	Revise eye sockets	24.48	NA	15.15	1.35	NA	40.42	$1,463.17	090	M			C+
21270	Augmentation, cheek bone	10.23	10.39	9.99	0.79	$772.85	20.95	$758.37	090	M			C+
21275	Revision, orbitofacial bones	11.24	NA	11.02	0.73	NA	23.29	$843.08	090	M			C+
21280	Revision of eyelid	6.03	NA	6.27	1.03	NA	12.57	$455.02	090	M	B	A+
21282	Revision of eyelid	3.49	NA	5.38	0.27	NA	9.08	$328.69	090	M	B	A

* **M** = multiple surgery adjustment applies
Me = multiple endoscopy rules may apply
B = bilateral surgery adjustment applies
A = assistant-at-surgery restriction

A+ = assistant-at-surgery restriction unless medical necessity established with documentation
C = cosurgeons payable
C+ = cosurgeons payable if medical necessity established with documentation

T = team surgeons permitted
T+ = team surgeons payable if medical necessity established with documentation
S = indicates services that are not covered by Medicare.

CPT five-digit codes, two-digit numeric modifiers, and descriptions only are © 2001 American Medical Association

Medicare RBRVS: The Physicians' Guide

Relative value units

CPT Code and Modifier	Description	Work RVU	Non Facility Practice Expense RVU	Facility Practice Expense RVU	PLI RVU	Total Non Facility RVUs	Medicare Payment Non Facility	Total Facility RVUs	Medicare Payment Facility	Global Period	Payment Policy Indicators*	
21295	Revision of jaw muscle/bone	1.53	NA	4.34	0.13	NA	NA	6.00	$217.20	090	M	A+
21296	Revision of jaw muscle/bone	4.25	NA	4.09	0.30	NA	NA	8.64	$312.76	090	M	A+
21299	Cranio/maxillofacial surgery	0.00	0.00	0.00	0.00	0.00	$0.00	0.00	$0.00	YYY	M	A+ C+ T+
21300	Treatment of skull fracture	0.72	2.77	0.30	0.09	3.58	$129.59	1.11	$40.18	000	M	A+
21310	Treatment of nose fracture	0.58	2.70	0.15	0.05	3.33	$120.54	0.78	$28.24	000	M	A
21315	Treatment of nose fracture	1.51	3.49	1.27	0.12	5.12	$185.34	2.90	$104.98	010	M	A
21320	Treatment of nose fracture	1.85	4.96	2.10	0.15	6.96	$251.95	4.10	$148.42	010	M	A
21325	Treatment of nose fracture	3.77	NA	3.73	0.31	NA	NA	7.81	$282.72	090	M	A+
21330	Treatment of nose fracture	5.38	NA	5.67	0.48	NA	NA	11.53	$417.38	090	M	A+
21335	Treatment of nose fracture	8.61	NA	7.34	0.64	NA	NA	16.59	$600.54	090	M	A
21336	Treat nasal septal fracture	5.72	NA	5.74	0.45	NA	NA	11.91	$431.13	090	M	A+
21337	Treat nasal septal fracture	2.70	5.24	3.42	0.22	8.16	$295.39	6.34	$229.50	090	M	A+
21338	Treat nasoethmoid fracture	6.46	NA	5.75	0.53	NA	NA	12.74	$461.18	090	M	A+
21339	Treat nasoethmoid fracture	8.09	NA	6.97	0.76	NA	NA	15.82	$572.67	090	M	C+
21340	Treatment of nose fracture	10.77	NA	8.78	0.85	NA	NA	20.40	$738.46	090	M	A+
21343	Treatment of sinus fracture	12.95	NA	9.48	1.06	NA	NA	23.49	$850.32	090	M	C+
21344	Treatment of sinus fracture	19.72	NA	13.82	1.72	NA	NA	35.26	$1,276.38	090	M	C
21345	Treat nose/jaw fracture	8.16	10.36	7.91	0.60	19.12	$692.13	16.67	$603.44	090	M	A+
21346	Treat nose/jaw fracture	10.61	NA	10.12	0.85	NA	NA	21.58	$781.18	090	M	A
21347	Treat nose/jaw fracture	12.69	NA	9.68	1.14	NA	NA	23.51	$851.04	090	M	C+
21348	Treat nose/jaw fracture	16.69	NA	11.57	1.50	NA	NA	29.76	$1,077.29	090	M	C
21355	Treat cheek bone fracture	3.77	3.89	2.54	0.29	7.95	$287.78	6.60	$238.91	010	M	A+
21356	Treat cheek bone fracture	4.15	NA	3.31	0.36	NA	NA	7.82	$283.08	010	M	A+
21360	Treat cheek bone fracture	6.46	NA	5.74	0.52	NA	NA	12.72	$460.45	090	M	
21365	Treat cheek bone fracture	14.95	NA	11.72	1.30	NA	NA	27.97	$1,012.49	090	M	C+
21366	Treat cheek bone fracture	17.77	NA	14.28	1.41	NA	NA	33.46	$1,211.23	090	M	C
21385	Treat eye socket fracture	9.16	NA	8.04	0.64	NA	NA	17.84	$645.79	090	M	C+

Code	Description									
21386	Treat eye socket fracture	9.16	NA	8.43	0.76	NA	NA	18.35	$664.26	090	M	
21387	Treat eye socket fracture	9.70	NA	8.55	0.78	NA	NA	19.03	$688.87	090	M	
21390	Treat eye socket fracture	10.13	NA	8.73	0.70	NA	NA	19.56	$708.06	090	M	C+
21395	Treat eye socket fracture	12.68	NA	9.24	1.09	NA	NA	23.01	$832.94	090	M	C+
21400	Treat eye socket fracture	1.40	3.29	1.05	0.12	4.81	$174.12	2.57	$93.03	090	M	A+
21401	Treat eye socket fracture	3.26	4.34	3.65	0.34	7.94	$287.42	7.25	$262.44	090	M	
21406	Treat eye socket fracture	7.01	NA	7.20	0.59	NA	NA	14.80	$535.75	090	M	C+
21407	Treat eye socket fracture	8.61	NA	7.99	0.67	NA	NA	17.27	$625.16	090	M	C+
21408	Treat eye socket fracture	12.38	NA	10.29	1.24	NA	NA	23.91	$865.52	090	M	C
21421	Treat mouth roof fracture	5.14	7.23	6.84	0.42	12.79	$462.99	12.40	$448.87	090	M	A+
21422	Treat mouth roof fracture	8.32	NA	7.93	0.69	NA	NA	16.94	$613.21	090	M	C+
21423	Treat mouth roof fracture	10.40	NA	8.63	0.95	NA	NA	19.98	$723.26	090	M	C
21431	Treat craniofacial fracture	7.05	NA	8.44	0.58	NA	NA	16.07	$581.72	090	M	
21432	Treat craniofacial fracture	8.61	NA	8.06	0.55	NA	NA	17.22	$623.35	090	M	
21433	Treat craniofacial fracture	25.35	NA	17.29	2.46	NA	NA	45.10	$1,632.58	090	M	C+
21435	Treat craniofacial fracture	17.25	NA	12.97	1.66	NA	NA	31.88	$1,154.03	090	M	
21436	Treat craniofacial fracture	28.04	NA	16.02	2.32	NA	NA	46.38	$1,678.92	090	M	C
21440	Treat dental ridge fracture	2.70	5.44	3.73	0.22	8.36	$302.63	6.65	$240.72	090	M	A+
21445	Treat dental ridge fracture	5.38	7.14	5.04	0.55	13.07	$473.12	10.97	$397.11	090	M	
21450	Treat lower jaw fracture	2.97	6.45	2.90	0.23	9.65	$349.32	6.10	$220.82	090	M	A+
21451	Treat lower jaw fracture	4.87	6.46	6.11	0.39	11.72	$424.25	11.37	$411.58	090	M	A+
21452	Treat lower jaw fracture	1.98	13.44	4.35	0.14	15.56	$563.26	6.47	$234.21	090	M	A+
21453	Treat lower jaw fracture	5.54	7.32	6.69	0.49	13.35	$483.26	12.72	$460.45	090	M	A+
21454	Treat lower jaw fracture	6.46	NA	5.72	0.55	NA	NA	12.73	$460.82	090	M	A+ C+
21461	Treat lower jaw fracture	8.09	8.40	8.26	0.73	17.22	$623.35	17.08	$618.28	090	M	C+
21462	Treat lower jaw fracture	9.79	10.06	8.18	0.80	20.65	$747.51	18.77	$679.46	090	M	C+
21465	Treat lower jaw fracture	11.91	NA	8.42	0.84	NA	NA	21.17	$766.34	090	M	C+
21470	Treat lower jaw fracture	15.34	NA	10.31	1.36	NA	NA	27.01	$977.74	090	M	C+

* **M** = multiple surgery adjustment applies
Me = multiple endoscopy rules may apply
B = bilateral surgery adjustment applies
A = assistant-at-surgery restriction

A+ = assistant-at-surgery restriction unless medical necessity established with documentation
C = cosurgeons payable
C+ = cosurgeons payable if medical necessity established with documentation

T = team surgeons permitted
T+ = team surgeons payable if medical necessity established with documentation
$ = indicates services that are not covered by Medicare.

149 CPT five-digit codes, two-digit numeric modifiers, and descriptions only are © 2001 American Medical Association

Medicare RBRVS: The Physicians' Guide

Relative value units

CPT Code and Modifier	Description	Work RVU	Non Facility Practice Expense RVU	Facility Practice Expense RVU	PLI RVU	Total Non Facility RVUs	Medicare Payment Non Facility	Total Facility RVUs	Medicare Payment Facility	Global Period	Payment Policy Indicators*			
21480	Reset dislocated jaw	0.61	1.62	0.18	0.05	2.28	$82.53	0.84	$30.41	000	M	B	A	
21485	Reset dislocated jaw	3.99	3.82	3.34	0.31	8.12	$293.94	7.64	$276.56	090	M	B	A+	
21490	Repair dislocated jaw	11.86	NA	7.69	1.31	NA	NA	20.86	$755.12	090	M	B		C+
21493	Treat hyoid bone fracture	1.27	NA	3.68	0.10	NA	NA	5.05	$182.81	090	M		A	C+
21494	Treat hyoid bone fracture	6.28	NA	4.21	0.44	NA	NA	10.93	$395.66	090	M			C+
21495	Treat hyoid bone fracture	5.69	NA	5.28	0.41	NA	NA	11.38	$411.95	090	M			
21497	Interdental wiring	3.86	4.68	3.81	0.31	8.85	$320.36	7.98	$288.87	090	M		A+	
21499	Head surgery procedure	0.00	0.00	0.00	0.00	0.00	$0.00	0.00	$0.00	YYY	M		A+	C+ T+
21501	Drain neck/chest lesion	3.81	4.50	3.64	0.36	8.67	$313.85	7.81	$282.72	090	M		A	
21502	Drain chest lesion	7.12	NA	7.05	0.79	NA	NA	14.96	$541.54	090	M			
21510	Drainage of bone lesion	5.74	NA	7.47	0.67	NA	NA	13.88	$502.44	090	M		A+	
21550	Biopsy of neck/chest	2.06	2.32	1.25	0.13	4.51	$163.26	3.44	$124.53	010	M		A	
21555	Remove lesion, neck/chest	4.35	4.25	2.43	0.41	9.01	$326.15	7.19	$260.27	090	M		A	
21556	Remove lesion, neck/chest	5.57	NA	3.29	0.51	NA	NA	9.37	$339.19	090	M		A	
21557	Remove tumor, neck/chest	8.88	NA	7.87	0.85	NA	NA	17.60	$637.11	090	M			C+
21600	Partial removal of rib	6.89	NA	7.80	0.81	NA	NA	15.50	$561.09	090	M			C+
21610	Partial removal of rib	14.61	NA	11.26	1.85	NA	NA	27.72	$1,003.44	090	M			
21615	Removal of rib	9.87	NA	7.90	1.20	NA	NA	18.97	$686.70	090	M	B		C+
21616	Removal of rib and nerves	12.04	NA	8.94	1.31	NA	NA	22.29	$806.88	090	M	B		
21620	Partial removal of sternum	6.79	NA	8.13	0.77	NA	NA	15.69	$567.97	090	M			C+
21627	Sternal debridement	6.81	NA	12.16	0.82	NA	NA	19.79	$716.38	090	M			
21630	Extensive sternum surgery	17.38	NA	14.03	1.95	NA	NA	33.36	$1,207.61	090	M			C+
21632	Extensive sternum surgery	18.14	NA	12.35	2.16	NA	NA	32.65	$1,181.90	090	M			C+
21700	Revision of neck muscle	6.19	8.63	7.19	0.31	15.13	$547.69	13.69	$495.57	090	M			
21705	Revision of neck muscle/rib	9.60	NA	7.87	0.92	NA	NA	18.39	$665.70	090	M			
21720	Revision of neck muscle	5.68	8.71	5.93	0.80	15.19	$549.87	12.41	$449.23	090	M			
21725	Revision of neck muscle	6.99	NA	7.28	0.90	NA	NA	15.17	$549.14	090	M			C+

Code	Description										
21740	Reconstruction of sternum	16.50	NA	12.85	2.03	NA	31.38	$1,135.93	090	M		C+
21750	Repair of sternum separation	10.77	NA	9.41	1.35	NA	21.53	$779.37	090	M		C+
21800	Treatment of rib fracture	0.96	2.31	1.11	0.09	3.36	2.16	$78.19	090	M	A	
21805	Treatment of rib fracture	2.75	NA	4.08	0.29	NA	7.12	$257.74	090	M	A+	
21810	Treatment of rib fracture(s)	6.86	NA	7.49	0.60	NA	14.95	$541.18	090	M		
21820	Treat sternum fracture	1.28	2.80	1.58	0.15	4.23	3.01	$108.96	090	M	A	
21825	Treat sternum fracture	7.41	NA	9.90	0.84	NA	18.15	$657.02	090	M		C+
21899	Neck/chest surgery procedure	0.00	0.00	0.00	0.00	0.00	0.00	$0.00	YYY	M	A+	C+ T+
21920	Biopsy soft tissue of back	2.06	2.40	0.77	0.12	4.58	2.95	$106.79	010	M	A	
21925	Biopsy soft tissue of back	4.49	10.19	4.79	0.44	15.12	9.72	$351.86	090	M	A	
21930	Remove lesion, back or flank	5.00	4.55	2.66	0.49	10.04	8.15	$295.02	090	M	A	
21935	Remove tumor, back	17.96	NA	13.53	1.87	NA	33.36	$1,207.61	090	M	A	C+
22100	Remove part of neck vertebra	9.73	NA	8.36	1.55	NA	19.64	$710.95	090	M		C+
22101	Remove part, thorax vertebra	9.81	NA	9.04	1.51	NA	20.36	$737.02	090	M		C+
22102	Remove part, lumbar vertebra	9.81	NA	9.18	1.46	NA	20.45	$740.27	090	M		C+
22103	Remove extra spine segment	2.34	NA	1.27	0.37	NA	3.98	$144.07	ZZZ	M		C+
22110	Remove part of neck vertebra	12.74	NA	11.06	2.20	NA	26.00	$941.18	090	M		C+
22112	Remove part, thorax vertebra	12.81	NA	10.95	1.96	NA	25.72	$931.04	090	M		C+
22114	Remove part, lumbar vertebra	12.81	NA	10.71	1.98	NA	25.50	$923.08	090	M		C+
22116	Remove extra spine segment	2.32	NA	1.26	0.40	NA	3.98	$144.07	ZZZ	M		C+
22210	Revision of neck spine	23.82	NA	17.42	4.23	NA	45.47	$1,645.98	090	M		C+
22212	Revision of thorax spine	19.42	NA	14.60	2.78	NA	36.80	$1,332.13	090	M		C+
22214	Revision of lumbar spine	19.45	NA	15.32	2.78	NA	37.55	$1,359.28	090	M		C+
22216	Revise, extra spine segment	6.04	NA	3.31	0.98	NA	10.33	$373.94	ZZZ	M	B	
22220	Revision of neck spine	21.37	NA	15.61	3.65	NA	40.63	$1,470.77	090	M		C+
22222	Revision of thorax spine	21.52	NA	15.08	3.08	NA	39.68	$1,436.38	090	M		C+
22224	Revision of lumbar spine	21.52	NA	15.70	3.20	NA	40.42	$1,463.17	090	M		C+
22226	Revise, extra spine segment	6.04	NA	3.22	1.01	NA	10.27	$371.77	ZZZ	M	B	C+

* **M** = multiple surgery adjustment applies
   Me = multiple endoscopy rules may apply
   B = bilateral surgery adjustment applies
   A = assistant-at-surgery restriction

A+ = assistant-at-surgery restriction unless medical necessity established with documentation
C = cosurgeons payable
C+ = cosurgeons payable if medical necessity established with documentation

T = team surgeons permitted
T+ = team surgeons payable if medical necessity established with documentation
§ = indicates services that are not covered by Medicare.

151 CPT five-digit codes, two-digit numeric modifiers, and descriptions only are © 2001 American Medical Association

Medicare RBRVS: The Physicians' Guide

Relative value units

CPT Code and Modifier	Description	Work RVU	Non Facility Practice Expense RVU	Facility Practice Expense RVU	PLI RVU	Total Non Facility RVUs	Medicare Payment Non Facility	Total Facility RVUs	Medicare Payment Facility	Global Period	Payment Policy Indicators*	
22305	Treat spine process fracture	2.05	3.25	2.01	0.29	5.59	$202.35	4.35	$157.47	090	M	A
22310	Treat spine fracture	2.61	4.77	3.54	0.37	7.75	$280.54	6.52	$236.02	090	M	A
22315	Treat spine fracture	8.84	NA	9.32	1.37	NA	NA	19.53	$706.97	090	M	A
22318	Treat odontoid fx w/o graft	21.50	NA	15.02	4.26	NA	NA	40.78	$1,476.20	090	M	C
22319	Treat odontoid fx w/graft	24.00	NA	17.42	4.76	NA	NA	46.18	$1,671.68	090	M	C
22325	Treat spine fracture	18.30	NA	14.94	2.61	NA	NA	35.85	$1,297.74	090	M	C+
22326	Treat neck spine fracture	19.59	NA	15.67	3.54	NA	NA	38.80	$1,404.53	090	M	C+
22327	Treat thorax spine fracture	19.20	NA	15.43	2.75	NA	NA	37.38	$1,353.13	090	M	C+
22328	Treat each add spine fx	4.61	NA	2.43	0.66	NA	NA	7.70	$278.73	ZZZ		C+
22505	Manipulation of spine	1.87	4.58	3.20	0.27	6.72	$243.26	5.34	$193.30	010	M	A
22520	Percut vertebroplasty thor	8.91	NA	4.15	0.99	NA	NA	14.05	$508.60	010	M	A
22521	Percut vertebroplasty lumb	8.34	NA	3.92	0.93	NA	NA	13.19	$477.47	010	M	A
22522	Percut vertebroplasty addl	4.31	NA	1.75	0.33	NA	NA	6.39	$231.31	ZZZ	M	A
22548	Neck spine fusion	25.82	NA	18.08	4.98	NA	NA	48.88	$1,769.42	090	M	C
22554	Neck spine fusion	18.62	NA	13.94	3.51	NA	NA	36.07	$1,305.71	090	M	C
22556	Thorax spine fusion	23.46	NA	16.80	3.78	NA	NA	44.04	$1,594.21	090	M	C
22558	Lumbar spine fusion	22.28	NA	15.27	3.18	NA	NA	40.73	$1,474.39	090	M	C
22585	Additional spinal fusion	5.53	NA	2.94	0.98	NA	NA	9.45	$342.08	ZZZ	M	C
22590	Spine & skull spinal fusion	20.51	NA	15.56	3.81	NA	NA	39.88	$1,443.62	090	M	C
22595	Neck spinal fusion	19.39	NA	14.58	3.62	NA	NA	37.59	$1,360.73	090	M	C
22600	Neck spine fusion	16.14	NA	12.66	2.89	NA	NA	31.69	$1,147.15	090	M	C
22610	Thorax spine fusion	16.02	NA	12.98	2.66	NA	NA	31.66	$1,146.07	090	M	C
22612	Lumbar spine fusion	21.00	NA	15.75	3.28	NA	NA	40.03	$1,449.05	090	M	C
22614	Spine fusion, extra segment	6.44	NA	3.54	1.04	NA	NA	11.02	$398.92	ZZZ	M	C
22630	Lumbar spine fusion	20.84	NA	16.01	3.79	NA	NA	40.64	$1,471.14	090	M	C
22632	Spine fusion, extra segment	5.23	NA	2.75	0.90	NA	NA	8.88	$321.45	ZZZ	M	C
22800	Fusion of spine	18.25	NA	14.30	2.71	NA	NA	35.26	$1,276.38	090	M	C+

Code	Description									
22802	Fusion of spine	30.88	NA	21.88	4.42	NA	57.18	$2,069.87	090	M	C+
22804	Fusion of spine	36.27	NA	24.48	5.23	NA	65.98	$2,388.42	090	M	C+
22808	Fusion of spine	26.27	NA	18.27	4.36	NA	48.90	$1,770.14	090	M	C+
22810	Fusion of spine	30.27	NA	19.63	4.49	NA	54.39	$1,968.87	090	M	C+
22812	Fusion of spine	32.70	NA	21.89	4.67	NA	59.26	$2,145.16	090	M	C+
22818	Kyphectomy, 1-2 segments	31.83	NA	21.69	5.01	NA	58.53	$2,118.74	090	M	C T
22819	Kyphectomy, 3 or more	36.44	NA	22.19	5.20	NA	63.83	$2,310.59	090	M	C T
22830	Exploration of spinal fusion	10.85	NA	10.05	1.73	NA	22.63	$819.19	090	M	C+
22840	Insert spine fixation device	12.54	NA	6.84	2.03	NA	21.41	$775.02	ZZZ		C+
22842	Insert spine fixation device	12.58	NA	6.83	2.04	NA	21.45	$776.47	ZZZ		C
22843	Insert spine fixation device	13.46	NA	7.39	2.10	NA	22.95	$830.77	ZZZ		C
22844	Insert spine fixation device	16.44	NA	9.26	2.42	NA	28.12	$1,017.92	ZZZ		C
22845	Insert spine fixation device	11.96	NA	6.38	2.22	NA	20.56	$744.26	ZZZ		C
22846	Insert spine fixation device	12.42	NA	6.70	2.26	NA	21.38	$773.94	ZZZ		C
22847	Insert spine fixation device	13.80	NA	7.08	2.36	NA	23.24	$841.27	ZZZ		C
22848	Insert pelv fixation device	6.00	NA	3.38	0.88	NA	10.26	$371.40	ZZZ		C
22849	Reinsert spinal fixation	18.51	NA	14.22	2.87	NA	35.60	$1,288.69	090	M	C+
22850	Remove spine fixation device	9.52	NA	8.89	1.51	NA	19.92	$721.09	090	M	C+
22851	Apply spine prosth device	6.71	NA	3.54	1.11	NA	11.36	$411.22	ZZZ		C
22852	Remove spine fixation device	9.01	NA	8.60	1.40	NA	19.01	$688.15	090	M	C+
22855	Remove spine fixation device	15.13	NA	11.67	2.74	NA	29.54	$1,069.32	090	M	C+
22899	Spine surgery procedure	0.00	0.00	0.00	0.00	$0.00	0.00	$0.00	YYY	M	C+ T+
22900	Remove abdominal wall lesion	5.80	NA	4.42	0.58	NA	10.80	$390.95	090	M	C+
22999	Abdomen surgery procedure	0.00	0.00	0.00	0.00	$0.00	0.00	$0.00	YYY	M	C+ T+ A+
23000	Removal of calcium deposits	4.36	9.04	6.97	0.50	$503.17	11.83	$428.24	090	M	C+
23020	Release shoulder joint	8.93	NA	10.53	1.23	NA	20.69	$748.96	090	M	B
23030	Drain shoulder lesion	3.43	6.40	4.44	0.42	$371.04	8.29	$300.09	010	M	A
23031	Drain shoulder bursa	2.74	5.80	4.16	0.33	$321.09	7.23	$261.72	010	M	B A

* **M** = multiple surgery adjustment applies
   Me = multiple endoscopy rules may apply
   B = bilateral surgery adjustment applies
   A = assistant-at-surgery restriction

A+ = assistant-at-surgery restriction unless medical necessity established with documentation
C = cosurgeons payable
C+ = cosurgeons payable if medical necessity established with documentation

T = team surgeons permitted
T+ = team surgeons payable if medical necessity established with documentation
§ = indicates services that are not covered by Medicare.

153   CPT five-digit codes, two-digit numeric modifiers, and descriptions only are © 2001 American Medical Association

Medicare RBRVS: The Physicians' Guide

Relative value units

CPT Code and Modifier	Description	Work RVU	Non Facility Practice Expense RVU	Facility Practice Expense RVU	PLI RVU	Total Non Facility RVUs	Medicare Payment Non Facility	Total Facility RVUs	Medicare Payment Facility	Global Period	Payment Policy Indicators*
23035	Drain shoulder bone lesion	8.61	NA	16.13	1.19	NA	NA	25.93	$938.65	090	M B
23040	Exploratory shoulder surgery	9.20	NA	11.71	1.28	NA	NA	22.19	$803.26	090	M B C+
23044	Exploratory shoulder surgery	7.12	NA	10.73	0.97	NA	NA	18.82	$681.27	090	M B A C+
23065	Biopsy shoulder tissues	2.27	2.61	1.34	0.14	5.02	$181.72	3.75	$135.75	010	M B A
23066	Biopsy shoulder tissues	4.16	8.34	6.16	0.50	13.00	$470.59	10.82	$391.68	090	M B A
23075	Removal of shoulder lesion	2.39	5.40	3.17	0.25	8.04	$291.04	5.81	$210.32	10	M B A
23076	Removal of shoulder lesion	7.63	NA	8.36	0.87	NA	NA	16.86	$610.32	090	M B A
23077	Remove tumor of shoulder	16.09	NA	14.41	1.81	NA	NA	32.31	$1,169.60	090	M B C+
23100	Biopsy of shoulder joint	6.03	NA	8.73	0.81	NA	NA	15.57	$563.62	090	M B C+
23101	Shoulder joint surgery	5.58	NA	8.63	0.77	NA	NA	14.98	$542.26	090	M B A C+
23105	Remove shoulder joint lining	8.23	NA	10.18	1.13	NA	NA	19.54	$707.33	090	M B A C+
23106	Incision of collarbone joint	5.96	NA	9.27	0.82	NA	NA	16.05	$581.00	090	M B A C+
23107	Explore treat shoulder joint	8.62	NA	10.41	1.19	NA	NA	20.22	$731.95	090	M B C+
23120	Partial removal, collar bone	7.11	NA	9.55	0.99	NA	NA	17.65	$638.92	090	M B C+
23125	Removal of collar bone	9.39	NA	10.78	1.27	NA	NA	21.44	$776.11	090	M B C+
23130	Remove shoulder bone, part	7.55	NA	9.82	1.06	NA	NA	18.43	$667.15	090	M B A C+
23140	Removal of bone lesion	6.89	NA	8.31	0.82	NA	NA	16.02	$579.91	090	M B A
23145	Removal of bone lesion	9.09	NA	10.87	1.24	NA	NA	21.20	$767.42	090	M B C+
23146	Removal of bone lesion	7.83	NA	10.70	1.11	NA	NA	19.64	$710.95	090	M B A+
23150	Removal of humerus lesion	8.48	NA	10.14	1.14	NA	NA	19.76	$715.30	090	M B C+
23155	Removal of humerus lesion	10.35	NA	12.33	1.20	NA	NA	23.88	$864.44	090	M B C+
23156	Removal of humerus lesion	8.68	NA	10.45	1.18	NA	NA	20.31	$735.21	090	M B A
23170	Remove collar bone lesion	6.86	NA	11.33	0.84	NA	NA	19.03	$688.87	090	M B A
23172	Remove shoulder blade lesion	6.90	NA	9.59	0.95	NA	NA	17.44	$631.31	090	M B
23174	Remove humerus lesion	9.51	NA	11.74	1.30	NA	NA	22.55	$816.29	090	M B C+
23180	Remove collar bone lesion	8.53	NA	16.16	1.18	NA	NA	25.87	$936.47	090	M B A C+
23182	Remove shoulder blade lesion	8.15	NA	16.18	1.08	NA	NA	25.41	$919.82	090	M B

Code	Description										
23184	Remove humerus lesion	9.38	NA	16.43	1.24	NA	27.05	$979.19	090	M	B	C+
23190	Partial removal of scapula	7.24	NA	8.74	0.97	NA	16.95	$613.58	090	M	B	C+
23195	Removal of head of humerus	9.81	NA	10.03	1.38	NA	21.22	$768.15	090	M	B	C+
23200	Removal of collar bone	12.08	NA	14.39	1.48	NA	27.95	$1,011.77	090	M	B	C+
23210	Removal of shoulder blade	12.49	NA	13.96	1.61	NA	28.06	$1,015.75	090	M	B	C+
23220	Partial removal of humerus	14.56	NA	15.57	2.03	NA	32.16	$1,164.17	090	M	B	C+
23221	Partial removal of humerus	17.74	NA	16.93	2.51	NA	37.18	$1,345.89	090	M	B	
23222	Partial removal of humerus	23.92	NA	20.66	3.37	NA	47.95	$1,735.75	090	M	B	C+
23330	Remove shoulder foreign body	1.85	6.15	3.49	0.18	$296.11	5.52	$199.82	010	M	B	A+
23331	Remove shoulder foreign body	7.38	NA	9.70	1.02	NA	18.10	$655.21	090	M	B	A+
23332	Remove shoulder foreign body	11.62	NA	12.12	1.62	NA	25.36	$918.01	090	M	B	C+
23350	Injection for shoulder x-ray	1.00	7.22	0.35	0.05	$299.37	1.40	$50.68	000	M	B	A
23395	Muscle transfer, shoulder/arm	16.85	NA	14.09	2.29	NA	33.23	$1,202.90	090	M		C+
23397	Muscle transfers	16.13	NA	13.86	2.24	NA	32.23	$1,166.70	090	M	B	C+
23400	Fixation of shoulder blade	13.54	NA	14.52	1.91	NA	29.97	$1,084.89	090	M	B	C+
23405	Incision of tendon & muscle	8.37	NA	9.66	1.12	NA	19.15	$693.21	090	M		
23406	Incise tendon(s) & muscle(s)	10.79	NA	11.55	1.48	NA	23.82	$862.26	090	M		
23410	Repair of tendon(s)	12.45	NA	12.55	1.72	NA	26.72	$967.24	090	M		C+
23412	Repair of tendon(s)	13.31	NA	13.05	1.86	NA	28.22	$1,021.54	090	M	B	C+
23415	Release of shoulder ligament	9.97	NA	10.22	1.39	NA	21.58	$1,084.89	090	M	B	A
23420	Repair of shoulder	13.30	NA	13.94	1.86	NA	29.10	$1,053.40	090	M	B	C+
23430	Repair biceps tendon	9.98	NA	11.15	1.40	NA	22.53	$815.57	090	M	B	C+
23440	Remove/transplant tendon	10.48	NA	11.54	1.47	NA	23.49	$850.32	090	M	B	C+
23450	Repair shoulder capsule	13.40	NA	13.02	1.86	NA	28.28	$1,023.71	090	M	B	C+
23455	Repair shoulder capsule	14.37	NA	13.62	2.01	NA	30.00	$1,085.98	090	M	B	C+
23460	Repair shoulder capsule	15.37	NA	14.21	2.17	NA	31.75	$1,149.32	090	M	B	C+
23462	Repair shoulder capsule	15.30	NA	13.68	2.16	NA	31.14	$1,127.24	090	M	B	C+
23465	Repair shoulder capsule	15.85	NA	14.47	1.61	NA	31.93	$1,155.84	090	M	B	C+

* **M** = multiple surgery adjustment applies
Me = multiple endoscopy rules may apply
B = bilateral surgery adjustment applies
A = assistant-at-surgery restriction

A+ = assistant-at-surgery restriction unless medical necessity established with documentation
C = cosurgeons payable
C+ = cosurgeons payable if medical necessity established with documentation

T = team surgeons permitted
T+ = team surgeons payable if medical necessity established with documentation
§ = indicates services that are not covered by Medicare.

CPT five-digit codes, two-digit numeric modifiers, and descriptions only are © 2001 American Medical Association

Medicare RBRVS: The Physicians' Guide

Relative value units

CPT Code and Modifier	Description	Work RVU	Non Facility Practice Expense RVU	Facility Practice Expense RVU	PLI RVU	Total Non Facility RVUs	Medicare Payment Non Facility	Total Facility RVUs	Medicare Payment Facility	Global Period	Payment Policy Indicators*			
23466	Repair shoulder capsule	14.22	NA	13.63	2.00	NA	NA	29.85	$1,080.55	090	M	B		C+
23470	Reconstruct shoulder joint	17.15	NA	15.16	2.40	NA	NA	34.71	$1,256.47	090	M	B		C+
23472	Reconstruct shoulder joint	21.10	NA	17.40	2.37	NA	NA	40.87	$1,479.46	090	M	B		C+
23480	Revision of collar bone	11.18	NA	11.94	1.56	NA	NA	24.68	$893.40	090	M	B	A	C+
23485	Revision of collar bone	13.43	NA	13.10	1.84	NA	NA	28.37	$1,026.97	090	M	B		C+
23490	Reinforce clavicle	11.86	NA	13.74	1.11	NA	NA	26.71	$966.88	090	M	B		
23491	Reinforce shoulder bones	14.21	NA	13.54	2.00	NA	NA	29.75	$1,076.93	090	M	B		C+
23500	Treat clavicle fracture	2.08	3.87	2.60	0.26	6.21	$224.80	4.94	$178.82	090	M	B	A	
23505	Treat clavicle fracture	3.69	5.98	4.02	0.50	10.17	$368.15	8.21	$297.20	090	M	B	A	
23515	Treat clavicle fracture	7.41	NA	8.24	1.03	NA	NA	16.68	$603.80	090	M	B		C+
23520	Treat clavicle dislocation	2.16	3.91	2.67	0.26	6.33	$229.14	5.09	$184.25	090	M	B	A+	
23525	Treat clavicle dislocation	3.60	7.16	4.08	0.44	11.20	$405.43	8.12	$293.94	090	M	B	A+	
23530	Treat clavicle dislocation	7.31	NA	7.94	0.85	NA	NA	16.10	$582.81	090	M	B		
23532	Treat clavicle dislocation	8.01	NA	8.67	1.13	NA	NA	17.81	$644.71	090	M	B		
23540	Treat clavicle dislocation	2.23	4.56	2.63	0.24	7.03	$254.48	5.10	$184.62	090	M	B	A	
23545	Treat clavicle dislocation	3.25	4.99	3.65	0.39	8.63	$312.40	7.29	$263.89	090	M	B	A+	
23550	Treat clavicle dislocation	7.24	NA	8.29	0.94	NA	NA	16.47	$596.20	090	M	B		C+
23552	Treat clavicle dislocation	8.45	NA	8.82	1.18	NA	NA	18.45	$667.88	090	M	B		C+
23570	Treat shoulder blade fx	2.23	3.84	2.70	0.29	6.36	$230.23	5.22	$188.96	090	M	B	A	
23575	Treat shoulder blade fx	4.06	6.22	4.18	0.53	10.81	$391.31	8.77	$317.47	090	M	B	A+	
23585	Treat scapula fracture	8.96	NA	9.31	1.25	NA	NA	19.52	$706.61	090	M	B		C+
23600	Treat humerus fracture	2.93	5.65	3.71	0.39	8.97	$324.71	7.03	$254.48	090	M	B	A	
23605	Treat humerus fracture	4.87	8.32	6.55	0.67	13.86	$501.72	12.09	$437.65	090	M	B	A	
23615	Treat humerus fracture	9.35	NA	10.19	1.31	NA	NA	20.85	$754.75	090	M	B		C+
23616	Treat humerus fracture	21.27	NA	16.26	2.98	NA	NA	40.51	$1,466.43	090	M	B		C
23620	Treat humerus fracture	2.40	5.35	3.43	0.32	8.07	$292.13	6.15	$222.63	090	M	B	A	
23625	Treat humerus fracture	3.93	7.35	5.57	0.53	11.81	$427.51	10.03	$363.08	090	M	B	A	

Code	Description											
23630	Treat humerus fracture	7.35	NA	8.20	1.03	NA	NA	16.58	$600.18	090	M	B		C+
23650	Treat shoulder dislocation	3.39	5.58	3.67	0.31	9.28	$335.93	7.37	$266.79	090	M	B	A
23655	Treat shoulder dislocation	4.57	NA	4.39	0.52	NA	NA	9.48	$343.17	090	M	B	A
23660	Treat shoulder dislocation	7.49	NA	8.27	1.01	NA	NA	16.77	$607.06	090	M	B		C+
23665	Treat dislocation/fracture	4.47	7.68	5.81	0.60	12.75	$461.54	10.88	$393.85	090	M	B	A
23670	Treat dislocation/fracture	7.90	NA	8.72	1.10	NA	NA	17.72	$641.45	090	M	B		C+
23675	Treat dislocation/fracture	6.05	8.22	6.71	0.83	15.10	$546.61	13.59	$491.95	090	M	B	A
23680	Treat dislocation/fracture	10.06	NA	9.89	1.39	NA	NA	21.34	$772.49	090	M	B		C+
23700	Fixation of shoulder	2.52	NA	3.48	0.35	NA	NA	6.35	$229.86	010	M		A
23800	Fusion of shoulder joint	14.16	NA	14.28	1.97	NA	NA	30.41	$1,100.82	090	M	B		C+
23802	Fusion of shoulder joint	16.60	NA	15.83	2.34	NA	NA	34.77	$1,258.65	090	M			C+
23900	Amputation of arm & girdle	19.72	NA	16.35	2.47	NA	NA	38.54	$1,395.12	090	M		
23920	Amputation at shoulder joint	14.61	NA	13.70	1.92	NA	NA	30.23	$1,094.30	090	M			C+
23921	Amputation follow-up surgery	5.49	NA	6.67	0.78	NA	NA	12.94	$468.42	090	M		A
23929	Shoulder surgery procedure	0.00	0.00	0.00	0.00	0.00	$0.00	0.00	$0.00	YYY	M			C+ T+
23930	Drainage of arm lesion	2.94	6.10	4.01	0.32	9.36	$338.82	7.27	$263.17	010	M	B	A
23931	Drainage of arm bursa	1.79	5.76	3.74	0.21	7.76	$280.91	5.74	$207.78	010	M	B	A
23935	Drain arm/elbow bone lesion	6.09	NA	12.90	0.84	NA	NA	19.83	$717.83	090	M	B	A+
24000	Exploratory elbow surgery	5.82	NA	6.06	0.77	NA	NA	12.65	$457.92	090	M	B	A+	C+
24006	Release elbow joint	9.31	NA	8.64	1.27	NA	NA	19.22	$695.75	090	M	B		C
24065	Biopsy arm/elbow soft tissue	2.08	5.50	3.25	0.14	7.72	$279.46	5.47	$198.01	010	M	B	A
24066	Biopsy arm/elbow soft tissue	5.21	8.48	6.40	0.61	14.30	$517.65	12.22	$442.35	090	M	B	A
24075	Remove arm/elbow lesion	3.92	7.80	5.91	0.43	12.15	$439.82	10.26	$371.40	090	M	B	A
24076	Remove arm/elbow lesion	6.30	NA	7.39	0.70	NA	NA	14.39	$520.91	090	M	B	A
24077	Remove tumor of arm/elbow	11.76	NA	14.23	1.32	NA	NA	27.31	$988.60	090	M	B		C+
24100	Biopsy elbow joint lining	4.93	NA	5.83	0.62	NA	NA	11.38	$411.95	090	M	B		C+
24101	Explore/treat elbow joint	6.13	NA	6.82	0.84	NA	NA	13.79	$499.19	090	M	B	
24102	Remove elbow joint lining	8.03	NA	7.81	1.09	NA	NA	16.93	$612.85	090	M	B		C+

* **M** = multiple surgery adjustment applies
Me = multiple endoscopy rules may apply
B = bilateral surgery adjustment applies
A = assistant-at-surgery restriction

A+ = assistant-at-surgery restriction unless medical necessity established with documentation
C = cosurgeons payable
C+ = cosurgeons payable if medical necessity established with documentation

T = team surgeons permitted
T+ = team surgeons payable if medical necessity established with documentation
§ = indicates services that are not covered by Medicare.

157   CPT five-digit codes, two-digit numeric modifiers, and descriptions only are © 2001 American Medical Association

Medicare RBRVS: The Physicians' Guide

Relative value units

CPT Code and Modifier	Description	Work RVU	Non Facility Practice Expense RVU	Facility Practice Expense RVU	PLI RVU	Total Non Facility RVUs	Medicare Payment Non Facility	Total Facility RVUs	Medicare Payment Facility	Global Period	Payment Policy Indicators*
24105	Removal of elbow bursa	3.61	NA	5.26	0.49	NA	NA	9.36	$338.82	090	M B A
24110	Remove humerus lesion	7.39	NA	9.75	0.99	NA	NA	18.13	$656.29	090	M B A C+
24115	Remove/graft bone lesion	9.63	NA	10.80	1.15	NA	NA	21.58	$781.18	090	M B C+
24116	Remove/graft bone lesion	11.81	NA	12.20	1.66	NA	NA	25.67	$929.23	090	M B
24120	Remove elbow lesion	6.65	NA	6.96	0.87	NA	NA	14.48	$524.16	090	M B A+
24125	Remove/graft bone lesion	7.89	NA	6.67	0.88	NA	NA	15.44	$558.92	090	M B C+
24126	Remove/graft bone lesion	8.31	NA	7.79	0.90	NA	NA	17.00	$615.39	090	M B
24130	Removal of head of radius	6.25	NA	6.91	0.87	NA	NA	14.03	$507.87	090	M B A C+
24134	Removal of arm bone lesion	9.73	NA	16.50	1.31	NA	NA	27.54	$996.93	090	M B
24136	Remove radius bone lesion	7.99	NA	7.09	0.85	NA	NA	15.93	$576.65	090	M B A
24138	Remove elbow bone lesion	8.05	NA	8.06	1.12	NA	NA	17.23	$623.71	090	M B
24140	Partial removal of arm bone	9.18	NA	16.67	1.23	NA	NA	27.08	$980.27	090	M B
24145	Partial removal of radius	7.58	NA	11.43	1.01	NA	NA	20.02	$724.71	090	M B A C+
24147	Partial removal of elbow	7.54	NA	11.40	1.04	NA	NA	19.98	$723.26	090	M B A C+
24149	Radical resection of elbow	14.20	NA	11.28	1.90	NA	NA	27.38	$991.13	090	M B C+
24150	Extensive humerus surgery	13.27	NA	14.92	1.81	NA	NA	30.00	$1,085.98	090	M B C+
24151	Extensive humerus surgery	15.58	NA	16.64	2.19	NA	NA	34.41	$1,245.61	090	M B C+
24152	Extensive radius surgery	10.06	NA	9.96	1.19	NA	NA	21.21	$767.79	090	M B C+
24153	Extensive radius surgery	11.54	NA	7.55	0.64	NA	NA	19.73	$714.21	090	M B A+ C+
24155	Removal of elbow joint	11.73	NA	9.66	1.42	NA	NA	22.81	$825.70	090	M B C+
24160	Remove elbow joint implant	7.83	NA	7.77	1.07	NA	NA	16.67	$603.44	090	M B A C+
24164	Remove radius head implant	6.23	NA	6.93	0.84	NA	NA	14.00	$506.79	090	M B A C+
24200	Removal of arm foreign body	1.76	5.80	3.25	0.15	7.71	$279.10	5.16	$186.79	010	M B A+
24201	Removal of arm foreign body	4.56	8.42	6.97	0.56	13.54	$490.14	12.09	$437.65	090	M B A
24220	Injection for elbow x-ray	1.31	11.16	0.47	0.07	12.54	$453.94	1.85	$66.97	000	M B A+
24300	Manipulate elbow w/anesth	3.75	NA	5.46	0.52	NA	NA	9.73	$352.22	090	M A
24301	Muscle/tendon transfer	10.20	NA	9.11	1.30	NA	NA	20.61	$746.07	090	M C+

Code	Description									
24305	Arm tendon lengthening	7.45	NA	7.70	0.98	NA	16.13	$583.89	090	M	A+
24310	Revision of arm tendon	5.98	NA	8.43	0.74	NA	15.15	$548.42	090	M	A+
24320	Repair of arm tendon	10.56	NA	11.29	1.00	NA	22.85	$827.15	090	M		C+
24330	Revision of arm muscles	9.60	NA	8.79	1.21	NA	19.60	$709.50	090	M	B
24331	Revision of arm muscles	10.65	NA	9.25	1.41	NA	21.31	$771.40	090	M	B
24332	Tenolysis, triceps	7.45	NA	5.23	0.77	NA	13.45	$486.88	090	M	A
24340	Repair of biceps tendon	7.89	NA	7.74	1.08	NA	16.71	$604.89	090	M	B	C+
24341	Repair arm tendon/muscle	7.90	NA	7.85	1.08	NA	16.83	$609.23	090	M	B	C+
24342	Repair of ruptured tendon	10.62	NA	9.37	1.48	NA	21.47	$777.20	090	M	B	C+
24343	Repr elbow lat ligmnt w/tiss	8.65	NA	7.91	1.21	NA	17.77	$643.26	090	M	B	C+
24344	Reconstruct elbow lat ligmnt	14.00	NA	10.87	1.95	NA	26.82	$970.86	090	M	B	C+
24345	Repr elbw med ligmnt w/tiss	8.65	NA	7.91	1.21	NA	17.77	$643.26	090	M	B	C+
24346	Reconstruct elbow med ligmnt	14.00	NA	10.87	1.95	NA	26.82	$970.86	090	M	B	C+
24350	Repair of tennis elbow	5.25	NA	6.25	0.72	NA	12.22	$442.35	090	M	B	A+
24351	Repair of tennis elbow	5.91	NA	6.72	0.82	NA	13.45	$486.88	090	M	B	A+
24352	Repair of tennis elbow	6.43	NA	7.01	0.90	NA	14.34	$519.10	090	M	B	C+
24354	Repair of tennis elbow	6.48	NA	6.85	0.88	NA	14.21	$514.39	090	M	B	A
24356	Revision of tennis elbow	6.68	NA	7.21	0.90	NA	14.79	$535.39	090	M	B	A+
24360	Reconstruct elbow joint	12.34	NA	10.26	1.69	NA	24.29	$879.28	090	M	B	C+
24361	Reconstruct elbow joint	14.08	NA	11.30	1.95	NA	27.33	$989.32	090	M	B	C+
24362	Reconstruct elbow joint	14.99	NA	11.30	1.92	NA	28.21	$1,021.18	090	M	B	C+
24363	Replace elbow joint	18.49	NA	13.80	2.52	NA	34.81	$1,260.09	090	M	B
24365	Reconstruct head of radius	8.39	NA	7.96	1.11	NA	17.46	$632.04	090	M	B	C+
24366	Reconstruct head of radius	9.13	NA	8.48	1.28	NA	18.89	$683.80	090	M	B	C+
24400	Revision of humerus	11.06	NA	12.48	1.53	NA	25.07	$907.51	090	M	B	C+
24410	Revision of humerus	14.82	NA	13.75	1.89	NA	30.46	$1,102.63	090	M	B	C+
24420	Revision of humerus	13.44	NA	16.08	1.82	NA	31.34	$1,134.48	090	M	B	C+
24430	Repair of humerus	12.81	NA	12.88	1.80	NA	27.49	$995.12	090	M	B	C+

* **M** = multiple surgery adjustment applies
Me = multiple endoscopy rules may apply
B = bilateral surgery adjustment applies
A = assistant-at-surgery restriction

A+ = assistant-at-surgery restriction unless medical necessity established with documentation
C = cosurgeons payable
C+ = cosurgeons payable if medical necessity established with documentation

T = team surgeons permitted
T+ = team surgeons payable if medical necessity established with documentation
$ = indicates services that are not covered by Medicare.

159 CPT five-digit codes, two-digit numeric modifiers, and descriptions only are © 2001 American Medical Association

Medicare RBRVS: The Physicians' Guide

Relative value units

CPT Code and Modifier	Description	Work RVU	Non Facility Practice Expense RVU	Facility Practice Expense RVU	PLI RVU	Total Non Facility RVUs	Medicare Payment Non Facility	Total Facility RVUs	Medicare Payment Facility	Global Period	Payment Policy Indicators*
24435	Repair humerus with graft	13.17	NA	13.98	1.84	NA	NA	28.99	$1,049.41	090	M B C+
24470	Revision of elbow joint	8.74	NA	6.59	1.23	NA	NA	16.56	$599.46	090	M B
24495	Decompression of forearm	8.12	NA	10.33	0.92	NA	NA	19.37	$701.18	090	M B A+
24498	Reinforce humerus	11.92	NA	12.31	1.67	NA	NA	25.90	$937.56	090	M B C+
24500	Treat humerus fracture	3.21	5.09	3.38	0.41	8.71	$315.30	7.00	$253.39	090	M B A
24505	Treat humerus fracture	5.17	8.88	6.81	0.72	14.77	$534.66	12.70	$459.73	090	M B A
24515	Treat humerus fracture	11.65	NA	11.40	1.63	NA	NA	24.68	$893.40	090	M B C+
24516	Treat humerus fracture	11.65	NA	11.85	1.63	NA	NA	25.13	$909.69	090	M B C
24530	Treat humerus fracture	3.50	6.19	4.86	0.47	10.16	$367.78	8.83	$319.64	090	M B A
24535	Treat humerus fracture	6.87	8.81	6.72	0.96	16.64	$602.35	14.55	$526.70	090	M B A
24538	Treat humerus fracture	9.43	NA	10.61	1.25	NA	NA	21.29	$770.68	090	M B A
24545	Treat humerus fracture	10.46	NA	10.18	1.47	NA	NA	22.11	$800.36	090	M B C+
24546	Treat humerus fracture	15.69	NA	13.69	2.18	NA	NA	31.56	$1,142.45	090	M B C
24560	Treat humerus fracture	2.80	4.87	3.23	0.35	8.02	$290.32	6.38	$230.95	090	M B A
24565	Treat humerus fracture	5.56	8.09	5.82	0.74	14.39	$520.91	12.12	$438.73	090	M B A
24566	Treat humerus fracture	7.79	NA	9.96	1.10	NA	NA	18.85	$682.35	090	M B A
24575	Treat humerus fracture	10.66	NA	8.49	1.44	NA	NA	20.59	$745.34	090	M B C+
24576	Treat humerus fracture	2.86	4.62	3.26	0.38	7.86	$284.53	6.50	$235.29	090	M B A
24577	Treat humerus fracture	5.79	8.22	6.13	0.81	14.82	$536.47	12.73	$460.82	090	M B A
24579	Treat humerus fracture	11.60	NA	11.32	1.62	NA	NA	24.54	$888.33	090	M B C+
24582	Treat humerus fracture	8.55	NA	10.46	1.20	NA	NA	20.21	$731.59	090	M B A
24586	Treat elbow fracture	15.21	NA	11.23	2.12	NA	NA	28.56	$1,033.85	090	M B C+
24587	Treat elbow fracture	15.16	NA	11.13	2.14	NA	NA	28.43	$1,029.14	090	M B C+
24600	Treat elbow dislocation	4.23	6.82	5.12	0.49	11.54	$417.74	9.84	$356.20	090	M B A
24605	Treat elbow dislocation	5.42	NA	5.02	0.72	NA	NA	11.16	$403.98	090	M B A
24615	Treat elbow dislocation	9.42	NA	7.94	1.31	NA	NA	18.67	$675.84	090	M B C+
24620	Treat elbow fracture	6.98	NA	6.63	0.90	NA	NA	14.51	$525.25	090	M B A+

Code	Description											
24635	Treat elbow fracture	13.19	NA	16.55	1.84	NA	31.58	$1,143.17	090	M	B		C+
24640	Treat elbow dislocation	1.20	3.35	1.88	0.11	4.66	3.19	$115.48	010	M	B	A+	
24650	Treat radius fracture	2.16	4.55	2.92	0.28	6.99	5.36	$194.03	090	M	B	A	
24655	Treat radius fracture	4.40	7.33	5.22	0.58	12.31	10.20	$369.23	090	M	B	A	
24665	Treat radius fracture	8.14	NA	9.40	1.13	$445.61	18.67	$675.84	090	M	B		C+
24666	Treat radius fracture	9.49	NA	10.18	1.32	NA	20.99	$759.82	090	M	B		C+
24670	Treat ulnar fracture	2.54	4.49	3.10	0.33	7.36	5.97	$216.11	090	M	B	A	
24675	Treat ulnar fracture	4.72	7.55	5.49	0.65	12.92	10.86	$393.12	090	M	B	A	
24685	Treat ulnar fracture	8.80	NA	9.79	1.23	$266.43	19.82	$717.47	090	M	B		C+
24800	Fusion of elbow joint	11.20	NA	9.90	1.41	$467.69	22.51	$814.84	090	M	B		C+
24802	Fusion/graft of elbow joint	13.69	NA	11.50	1.89	NA	27.08	$980.27	090	M	B		
24900	Amputation of upper arm	9.60	NA	11.37	1.18	NA	22.15	$801.81	090	M	B		C+
24920	Amputation of upper arm	9.54	NA	13.96	1.22	NA	24.72	$894.84	090	M	B		C+
24925	Amputation follow-up surgery	7.07	NA	9.64	0.95	NA	17.66	$639.28	090	M	B		
24930	Amputation follow-up surgery	10.25	NA	10.86	1.23	NA	22.34	$808.69	090	M	B		
24931	Amputate upper arm & implant	12.72	NA	11.63	1.56	NA	25.91	$937.92	090	M	B		
24935	Revision of amputation	15.56	NA	13.22	1.58	NA	30.36	$1,099.01	090	M	B	A+	
24940	Revision of upper arm	0.00	0.00	0.00	0.00	0.00	0.00	$0.00	090	M	B		
24999	Upper arm/elbow surgery	0.00	0.00	0.00	0.00	$0.00	0.00	$0.00	YYY	M	B		T+
25000	Incision of tendon sheath	3.38	NA	7.49	0.45	NA	11.32	$409.77	090	M	B	A+	C+
25001	Incise flexor carpi radialis	3.38	NA	4.30	0.45	NA	8.13	$294.30	090	M	B	A	
25020	Decompress forearm 1 space	5.92	NA	11.49	0.75	NA	18.16	$657.38	090	M	B	A	
25023	Decompress forearm 1 space	12.96	NA	17.50	1.50	NA	31.96	$1,156.93	090	M	B	A+	
25024	Decompress forearm 2 spaces	9.50	NA	8.17	1.20	NA	18.87	$683.08	090	M	B	A	
25025	Decompress forearm 2 spaces	16.54	NA	12.05	1.91	NA	30.50	$1,104.08	090	M	B	A+	
25028	Drainage of forearm lesion	5.25	NA	10.20	0.61	NA	16.06	$581.36	090	M	B	A	
25031	Drainage of forearm bursa	4.14	NA	10.24	0.50	NA	14.88	$538.64	090	M	B	A+	
25035	Treat forearm bone lesion	7.36	NA	16.18	0.98	NA	24.52	$887.60	090	M	B	A+	

* **M** = multiple surgery adjustment applies
Me = multiple endoscopy rules may apply
B = bilateral surgery adjustment applies
A = assistant-at-surgery restriction

A+ = assistant-at-surgery restriction unless medical necessity established with documentation
C = cosurgeons payable
C+ = cosurgeons payable if medical necessity established with documentation

T = team surgeons permitted
T+ = team surgeons payable if medical necessity established with documentation
S = indicates services that are not covered by Medicare.

161 CPT five-digit codes, two-digit numeric modifiers, and descriptions only are © 2001 American Medical Association

Medicare RBRVS: The Physicians' Guide

Relative value units

CPT Code and Modifier	Description	Work RVU	Non Facility Practice Expense RVU	Facility Practice Expense RVU	PLI RVU	Total Non Facility RVUs	Medicare Payment Non Facility	Total Facility RVUs	Medicare Payment Facility	Global Period	Payment Policy Indicators*
25040	Explore/treat wrist joint	7.18	NA	9.40	0.96	NA	NA	17.54	$634.93	090	M B A+
25065	Biopsy forearm soft tissues	1.99	2.53	2.53	0.12	4.64	$167.96	4.64	$167.96	010	M B A
25066	Biopsy forearm soft tissues	4.13	NA	8.40	0.49	NA	NA	13.02	$471.31	090	M B A
25075	Remove forearm lesion subcut	3.74	NA	7.13	0.40	NA	NA	11.27	$407.96	090	M B A
25076	Remove forearm lesion deep	4.92	NA	12.68	0.59	NA	NA	18.19	$658.46	090	M B A
25077	Remove tumor, forearm/wrist	9.76	NA	15.66	1.10	NA	NA	26.52	$960.00	090	M B A
25085	Incision of wrist capsule	5.50	NA	11.29	0.71	NA	NA	17.50	$633.49	090	M B
25100	Biopsy of wrist joint	3.90	NA	7.99	0.50	NA	NA	12.39	$448.51	090	M B A+
25101	Explore/treat wrist joint	4.69	NA	7.75	0.60	NA	NA	13.04	$472.04	090	M B A+
25105	Remove wrist joint lining	5.85	NA	11.22	0.77	NA	NA	17.84	$645.79	090	M B A+ C+
25107	Remove wrist joint cartilage	6.43	NA	11.41	0.82	NA	NA	18.66	$675.48	090	M B C+
25110	Remove wrist tendon lesion	3.92	NA	8.94	0.48	NA	NA	13.34	$482.90	090	M B A
25111	Remove wrist tendon lesion	3.39	NA	6.70	0.42	NA	NA	10.51	$380.45	090	M B A
25112	Reremove wrist tendon lesion	4.53	NA	7.43	0.54	NA	NA	12.50	$452.49	090	M B A
25115	Remove wrist/forearm lesion	8.82	NA	17.19	1.11	NA	NA	27.12	$981.72	090	M B A
25116	Remove wrist/forearm lesion	7.11	NA	16.20	0.90	NA	NA	24.21	$876.38	090	M B A+ C+
25118	Excise wrist tendon sheath	4.37	NA	7.93	0.55	NA	NA	12.85	$465.16	090	M B A
25119	Partial removal of ulna	6.04	NA	11.45	0.80	NA	NA	18.29	$662.08	090	M B C+
25120	Removal of forearm lesion	6.10	NA	14.87	0.81	NA	NA	21.78	$788.42	090	M B A+
25125	Remove/graft forearm lesion	7.48	NA	16.11	1.02	NA	NA	24.61	$890.86	090	M B A+
25126	Remove/graft forearm lesion	7.55	NA	15.76	1.00	NA	NA	24.31	$880.00	090	M B
25130	Removal of wrist lesion	5.26	NA	8.33	0.66	NA	NA	14.25	$515.84	090	M B A+
25135	Remove & graft wrist lesion	6.89	NA	9.00	0.89	NA	NA	16.78	$607.42	090	M B C+
25136	Remove & graft wrist lesion	5.97	NA	9.26	0.58	NA	NA	15.81	$572.31	090	M B C+
25145	Remove forearm bone lesion	6.37	NA	15.43	0.82	NA	NA	22.62	$818.83	090	M B
25150	Partial removal of ulna	7.09	NA	12.00	0.96	NA	NA	20.05	$725.79	090	M B A C+
25151	Partial removal of radius	7.39	NA	16.22	0.93	NA	NA	24.54	$888.33	090	M B C+

Code	Description											
25170	Extensive forearm surgery	11.09	NA	17.56	1.52	NA	30.17	$1,092.13	090	M	B	A+	C+
25210	Removal of wrist bone	5.95	NA	8.71	0.73	NA	15.39	$557.11	090	M		A+	C+
25215	Removal of wrist bones	7.89	NA	12.27	1.02	NA	21.18	$766.70	090	M		A	C+
25230	Partial removal of radius	5.23	NA	8.23	0.66	NA	14.12	$511.13	090	M	B	A	C+
25240	Partial removal of ulna	5.17	NA	10.78	0.69	NA	16.64	$602.35	090	M	B	A+	C+
25246	Injection for wrist x-ray	1.45	10.20	0.52	0.07	11.72	2.04	$73.85	000	M	B	A	
25248	Remove forearm foreign body	5.14	NA	10.66	0.54	NA	16.34	$591.49	090	M	B	A	
25250	Removal of wrist prosthesis	6.60	NA	8.91	0.84	NA	16.35	$591.86	090	M	B	A	
25251	Removal of wrist prosthesis	9.57	NA	12.52	1.15	NA	23.24	$841.27	090	M	B		
25259	Manipulate wrist w/anesthes	3.75	NA	5.35	0.52	NA	9.62	$348.24	090	M		A	
25260	Repair forearm tendon/muscle	7.80	NA	17.11	0.97	NA	25.88	$936.84	090	M		A	
25263	Repair forearm tendon/muscle	7.82	NA	15.65	0.94	NA	24.41	$883.62	090	M			
25265	Repair forearm tendon/muscle	9.88	NA	17.11	1.19	NA	28.18	$1,020.09	090	M		A+	
25270	Repair forearm tendon/muscle	6.00	NA	16.04	0.76	NA	22.80	$825.34	090	M		A+	
25272	Repair forearm tendon/muscle	7.04	NA	16.50	0.89	NA	24.43	$884.35	090	M		A+	C+
25274	Repair forearm tendon/muscle	8.75	NA	17.36	1.11	NA	27.22	$985.34	090	M		A+	C+
25275	Repair forearm tendon sheath	8.50	NA	7.53	1.11	NA	17.14	$620.45	090	M		A+	
25280	Revise wrist/forearm tendon	7.22	NA	15.80	0.91	NA	23.93	$866.25	090	M		A+	C+
25290	Incise wrist/forearm tendon	5.29	NA	18.17	0.66	NA	24.12	$873.12	090	M		A	
25295	Release wrist/forearm tendon	6.55	NA	15.16	0.84	NA	22.55	$816.29	090	M		A	
25300	Fusion of tendons at wrist	8.80	NA	10.02	1.07	NA	19.89	$720.00	090	M	B		
25301	Fusion of tendons at wrist	8.40	NA	10.15	1.08	NA	19.63	$710.59	090	M	B		
25310	Transplant forearm tendon	8.14	NA	16.47	1.01	NA	25.62	$927.42	090	M			C+
25312	Transplant forearm tendon	9.57	NA	17.24	1.22	NA	28.03	$1,014.66	090	M			C+
25315	Revise palsy hand tendon(s)	10.20	NA	18.59	1.26	NA	30.05	$1,087.79	090	M	B		
25316	Revise palsy hand tendon(s)	12.33	NA	18.40	1.74	NA	32.47	$1,175.39	090	M	B		
25320	Repair/revise wrist joint	10.77	NA	11.53	1.32	NA	23.62	$855.03	090	M	B		
25332	Revise wrist joint	11.41	NA	11.89	1.46	NA	24.76	$896.29	090	M	B		

* **M** = multiple surgery adjustment applies
Me = multiple endoscopy rules may apply
B = bilateral surgery adjustment applies
A = assistant-at-surgery restriction

A+ = assistant-at-surgery restriction unless medical necessity established with documentation
C = cosurgeons payable
C+ = cosurgeons payable if medical necessity established with documentation

T = team surgeons permitted
T+ = team surgeons payable if medical necessity established with documentation
§ = indicates services that are not covered by Medicare.

163 CPT five-digit codes, two-digit numeric modifiers, and descriptions only are © 2001 American Medical Association

Medicare RBRVS: The Physicians' Guide

Relative value units

CPT Code and Modifier	Description	Work RVU	Non Facility Practice Expense RVU	Facility Practice Expense RVU	PLI RVU	Total Non Facility RVUs	Medicare Payment Non Facility	Total Facility RVUs	Medicare Payment Facility	Global Period	Payment Policy Indicators*
25335	Realignment of hand	12.88	NA	13.60	1.66	NA	NA	28.14	$1,018.65	090	M B
25337	Reconstruct ulna/radioulnar	10.17	NA	13.80	1.31	NA	NA	25.28	$915.12	090	M B A
25350	Revision of radius	8.78	NA	16.68	1.17	NA	NA	26.63	$963.98	090	M B
25355	Revision of radius	10.17	NA	17.17	1.44	NA	NA	28.78	$1,041.81	090	M B
25360	Revision of ulna	8.43	NA	16.86	1.17	NA	NA	26.46	$957.83	090	M B C+
25365	Revise radius & ulna	12.40	NA	18.74	1.67	NA	NA	32.81	$1,187.70	090	M B
25370	Revise radius or ulna	13.36	NA	17.84	1.88	NA	NA	33.08	$1,197.47	090	M B
25375	Revise radius & ulna	13.04	NA	16.44	1.84	NA	NA	31.32	$1,133.76	090	M B C+
25390	Shorten radius or ulna	10.40	NA	17.38	1.38	NA	NA	29.16	$1,055.57	090	M B C+
25391	Lengthen radius or ulna	13.65	NA	19.01	1.73	NA	NA	34.39	$1,244.89	090	M B C+
25392	Shorten radius & ulna	13.95	NA	15.59	1.73	NA	NA	31.27	$1,131.95	090	M B
25393	Lengthen radius & ulna	15.87	NA	21.72	1.87	NA	NA	39.46	$1,428.42	090	M B C+
25394	Repair carpal bone, shorten	10.40	NA	8.43	1.15	NA	NA	19.98	$723.26	090	M B C+
25400	Repair radius or ulna	10.92	NA	17.98	1.50	NA	NA	30.40	$1,100.46	090	M B C+
25405	Repair/graft radius or ulna	14.38	NA	20.38	1.95	NA	NA	36.71	$1,328.87	090	M B C+
25415	Repair radius & ulna	13.35	NA	19.14	1.87	NA	NA	34.36	$1,243.80	090	M B C+
25420	Repair/graft radius & ulna	16.33	NA	21.72	2.20	NA	NA	40.25	$1,457.02	090	M B C+
25425	Repair/graft radius or ulna	13.21	NA	24.75	1.61	NA	NA	39.57	$1,432.40	090	M B C+
25426	Repair/graft radius & ulna	15.82	NA	18.15	2.23	NA	NA	36.20	$1,310.41	090	M B C+
25430	Vasc graft into carpal bone	9.25	NA	7.82	0.56	NA	NA	17.63	$638.19	090	M A
25431	Repair nonunion carpal bone	10.44	NA	6.42	0.56	NA	NA	17.42	$630.59	090	M B C+
25440	Repair/graft wrist bone	10.44	NA	11.05	1.41	NA	NA	22.90	$828.96	090	M B C+
25441	Reconstruct wrist joint	12.90	NA	12.24	1.83	NA	NA	26.97	$976.29	090	M B C+
25442	Reconstruct wrist joint	10.85	NA	11.46	1.24	NA	NA	23.55	$852.49	090	M B C+
25443	Reconstruct wrist joint	10.39	NA	13.29	1.30	NA	NA	24.98	$904.26	090	M B C+
25444	Reconstruct wrist joint	11.15	NA	14.29	1.43	NA	NA	26.87	$972.67	090	M B
25445	Reconstruct wrist joint	9.69	NA	13.50	1.26	NA	NA	24.45	$885.07	090	M B A C+

Code	Description										
25446	Wrist replacement	16.55	NA	14.45	2.20	NA	33.20	$1,201.81	090	M	B	C+
25447	Repair wrist joint(s)	10.37	NA	11.27	1.34	NA	22.98	$831.86	090	M	B	C+
25449	Remove wrist joint implant	14.49	NA	16.20	1.77	NA	32.46	$1,175.03	090	M	B	C+
25450	Revision of wrist joint	7.87	NA	13.91	0.88	NA	22.66	$820.27	090	M	B	A
25455	Revision of wrist joint	9.49	NA	15.22	1.07	NA	25.78	$933.22	090	M	B	A
25490	Reinforce radius	9.54	NA	16.70	1.19	NA	27.43	$992.94	090	M	B	
25491	Reinforce ulna	9.96	NA	16.98	1.41	NA	28.35	$1,026.25	090	M	B	
25492	Reinforce radius and ulna	12.33	NA	16.09	1.62	NA	30.04	$1,087.42	090	M	B	A
25500	Treat fracture of radius	2.45	4.27	2.94	0.28	7.00	5.67	$205.25	090	M	B	A
25505	Treat fracture of radius	5.21	7.87	5.65	0.69	13.77	11.55	$418.10	090	M	B	A
25515	Treat fracture of radius	9.18	NA	10.00	1.22	NA	20.40	$738.46	090	M	B	C+
25520	Treat fracture of radius	6.26	8.00	6.28	0.85	15.11	13.39	$484.71	090	M	B	A
25525	Treat fracture of radius	12.24	NA	11.65	1.68	NA	25.57	$925.61	090	M	B	C
25526	Treat fracture of radius	12.98	NA	15.01	1.80	NA	29.79	$1,078.37	090	M	B	C
25530	Treat fracture of ulna	2.09	4.21	2.87	0.27	6.57	5.23	$189.32	090	M	B	A
25535	Treat fracture of ulna	5.14	7.74	5.72	0.68	13.56	11.54	$417.74	090	M	B	A
25545	Treat fracture of ulna	8.90	NA	9.88	1.23	NA	20.01	$724.35	090	M	B	C+
25560	Treat fracture radius & ulna	2.44	4.28	2.93	0.27	6.99	5.64	$204.16	090	M	B	A
25565	Treat fracture radius & ulna	5.63	8.02	5.94	0.76	14.41	12.33	$446.34	090	M	B	A
25574	Treat fracture radius & ulna	7.01	NA	8.72	0.96	NA	16.69	$604.16	090	M	B	C
25575	Treat fracture radius/ulna	10.45	NA	10.74	1.46	NA	22.65	$819.91	090	M	B	C+
25600	Treat fracture radius/ulna	2.63	4.53	3.10	0.34	7.50	6.07	$219.73	090	M	B	A
25605	Treat fracture radius/ulna	5.81	8.18	6.11	0.81	14.80	12.73	$460.82	090	M	B	A
25611	Treat fracture radius/ulna	7.77	NA	10.04	1.08	NA	18.89	$683.80	090	M	B	A
25620	Treat fracture radius/ulna	8.55	NA	9.67	1.17	NA	19.39	$701.90	090	M	B	
25622	Treat wrist bone fracture	2.61	4.48	3.10	0.33	7.42	6.04	$218.64	090	M	B	A
25624	Treat wrist bone fracture	4.53	7.40	5.34	0.61	12.54	10.48	$379.37	090	M	B	A+
25628	Treat wrist bone fracture	8.43	NA	9.68	1.14	NA	19.25	$696.83	090	M	B	

* **M** = multiple surgery adjustment applies
Me = multiple endoscopy rules may apply
B = bilateral surgery adjustment applies
A = assistant-at-surgery restriction

A+ = assistant-at-surgery restriction unless medical necessity established with documentation
C = cosurgeons payable
C+ = cosurgeons payable if medical necessity established with documentation

T = team surgeons permitted
T+ = team surgeons payable if medical necessity established with documentation
$ = indicates services that are not covered by Medicare.

165 CPT five-digit codes, two-digit numeric modifiers, and descriptions only are © 2001 American Medical Association

Medicare RBRVS: The Physicians' Guide

Relative value units

CPT Code and Modifier	Description	Work RVU	Non Facility Practice Expense RVU	Facility Practice Expense RVU	PLI RVU	Total Non Facility RVUs	Medicare Payment Non Facility	Total Facility RVUs	Medicare Payment Facility	Global Period	Payment Policy Indicators*
25630	Treat wrist bone fracture	2.88	4.66	3.20	0.37	7.91	$286.34	6.45	$233.48	090	M B A
25635	Treat wrist bone fracture	4.39	7.45	5.11	0.39	12.23	$442.72	9.89	$358.01	090	M B A+
25645	Treat wrist bone fracture	7.25	NA	9.56	0.93	NA	NA	17.74	$642.17	090	M B
25650	Treat wrist bone fracture	3.05	4.75	3.24	0.37	8.17	$295.75	6.66	$241.09	090	M B A
25651	Pin ulnar styloid fracture	5.36	NA	4.39	0.73	NA	NA	10.48	$379.37	090	M B A+
25652	Treat fracture ulnar styloid	7.60	NA	6.90	0.97	NA	NA	15.47	$560.00	090	M B A C+
25660	Treat wrist dislocation	4.76	NA	5.45	0.59	NA	NA	10.80	$390.95	090	M B A+
25670	Treat wrist dislocation	7.92	NA	9.54	1.07	NA	NA	18.53	$670.77	090	M B C+
25671	Pin radioulnar dislocation	6.00	NA	6.02	0.75	NA	NA	12.77	$462.26	090	M B A
25675	Treat wrist dislocation	4.67	7.57	5.39	0.57	12.81	$463.71	10.63	$384.80	090	M B A+
25676	Treat wrist dislocation	8.04	NA	9.52	1.10	NA	NA	18.66	$675.48	090	M B
25680	Treat wrist fracture	5.99	NA	6.45	0.61	NA	NA	13.05	$472.40	090	M B A+
25685	Treat wrist fracture	9.78	NA	10.20	1.25	NA	NA	21.23	$768.51	090	M B
25690	Treat wrist dislocation	5.50	NA	7.00	0.78	NA	NA	13.28	$480.73	090	M B A+
25695	Treat wrist dislocation	8.34	NA	9.68	1.07	NA	NA	19.09	$691.04	090	M B C+
25800	Fusion of wrist joint	9.76	NA	10.87	1.30	NA	NA	21.93	$793.85	090	M B C+
25805	Fusion/graft of wrist joint	11.28	NA	11.61	1.51	NA	NA	24.40	$883.26	090	M B C+
25810	Fusion/graft of wrist joint	10.57	NA	11.33	1.37	NA	NA	23.27	$842.36	090	M B C+
25820	Fusion of hand bones	7.45	NA	9.54	0.96	NA	NA	17.95	$649.78	090	M B C+
25825	Fuse hand bones with graft	9.27	NA	10.51	1.20	NA	NA	20.98	$759.46	090	M B C+
25830	Fusion, radioulnar jnt/ulna	10.06	NA	16.99	1.27	NA	NA	28.32	$1,025.16	090	M B C+
25900	Amputation of forearm	9.01	NA	15.04	1.08	NA	NA	25.13	$909.69	090	M B A+
25905	Amputation of forearm	9.12	NA	14.25	1.06	NA	NA	24.43	$884.35	090	M B
25907	Amputation follow-up surgery	7.80	NA	15.26	1.01	NA	NA	24.07	$871.31	090	M B
25909	Amputation follow-up surgery	8.96	NA	14.51	1.07	NA	NA	24.54	$888.33	090	M B
25915	Amputation of forearm	17.08	NA	15.11	2.41	NA	NA	34.60	$1,252.49	090	M B
25920	Amputate hand at wrist	8.68	NA	10.12	1.06	NA	NA	19.86	$718.92	090	M B A+

Code	Description										
25922	Amputate hand at wrist	7.42	NA	7.58	0.93	NA	NA	15.93	$576.65	090	M	B
25924	Amputation follow-up surgery	8.46	NA	10.19	1.07	NA	NA	19.72	$713.85	090	M	B
25927	Amputation of hand	8.80	NA	14.11	1.02	NA	NA	23.93	$866.25	090	M	B	A+
25929	Amputation follow-up surgery	7.59	NA	7.42	0.89	NA	NA	15.90	$575.57	090	M	B
25931	Amputation follow-up surgery	7.81	NA	15.79	0.88	NA	NA	24.48	$886.16	090	M	B	A
25999	Forearm or wrist surgery	0.00	0.00	0.00	0.00	0.00	$0.00	0.00	$0.00	YYY	M	B	C+	T+
26010	Drainage of finger abscess	1.54	5.24	3.94	0.14	6.92	$250.50	5.62	$203.44	010	M	A+
26011	Drainage of finger abscess	2.19	7.48	6.50	0.25	9.92	$359.10	8.94	$323.62	010	M	A
26020	Drain hand tendon sheath	4.67	NA	13.10	0.59	NA	NA	18.36	$664.62	090	M	A
26025	Drainage of palm bursa	4.82	NA	13.26	0.60	NA	NA	18.68	$676.20	090	M	A+
26030	Drainage of palm bursa(s)	5.93	NA	14.02	0.72	NA	NA	20.67	$748.24	090	M	A+
26034	Treat hand bone lesion	6.23	NA	14.84	0.79	NA	NA	21.86	$791.31	090	M	A
26035	Decompress fingers/hand	9.51	NA	15.17	1.12	NA	NA	25.80	$933.94	090	M	A+
26037	Decompress fingers/hand	7.25	NA	12.67	0.87	NA	NA	20.79	$752.58	090	M	A+
26040	Release palm contracture	3.33	NA	12.87	0.45	NA	NA	16.65	$602.72	090	M	B	A
26045	Release palm contracture	5.56	NA	14.17	0.74	NA	NA	20.47	$741.00	090	M	B	A
26055	Incise finger tendon sheath	2.69	8.12	7.69	0.36	11.17	$404.35	10.74	$388.78	090	M	A
26060	Incision of finger tendon	2.81	NA	7.57	0.35	NA	NA	10.73	$388.42	090	M	A+
26070	Explore/treat hand joint	3.69	NA	11.69	0.35	NA	NA	15.73	$569.41	090	M	B	A
26075	Explore/treat finger joint	3.79	NA	12.47	0.40	NA	NA	16.66	$603.08	090	M	B	A
26080	Explore/treat finger joint	4.24	NA	13.09	0.52	NA	NA	17.85	$646.16	090	M	B	A
26100	Biopsy hand joint lining	3.67	NA	8.43	0.45	NA	NA	12.55	$454.30	090	M	B	A+
26105	Biopsy finger joint lining	3.71	NA	12.95	0.45	NA	NA	17.11	$619.37	090	M	B	A+
26110	Biopsy finger joint lining	3.53	NA	12.46	0.44	NA	NA	16.43	$594.75	090	M	A
26115	Remove hand lesion subcut	3.86	7.66	7.66	0.48	12.00	$434.39	12.00	$434.39	090	M	A
26116	Remove hand lesion, deep	5.53	NA	13.91	0.69	NA	NA	20.13	$728.69	090	M	A
26117	Remove tumor, hand/finger	8.55	NA	15.41	1.01	NA	NA	24.97	$903.89	090	M	A
26121	Release palm contracture	7.54	NA	15.80	0.94	NA	NA	24.28	$878.92	090	M	B	A

* **M** = multiple surgery adjustment applies
   Me = multiple endoscopy rules may apply
   B = bilateral surgery adjustment applies
   A = assistant-at-surgery restriction

A+ = assistant-at-surgery restriction unless medical necessity established with documentation
C = cosurgeons payable
C+ = cosurgeons payable if medical necessity established with documentation

T = team surgeons permitted
T+ = team surgeons payable if medical necessity established with documentation
$ = indicates services that are not covered by Medicare.

CPT five-digit codes, two-digit numeric modifiers, and descriptions only are © 2001 American Medical Association

Medicare RBRVS: The Physicians' Guide

Relative value units

CPT Code and Modifier	Description	Work RVU	Non Facility Practice Expense RVU	Facility Practice Expense RVU	PLI RVU	Total Non Facility RVUs	Medicare Payment Non Facility	Total Facility RVUs	Medicare Payment Facility	Global Period	Payment Policy Indicators*
26123	Release palm contracture	9.29	NA	16.73	1.17	NA	NA	27.19	$984.26	090	M B A
26125	Release palm contracture	4.61	NA	2.60	0.57	NA	NA	7.78	$281.63	ZZZ	A
26130	Remove wrist joint lining	5.42	NA	15.62	0.65	NA	NA	21.69	$785.16	090	M B A
26135	Revise finger joint, each	6.96	NA	17.04	0.87	NA	NA	24.87	$900.27	090	M A+
26140	Revise finger joint, each	6.17	NA	16.33	0.76	NA	NA	23.26	$841.99	090	M A
26145	Tendon excision, palm/finger	6.32	NA	16.86	0.77	NA	NA	23.95	$866.97	090	M A
26160	Remove tendon sheath lesion	3.15	7.93	7.88	0.39	11.47	$415.20	11.42	$413.39	090	M A
26170	Removal of palm tendon, each	4.77	NA	8.53	0.60	NA	NA	13.90	$503.17	090	M A+
26180	Removal of finger tendon	5.18	NA	9.19	0.64	NA	NA	15.01	$543.35	090	M A+
26185	Remove finger bone	5.25	NA	8.76	0.67	NA	NA	14.68	$531.40	090	M B C+
26200	Remove hand bone lesion	5.51	NA	13.97	0.71	NA	NA	20.19	$730.86	090	M A+
26205	Remove/graft bone lesion	7.70	NA	15.35	0.95	NA	NA	24.00	$868.78	090	M A
26210	Removal of finger lesion	5.15	NA	14.32	0.64	NA	NA	20.11	$727.97	090	M A
26215	Remove/graft finger lesion	7.10	NA	14.89	0.77	NA	NA	22.76	$823.89	090	M A
26230	Partial removal of hand bone	6.33	NA	12.87	0.84	NA	NA	20.04	$725.43	090	M A+
26235	Partial removal, finger bone	6.19	NA	12.56	0.78	NA	NA	19.53	$706.97	090	M A+
26236	Partial removal, finger bone	5.32	NA	12.62	0.66	NA	NA	18.60	$673.31	090	M A
26250	Extensive hand surgery	7.55	NA	17.33	0.92	NA	NA	25.80	$933.94	090	M A+
26255	Extensive hand surgery	12.43	NA	18.74	1.05	NA	NA	32.22	$1,166.34	090	M C+
26260	Extensive finger surgery	7.03	NA	16.39	0.83	NA	NA	24.25	$877.83	090	M
26261	Extensive finger surgery	9.09	NA	16.10	0.84	NA	NA	26.03	$942.27	090	M
26262	Partial removal of finger	5.67	NA	14.81	0.70	NA	NA	21.18	$766.70	090	M
26320	Removal of implant from hand	3.98	NA	13.08	0.49	NA	NA	17.55	$635.30	090	M A
26340	Manipulate finger w/anesth	2.50	NA	4.53	0.32	NA	NA	7.35	$266.06	090	M A
26350	Repair finger/hand tendon	5.99	NA	20.24	0.73	NA	NA	26.96	$975.93	090	M A
26352	Repair/graft hand tendon	7.68	NA	19.74	0.93	NA	NA	28.35	$1,026.25	090	M C+
26356	Repair finger/hand tendon	8.07	NA	21.55	0.99	NA	NA	30.61	$1,108.06	090	M A

Code	Description								
26357	Repair finger/hand tendon	8.58	NA	21.30	1.02	NA	30.90	$1,118.56	090	M	
26358	Repair/graft hand tendon	9.14	NA	22.43	1.07	NA	32.64	$1,181.54	090	M	
26370	Repair finger/hand tendon	7.11	NA	20.61	0.90	NA	28.62	$1,036.02	090	M	A+
26372	Repair/graft hand tendon	8.76	NA	20.46	1.06	NA	30.28	$1,096.11	090	M	
26373	Repair finger/graft tendon	8.16	NA	22.61	0.98	NA	31.75	$1,149.32	090	M	
26390	Revise hand/finger tendon	9.19	NA	16.93	1.09	NA	27.21	$984.98	090	M	C+
26392	Repair/graft hand tendon	10.26	NA	23.05	1.26	NA	34.57	$1,251.41	090	M	C+
26410	Repair hand tendon	4.63	NA	16.26	0.57	NA	21.46	$776.83	090	M	A
26412	Repair/graft hand tendon	6.31	NA	16.83	0.80	NA	23.94	$866.61	090	M	A+
26415	Excision, hand/finger tendon	8.34	NA	18.14	0.77	NA	27.25	$986.43	090	M	A+
26416	Graft hand or finger tendon	9.37	NA	18.95	1.20	NA	29.52	$1,068.60	090	M	A
26418	Repair finger tendon	4.25	NA	16.34	0.50	NA	21.09	$763.44	090	M	A
26420	Repair/graft finger tendon	6.77	NA	17.92	0.83	NA	25.52	$923.80	090	M	
26426	Repair finger/hand tendon	6.15	NA	17.05	0.77	NA	23.97	$867.69	090	M	A
26428	Repair/graft finger tendon	7.21	NA	16.05	0.84	NA	24.10	$872.40	090	M	A+
26432	Repair finger tendon	4.02	NA	13.49	0.48	NA	17.99	$651.22	090	M	A
26433	Repair finger tendon	4.56	NA	14.42	0.56	NA	19.54	$707.33	090	M	A
26434	Repair/graft finger tendon	6.09	NA	15.34	0.71	NA	22.14	$801.45	090	M	
26437	Realignment of tendons	5.82	NA	14.16	0.74	NA	20.72	$750.05	090	M	A
26440	Release palm/finger tendon	5.02	NA	18.48	0.62	NA	24.12	$873.12	090	M	A
26442	Release palm & finger tendon	8.16	NA	19.40	0.94	NA	28.50	$1,031.68	090	M	A
26445	Release hand/finger tendon	4.31	NA	18.27	0.54	NA	23.12	$836.93	090	M	A
26449	Release forearm/hand tendon	7.00	NA	20.16	0.84	NA	28.00	$1,013.58	090	M	A+
26450	Incision of palm tendon	3.67	NA	8.71	0.46	NA	12.84	$464.80	090	M	A+
26455	Incision of finger tendon	3.64	NA	8.38	0.47	NA	12.49	$452.13	090	M	A+
26460	Incise hand/finger tendon	3.46	NA	8.06	0.44	NA	11.96	$432.94	090	M	A
26471	Fusion of finger tendons	5.73	NA	13.93	0.73	NA	20.39	$738.10	090	M	A+
26474	Fusion of finger tendons	5.32	NA	13.30	0.69	NA	19.31	$699.01	090	M	

* **M** = multiple surgery adjustment applies
   Me = multiple endoscopy rules may apply
   B = bilateral surgery adjustment applies
   A = assistant-at-surgery restriction

A+ = assistant-at-surgery restriction unless medical necessity established with documentation
C = cosurgeons payable
C+ = cosurgeons payable if medical necessity established with documentation

T = team surgeons permitted
T+ = team surgeons payable if medical necessity established with documentation
§ = indicates services that are not covered by Medicare.

CPT five-digit codes, two-digit numeric modifiers, and descriptions only are © 2001 American Medical Association

Relative value units

CPT Code and Modifier	Description	Work RVU	Non Facility Practice Expense RVU	Facility Practice Expense RVU	PLI RVU	Total Non Facility RVUs	Medicare Payment Non Facility	Total Facility RVUs	Medicare Payment Facility	Global Period	Payment Policy Indicators*
26476	Tendon lengthening	5.18	NA	12.72	0.62	NA	NA	18.52	$670.41	090	M A
26477	Tendon shortening	5.15	NA	13.73	0.60	NA	NA	19.48	$705.16	090	M A C+
26478	Lengthening of hand tendon	5.80	NA	14.73	0.77	NA	NA	21.30	$771.04	090	M A+
26479	Shortening of hand tendon	5.74	NA	13.71	0.76	NA	NA	20.21	$731.59	090	M
26480	Transplant hand tendon	6.69	NA	19.63	0.84	NA	NA	27.16	$983.17	090	M A+
26483	Transplant/graft hand tendon	8.29	NA	19.79	1.03	NA	NA	29.11	$1,053.76	090	M C+
26485	Transplant palm tendon	7.70	NA	20.08	0.94	NA	NA	28.72	$1,039.64	090	M C+
26489	Transplant/graft palm tendon	9.55	NA	17.34	0.98	NA	NA	27.87	$1,008.87	090	M A+
26490	Revise thumb tendon	8.41	NA	14.87	1.05	NA	NA	24.33	$880.73	090	M A+
26492	Tendon transfer with graft	9.62	NA	15.84	1.19	NA	NA	26.65	$964.71	090	M C+
26494	Hand tendon/muscle transfer	8.47	NA	13.52	1.13	NA	NA	23.12	$836.93	090	M C+
26496	Revise thumb tendon	9.59	NA	15.53	1.17	NA	NA	26.29	$951.68	090	M A+
26497	Finger tendon transfer	9.57	NA	16.42	1.17	NA	NA	27.16	$983.17	090	M
26498	Finger tendon transfer	14.00	NA	18.19	1.74	NA	NA	33.93	$1,228.24	090	M C+
26499	Revision of finger	8.98	NA	14.61	0.94	NA	NA	24.53	$887.97	090	M C+
26500	Hand tendon reconstruction	5.96	NA	15.16	0.66	NA	NA	21.78	$788.42	090	M A+
26502	Hand tendon reconstruction	7.14	NA	15.14	0.87	NA	NA	23.15	$838.01	090	M
26504	Hand tendon reconstruction	7.47	NA	14.31	0.84	NA	NA	22.62	$818.83	090	M
26508	Release thumb contracture	6.01	NA	14.11	0.76	NA	NA	20.88	$755.84	090	M A+
26510	Thumb tendon transfer	5.43	NA	14.18	0.71	NA	NA	20.32	$735.57	090	M A+
26516	Fusion of knuckle joint	7.15	NA	15.06	0.90	NA	NA	23.11	$836.56	090	M A+
26517	Fusion of knuckle joints	8.83	NA	15.89	0.96	NA	NA	25.68	$929.60	090	M
26518	Fusion of knuckle joints	9.02	NA	15.91	1.13	NA	NA	26.06	$943.35	090	M C+
26520	Release knuckle contracture	5.30	NA	18.59	0.65	NA	NA	24.54	$888.33	090	M A
26525	Release finger contracture	5.33	NA	18.67	0.66	NA	NA	24.66	$892.67	090	M A C+
26530	Revise knuckle joint	6.69	NA	19.35	0.86	NA	NA	26.90	$973.76	090	M
26531	Revise knuckle with implant	7.91	NA	19.41	1.01	NA	NA	28.33	$1,025.52	090	M C+

Code	Description									
26535	Revise finger joint	5.24	NA	11.10	0.66	NA	17.00	$615.39	090	M	A
26536	Revise/implant finger joint	6.37	NA	17.97	0.80	NA	25.14	$910.05	090	M	A+
26540	Repair hand joint	6.43	NA	14.54	0.81	NA	21.78	$788.42	090	M	A+ C+
26541	Repair hand joint with graft	8.62	NA	16.36	1.12	NA	26.10	$944.80	090	M	C+
26542	Repair hand joint with graft	6.78	NA	14.51	0.87	NA	22.16	$802.17	090	M	A+
26545	Reconstruct finger joint	6.92	NA	16.16	0.79	NA	23.87	$864.07	090	M	A+
26546	Repair nonunion hand	8.92	NA	15.95	1.14	NA	26.01	$941.54	090	M	B
26548	Reconstruct finger joint	8.03	NA	16.13	0.98	NA	25.14	$910.05	090	M	A+
26550	Construct thumb replacement	21.24	NA	30.36	1.80	NA	53.40	$1,933.04	090	M	
26551	Great toe-hand transfer	46.58	NA	29.35	6.57	NA	82.50	$2,986.43	090	M	
26553	Single transfer, toe-hand	46.27	NA	29.23	1.99	NA	77.49	$2,805.08	090	M	C+
26554	Double transfer, toe-hand	54.95	NA	32.69	7.76	NA	95.40	$3,453.40	090	M	C+
26555	Positional change of finger	16.63	NA	24.00	2.13	NA	42.76	$1,547.88	090	M	
26556	Toe joint transfer	47.26	NA	29.62	6.67	NA	83.55	$3,024.44	090	M	C+
26560	Repair of web finger	5.38	NA	12.55	0.60	NA	18.53	$670.77	090	M	
26561	Repair of web finger	10.92	NA	18.61	0.69	NA	30.22	$1,093.94	090	M	C+
26562	Repair of web finger	15.00	NA	13.44	0.98	NA	29.42	$1,064.98	090	M	
26565	Correct metacarpal flaw	6.74	NA	14.77	0.84	NA	22.35	$809.05	090	M	
26567	Correct finger deformity	6.82	NA	15.10	0.84	NA	22.76	$823.89	090	M	A+
26568	Lengthen metacarpal/finger	9.08	NA	19.48	1.10	NA	29.66	$1,073.67	090	M	
26580	Repair hand deformity	18.18	NA	17.22	1.46	NA	36.86	$1,334.30	090	M	
26587	Reconstruct extra finger	14.05	4.67	4.67	1.08	19.80	19.80	$716.74	090	M	
26590	Repair finger deformity	17.96	NA	14.62	1.32	NA	33.90	$1,227.15	090	M	
26591	Repair muscles of hand	3.25	NA	14.22	0.37	NA	17.84	$645.79	090	M	A+
26593	Release muscles of hand	5.31	NA	13.33	0.64	NA	19.28	$697.92	090	M	A
26596	Excision constricting tissue	8.95	NA	10.26	0.87	NA	20.08	$726.88	090	M	
26600	Treat metacarpal fracture	1.96	4.15	2.83	0.25	6.36	5.04	$182.44	090	M	A
26605	Treat metacarpal fracture	2.85	6.05	4.29	0.38	9.28	7.52	$272.22	090	M	A

* **M** = multiple surgery adjustment applies
Me = multiple endoscopy rules may apply
B = bilateral surgery adjustment applies
A = assistant-at-surgery restriction

A+ = assistant-at-surgery restriction unless medical necessity established with documentation
C = cosurgeons payable
C+ = cosurgeons payable if medical necessity established with documentation

T = team surgeons permitted
T+ = team surgeons payable if medical necessity established with documentation
§ = indicates services that are not covered by Medicare.

171   CPT five-digit codes, two-digit numeric modifiers, and descriptions only are © 2001 American Medical Association

Medicare RBRVS: The Physicians' Guide

Relative value units

CPT Code and Modifier	Description	Work RVU	Non Facility Practice Expense RVU	Facility Practice Expense RVU	PLI RVU	Total Non Facility RVUs	Medicare Payment Non Facility	Total Facility RVUs	Medicare Payment Facility	Global Period	Payment Policy Indicators*
26607	Treat metacarpal fracture	5.36	NA	8.33	0.70	NA	NA	14.39	$520.91	090	M A+
26608	Treat metacarpal fracture	5.36	NA	8.85	0.73	NA	NA	14.94	$540.82	090	M A+
26615	Treat metacarpal fracture	5.33	NA	8.43	0.70	NA	NA	14.46	$523.44	090	M A
26641	Treat thumb dislocation	3.94	6.58	4.99	0.42	10.94	$396.02	9.35	$338.46	090	M A+
26645	Treat thumb fracture	4.41	7.33	5.30	0.54	12.28	$444.53	10.25	$371.04	090	M A+
26650	Treat thumb fracture	5.72	NA	9.02	0.77	NA	NA	15.51	$561.45	090	M A
26665	Treat thumb fracture	7.60	NA	9.24	0.97	NA	NA	17.81	$644.71	090	M A C+
26670	Treat hand dislocation	3.69	6.46	4.93	0.36	10.51	$380.45	8.98	$325.07	090	M A+
26675	Treat hand dislocation	4.64	6.82	4.71	0.56	12.02	$435.11	9.91	$358.73	090	M A+
26676	Pin hand dislocation	5.52	NA	9.36	0.76	NA	NA	15.64	$566.16	090	M A
26685	Treat hand dislocation	6.98	NA	8.88	0.95	NA	NA	16.81	$608.51	090	M A C+
26686	Treat hand dislocation	7.94	NA	9.84	1.05	NA	NA	18.83	$681.63	090	M A
26700	Treat knuckle dislocation	3.69	5.01	3.02	0.35	9.05	$327.60	7.06	$255.57	090	M A
26705	Treat knuckle dislocation	4.19	6.26	4.33	0.50	10.95	$396.38	9.02	$326.52	090	M A+
26706	Pin knuckle dislocation	5.12	NA	5.87	0.64	NA	NA	11.63	$421.00	090	M A
26715	Treat knuckle dislocation	5.74	NA	8.62	0.75	NA	NA	15.11	$546.97	090	M A+
26720	Treat finger fracture, each	1.66	3.06	1.72	0.20	4.92	$178.10	3.58	$129.59	090	M A
26725	Treat finger fracture, each	3.33	5.27	3.26	0.43	9.03	$326.88	7.02	$254.12	090	M A
26727	Treat finger fracture, each	5.23	NA	8.88	0.69	NA	NA	14.80	$535.75	090	M A
26735	Treat finger fracture, each	5.98	NA	8.99	0.77	NA	NA	15.74	$569.78	090	M A
26740	Treat finger fracture, each	1.94	3.86	2.67	0.24	6.04	$218.64	4.85	$175.57	090	M A
26742	Treat finger fracture, each	3.85	7.21	5.13	0.49	11.55	$418.10	9.47	$342.81	090	M A
26746	Treat finger fracture, each	5.81	NA	8.93	0.74	NA	NA	15.48	$560.36	090	M A
26750	Treat finger fracture, each	1.70	3.66	2.47	0.19	5.55	$200.91	4.36	$157.83	090	M A
26755	Treat finger fracture, each	3.10	5.08	3.27	0.37	8.55	$309.50	6.74	$243.98	090	M A
26756	Pin finger fracture, each	4.39	NA	8.74	0.56	NA	NA	13.69	$495.57	090	M A+
26765	Treat finger fracture, each	4.17	NA	8.02	0.51	NA	NA	12.70	$459.73	090	M A

Code	Description										
26770	Treat finger dislocation	3.02	4.87	2.80	0.27	8.16	$295.39	6.09	$220.45	090	M	A
26775	Treat finger dislocation	3.71	6.07	4.09	0.43	10.21	$369.59	8.23	$297.92	090	M	A
26776	Pin finger dislocation	4.80	NA	8.61	0.63	NA	NA	14.04	$508.24	090	M	A
26785	Treat finger dislocation	4.21	NA	7.95	0.54	NA	NA	12.70	$459.73	090	M	A
26820	Thumb fusion with graft	8.26	NA	15.80	1.11	NA	NA	25.17	$911.13	090	M	C+
26841	Fusion of thumb	7.13	NA	15.37	0.97	NA	NA	23.47	$849.60	090	M	A+
26842	Thumb fusion with graft	8.24	NA	15.49	1.10	NA	NA	24.83	$898.83	090	M	C+
26843	Fusion of hand joint	7.61	NA	13.91	0.99	NA	NA	22.51	$814.84	090	M	C+
26844	Fusion/graft of hand joint	8.73	NA	15.63	1.12	NA	NA	25.48	$922.36	090	M	C+
26850	Fusion of knuckle	6.97	NA	14.63	0.89	NA	NA	22.49	$814.12	090	M	A+
26852	Fusion of knuckle with graft	8.46	NA	15.19	1.05	NA	NA	24.70	$894.12	090	M	C+
26860	Fusion of finger joint	4.69	NA	13.45	0.60	NA	NA	18.74	$678.37	090	M	A
26861	Fusion of finger jnt, add-on	1.74	NA	0.99	0.22	NA	NA	2.95	$106.79	ZZZ	M	A
26862	Fusion/graft of finger joint	7.37	NA	15.18	0.92	NA	NA	23.47	$849.60	090	M	C+
26863	Fuse/graft added joint	3.90	NA	2.25	0.51	NA	NA	6.66	$241.09	ZZZ		
26910	Amputate metacarpal bone	7.60	NA	13.98	0.90	NA	NA	22.48	$813.76	090	M	A
26951	Amputation of finger/thumb	4.59	NA	13.06	0.56	NA	NA	18.21	$659.19	090	M	A
26952	Amputation of finger/thumb	6.31	NA	14.47	0.74	NA	NA	21.52	$779.01	090	M	A
26989	Hand/finger surgery	0.00	0.00	0.00	0.00	0.00	$0.00	0.00	$0.00	YYY	M	A	T+
26990	Drainage of pelvis lesion	7.48	NA	15.92	0.92	NA	NA	24.32	$880.36	090	M	A
26991	Drainage of pelvis bursa	6.68	11.32	9.39	0.85	18.85	$682.35	16.92	$612.49	090	M	A+
26992	Drainage of bone lesion	13.02	NA	19.95	1.75	NA	NA	34.72	$1,256.84	090	M	A+
27000	Incision of hip tendon	5.62	NA	7.48	0.76	NA	NA	13.86	$501.72	090	M	B	A	C+
27001	Incision of hip tendon	6.94	NA	8.42	0.95	NA	NA	16.31	$590.41	090	M	B	B	C+
27003	Incision of hip tendon	7.34	NA	9.01	0.93	NA	NA	17.28	$625.52	090	M	B	B	C+
27005	Incision of hip tendon	9.66	NA	10.50	1.36	NA	NA	21.52	$779.01	090	M	B	B	C+
27006	Incision of hip tendons	9.68	NA	10.59	1.33	NA	NA	21.60	$781.90	090	M	B	B	C+
27025	Incision of hip/thigh fascia	11.16	NA	10.53	1.38	NA	NA	23.07	$835.12	090	M	B	A+	C+

* **M** = multiple surgery adjustment applies
Me = multiple endoscopy rules may apply
B = bilateral surgery adjustment applies
A = assistant-at-surgery restriction

A+ = assistant-at-surgery restriction unless medical necessity established with documentation
C = cosurgeons payable
C+ = cosurgeons payable if medical necessity established with documentation

T = team surgeons permitted
T+ = team surgeons payable if medical necessity established with documentation
$ = indicates services that are not covered by Medicare.

173 CPT five-digit codes, two-digit numeric modifiers, and descriptions only are © 2001 American Medical Association

Medicare RBRVS: The Physicians' Guide

Relative value units

CPT Code and Modifier	Description	Work RVU	Non Facility Practice Expense RVU	Facility Practice Expense RVU	PLI RVU	Total Non Facility RVUs	Medicare Payment Non Facility	Total Facility RVUs	Medicare Payment Facility	Global Period	Payment Policy Indicators*
27030	Drainage of hip joint	13.01	NA	12.45	1.81	NA	NA	27.27	$987.15	090	M B C+
27033	Exploration of hip joint	13.39	NA	12.62	1.87	NA	NA	27.88	$1,009.23	090	M B C+
27035	Denervation of hip joint	16.69	NA	19.67	1.70	NA	NA	38.06	$1,377.74	090	M B C+
27036	Excision of hip joint/muscle	12.88	NA	14.03	1.80	NA	NA	28.71	$1,039.28	090	M B C+
27040	Biopsy of soft tissues	2.87	6.23	4.00	0.21	9.31	$337.01	7.08	$256.29	010	M B A
27041	Biopsy of soft tissues	9.89	NA	8.60	1.01	NA	NA	19.50	$705.88	090	M B A
27047	Remove hip/pelvis lesion	7.45	9.26	7.03	0.79	17.50	$633.49	15.27	$552.76	090	M B A
27048	Remove hip/pelvis lesion	6.25	NA	7.94	0.73	NA	NA	14.92	$540.09	090	M B C+
27049	Remove tumor, hip/pelvis	13.66	NA	13.77	1.60	NA	NA	29.03	$1,050.86	090	M B C+
27050	Biopsy of sacroiliac joint	4.36	NA	7.52	0.53	NA	NA	12.41	$449.23	090	M B A+
27052	Biopsy of hip joint	6.23	NA	8.24	0.85	NA	NA	15.32	$554.57	090	M B C+
27054	Removal of hip joint lining	8.54	NA	10.67	1.17	NA	NA	20.38	$737.74	090	M B C+
27060	Removal of ischial bursa	5.43	NA	7.21	0.60	NA	NA	13.24	$479.28	090	M B A
27062	Remove femur lesion/bursa	5.37	NA	7.32	0.74	NA	NA	13.43	$486.16	090	M B A
27065	Removal of hip bone lesion	5.90	NA	8.65	0.76	NA	NA	15.31	$554.21	090	M B C+
27066	Removal of hip bone lesion	10.33	NA	12.53	1.42	NA	NA	24.28	$878.92	090	M B C+
27067	Remove/graft hip bone lesion	13.83	NA	14.54	1.95	NA	NA	30.32	$1,097.56	090	M B
27070	Partial removal of hip bone	10.72	NA	17.71	1.36	NA	NA	29.79	$1,078.37	090	M B C+
27071	Partial removal of hip bone	11.46	NA	18.67	1.51	NA	NA	31.64	$1,145.34	090	M B C+
27075	Extensive hip surgery	35.00	NA	25.75	2.22	NA	NA	62.97	$2,279.46	090	M C+
27076	Extensive hip surgery	22.12	NA	20.08	2.86	NA	NA	45.06	$1,631.14	090	M C+
27077	Extensive hip surgery	40.00	NA	30.55	3.18	NA	NA	73.73	$2,668.97	090	M C+
27078	Extensive hip surgery	13.44	NA	16.30	1.67	NA	NA	31.41	$1,137.02	090	M C+
27079	Extensive hip surgery	13.75	NA	13.43	1.86	NA	NA	29.04	$1,051.22	090	M C+
27080	Removal of tail bone	6.39	NA	7.64	0.80	NA	NA	14.83	$536.83	090	M C+
27086	Remove hip foreign body	1.87	5.85	3.70	0.17	7.89	$285.61	5.74	$207.78	010	M B A+
27087	Remove hip foreign body	8.54	NA	9.04	1.09	NA	NA	18.67	$675.84	090	M B C+

Code	Description										
27090	Removal of hip prosthesis	11.15	NA	11.37	1.55	NA	24.07	$871.31	090	M	B		C+
27091	Removal of hip prosthesis	22.14	NA	15.14	3.11	NA	40.39	$1,462.09	090	M	B		C+
27093	Injection for hip x-ray	1.30	13.59	0.53	0.09	$542.26	1.92	$69.50	000	M	B	A	
27095	Injection for hip x-ray	1.50	11.00	0.60	0.10	$456.11	2.20	$79.64	000	M	B	A	
27096	Inject sacroiliac joint	1.40	8.86	0.35	0.08	$374.30	1.83	$66.24	000	M	B	A	
27097	Revision of hip tendon	8.80	NA	8.13	1.22	NA	18.15	$657.02	090	M	B		C+
27098	Transfer tendon to pelvis	8.83	NA	9.18	1.24	NA	19.25	$696.83	090	M	B		
27100	Transfer of abdominal muscle	11.08	NA	13.03	1.57	NA	25.68	$929.60	090	M	B		C+
27105	Transfer of spinal muscle	11.77	NA	12.14	1.66	NA	25.57	$925.61	090	M	B		
27110	Transfer of iliopsoas muscle	13.26	NA	12.99	1.38	NA	27.63	$1,000.18	090	M	B		C+
27111	Transfer of iliopsoas muscle	12.15	NA	11.77	1.48	NA	25.40	$919.46	090	M	B		C+
27120	Reconstruction of hip socket	18.01	NA	14.28	2.45	NA	34.74	$1,257.56	090	M	B		C+
27122	Reconstruction of hip socket	14.98	NA	14.48	2.08	NA	31.54	$1,141.72	090	M	B		C+
27125	Partial hip replacement	14.69	NA	14.02	2.05	NA	30.76	$1,113.49	090	M	B		C+
27130	Total hip arthroplasty	20.12	NA	17.18	2.82	NA	40.12	$1,452.31	090	M	B		C+
27132	Total hip arthroplasty	23.30	NA	19.00	3.26	NA	45.56	$1,649.24	090	M	B		C+
27134	Revise hip joint replacement	28.52	NA	21.82	3.97	NA	54.31	$1,965.98	090	M	B		C+
27137	Revise hip joint replacement	21.17	NA	17.54	2.97	NA	41.68	$1,508.78	090	M	B		C+
27138	Revise hip joint replacement	22.17	NA	17.94	3.11	NA	43.22	$1,564.53	090	M	B		C+
27140	Transplant femur ridge	12.24	NA	11.98	1.67	NA	25.89	$937.20	090	M	B		C+
27146	Incision of hip bone	17.43	NA	15.87	2.27	NA	35.57	$1,287.61	090	M	B		C+
27147	Revision of hip bone	20.58	NA	17.87	2.61	NA	41.06	$1,486.34	090	M	B		C+
27151	Incision of hip bones	22.51	NA	18.97	3.12	NA	44.60	$1,614.48	090	M	B		C+
27156	Revision of hip bones	24.63	NA	19.84	3.48	NA	47.95	$1,735.75	090	M	B		C+
27158	Revision of pelvis	19.74	NA	15.58	2.60	NA	37.92	$1,372.67	090	M	B		
27161	Incision of neck of femur	16.71	NA	14.47	2.32	NA	33.50	$1,212.67	090	M	B		C+
27165	Incision/fixation of femur	17.91	NA	14.92	2.51	NA	35.34	$1,279.28	090	M	B		C+
27170	Repair/graft femur head/neck	16.07	NA	14.16	2.20	NA	32.43	$1,173.94	090	M	B		C+

* **M** = multiple surgery adjustment applies
Me = multiple endoscopy rules may apply
B = bilateral surgery adjustment applies
A = assistant-at-surgery restriction

A+ = assistant-at-surgery restriction unless medical necessity established with documentation
C = cosurgeons payable
C+ = cosurgeons payable if medical necessity established with documentation

T = team surgeons permitted
T+ = team surgeons payable if medical necessity established with documentation
§ = indicates services that are not covered by Medicare.

CPT five-digit codes, two-digit numeric modifiers, and descriptions only are © 2001 American Medical Association

Medicare RBRVS: The Physicians' Guide

Relative value units

CPT Code and Modifier	Description	Work RVU	Non Facility Practice Expense RVU	Facility Practice Expense RVU	PLI RVU	Total Non Facility RVUs	Medicare Payment Non Facility	Total Facility RVUs	Medicare Payment Facility	Global Period	Payment Policy Indicators*			
27175	Treat slipped epiphysis	8.46	NA	7.26	1.19	NA	NA	16.91	$612.13	090	M	B	A+	
27176	Treat slipped epiphysis	12.05	NA	10.23	1.68	NA	NA	23.96	$867.33	090	M	B		C+
27177	Treat slipped epiphysis	15.08	NA	12.22	2.11	NA	NA	29.41	$1,064.62	090	M	B		C+
27178	Treat slipped epiphysis	11.99	NA	10.13	1.68	NA	NA	23.80	$861.54	090	M	B		C+
27179	Revise head/neck of femur	12.98	NA	10.90	1.84	NA	NA	25.72	$931.04	090	M	B		
27181	Treat slipped epiphysis	14.68	NA	11.92	1.74	NA	NA	28.34	$1,025.89	090	M	B		
27185	Revision of femur epiphysis	9.18	NA	10.04	1.29	NA	NA	20.51	$742.45	090	M	B	A	C+
27187	Reinforce hip bones	13.54	NA	13.53	1.89	NA	NA	28.96	$1,048.33	090	M	B		C+
27193	Treat pelvic ring fracture	5.56	7.14	5.36	0.77	13.47	$487.60	11.69	$423.17	090	M	B	A	
27194	Treat pelvic ring fracture	9.65	9.20	7.69	1.32	20.17	$730.14	18.66	$675.48	090	M	B	A+	C
27200	Treat tail bone fracture	1.84	3.13	1.84	0.22	5.19	$187.87	3.90	$141.18	090	M	B	A	
27202	Treat tail bone fracture	7.04	NA	21.62	0.69	NA	NA	29.35	$1,062.45	090	M	B		
27215	Treat pelvic fracture(s)	10.05	NA	10.60	1.37	NA	NA	22.02	$797.11	090	M	B		C
27216	Treat pelvic ring fracture	15.19	NA	15.51	2.15	NA	NA	32.85	$1,189.14	090	M	B		C
27217	Treat pelvic ring fracture	14.11	NA	12.83	1.95	NA	NA	28.89	$1,045.79	090	M	B		C
27218	Treat pelvic ring fracture	20.15	NA	16.68	2.85	NA	NA	39.68	$1,436.38	090	M	B		C
27220	Treat hip socket fracture	6.18	7.48	5.72	0.85	14.51	$525.25	12.75	$461.54	090	M	B	A	
27222	Treat hip socket fracture	12.70	NA	10.37	1.77	NA	NA	24.84	$899.19	090	M	B	A	
27226	Treat hip wall fracture	14.91	NA	10.36	2.07	NA	NA	27.34	$989.69	090	M	B		C
27227	Treat hip fracture(s)	23.45	NA	17.22	3.24	NA	NA	43.91	$1,589.51	090	M	B		C
27228	Treat hip fracture(s)	27.16	NA	19.67	3.77	NA	NA	50.60	$1,831.68	090	M	B		C
27230	Treat thigh fracture	5.50	7.62	6.30	0.73	13.85	$501.36	12.53	$453.58	090	M	B	A	
27232	Treat thigh fracture	10.68	NA	9.31	1.45	NA	NA	21.44	$776.11	090	M	B	A	
27235	Treat thigh fracture	12.16	NA	11.24	1.71	NA	NA	25.11	$908.96	090	M	B	A	C+
27236	Treat thigh fracture	15.60	NA	12.99	2.18	NA	NA	30.77	$1,113.85	090	M	B		C+
27238	Treat thigh fracture	5.52	NA	6.36	0.76	NA	NA	12.64	$457.56	090	M	B	A	
27240	Treat thigh fracture	12.50	NA	10.38	1.69	NA	NA	24.57	$889.41	090	M	B	A	

Code	Description										
27244	Treat thigh fracture	15.94	NA	13.25	2.23	NA	31.42	$1,137.38	090	M	B		C+
27245	Treat thigh fracture	20.31	NA	15.61	2.85	NA	38.77	$1,403.44	090	M	B		C
27246	Treat thigh fracture	4.71	7.31	5.93	0.66	12.68	11.30	$409.05	090	M	B	A	
27248	Treat thigh fracture	10.45	NA	10.20	1.45	NA	22.10	$800.00	090	M	B		C+
27250	Treat hip dislocation	6.95	NA	6.55	0.68	NA	14.18	$513.30	090	M	B	A	
27252	Treat hip dislocation	10.39	NA	8.31	1.37	NA	20.07	$726.52	090	M	B	A	
27253	Treat hip dislocation	12.92	NA	11.10	1.81	NA	25.83	$935.03	090	M	B		C+
27254	Treat hip dislocation	18.26	NA	14.29	2.52	NA	35.07	$1,269.51	090	M	B		C+
27256	Treat hip dislocation	4.12	NA	4.31	0.49	NA	8.92	$322.90	010	M	B	A+	
27257	Treat hip dislocation	5.22	NA	4.59	0.56	NA	10.37	$375.39	010	M	B	A+	
27258	Treat hip dislocation	15.43	NA	13.93	2.06	NA	31.42	$1,137.38	090	M	B		C+
27259	Treat hip dislocation	21.55	NA	18.02	2.99	NA	42.56	$1,540.64	090	M	B		
27265	Treat hip dislocation	5.05	NA	6.09	0.65	NA	11.79	$426.79	090	M	B	A	
27266	Treat hip dislocation	7.49	NA	7.50	1.04	NA	16.03	$580.27	090	M	B	A	
27275	Manipulation of hip joint	2.27	NA	3.62	0.31	NA	6.20	$224.44	010	M		A	
27280	Fusion of sacroiliac joint	13.39	NA	13.95	1.98	NA	29.32	$1,061.36	090	M	B		C+
27282	Fusion of pubic bones	11.34	NA	12.33	1.14	NA	24.81	$898.10	090	M			C+
27284	Fusion of hip joint	23.45	NA	18.86	2.36	NA	44.67	$1,617.02	090	M	B		C+
27286	Fusion of hip joint	23.45	NA	19.13	2.37	NA	44.95	$1,627.15	090	M	B		C+
27290	Amputation of leg at hip	23.28	NA	17.37	2.94	NA	43.59	$1,577.92	090	M	B		C+
27295	Amputation of leg at hip	18.65	NA	14.65	2.35	NA	35.65	$1,290.50	090	M	B		C+
27299	Pelvis/hip joint surgery	0.00	0.00	0.00	0.00	0.00	0.00	$0.00	YYY	M	B		C+ T+
27301	Drain thigh/knee lesion	6.49	15.30	14.04	0.80	22.59	21.33	$772.13	090	M	B	A	
27303	Drainage of bone lesion	8.28	NA	14.63	1.14	NA	24.05	$870.59	090	M	B		C+
27305	Incise thigh tendon & fascia	5.92	NA	8.88	0.77	NA	15.57	$563.62	090	M	B		C+
27306	Incision of thigh tendon	4.62	NA	7.54	0.62	NA	12.78	$462.63	090	M	B		
27307	Incision of thigh tendons	5.80	NA	8.15	0.78	NA	14.73	$533.21	090	M	B	A+	C+
27310	Exploration of knee joint	9.27	NA	10.14	1.29	NA	20.70	$749.32	090	M	B		C+

* **M** = multiple surgery adjustment applies
Me = multiple endoscopy rules may apply
B = bilateral surgery adjustment applies
A = assistant-at-surgery restriction

A+ = assistant-at-surgery restriction unless medical necessity established with documentation
C = cosurgeons payable
C+ = cosurgeons payable if medical necessity established with documentation

T = team surgeons permitted
T+ = team surgeons payable if medical necessity established with documentation
$ = indicates services that are not covered by Medicare.

177 CPT five-digit codes, two-digit numeric modifiers, and descriptions only are © 2001 American Medical Association

Medicare RBRVS: The Physicians' Guide

Relative value units

CPT Code and Modifier	Description	Work RVU	Non Facility Practice Expense RVU	Facility Practice Expense RVU	PLI RVU	Total Non Facility RVUs	Medicare Payment Non Facility	Total Facility RVUs	Medicare Payment Facility	Global Period	Payment Policy Indicators*		
27315	Partial removal, thigh nerve	6.97	NA	4.04	0.79	NA	NA	11.80	$427.15	090	M	B	
27320	Partial removal, thigh nerve	6.30	NA	5.07	0.78	NA	NA	12.15	$439.82	090	M	B	C+
27323	Biopsy, thigh soft tissues	2.28	5.57	3.49	0.17	8.02	$290.32	5.94	$215.02	010	M	B	A
27324	Biopsy, thigh soft tissues	4.90	NA	6.79	0.59	NA	NA	12.28	$444.53	090	M	B	A
27327	Removal of thigh lesion	4.47	8.47	6.35	0.50	13.44	$486.52	11.32	$409.77	090	M	B	A
27328	Removal of thigh lesion	5.57	NA	7.19	0.66	NA	NA	13.42	$485.79	090	M	B	A
27329	Remove tumor, thigh/knee	14.14	NA	15.02	1.68	NA	NA	30.84	$1,116.38	090	M	B	C+
27330	Biopsy, knee joint lining	4.97	NA	6.42	0.66	NA	NA	12.05	$436.20	090	M	B	A
27331	Explore/treat knee joint	5.88	NA	7.56	0.81	NA	NA	14.25	$515.84	090	M	B	C+
27332	Removal of knee cartilage	8.27	NA	8.84	1.15	NA	NA	18.26	$661.00	090	M	B	C+
27333	Removal of knee cartilage	7.30	NA	8.49	1.03	NA	NA	16.82	$608.87	090	M	B	C+
27334	Remove knee joint lining	8.70	NA	9.80	1.21	NA	NA	19.71	$713.49	090	M	B	C+
27335	Remove knee joint lining	10.00	NA	10.58	1.41	NA	NA	21.99	$796.02	090	M	B	C+
27340	Removal of kneecap bursa	4.18	NA	6.03	0.58	NA	NA	10.79	$390.59	090	M	B	A
27345	Removal of knee cyst	5.92	NA	7.49	0.81	NA	NA	14.22	$514.75	090	M	B	C+
27347	Remove knee cyst	5.78	2.64	2.64	0.76	9.18	$332.31	9.18	$332.31	090	M	B	C+
27350	Removal of kneecap	8.17	NA	8.95	1.15	NA	NA	18.27	$661.36	090	M	B	C+
27355	Remove femur lesion	7.65	NA	10.36	1.07	NA	NA	19.08	$690.68	090	M	B	C+
27356	Remove femur lesion/graft	9.48	NA	11.32	1.29	NA	NA	22.09	$799.64	090	M	B	C+
27357	Remove femur lesion/graft	10.53	NA	11.75	1.48	NA	NA	23.76	$860.09	090	M	B	C+
27358	Remove femur lesion/fixation	4.74	NA	2.69	0.67	NA	NA	8.10	$293.21	ZZZ		B	
27360	Partial removal, leg bone(s)	10.50	NA	18.43	1.42	NA	NA	30.35	$1,098.65	090	M	B	C+
27365	Extensive leg surgery	16.27	NA	14.69	2.26	NA	NA	33.22	$1,202.54	090	M	B	C+
27370	Injection for knee x-ray	0.96	11.10	0.35	0.06	12.12	$438.73	1.37	$49.59	000	M	B	A
27372	Removal of foreign body	5.07	8.66	6.28	0.62	14.35	$519.46	11.97	$433.30	090	M	B	A+
27380	Repair of kneecap tendon	7.16	NA	8.57	1.00	NA	NA	16.73	$605.61	090	M	B	C+
27381	Repair/graft kneecap tendon	10.34	NA	10.34	1.44	NA	NA	22.12	$800.73	090	M	B	C+

Code	Description										
27385	Repair of thigh muscle	7.76	NA	8.93	1.09	NA	NA	17.78	$643.62	090	M	B	C+
27386	Repair/graft of thigh muscle	10.56	NA	11.12	1.49	NA	NA	23.17	$838.74	090	M	B	C+
27390	Incision of thigh tendon	5.33	NA	8.22	0.69	NA	NA	14.24	$515.48	090	M		
27391	Incision of thigh tendons	7.20	NA	9.08	0.99	NA	NA	17.27	$625.16	090	M		A+	C+
27392	Incision of thigh tendons	9.20	NA	11.15	1.23	NA	NA	21.58	$781.18	090	M			C+
27393	Lengthening of thigh tendon	6.39	NA	8.45	0.90	NA	NA	15.74	$569.78	090	M			C+
27394	Lengthening of thigh tendons	8.50	NA	10.51	1.17	NA	NA	20.18	$730.50	090	M			
27395	Lengthening of thigh tendons	11.73	NA	13.19	1.63	NA	NA	26.55	$961.09	090	M			C+
27396	Transplant of thigh tendon	7.86	NA	9.65	1.11	NA	NA	18.62	$674.03	090	M			C+
27397	Transplants of thigh tendons	11.28	NA	11.71	1.58	NA	NA	24.57	$889.41	090	M			
27400	Revise thigh muscles/tendons	9.02	NA	10.67	1.18	NA	NA	20.87	$755.48	090	M	B		C+
27403	Repair of knee cartilage	8.33	NA	8.88	1.16	NA	NA	18.37	$664.98	090	M	B		C+
27405	Repair of knee ligament	8.65	NA	9.81	1.21	NA	NA	19.67	$712.04	090	M	B		C+
27407	Repair of knee ligament	10.28	NA	10.67	1.38	NA	NA	22.33	$808.33	090	M	B		C+
27409	Repair of knee ligaments	12.90	NA	12.11	1.75	NA	NA	26.76	$968.69	090	M	B		C+
27418	Repair degenerated kneecap	10.85	NA	10.99	1.51	NA	NA	23.35	$845.25	090	M	B		C+
27420	Revision of unstable kneecap	9.83	NA	9.87	1.38	NA	NA	21.08	$763.08	090	M	B		C+
27422	Revision of unstable kneecap	9.78	NA	9.83	1.37	NA	NA	20.98	$759.46	090	M	B		C+
27424	Revision/removal of kneecap	9.81	NA	9.75	1.38	NA	NA	20.94	$758.01	090	M	B		C+
27425	Lateral retinacular release	5.22	NA	7.29	0.73	NA	NA	13.24	$479.28	090	M	B	A	C+
27427	Reconstruction, knee	9.36	NA	9.57	1.29	NA	NA	20.22	$731.95	090	M	B		C+
27428	Reconstruction, knee	14.00	NA	12.85	1.95	NA	NA	28.80	$1,042.54	090	M	B		C+
27429	Reconstruction, knee	15.52	NA	13.69	2.18	NA	NA	31.39	$1,136.29	090	M	B		C+
27430	Revision of thigh muscles	9.67	NA	9.90	1.35	NA	NA	20.92	$757.29	090	M	B		C+
27435	Incision of knee joint	9.49	NA	9.68	1.33	NA	NA	20.50	$742.08	090	M	B		C+
27437	Revise kneecap	8.46	NA	10.06	1.18	NA	NA	19.70	$713.12	090	M	B	A	
27438	Revise kneecap with implant	11.23	NA	11.34	1.56	NA	NA	24.13	$873.49	090	M	B		C+
27440	Revision of knee joint	10.43	NA	10.92	1.42	NA	NA	22.77	$824.26	090	M	B		C+

* **M** = multiple surgery adjustment applies
Me = multiple endoscopy rules may apply
B = bilateral surgery adjustment applies
A = assistant-at-surgery restriction

A+ = assistant-at-surgery restriction unless medical necessity established with documentation
C = cosurgeons payable
C+ = cosurgeons payable if medical necessity established with documentation

T = team surgeons permitted
T+ = team surgeons payable if medical necessity established with documentation
S = indicates services that are not covered by Medicare.

CPT five-digit codes, two-digit numeric modifiers, and descriptions only are © 2001 American Medical Association

Medicare RBRVS: The Physicians' Guide

Relative value units

CPT Code and Modifier	Description	Work RVU	Non Facility Practice Expense RVU	Facility Practice Expense RVU	PLI RVU	Total Non Facility RVUs	Medicare Payment Non Facility	Total Facility RVUs	Medicare Payment Facility	Global Period	Payment Policy Indicators*
27441	Revision of knee joint	10.82	NA	11.24	1.49	NA	NA	23.55	$852.49	090	M B C+
27442	Revision of knee joint	11.89	NA	11.77	1.68	NA	NA	25.34	$917.29	090	M B C+
27443	Revision of knee joint	10.93	NA	11.56	1.52	NA	NA	24.01	$869.14	090	M B C+
27445	Revision of knee joint	17.68	NA	14.98	2.49	NA	NA	35.15	$1,272.40	090	M B C+
27446	Revision of knee joint	15.84	NA	14.26	2.22	NA	NA	32.32	$1,169.96	090	M B C+
27447	Total knee arthroplasty	21.48	NA	17.35	3.00	NA	NA	41.83	$1,514.21	090	M B C+
27448	Incision of thigh	11.06	NA	11.98	1.51	NA	NA	24.55	$888.69	090	M B C+
27450	Incision of thigh	13.98	NA	13.83	1.96	NA	NA	29.77	$1,077.65	090	M B C+
27454	Realignment of thigh bone	17.56	NA	15.83	2.46	NA	NA	35.85	$1,297.74	090	M B C+
27455	Realignment of knee	12.82	NA	12.57	1.78	NA	NA	27.17	$983.53	090	M B C+
27457	Realignment of knee	13.45	NA	11.73	1.88	NA	NA	27.06	$979.55	090	M B C+
27465	Shortening of thigh bone	13.87	NA	14.09	1.86	NA	NA	29.82	$1,079.46	090	M B C+
27466	Lengthening of thigh bone	16.33	NA	16.19	1.92	NA	NA	34.44	$1,246.70	090	M B C+
27468	Shorten/lengthen thighs	18.97	NA	14.57	2.68	NA	NA	36.22	$1,311.14	090	M B C+
27470	Repair of thigh	16.07	NA	16.07	2.24	NA	NA	34.38	$1,244.53	090	M B C+
27472	Repair/graft of thigh	17.72	NA	16.98	2.49	NA	NA	37.19	$1,346.25	090	M B C+
27475	Surgery to stop leg growth	8.64	NA	9.51	1.13	NA	NA	19.28	$697.92	090	M B A C+
27477	Surgery to stop leg growth	9.85	NA	10.10	1.31	NA	NA	21.26	$769.59	090	M B A C+
27479	Surgery to stop leg growth	12.80	NA	12.09	1.81	NA	NA	26.70	$966.52	090	M B
27485	Surgery to stop leg growth	8.84	NA	9.40	1.24	NA	NA	19.48	$705.16	090	M B A
27486	Revise/replace knee joint	19.27	NA	16.13	2.70	NA	NA	38.10	$1,379.19	090	M B C+
27487	Revise/replace knee joint	25.27	NA	19.26	3.54	NA	NA	48.07	$1,740.10	090	M B C+
27488	Removal of knee prosthesis	15.74	NA	14.21	2.21	NA	NA	32.16	$1,164.17	090	M B C+
27495	Reinforce thigh	15.55	NA	15.78	2.18	NA	NA	33.51	$1,213.04	090	M B C+
27496	Decompression of thigh/knee	6.11	NA	7.96	0.77	NA	NA	14.84	$537.20	090	M B A
27497	Decompression of thigh/knee	7.17	NA	8.16	0.84	NA	NA	16.17	$585.34	090	M B A+ C
27498	Decompression of thigh/knee	7.99	NA	8.37	0.97	NA	NA	17.33	$627.33	090	M B C

Code	Description											
27499	Decompression of thigh/knee	9.00	NA	9.42	1.18	NA	19.60	$709.50	090	M	B		C
27500	Treatment of thigh fracture	5.92	9.84	7.57	0.80	16.56	14.29	$517.29	090	M	B	A	
27501	Treatment of thigh fracture	5.92	10.92	8.62	0.83	17.67	15.37	$556.38	090	M	B	A+	
27502	Treatment of thigh fracture	10.58	NA	11.27	1.49	NA	23.34	$844.89	090	M	B	A	
27503	Treatment of thigh fracture	10.58	NA	11.26	1.49	NA	23.33	$844.53	090	M	B	A+	
27506	Treatment of thigh fracture	17.45	NA	14.57	2.33	NA	34.35	$1,243.44	090	M	B		C+
27507	Treatment of thigh fracture	13.99	NA	12.58	1.95	NA	28.52	$1,032.40	090	M	B		C
27508	Treatment of thigh fracture	5.83	7.17	5.43	0.80	13.80	12.06	$436.56	090	M	B	A	
27509	Treatment of thigh fracture	7.71	NA	9.44	1.08	NA	18.23	$659.91	090	M	B	A+	
27510	Treatment of thigh fracture	9.13	NA	7.37	1.26	NA	17.76	$642.90	090	M	B	A	
27511	Treatment of thigh fracture	13.64	NA	13.38	1.91	NA	28.93	$1,047.24	090	M	B		C
27513	Treatment of thigh fracture	17.92	NA	15.80	2.51	NA	36.23	$1,311.50	090	M	B		C
27514	Treatment of thigh fracture	17.30	NA	14.55	2.41	NA	34.26	$1,240.18	090	M	B		C+
27516	Treat thigh fx growth plate	5.37	7.98	5.85	0.74	14.09	11.96	$432.94	090	M	B	A	
27517	Treat thigh fx growth plate	8.78	9.94	7.90	1.22	19.94	17.90	$647.97	090	M	B	A+	
27519	Treat thigh fx growth plate	15.02	NA	13.11	2.09	NA	30.22	$1,093.94	090	M	B		C+
27520	Treat kneecap fracture	2.86	5.48	3.82	0.38	8.72	7.06	$255.57	090	M	B	A	
27524	Treat kneecap fracture	10.00	NA	8.98	1.40	NA	20.38	$737.74	090	M	B		C+
27530	Treat knee fracture	3.78	6.00	4.33	0.51	10.29	8.62	$312.04	090	M	B	A	
27532	Treat knee fracture	7.30	7.65	5.84	1.02	15.97	14.16	$512.58	090	M	B	A	
27535	Treat knee fracture	11.50	NA	12.15	1.61	NA	25.26	$914.39	090	M	B		C
27536	Treat knee fracture	15.65	NA	12.16	2.19	NA	30.00	$1,085.98	090	M	B		C+
27538	Treat knee fracture(s)	4.87	7.64	5.60	0.67	13.18	11.14	$403.26	090	M	B	A+	
27540	Treat knee fracture	13.10	NA	10.75	1.80	NA	25.65	$928.51	090	M	B		C+
27550	Treat knee dislocation	5.76	7.60	5.79	0.68	14.04	12.23	$442.72	090	M	B	A+	
27552	Treat knee dislocation	7.90	NA	8.04	1.10	NA	17.04	$616.83	090	M	B	A+	
27556	Treat knee dislocation	14.41	NA	14.45	2.01	NA	30.87	$1,117.47	090	M	B		C+
27557	Treat knee dislocation	16.77	NA	15.78	2.37	NA	34.92	$1,264.08	090	M	B		C+

* **M** = multiple surgery adjustment applies
Me = multiple endoscopy rules may apply
B = bilateral surgery adjustment applies
A = assistant-at-surgery restriction

A+ = assistant-at-surgery restriction unless medical necessity established with documentation
C = cosurgeons payable
C+ = cosurgeons payable if medical necessity established with documentation

T = team surgeons permitted
T+ = team surgeons payable if medical necessity established with documentation
S = indicates services that are not covered by Medicare.

181   CPT five-digit codes, two-digit numeric modifiers, and descriptions only are © 2001 American Medical Association

Medicare RBRVS: The Physicians' Guide

Relative value units

CPT Code and Modifier	Description	Work RVU	Non Facility Practice Expense RVU	Facility Practice Expense RVU	PLI RVU	Total Non Facility RVUs	Medicare Payment Non Facility	Total Facility RVUs	Medicare Payment Facility	Global Period	Payment Policy Indicators*			
27558	Treat knee dislocation	17.72	NA	15.91	2.51	NA	NA	36.14	$1,308.24	090	M	B	C	
27560	Treat kneecap dislocation	3.82	5.89	4.04	0.40	10.11	$365.97	8.26	$299.01	090	M	B	A	
27562	Treat kneecap dislocation	5.79	NA	5.67	0.69	NA	NA	12.15	$439.82	090	M	B	A+	
27566	Treat kneecap dislocation	12.23	NA	10.09	1.73	NA	NA	24.05	$870.59	090	M	B	C+	
27570	Fixation of knee joint	1.74	NA	3.24	0.24	NA	NA	5.22	$188.96	010	M	B	A	
27580	Fusion of knee	19.37	NA	16.63	2.70	NA	NA	38.70	$1,400.91	090	M	B	C+	
27590	Amputate leg at thigh	12.03	NA	12.67	1.35	NA	NA	26.05	$942.99	090	M	B	C+	
27591	Amputate leg at thigh	12.68	NA	14.01	1.63	NA	NA	28.32	$1,025.16	090	M	B	C+	
27592	Amputate leg at thigh	10.02	NA	12.55	1.17	NA	NA	23.74	$859.37	090	M	B	C+	
27594	Amputation follow-up surgery	6.92	NA	9.05	0.82	NA	NA	16.79	$607.78	090	M	B	A	
27596	Amputation follow-up surgery	10.60	NA	12.64	1.24	NA	NA	24.48	$886.16	090	M	B	A	
27598	Amputate lower leg at knee	10.53	NA	11.69	1.24	NA	NA	23.46	$849.23	090	M	B	C+	
27599	Leg surgery procedure	0.00	0.00	0.00	0.00	0.00	$0.00	0.00	$0.00	YYY	M	B	C+	T+
27600	Decompression of lower leg	5.65	NA	7.67	0.68	NA	NA	14.00	$506.79	090	M	B	A	
27601	Decompression of lower leg	5.64	NA	7.68	0.69	NA	NA	14.01	$507.15	090	M	B	A	
27602	Decompression of lower leg	7.35	NA	8.08	0.85	NA	NA	16.28	$589.32	090	M	B	C+	
27603	Drain lower leg lesion	4.94	16.03	10.54	0.56	21.53	$779.37	16.04	$580.64	090	M	B	A	
27604	Drain lower leg bursa	4.47	11.01	8.47	0.54	16.02	$579.91	13.48	$487.97	090	M	B	A+	
27605	Incision of achilles tendon	2.87	9.81	3.67	0.38	13.06	$472.76	6.92	$250.50	010	M	B	A+	
27606	Incision of achilles tendon	4.14	13.19	5.08	0.57	17.90	$647.97	9.79	$354.39	010	M	B	A	
27607	Treat lower leg bone lesion	7.97	NA	12.78	1.08	NA	NA	21.83	$790.23	090	M	B	A	
27610	Explore/treat ankle joint	8.34	NA	10.43	1.15	NA	NA	19.92	$721.09	090	M	B	A	
27612	Exploration of ankle joint	7.33	NA	8.32	1.01	NA	NA	16.66	$603.08	090	M	B	C+	
27613	Biopsy lower leg soft tissue	2.17	5.38	2.96	0.16	7.71	$279.10	5.29	$191.49	010	M	B	A	
27614	Biopsy lower leg soft tissue	5.66	10.88	7.17	0.62	17.16	$621.18	13.45	$486.88	090	M	B	A	
27615	Remove tumor, lower leg	12.56	NA	17.07	1.39	NA	NA	31.02	$1,122.90	090	M	B	A+	
27618	Remove lower leg lesion	5.09	11.72	6.72	0.54	17.35	$628.06	12.35	$447.06	090	M	B	A	

Code	Description										
27619	Remove lower leg lesion	8.40	12.63	9.55	1.01	22.04	$797.83	18.96	$686.34	090	M	B	A	
27620	Explore/treat ankle joint	5.98	NA	8.20	0.83	NA	NA	15.01	$543.35	090	M	B		C+
27625	Remove ankle joint lining	8.30	NA	9.57	1.16	NA	NA	19.03	$688.87	090	M	B		C+
27626	Remove ankle joint lining	8.91	NA	10.39	1.23	NA	NA	20.53	$743.17	090	M	B		
27630	Removal of tendon lesion	4.80	10.70	6.87	0.60	16.10	$582.81	12.27	$444.16	090	M	B	A	
27635	Remove lower leg bone lesion	7.78	NA	11.13	1.06	NA	NA	19.97	$722.90	090	M	B	A	C+
27637	Remove/graft leg bone lesion	9.85	NA	12.36	1.38	NA	NA	23.59	$853.94	090	M	B		C+
27638	Remove/graft leg bone lesion	10.57	NA	12.55	1.47	NA	NA	24.59	$890.14	090	M	B		C+
27640	Partial removal of tibia	11.37	NA	18.46	1.54	NA	NA	31.37	$1,135.57	090	M	B	A	C+
27641	Partial removal of fibula	9.24	NA	16.52	1.22	NA	NA	26.98	$976.65	090	M	B	A	C+
27645	Extensive lower leg surgery	14.17	NA	18.78	1.98	NA	NA	34.93	$1,264.44	090	M	B		C+
27646	Extensive lower leg surgery	12.66	NA	18.50	1.55	NA	NA	32.71	$1,184.08	090	M	B		C+
27647	Extensive ankle/heel surgery	12.24	NA	11.31	1.64	NA	NA	25.19	$911.86	090	M	B		
27648	Injection for ankle x-ray	0.96	9.49	0.36	0.05	10.50	$380.09	1.37	$49.59	000	M	B	A+	
27650	Repair achilles tendon	9.69	NA	9.60	1.35	NA	NA	20.64	$747.15	090	M	B		C+
27652	Repair/graft achilles tendon	10.33	NA	9.90	1.45	NA	NA	21.68	$784.80	090	M	B	A	C+
27654	Repair of achilles tendon	10.02	NA	10.34	1.41	NA	NA	21.77	$788.06	090	M	B		C+
27656	Repair leg fascia defect	4.57	11.38	7.06	0.48	16.43	$594.75	12.11	$438.37	090	M	B		
27658	Repair of leg tendon, each	4.98	10.63	9.14	0.68	16.29	$589.68	14.80	$535.75	090	M			C+
27659	Repair of leg tendon, each	6.81	12.77	9.97	0.96	20.54	$743.53	17.74	$642.17	090	M			C+
27664	Repair of leg tendon, each	4.59	17.85	9.17	0.63	23.07	$835.12	14.39	$520.91	090	M		A+	
27665	Repair of leg tendon, each	5.40	8.95	8.95	0.75	15.10	$546.61	15.10	$546.61	090	M			C+
27675	Repair lower leg tendons	7.18	NA	8.48	1.01	NA	NA	16.67	$603.44	090	M	B		C+
27676	Repair lower leg tendons	8.42	NA	9.72	1.15	NA	NA	19.29	$698.28	090	M	B		
27680	Release of lower leg tendon	5.74	NA	8.27	0.80	NA	NA	14.81	$536.11	090	M		A	C+
27681	Release of lower leg tendons	6.82	NA	8.88	0.92	NA	NA	16.62	$601.63	090	M		A	C+
27685	Revision of lower leg tendon	6.50	10.37	8.45	0.91	17.78	$643.62	15.86	$574.12	090	M			C+
27686	Revise lower leg tendons	7.46	15.30	9.89	1.05	23.81	$861.90	18.40	$666.07	090	M		A	C+

*M = multiple surgery adjustment applies
Me = multiple endoscopy rules may apply
B = bilateral surgery adjustment applies
A = assistant-at-surgery restriction

A+ = assistant-at-surgery restriction unless medical necessity established with documentation
C = cosurgeons payable
C+ = cosurgeons payable if medical necessity established with documentation

T = team surgeons permitted
T+ = team surgeons payable if medical necessity established with documentation
§ = indicates services that are not covered by Medicare.

Medicare RBRVS: The Physicians' Guide

Relative value units

CPT Code and Modifier	Description	Work RVU	Non Facility Practice Expense RVU	Facility Practice Expense RVU	PLI RVU	Total Non Facility RVUs	Medicare Payment Non Facility	Total Facility RVUs	Medicare Payment Facility	Global Period	Payment Policy Indicators*
27687	Revision of calf tendon	6.24	NA	8.70	0.88	NA	NA	15.82	$572.67	090	M B C+
27690	Revise lower leg tendon	8.71	NA	9.61	1.22	NA	NA	19.54	$707.33	090	M B C+
27691	Revise lower leg tendon	9.96	NA	11.10	1.40	NA	NA	22.46	$813.03	090	M B C+
27692	Revise additional leg tendon	1.87	NA	0.99	0.26	NA	NA	3.12	$112.94	ZZZ	M B C+
27695	Repair of ankle ligament	6.51	NA	9.20	0.90	NA	NA	16.61	$601.27	090	M B A C+
27696	Repair of ankle ligaments	8.27	NA	9.54	1.16	NA	NA	18.97	$686.70	090	M B A C+
27698	Repair of ankle ligament	9.36	NA	9.72	1.31	NA	NA	20.39	$738.10	090	M B C+
27700	Revision of ankle joint	9.29	NA	7.95	1.24	NA	NA	18.48	$668.96	090	M B C+
27702	Reconstruct ankle joint	13.67	NA	13.02	1.92	NA	NA	28.61	$1,035.66	090	M B C+
27703	Reconstruction, ankle joint	15.87	NA	13.31	2.24	NA	NA	31.42	$1,137.38	090	M B
27704	Removal of ankle implant	7.62	NA	9.40	0.61	NA	NA	17.63	$638.19	090	M B A C+
27705	Incision of tibia	10.38	NA	11.55	1.44	NA	NA	23.37	$845.98	090	M B C+
27707	Incision of fibula	4.37	NA	8.48	0.60	NA	NA	13.45	$486.88	090	M B A C+
27709	Incision of tibia & fibula	9.95	NA	11.48	1.39	NA	NA	22.82	$826.07	090	M B C+
27712	Realignment of lower leg	14.25	NA	13.92	2.00	NA	NA	30.17	$1,092.13	090	M B C+
27715	Revision of lower leg	14.39	NA	15.22	2.00	NA	NA	31.61	$1,144.26	090	M B C+
27720	Repair of tibia	11.79	NA	13.67	1.66	NA	NA	27.12	$981.72	090	M B C+
27722	Repair/graft of tibia	11.82	NA	13.46	1.65	NA	NA	26.93	$974.84	090	M B C+
27724	Repair/graft of tibia	18.20	NA	17.28	2.10	NA	NA	37.58	$1,360.37	090	M B C+
27725	Repair of lower leg	15.59	NA	15.62	2.20	NA	NA	33.41	$1,209.42	090	M B C+
27727	Repair of lower leg	14.01	NA	14.43	1.84	NA	NA	30.28	$1,096.11	090	M B C+
27730	Repair of tibia epiphysis	7.41	21.54	10.22	0.75	29.70	$1,075.12	18.38	$665.34	090	M B A C+
27732	Repair of fibula epiphysis	5.32	14.45	7.22	0.63	20.40	$738.46	13.17	$476.74	090	M B A
27734	Repair lower leg epiphysis	8.48	NA	10.84	0.85	NA	NA	20.17	$730.14	090	M B A C+
27740	Repair of leg epiphyses	9.30	16.04	9.72	1.31	26.65	$964.71	20.33	$735.93	090	M B
27742	Repair of leg epiphyses	10.30	16.44	9.27	1.55	28.29	$1,024.08	21.12	$764.53	090	M B C+
27745	Reinforce tibia	10.07	NA	11.60	1.38	NA	NA	23.05	$834.39	090	M B C+

Code	Description												
27750	Treatment of tibia fracture	3.19	5.65	4.00	0.43	9.27	$335.57	7.62	$275.84	090	M	B	A
27752	Treatment of tibia fracture	5.84	8.20	6.17	0.82	14.86	$537.92	12.83	$464.44	090	M	B	A
27756	Treatment of tibia fracture	6.78	NA	10.84	0.94	NA	NA	18.56	$671.86	090	M	B	C+
27758	Treatment of tibia fracture	11.67	NA	12.22	1.52	NA	NA	25.41	$919.82	090	M	B	C+
27759	Treatment of tibia fracture	13.76	NA	13.46	1.93	NA	NA	29.15	$1,055.21	090	M	B	C
27760	Treatment of ankle fracture	3.01	5.42	3.87	0.39	8.82	$319.28	7.27	$263.17	090	M	B	A
27762	Treatment of ankle fracture	5.25	7.57	5.75	0.71	13.53	$489.78	11.71	$423.89	090	M	B	A
27766	Treatment of ankle fracture	8.36	NA	8.26	1.17	NA	NA	17.79	$643.98	090	M	B	C+
27780	Treatment of fibula fracture	2.65	5.37	3.69	0.33	8.35	$302.26	6.67	$241.45	090	M	B	A
27781	Treatment of fibula fracture	4.40	6.38	4.62	0.57	11.35	$410.86	9.59	$347.15	090	M	B	A
27784	Treatment of fibula fracture	7.11	NA	8.63	0.98	NA	NA	16.72	$605.25	090	M	B	C+
27786	Treatment of ankle fracture	2.84	5.38	3.78	0.37	8.59	$310.95	6.99	$253.03	090	M	B	A
27788	Treatment of ankle fracture	4.45	6.65	4.62	0.61	11.71	$423.89	9.68	$350.41	090	M	B	A
27792	Treatment of ankle fracture	7.66	NA	8.18	1.07	NA	NA	16.91	$612.13	090	M	B	C+
27808	Treatment of ankle fracture	2.83	6.44	4.50	0.38	9.65	$349.32	7.71	$279.10	090	M	B	A
27810	Treatment of ankle fracture	5.13	7.77	5.71	0.71	13.61	$492.67	11.55	$418.10	090	M	B	A
27814	Treatment of ankle fracture	10.68	NA	10.93	1.50	NA	NA	23.11	$836.56	090	M	B	C+
27816	Treatment of ankle fracture	2.89	5.97	4.55	0.37	9.23	$334.12	7.81	$282.72	090	M	B	A
27818	Treatment of ankle fracture	5.50	7.89	5.88	0.74	14.13	$511.49	12.12	$438.73	090	M	B	A
27822	Treatment of ankle fracture	11.00	NA	13.18	1.29	NA	NA	25.47	$921.99	090	M	B	C+
27823	Treatment of ankle fracture	13.00	NA	14.39	1.65	NA	NA	29.04	$1,051.22	090	M	B	C+
27824	Treat lower leg fracture	2.89	6.43	4.50	0.39	9.71	$351.49	7.78	$281.63	090	M	B	A
27825	Treat lower leg fracture	6.19	8.30	6.32	0.85	15.34	$555.30	13.36	$483.62	090	M	B	A+
27826	Treat lower leg fracture	8.54	NA	11.88	1.19	NA	NA	21.61	$782.26	090	M	B	C
27827	Treat lower leg fracture	14.06	NA	15.00	1.96	NA	NA	31.02	$1,122.90	090	M	B	C
27828	Treat lower leg fracture	16.23	NA	15.03	2.27	NA	NA	33.53	$1,213.76	090	M	B	C
27829	Treat lower leg joint	5.49	NA	8.67	0.77	NA	NA	14.93	$540.45	090	M	B	C
27830	Treat lower leg dislocation	3.79	5.82	4.36	0.44	10.05	$363.80	8.59	$310.95	090	M	B	A+

*M = multiple surgery adjustment applies
Me = multiple endoscopy rules may apply
B = bilateral surgery adjustment applies
A = assistant-at-surgery restriction

A+ = assistant-at-surgery restriction unless medical necessity established with documentation
C = cosurgeons payable
C+ = cosurgeons payable if medical necessity established with documentation

T = team surgeons permitted
T+ = team surgeons payable if medical necessity established with documentation
§ = indicates services that are not covered by Medicare.

185 CPT five-digit codes, two-digit numeric modifiers, and descriptions only are © 2001 American Medical Association

Medicare RBRVS: The Physicians' Guide

Relative value units

CPT Code and Modifier	Description	Work RVU	Non Facility Practice Expense RVU	Facility Practice Expense RVU	PLI RVU	Total Non Facility RVUs	Medicare Payment Non Facility	Total Facility RVUs	Medicare Payment Facility	Global Period	Payment Policy Indicators*
27831	Treat lower leg dislocation	4.56	NA	4.94	0.61	NA	NA	10.11	$365.97	090	M B A+
27832	Treat lower leg dislocation	6.49	NA	8.06	0.91	NA	NA	15.46	$559.64	090	M B C+
27840	Treat ankle dislocation	4.58	NA	6.21	0.47	NA	NA	11.26	$407.60	090	M B A
27842	Treat ankle dislocation	6.21	NA	5.25	0.76	NA	NA	12.22	$442.35	090	M B A
27846	Treat ankle dislocation	9.79	NA	10.46	1.36	NA	NA	21.61	$782.26	090	M B C+
27848	Treat ankle dislocation	11.20	NA	11.70	1.55	NA	NA	24.45	$885.07	090	M B C+
27860	Fixation of ankle joint	2.34	NA	3.78	0.31	NA	NA	6.43	$232.76	010	M A+
27870	Fusion of ankle joint	13.91	NA	13.76	1.95	NA	NA	29.62	$1,072.22	090	M B C+
27871	Fusion of tibiofibular joint	9.17	NA	11.03	1.29	NA	NA	21.49	$777.92	090	M B C+
27880	Amputation of lower leg	11.85	NA	11.95	1.38	NA	NA	25.18	$911.50	090	M B C+
27881	Amputation of lower leg	12.34	NA	13.44	1.59	NA	NA	27.37	$990.77	090	M B C+
27882	Amputation of lower leg	8.94	NA	13.13	1.03	NA	NA	23.10	$836.20	090	M B A+
27884	Amputation follow-up surgery	8.21	NA	10.78	0.95	NA	NA	19.94	$721.81	090	M B A
27886	Amputation follow-up surgery	9.32	NA	11.26	1.13	NA	NA	21.71	$785.88	090	M B C+
27888	Amputation of foot at ankle	9.67	NA	11.11	1.26	NA	NA	22.04	$797.83	090	M B C+
27889	Amputation of foot at ankle	9.98	NA	10.45	1.19	NA	NA	21.62	$782.63	090	M B A
27892	Decompression of leg	7.39	NA	8.41	0.86	NA	NA	16.66	$603.08	090	M B A+
27893	Decompression of leg	7.35	NA	8.58	0.90	NA	NA	16.83	$609.23	090	M B A+
27894	Decompression of leg	10.49	NA	10.09	1.25	NA	NA	21.83	$790.23	090	M B
27899	Leg/ankle surgery procedure	0.00	0.00	0.00	0.00	0.00	$0.00	0.00	$0.00	YYY	M B A+ C+ T+
28001	Drainage of bursa of foot	2.73	5.62	3.09	0.31	8.66	$313.49	6.13	$221.90	010	M A
28002	Treatment of foot infection	4.62	6.78	4.22	0.56	11.96	$432.94	9.40	$340.27	010	M A
28003	Treatment of foot infection	8.41	11.40	10.63	1.03	20.84	$754.39	20.07	$726.52	090	M A
28005	Treat foot bone lesion	8.68	NA	10.26	1.14	NA	NA	20.08	$726.88	090	M A
28008	Incision of foot fascia	4.45	8.17	6.38	0.56	13.18	$477.11	11.39	$412.31	090	M A
28010	Incision of toe tendon	2.84	7.64	5.37	0.39	10.87	$393.49	8.60	$311.31	090	M A
28011	Incision of toe tendons	4.14	9.36	6.79	0.58	14.08	$509.68	11.51	$416.65	090	M A

Code	Description											
28020	Exploration of foot joint	5.01	8.12	6.81	0.64	13.77	$498.46	12.46	$451.04	090	M	A	C+
28022	Exploration of foot joint	4.67	7.90	6.26	0.62	13.19	$477.47	11.55	$418.10	090	M	A	
28024	Exploration of toe joint	4.38	8.55	6.64	0.50	13.43	$486.16	11.52	$417.01	090	M	A	
28030	Removal of foot nerve	6.15	NA	3.50	0.85	NA	NA	10.50	$380.09	090	M	A+	
28035	Decompression of tibia nerve	5.09	8.80	5.35	0.71	14.60	$528.51	11.15	$403.62	090	M	A	C+
28043	Excision of foot lesion	3.54	7.47	4.96	0.45	11.46	$414.84	8.95	$323.98	090	M	B	A
28045	Excision of foot lesion	4.72	8.18	5.81	0.62	13.52	$489.41	11.15	$403.62	090	M	B	A+
28046	Resection of tumor, foot	10.18	13.58	11.38	1.13	24.89	$901.00	22.69	$821.36	090	M	B	A	C+
28050	Biopsy of foot joint lining	4.25	9.52	6.11	0.55	14.32	$518.37	10.91	$394.93	090	M	B	A	C+
28052	Biopsy of foot joint lining	3.94	8.01	5.76	0.51	12.46	$451.04	10.21	$369.59	090	M	B	A	C+
28054	Biopsy of toe joint lining	3.45	7.70	5.50	0.45	11.60	$419.91	9.40	$340.27	090	M	B	A+	
28060	Partial removal, foot fascia	5.23	8.72	6.51	0.69	14.64	$529.96	12.43	$449.96	090	M	B	A	
28062	Removal of foot fascia	6.52	9.27	6.87	0.85	16.64	$602.35	14.24	$515.48	090	M	B	A	C+
28070	Removal of foot joint lining	5.10	7.98	6.12	0.68	13.76	$498.10	11.90	$430.77	090	M	B	A	
28072	Removal of foot joint lining	4.58	8.84	6.67	0.64	14.06	$508.96	11.89	$430.41	090	M	B	A	
28080	Removal of foot lesion	3.58	7.82	5.51	0.50	11.90	$430.77	9.59	$347.15	090	M	B	A+	
28086	Excise foot tendon sheath	4.78	11.87	7.11	0.66	17.31	$626.61	12.55	$454.30	090	M	B	A	C+
28088	Excise foot tendon sheath	3.86	9.97	6.62	0.52	14.35	$519.46	11.00	$398.19	090	M	B	A+	
28090	Removal of foot lesion	4.41	8.12	5.64	0.57	13.10	$474.21	10.62	$384.44	090	M	B	A	
28092	Removal of toe lesions	3.64	8.17	6.08	0.46	12.27	$444.16	10.18	$368.51	090	M	B	A	
28100	Removal of ankle/heel lesion	5.66	13.07	7.70	0.76	19.49	$705.52	14.12	$511.13	090	M	B	A	C+
28102	Remove/graft foot lesion	7.73	NA	9.00	0.97	NA	NA	17.70	$640.73	090	M	B		
28103	Remove/graft foot lesion	6.50	8.76	6.93	0.89	16.15	$584.62	14.32	$518.37	090	M	B	A	
28104	Remove/graft foot lesion	5.12	8.49	6.76	0.69	14.30	$517.65	12.57	$455.02	090	M	B	A	C+
28106	Remove/graft foot lesion	7.16	NA	6.97	1.01	NA	NA	15.14	$548.06	090	M	B		
28107	Remove/graft foot lesion	5.56	9.96	7.13	0.74	16.26	$588.60	13.43	$486.16	090	M	B	A	C+
28108	Removal of toe lesions	4.16	7.49	5.36	0.52	12.17	$440.54	10.04	$363.44	090	M		A	
28110	Part removal of metatarsal	4.08	8.80	6.87	0.49	13.37	$483.98	11.44	$414.12	090	M	B	A	C+

* **M** = multiple surgery adjustment applies
Me = multiple endoscopy rules may apply
B = bilateral surgery adjustment applies
A = assistant-at-surgery restriction

A+ = assistant-at-surgery restriction unless medical necessity established with documentation
C = cosurgeons payable
C+ = cosurgeons payable if medical necessity established with documentation

T = team surgeons permitted
T+ = team surgeons payable if medical necessity established with documentation
$ = indicates services that are not covered by Medicare.

187   CPT five-digit codes, two-digit numeric modifiers, and descriptions only are © 2001 American Medical Association

Medicare RBRVS: The Physicians' Guide

Relative value units

CPT Code and Modifier	Description	Work RVU	Non Facility Practice Expense RVU	Facility Practice Expense RVU	PLI RVU	Total Non Facility RVUs	Medicare Payment Non Facility	Total Facility RVUs	Medicare Payment Facility	Global Period	Payment Policy Indicators*			
28111	Part removal of metatarsal	5.01	9.09	7.69	0.63	14.73	$533.21	13.33	$482.54	090	M	B	A	C+
28112	Part removal of metatarsal	4.49	8.89	7.47	0.60	13.98	$506.06	12.56	$454.66	090	M	B	A	C+
28113	Part removal of metatarsal	4.79	8.92	7.13	0.63	14.34	$519.10	12.55	$454.30	090	M	B	A+	
28114	Removal of metatarsal heads	9.79	12.36	10.85	1.36	23.51	$851.04	22.00	$796.38	090	M	B	A	C+
28116	Revision of foot	7.75	9.27	6.38	1.03	18.05	$653.40	15.16	$548.78	090	M	B	A	
28118	Removal of heel bone	5.96	9.37	7.24	0.79	16.12	$583.53	13.99	$506.43	090	M	B	A	C+
28119	Removal of heel spur	5.39	8.58	6.15	0.74	14.71	$532.49	12.28	$444.53	090	M	B	A	C+
28120	Part removal of ankle/heel	5.40	11.28	9.83	0.69	17.37	$628.78	15.92	$576.29	090	M	B	A	C+
28122	Partial removal of foot bone	7.29	10.94	9.50	0.96	19.19	$694.66	17.75	$642.54	090	M	B	A	C+
28124	Partial removal of toe	4.81	9.61	7.61	0.65	15.07	$545.52	13.07	$473.12	090	M	B	A	
28126	Partial removal of toe	3.52	8.37	6.76	0.49	12.38	$448.15	10.77	$389.87	090	M	B	A	
28130	Removal of ankle bone	8.11	NA	8.77	1.11	NA	NA	17.99	$651.22	090	M	B		
28140	Removal of metatarsal	6.91	10.40	7.92	0.84	18.15	$657.02	15.67	$567.24	090	M		A	C+
28150	Removal of toe	4.09	8.75	7.07	0.52	13.36	$483.62	11.68	$422.81	090	M		A	
28153	Partial removal of toe	3.66	8.39	6.22	0.49	12.54	$453.94	10.37	$375.39	090	M		A	
28160	Partial removal of toe	3.74	8.55	7.22	0.51	12.80	$463.35	11.47	$415.20	090	M		A	
28171	Extensive foot surgery	9.60	NA	8.27	1.13	NA	NA	19.00	$687.78	090	M			
28173	Extensive foot surgery	8.80	10.83	8.88	1.04	20.67	$748.24	18.72	$677.65	090	M		A	C+
28175	Extensive foot surgery	6.05	9.54	6.99	0.75	16.34	$591.49	13.79	$499.19	090	M		A	C+
28190	Removal of foot foreign body	1.96	6.54	3.53	0.16	8.66	$313.49	5.65	$204.53	010	M	B	A	
28192	Removal of foot foreign body	4.64	8.20	5.44	0.52	13.36	$483.62	10.60	$383.71	90	M	B	A	
28193	Removal of foot foreign body	5.73	8.94	6.67	0.63	15.30	$553.85	13.03	$471.68	090	M	B	A	
28200	Repair of foot tendon	4.60	8.47	6.32	0.59	13.66	$494.48	11.51	$416.65	090	M		A	C+
28202	Repair/graft of foot tendon	6.84	12.63	6.83	0.86	20.33	$735.93	14.53	$525.97	090	M			C+
28208	Repair of foot tendon	4.37	8.17	6.03	0.59	13.13	$475.30	10.99	$397.83	090	M		A	C+
28210	Repair/graft of foot tendon	6.35	9.83	6.38	0.77	16.95	$613.58	13.50	$488.69	090	M			
28220	Release of foot tendon	4.53	8.12	6.41	0.63	13.28	$480.73	11.57	$418.82	090	M		A	

Code	Description										
28222	Release of foot tendons	5.62	8.40	6.77	0.77	14.79	$535.39	13.16	$476.38	090	M	A
28225	Release of foot tendon	3.66	7.76	5.57	0.50	11.92	$431.49	9.73	$352.22	090	M	A	C+
28226	Release of foot tendons	4.53	8.30	6.66	0.62	13.45	$486.88	11.81	$427.51	090	M	A
28230	Incision of foot tendon(s)	4.24	8.26	6.83	0.59	13.09	$473.85	11.66	$422.08	090	M	A
28232	Incision of toe tendon	3.39	8.12	6.53	0.48	11.99	$434.03	10.40	$376.47	090	M	A
28234	Incision of foot tendon	3.37	7.98	6.11	0.46	11.81	$427.51	9.94	$359.82	090	M	A
28238	Revision of foot tendon	7.73	9.77	7.60	1.08	18.58	$672.58	16.41	$594.03	090	M	B	C+
28240	Release of big toe	4.36	8.17	6.40	0.61	13.14	$475.66	11.37	$411.58	090	M	B	A
28250	Revision of foot fascia	5.92	9.05	7.12	0.81	15.78	$571.22	13.85	$501.36	090	M	B	C+
28260	Release of midfoot joint	7.96	11.04	8.08	1.08	20.08	$726.88	17.12	$619.73	090	M	B	C+
28261	Revision of foot tendon	11.73	11.16	9.64	1.66	24.55	$888.69	23.03	$833.67	090	M	B	A+
28262	Revision of foot and ankle	15.83	15.66	15.09	2.22	33.71	$1,220.28	33.14	$1,199.64	090	M	B	C+
28264	Release of midfoot joint	10.35	10.98	10.98	1.46	22.79	$824.98	22.79	$824.98	090	M	B
28270	Release of foot contracture	4.76	8.75	7.43	0.67	14.18	$513.30	12.86	$465.52	090	M	B	A
28272	Release of toe joint, each	3.80	7.70	5.50	0.52	12.02	$435.11	9.82	$355.48	090	M	B	A
28280	Fusion of toes	5.19	8.39	6.77	0.72	14.30	$517.65	12.68	$459.01	090	M	B	A+
28285	Repair of hammertoe	4.59	8.79	6.76	0.64	14.02	$507.51	11.99	$434.03	090	M	A	C+
28286	Repair of hammertoe	4.56	8.78	6.75	0.64	13.98	$506.06	11.95	$432.58	090	M	A
28288	Partial removal of foot bone	4.74	9.00	8.02	0.65	14.39	$520.91	13.41	$485.43	090	M	A
28289	Repair hallux rigidus	7.04	10.54	9.75	0.96	18.54	$671.13	17.75	$642.54	090	M	B	C+
28290	Correction of bunion	5.66	9.55	8.81	0.79	16.00	$579.19	15.26	$552.40	090	M	B	A
28292	Correction of bunion	7.04	9.82	7.69	0.98	17.84	$645.79	15.71	$568.69	090	M	B	C+
28293	Correction of bunion	9.15	10.67	8.02	1.28	21.10	$763.80	18.45	$667.88	090	M	B	C+
28294	Correction of bunion	8.56	10.52	8.30	1.16	20.24	$732.67	18.02	$652.31	090	M	B	C+
28296	Correction of bunion	9.18	10.84	8.65	1.28	21.30	$771.04	19.11	$691.77	090	M	B	C+
28297	Correction of bunion	9.18	12.80	10.25	1.31	23.29	$843.08	20.74	$750.77	090	M	B	C+
28298	Correction of bunion	7.94	10.10	8.48	1.12	19.16	$693.58	17.54	$634.93	090	M	B	C+
28299	Correction of bunion	10.58	11.55	9.21	1.24	23.37	$845.98	21.03	$761.27	090	M	B	C+

* **M** = multiple surgery adjustment applies
Me = multiple endoscopy rules may apply
B = bilateral surgery adjustment applies
A = assistant-at-surgery restriction

A+ = assistant-at-surgery restriction unless medical necessity established with documentation
C = cosurgeons payable
C+ = cosurgeons payable if medical necessity established with documentation

T = team surgeons permitted
T+ = team surgeons payable if medical necessity established with documentation
$ = indicates services that are not covered by Medicare.

CPT five-digit codes, two-digit numeric modifiers, and descriptions only are © 2001 American Medical Association

Medicare RBRVS: The Physicians' Guide

Relative value units

CPT Code and Modifier	Description	Work RVU	Non Facility Practice Expense RVU	Facility Practice Expense RVU	PLI RVU	Total Non Facility RVUs	Medicare Payment Non Facility	Total Facility RVUs	Medicare Payment Facility	Global Period	Payment Policy Indicators*
28300	Incision of heel bone	9.54	14.15	9.43	1.31	25.00	$904.98	20.28	$734.12	090	M B C+
28302	Incision of ankle bone	9.55	9.55	9.22	1.15	20.25	$733.03	19.92	$721.09	090	M B C+
28304	Incision of midfoot bones	9.16	9.53	7.88	1.00	19.69	$712.76	18.04	$653.03	090	M C+
28305	Incise/graft midfoot bones	10.50	14.52	10.07	0.55	25.57	$925.61	21.12	$764.53	090	M C+
28306	Incision of metatarsal	5.86	8.84	6.51	0.81	15.51	$561.45	13.18	$477.11	090	M C+
28307	Incision of metatarsal	6.33	13.70	7.74	0.71	20.74	$750.77	14.78	$535.02	090	M A+
28308	Incision of metatarsal	5.29	7.97	5.60	0.74	14.00	$506.79	11.63	$421.00	090	M C+
28309	Incision of metatarsals	12.78	NA	11.08	1.64	NA	NA	25.50	$923.08	090	M A+
28310	Revision of big toe	5.43	9.00	6.93	0.76	15.19	$549.87	13.12	$474.93	090	M A C+
28312	Revision of toe	4.55	8.66	7.87	0.62	13.83	$500.63	13.04	$472.04	090	M A C+
28313	Repair deformity of toe	5.01	9.06	9.06	0.68	14.75	$533.94	14.75	$533.94	090	M A
28315	Removal of sesamoid bone	4.86	7.95	5.82	0.66	13.47	$487.60	11.34	$410.50	090	M B A C+
28320	Repair of foot bones	9.18	NA	9.02	1.27	NA	NA	19.47	$704.80	090	M A C+
28322	Repair of metatarsals	8.34	11.71	8.38	1.17	21.22	$768.15	17.89	$647.60	090	M A C+
28340	Resect enlarged toe tissue	6.98	8.96	6.28	0.98	16.92	$612.49	14.24	$515.48	090	M A
28341	Resect enlarged toe	8.41	9.55	6.88	1.18	19.14	$692.85	16.47	$596.20	090	M A
28344	Repair extra toe(s)	4.26	7.38	4.86	0.60	12.24	$443.08	9.72	$351.86	090	M B A C+
28345	Repair webbed toe(s)	5.92	9.48	7.58	0.84	16.24	$587.88	14.34	$519.10	090	M A+
28360	Reconstruct cleft foot	13.34	NA	12.22	1.88	NA	NA	27.44	$993.31	090	M
28400	Treatment of heel fracture	2.16	5.76	4.74	0.29	8.21	$297.20	7.19	$260.27	090	M B A
28405	Treatment of heel fracture	4.57	6.66	5.87	0.63	11.86	$429.32	11.07	$400.73	090	M B A+
28406	Treatment of heel fracture	6.31	NA	8.69	0.87	NA	NA	15.87	$574.48	090	M B A+
28415	Treat heel fracture	15.97	NA	15.72	2.24	NA	NA	33.93	$1,228.24	090	M B C+
28420	Treat/graft heel fracture	16.64	NA	15.95	2.29	NA	NA	34.88	$1,262.63	090	M B C+
28430	Treatment of ankle fracture	2.09	5.25	4.26	0.27	7.61	$275.48	6.62	$239.64	090	M B A
28435	Treatment of ankle fracture	3.40	5.41	4.57	0.47	9.28	$335.93	8.44	$305.52	090	M B A+
28436	Treatment of ankle fracture	4.71	NA	7.86	0.66	NA	NA	13.23	$478.92	090	M A

Code	Description										
28445	Treat ankle fracture	15.62	NA	13.94	1.29	NA	30.85	$1,116.75	090	M	B	C+
28450	Treat midfoot fracture, each	1.90	5.28	4.07	0.25	7.43	6.22	$225.16	090	M	A
28455	Treat midfoot fracture, each	3.09	5.51	4.94	0.43	9.03	8.46	$306.25	090	M	A+
28456	Treat midfoot fracture	2.68	NA	6.27	0.36	NA	9.31	$337.01	090	M	A
28465	Treat midfoot fracture, each	7.01	NA	8.25	0.87	NA	16.13	$583.89	090	M	A
28470	Treat metatarsal fracture	1.99	4.52	3.41	0.26	6.77	5.66	$204.89	090	M	A
28475	Treat metatarsal fracture	2.97	5.18	4.38	0.41	8.56	7.76	$280.91	090	M	A
28476	Treat metatarsal fracture	3.38	NA	6.71	0.46	NA	10.55	$381.90	090	M	A+
28485	Treat metatarsal fracture	5.71	NA	8.16	0.80	NA	14.67	$531.04	090	M	A	C+
28490	Treat big toe fracture	1.09	2.76	2.21	0.13	3.98	3.43	$124.16	090	M	A
28495	Treat big toe fracture	1.58	2.82	2.31	0.19	4.59	4.08	$147.69	090	M	A
28496	Treat big toe fracture	2.33	11.10	4.58	0.32	13.75	7.23	$261.72	090	M	A
28505	Treat big toe fracture	3.81	11.46	6.74	0.50	15.77	11.05	$400.00	090	M	A
28510	Treatment of toe fracture	1.09	2.51	2.23	0.13	3.73	3.45	$124.89	090	M	A
28515	Treatment of toe fracture	1.46	2.83	2.30	0.17	4.46	3.93	$142.26	090	M	A
28525	Treat toe fracture	3.32	10.82	6.16	0.44	14.58	9.92	$359.10	090	M	A+
28530	Treat sesamoid bone fracture	1.06	2.91	2.91	0.13	4.10	4.10	$148.42	090	M	A+
28531	Treat sesamoid bone fracture	2.35	11.91	4.73	0.33	14.59	7.41	$268.24	090	M	A	C
28540	Treat foot dislocation	2.04	3.75	3.75	0.24	6.03	6.03	$218.28	090	M	A+
28545	Treat foot dislocation	2.45	4.76	4.76	0.33	7.54	7.54	$272.94	090	M	A+
28546	Treat foot dislocation	3.20	12.55	6.31	0.46	16.21	9.97	$360.91	090	M	A+
28555	Repair foot dislocation	6.30	13.49	8.36	0.88	20.67	15.54	$562.54	090	M	A+	C+
28570	Treat foot dislocation	1.66	3.67	3.67	0.22	5.55	5.55	$200.91	090	M	A+
28575	Treat foot dislocation	3.31	5.19	5.19	0.45	8.95	8.95	$323.98	090	M	A+
28576	Treat foot dislocation	4.17	12.06	6.85	0.56	16.79	11.58	$419.19	090	M	A+
28585	Repair foot dislocation	7.99	8.75	8.32	1.13	17.87	17.44	$631.31	090	M	A+	C+
28600	Treat foot dislocation	1.89	4.32	3.89	0.24	6.45	6.02	$217.92	090	M	A+
28605	Treat foot dislocation	2.71	4.40	4.40	0.35	7.46	7.46	$270.05	090	M	A+

* **M** = multiple surgery adjustment applies
Me = multiple endoscopy rules may apply
B = bilateral surgery adjustment applies
A = assistant-at-surgery restriction

A+ = assistant-at-surgery restriction unless medical necessity established with documentation
C = cosurgeons payable
C+ = cosurgeons payable if medical necessity established with documentation

T = team surgeons permitted
T+ = team surgeons payable if medical necessity established with documentation
§ = indicates services that are not covered by Medicare.

191   CPT five-digit codes, two-digit numeric modifiers, and descriptions only are © 2001 American Medical Association

Medicare RBRVS: The Physicians' Guide

Relative value units

CPT Code and Modifier	Description	Work RVU	Non Facility Practice Expense RVU	Facility Practice Expense RVU	PLI RVU	Total Non Facility RVUs	Medicare Payment Non Facility	Total Facility RVUs	Medicare Payment Facility	Global Period	Payment Policy Indicators*			
28606	Treat foot dislocation	4.90	16.14	7.09	0.68	21.72	$786.25	12.67	$458.64	090	M		A	
28615	Repair foot dislocation	7.77	NA	9.45	1.09	NA	NA	18.31	$662.81	090	M			C+
28630	Treat toe dislocation	1.70	2.35	2.35	0.17	4.22	$152.76	4.22	$152.76	010	M		A+	
28635	Treat toe dislocation	1.91	2.49	2.49	0.24	4.64	$167.96	4.64	$167.96	010	M		A+	
28636	Treat toe dislocation	2.77	4.81	3.22	0.39	7.97	$288.51	6.38	$230.95	010	M		A	C
28645	Repair toe dislocation	4.22	6.69	4.34	0.58	11.49	$415.93	9.14	$330.86	090	M		A	C+
28660	Treat toe dislocation	1.23	3.11	2.60	0.11	4.45	$161.09	3.94	$142.62	010	M		A	
28665	Treat toe dislocation	1.92	2.47	2.47	0.24	4.63	$167.60	4.63	$167.60	010	M		A+	
28666	Treat toe dislocation	2.66	13.30	3.00	0.38	16.34	$591.49	6.04	$218.64	010	M		A	C
28675	Repair of toe dislocation	2.92	9.48	4.90	0.41	12.81	$463.71	8.23	$297.92	090	M		A	
28705	Fusion of foot bones	18.80	NA	15.67	2.13	NA	NA	36.60	$1,324.89	090	M			C+
28715	Fusion of foot bones	13.10	NA	12.57	1.84	NA	NA	27.51	$995.84	090	M			C+
28725	Fusion of foot bones	11.61	NA	11.48	1.63	NA	NA	24.72	$894.84	090	M			C+
28730	Fusion of foot bones	10.76	NA	10.76	1.51	NA	NA	23.03	$833.67	090	M			C+
28735	Fusion of foot bones	10.85	NA	10.45	1.51	NA	NA	22.81	$825.70	090	M			C+
28737	Revision of foot bones	9.64	NA	9.04	1.36	NA	NA	20.04	$725.43	090	M			C+
28740	Fusion of foot bones	8.02	13.03	8.94	1.13	22.18	$802.90	18.09	$654.84	090	M			C+
28750	Fusion of big toe joint	7.30	12.48	9.13	1.03	20.81	$753.31	17.46	$632.04	090	M	B	A+	
28755	Fusion of big toe joint	4.74	8.52	6.42	0.66	13.92	$503.89	11.82	$427.87	090	M	B	A	C+
28760	Fusion of big toe joint	7.75	10.39	7.82	1.07	19.21	$695.39	16.64	$602.35	090	M	B		C+
28800	Amputation of midfoot	8.21	NA	8.90	0.98	NA	NA	18.09	$654.84	090	M	B		C+
28805	Amputation thru metatarsal	8.39	NA	9.00	0.97	NA	NA	18.36	$664.62	090	M	B	A+	
28810	Amputation toe & metatarsal	6.21	NA	7.97	0.70	NA	NA	14.88	$538.64	090	M		A+	
28820	Amputation of toe	4.41	9.91	7.16	0.51	14.83	$536.83	12.08	$437.29	090	M		A	
28825	Partial amputation of toe	3.59	10.12	6.95	0.43	14.14	$511.86	10.97	$397.11	090	M		A	
28899	Foot/toes surgery procedure	0.00	0.00	0.00	0.00	0.00	$0.00	0.00	$0.00	YYY	M		A+	C+ T+
29000	Application of body cast	2.25	2.71	1.67	0.30	5.26	$190.41	4.22	$152.76	000	M		A+	

Code	Description									
29010	Application of body cast	2.06	2.98	1.72	0.27	5.31	4.05	$146.61	000	M	A+
29015	Application of body cast	2.41	3.17	1.93	0.21	5.79	4.55	$164.71	000	M	A+
29020	Application of body cast	2.11	3.33	1.47	0.16	5.60	3.74	$135.39	000	M	A+
29025	Application of body cast	2.40	3.32	1.86	0.26	5.98	4.52	$163.62	000	M	A+
29035	Application of body cast	1.77	3.05	1.56	0.24	5.06	3.57	$129.23	000	M	A+
29040	Application of body cast	2.22	2.54	1.49	0.35	5.11	4.06	$146.97	000	M	A+
29044	Application of body cast	2.12	3.20	1.81	0.29	5.61	4.22	$152.76	000	M	A+
29046	Application of body cast	2.41	3.31	2.04	0.34	6.06	4.79	$173.39	000	M	A+
29049	Application of figure eight	0.89	1.07	0.57	0.12	2.08	1.58	$57.19	000	M	A+
29055	Application of shoulder cast	1.78	2.40	1.42	0.24	4.42	3.44	$124.53	000	M	A+
29058	Application of shoulder cast	1.31	1.33	0.73	0.14	2.78	2.18	$78.91	000	M	A+
29065	Application of long arm cast	0.87	1.10	0.69	0.12	2.09	1.68	$60.81	000	M	A B
29075	Application of forearm cast	0.77	1.05	0.63	0.11	1.93	1.51	$54.66	000	M	A B
29085	Apply hand/wrist cast	0.87	1.10	0.62	0.11	2.08	1.60	$57.92	000	M	A B
29086	Apply finger cast	0.62	0.81	0.50	0.07	1.50	1.19	$43.08	000	M	A B
29105	Apply long arm splint	0.87	1.05	0.52	0.11	2.03	1.50	$54.30	000	M	A B
29125	Apply forearm splint	0.59	0.88	0.41	0.06	1.53	1.06	$38.37	000	M	A B
29126	Apply forearm splint	0.77	1.21	0.47	0.06	2.04	1.30	$47.06	000	M	A B
29130	Application of finger splint	0.50	0.44	0.18	0.05	0.99	0.73	$26.43	000	M	A B
29131	Application of finger splint	0.55	0.71	0.23	0.03	1.29	0.81	$29.32	000	M	A B
29200	Strapping of chest	0.65	0.85	0.37	0.04	1.54	1.06	$38.37	000	M	A
29220	Strapping of low back	0.64	0.96	0.41	0.07	1.67	1.12	$40.54	000	M	A
29240	Strapping of shoulder	0.71	0.92	0.39	0.05	1.68	1.15	$41.63	000	M	A
29260	Strapping of elbow or wrist	0.55	0.85	0.35	0.04	1.44	0.94	$34.03	000	M	A B
29280	Strapping of hand or finger	0.51	0.91	0.39	0.04	1.46	0.94	$34.03	000	M	A B
29305	Application of hip cast	2.03	2.74	1.60	0.29	5.06	3.92	$141.90	000	M	A+
29325	Application of hip casts	2.32	3.05	1.79	0.31	5.68	4.42	$160.00	000	M	A+
29345	Application of long leg cast	1.40	1.51	1.02	0.19	3.10	2.61	$94.48	000	M	A B

* **M** = multiple surgery adjustment applies
Me = multiple endoscopy rules may apply
B = bilateral surgery adjustment applies
A = assistant-at-surgery restriction

A+ = assistant-at-surgery restriction unless medical necessity established with documentation
C = cosurgeons payable
C+ = cosurgeons payable if medical necessity established with documentation

T = team surgeons permitted
T+ = team surgeons payable if medical necessity established with documentation
§ = indicates services that are not covered by Medicare.

193   CPT five-digit codes, two-digit numeric modifiers, and descriptions only are © 2001 American Medical Association

Medicare RBRVS: The Physicians' Guide

Relative value units

CPT Code and Modifier	Description	Work RVU	Non Facility Practice Expense RVU	Facility Practice Expense RVU	PLI RVU	Total Non Facility RVUs	Medicare Payment Non Facility	Total Facility RVUs	Medicare Payment Facility	Global Period	Payment Policy Indicators*
29355	Application of long leg cast	1.53	1.47	1.11	0.20	3.20	$115.84	2.84	$102.81	000	M B A
29358	Apply long leg cast brace	1.43	1.72	1.07	0.19	3.34	$120.91	2.69	$97.38	000	M B A
29365	Application of long leg cast	1.18	1.38	0.90	0.17	2.73	$98.82	2.25	$81.45	000	M B A
29405	Apply short leg cast	0.86	1.03	0.66	0.12	2.01	$72.76	1.64	$59.37	000	M B A
29425	Apply short leg cast	1.01	1.05	0.68	0.14	2.20	$79.64	1.83	$66.24	000	M B A
29435	Apply short leg cast	1.18	1.35	0.88	0.17	2.70	$97.74	2.23	$80.72	000	M B A
29440	Addition of walker to cast	0.57	0.61	0.26	0.07	1.25	$45.25	0.90	$32.58	000	M B A
29445	Apply rigid leg cast	1.78	1.58	0.96	0.24	3.60	$130.32	2.98	$107.87	000	M B A
29450	Application of leg cast	2.08	1.40	1.11	0.13	3.61	$130.68	3.32	$120.18	000	M B A
29505	Application, long leg splint	0.69	1.10	0.48	0.06	1.85	$66.97	1.23	$44.53	000	M B A
29515	Application lower leg splint	0.73	0.78	0.48	0.07	1.58	$57.19	1.28	$46.33	000	M B A
29520	Strapping of hip	0.54	0.93	0.44	0.02	1.49	$53.94	1.00	$36.20	000	M A+
29530	Strapping of knee	0.57	0.83	0.36	0.04	1.44	$52.13	0.97	$35.11	000	M A
29540	Strapping of ankle	0.51	0.40	0.32	0.04	0.95	$34.39	0.87	$31.49	000	M A
29550	Strapping of toes	0.47	0.40	0.29	0.05	0.92	$33.30	0.81	$29.32	000	M A
29580	Application of paste boot	0.57	0.61	0.36	0.05	1.23	$44.53	0.98	$35.48	000	M B A
29590	Application of foot splint	0.76	0.50	0.30	0.06	1.32	$47.78	1.12	$40.54	000	M A
29700	Removal/revision of cast	0.57	0.81	0.28	0.07	1.45	$52.49	0.92	$33.30	000	M A
29705	Removal/revision of cast	0.76	0.73	0.39	0.10	1.59	$57.56	1.25	$45.25	000	M B A
29710	Removal/revision of cast	1.34	1.50	0.66	0.17	3.01	$108.96	2.17	$78.55	000	M B A+
29715	Removal/revision of cast	0.94	0.98	0.29	0.08	2.00	$72.40	1.31	$47.42	000	M A+
29720	Repair of body cast	0.68	0.95	0.36	0.10	1.73	$62.62	1.14	$41.27	000	M A
29730	Windowing of cast	0.75	0.71	0.36	0.10	1.56	$56.47	1.21	$43.80	000	M A
29740	Wedging of cast	1.12	1.02	0.46	0.15	2.29	$82.90	1.73	$62.62	000	M A
29750	Wedging of clubfoot cast	1.26	1.13	0.62	0.16	2.55	$92.31	2.04	$73.85	000	M B A+
29799	Casting/strapping procedure	0.00	0.00	0.00	0.00	0.00	$0.00	0.00	$0.00	YYY	M A+ C+
29800	Jaw arthroscopy/surgery	6.43	NA	9.15	0.84	NA	NA	16.42	$594.39	090	M B A+ T+

Code	Description											
29804	Jaw arthroscopy/surgery	8.14	NA	8.73	0.66	NA	NA	17.53	$634.57	090	M	B	C+
29805	Shoulder arthroscopy, dx	5.89	3.23	3.23	0.83	9.95	$360.18	9.95	$360.18	090	M	B	A	C+
29806	Shoulder arthroscopy/surgery	14.37	NA	11.33	2.01	NA	NA	27.71	$1,003.08	090	M	B	A	C+
29807	Shoulder arthroscopy/surgery	13.90	NA	11.06	2.01	NA	NA	26.97	$976.29	090	M	B	A	C+
29819	Shoulder arthroscopy/surgery	7.62	NA	9.82	1.07	NA	NA	18.51	$670.05	090	Me	B	A	C+
29820	Shoulder arthroscopy/surgery	7.07	NA	9.55	0.99	NA	NA	17.61	$637.47	090	Me	B		C+
29821	Shoulder arthroscopy/surgery	7.72	NA	9.84	1.08	NA	NA	18.64	$674.75	090	Me	B		C+
29822	Shoulder arthroscopy/surgery	7.43	NA	9.75	1.04	NA	NA	18.22	$659.55	090	Me	B		
29823	Shoulder arthroscopy/surgery	8.17	NA	10.14	1.15	NA	NA	19.46	$704.44	090	Me	B		C+
29824	Shoulder arthroscopy/surgery	8.25	NA	7.48	1.16	NA	NA	16.89	$611.40	090	M	B		C+
29825	Shoulder arthroscopy/surgery	7.62	NA	9.80	1.06	NA	NA	18.48	$668.96	090	Me	B		C+
29826	Shoulder arthroscopy/surgery	8.99	NA	10.65	1.26	NA	NA	20.90	$756.56	090	Me	B		C+
29830	Elbow arthroscopy	5.76	NA	6.14	0.79	NA	NA	12.69	$459.37	090	M	B	A	
29834	Elbow arthroscopy/surgery	6.28	NA	6.94	0.86	NA	NA	14.08	$509.68	090	Me	B		C+
29835	Elbow arthroscopy/surgery	6.48	NA	6.95	0.88	NA	NA	14.31	$518.01	090	Me	B		C+
29836	Elbow arthroscopy/surgery	7.55	NA	7.62	1.06	NA	NA	16.23	$587.51	090	Me	B		C+
29837	Elbow arthroscopy/surgery	6.87	NA	7.30	0.96	NA	NA	15.13	$547.69	090	Me	B		C+
29838	Elbow arthroscopy/surgery	7.71	NA	7.73	1.07	NA	NA	16.51	$597.65	090	Me	B	A+	
29840	Wrist arthroscopy	5.54	NA	8.38	0.69	NA	NA	14.61	$528.87	090	M	B	A+	
29843	Wrist arthroscopy/surgery	6.01	NA	8.70	0.82	NA	NA	15.53	$562.17	090	Me	B		C+
29844	Wrist arthroscopy/surgery	6.37	NA	8.96	0.86	NA	NA	16.19	$586.07	090	Me	B		
29845	Wrist arthroscopy/surgery	7.52	NA	9.56	0.84	NA	NA	17.92	$648.69	090	Me	B		C+
29846	Wrist arthroscopy/surgery	6.75	NA	11.67	0.89	NA	NA	19.31	$699.01	090	Me	B	A+	
29847	Wrist arthroscopy/surgery	7.08	NA	11.85	0.91	NA	NA	19.84	$718.19	090	Me	B		
29848	Wrist endoscopy/surgery	5.44	NA	8.46	0.72	NA	NA	14.62	$529.23	090	M	B	A	
29850	Knee arthroscopy/surgery	8.19	NA	7.49	0.74	NA	NA	16.42	$594.39	090	M	B	A+	C
29851	Knee arthroscopy/surgery	13.10	NA	12.00	1.81	NA	NA	26.91	$974.12	090	M	B		C
29855	Tibial arthroscopy/surgery	10.62	NA	10.55	1.50	NA	NA	22.67	$820.64	090	M	B		C

*M = multiple surgery adjustment applies
Me = multiple endoscopy rules may apply
B = bilateral surgery adjustment applies
A = assistant-at-surgery restriction

A+ = assistant-at-surgery restriction unless medical necessity established with documentation
C = cosurgeons payable
C+ = cosurgeons payable if medical necessity established with documentation

T = team surgeons permitted
T+ = team surgeons payable if medical necessity established with documentation
S = indicates services that are not covered by Medicare.

195 CPT five-digit codes, two-digit numeric modifiers, and descriptions only are © 2001 American Medical Association

Medicare RBRVS: The Physicians' Guide

Relative value units

CPT Code and Modifier	Description	Work RVU	Non Facility Practice Expense RVU	Facility Practice Expense RVU	PLI RVU	Total Non Facility RVUs	Medicare Payment Non Facility	Total Facility RVUs	Medicare Payment Facility	Global Period	Payment Policy Indicators*
29856	Tibial arthroscopy/surgery	14.14	NA	12.49	2.00	NA	NA	28.63	$1,036.38	090	M B C
29860	Hip arthroscopy, dx	8.05	NA	8.05	1.14	NA	NA	17.24	$624.07	090	M B C+
29861	Hip arthroscopy/surgery	9.15	NA	8.71	1.29	NA	NA	19.15	$693.21	090	Me B C+
29862	Hip arthroscopy/surgery	9.90	NA	9.75	1.39	NA	NA	21.04	$761.63	090	Me B C+
29863	Hip arthroscopy/surgery	9.90	NA	10.31	1.40	NA	NA	21.61	$782.26	090	Me B C+
29870	Knee arthroscopy, dx	5.07	NA	6.27	0.67	NA	NA	12.01	$434.75	090	M B C+
29871	Knee arthroscopy/drainage	6.55	NA	8.38	0.88	NA	NA	15.81	$572.31	090	Me A B
29874	Knee arthroscopy/surgery	7.05	NA	8.15	0.87	NA	NA	16.07	$581.72	090	Me A B
29875	Knee arthroscopy/surgery	6.31	NA	7.69	0.88	NA	NA	14.88	$538.64	090	Me A+ B
29876	Knee arthroscopy/surgery	7.92	NA	9.19	1.11	NA	NA	18.22	$659.55	090	Me A+ B
29877	Knee arthroscopy/surgery	7.35	NA	8.29	1.03	NA	NA	16.67	$603.44	090	Me A B
29879	Knee arthroscopy/surgery	8.04	NA	8.68	1.13	NA	NA	17.85	$646.16	090	Me A+ B
29880	Knee arthroscopy/surgery	8.50	NA	8.95	1.19	NA	NA	18.64	$674.75	090	Me A+ B C+
29881	Knee arthroscopy/surgery	7.76	NA	8.53	1.09	NA	NA	17.38	$629.14	090	Me A+ B
29882	Knee arthroscopy/surgery	8.65	NA	9.01	1.09	NA	NA	18.75	$678.74	090	Me A B
29883	Knee arthroscopy/surgery	11.05	NA	10.41	1.33	NA	NA	22.79	$824.98	090	Me A+ B
29884	Knee arthroscopy/surgery	7.33	NA	8.87	1.03	NA	NA	17.23	$623.71	090	Me B C+
29885	Knee arthroscopy/surgery	9.09	NA	9.85	1.27	NA	NA	20.21	$731.59	090	Me B C+
29886	Knee arthroscopy/surgery	7.54	NA	8.99	1.06	NA	NA	17.59	$636.74	090	Me A B
29887	Knee arthroscopy/surgery	9.04	NA	9.83	1.27	NA	NA	20.14	$729.05	090	Me B C+
29888	Knee arthroscopy/surgery	13.90	NA	12.50	1.95	NA	NA	28.35	$1,026.25	090	M B C+
29889	Knee arthroscopy/surgery	16.00	NA	13.71	2.11	NA	NA	31.82	$1,151.86	090	M B C+
29891	Ankle arthroscopy/surgery	8.40	NA	8.92	1.17	NA	NA	18.49	$669.32	090	M B
29892	Ankle arthroscopy/surgery	9.00	NA	9.04	1.26	NA	NA	19.30	$698.64	090	M B
29893	Scope, plantar fasciotomy	5.22	NA	5.56	0.74	NA	NA	11.52	$417.01	090	M B C+
29894	Ankle arthroscopy/surgery	7.21	NA	8.04	1.01	NA	NA	16.26	$588.60	090	M B C+
29895	Ankle arthroscopy/surgery	6.99	NA	8.01	0.97	NA	NA	15.97	$578.10	090	M B C+

29897	Ankle arthroscopy/surgery	7.18	NA	8.73	1.01	NA	16.92	$612.49	090	M	B
29898	Ankle arthroscopy/surgery	8.32	NA	8.79	1.14	NA	18.25	$660.64	090	M	B C+
29900	Mcp joint arthroscopy, dx	5.42	NA	5.88	0.69	NA	11.99	$434.03	090	M	B A+
29901	Mcp joint arthroscopy, surg	6.13	NA	6.28	0.81	NA	13.22	$478.55	090	M	B A+
29902	Mcp joint arthroscopy, surg	6.70	NA	6.60	0.89	NA	14.19	$513.67	090	M	B A+
29999	Arthroscopy of joint	0.00	0.00	0.00	0.00	0.00	0.00	$0.00	YYY	M	B C+

Surgery: Respiratory system

30000	Drainage of nose lesion	1.43	2.53	1.51	0.10	4.06	3.04	$110.05	010	M	A+
30020	Drainage of nose lesion	1.43	2.64	1.57	0.08	4.15	3.08	$111.49	010	M	A
30100	Intranasal biopsy	0.94	1.34	0.53	0.06	2.34	1.53	$55.38	000	M	A
30110	Removal of nose polyp(s)	1.63	2.80	0.88	0.12	4.55	2.63	$95.20	010	M	B A
30115	Removal of nose polyp(s)	4.35	NA	4.54	0.31	NA	9.20	$333.03	090	M	B A
30117	Removal of intranasal lesion	3.16	4.95	3.20	0.22	8.33	6.58	$238.19	090	M	A
30118	Removal of intranasal lesion	9.69	NA	8.55	0.66	NA	18.90	$684.16	090	M	C+
30120	Revision of nose	5.27	5.71	5.71	0.41	11.39	11.39	$412.31	090	M	A
30124	Removal of nose lesion	3.10	NA	3.31	0.20	NA	6.61	$239.28	090	M	A
30125	Removal of nose lesion	7.16	NA	6.61	0.54	NA	14.31	$518.01	090	M	A
30130	Removal of turbinate bones	3.38	NA	3.99	0.22	NA	7.59	$274.75	090	M	B A
30140	Removal of turbinate bones	3.43	NA	4.61	0.24	NA	8.28	$299.73	090	M	B A
30150	Partial removal of nose	9.14	NA	8.83	0.76	NA	18.73	$678.01	090	M	A C+
30160	Removal of nose	9.58	NA	8.79	0.78	NA	19.15	$693.21	090	M	A C+
30200	Injection treatment of nose	0.78	1.23	0.46	0.06	2.07	1.30	$47.06	000	M	A
30210	Nasal sinus therapy	1.08	2.15	0.61	0.08	3.31	1.77	$64.07	010	M	A
30220	Insert nasal septal button	1.54	2.52	0.84	0.11	4.17	2.49	$90.14	010	M	A
30300	Remove nasal foreign body	1.04	2.62	0.37	0.07	3.73	1.48	$53.57	010	M	A
30310	Remove nasal foreign body	1.96	NA	1.92	0.14	NA	4.02	$145.52	010	M	A+
30320	Remove nasal foreign body	4.52	NA	5.26	0.36	NA	10.14	$367.06	090	M	A+
30400	Reconstruction of nose	9.83	NA	8.95	0.80	NA	19.58	$708.78	090	M	A+

* **M** = multiple surgery adjustment applies
Me = multiple endoscopy rules may apply
B = bilateral surgery adjustment applies
A = assistant-at-surgery restriction

A+ = assistant-at-surgery restriction unless medical necessity established with documentation
C = cosurgeons payable
C+ = cosurgeons payable if medical necessity established with documentation

T = team surgeons permitted
T+ = team surgeons payable if medical necessity established with documentation
S = indicates services that are not covered by Medicare.

197 CPT five-digit codes, two-digit numeric modifiers, and descriptions only are © 2001 American Medical Association

Medicare RBRVS: The Physicians' Guide

Relative value units

CPT Code and Modifier	Description	Work RVU	Non Facility Practice Expense RVU	Facility Practice Expense RVU	PLI RVU	Total Non Facility RVUs	Medicare Payment Non Facility	Total Facility RVUs	Medicare Payment Facility	Global Period	Payment Policy Indicators*
30410	Reconstruction of nose	12.98	NA	10.45	1.08	NA	NA	24.51	$887.24	090	M
30420	Reconstruction of nose	15.88	NA	12.50	1.24	NA	NA	29.62	$1,072.22	090	M A
30430	Revision of nose	7.21	NA	7.40	0.62	NA	NA	15.23	$551.31	090	M
30435	Revision of nose	11.71	NA	10.68	1.10	NA	NA	23.49	$850.32	090	M
30450	Revision of nose	18.65	NA	14.37	1.53	NA	NA	34.55	$1,250.68	090	M
30460	Revision of nose	9.96	NA	9.16	0.85	NA	NA	19.97	$722.90	090	M C
30462	Revision of nose	19.57	NA	14.30	1.92	NA	NA	35.79	$1,295.57	090	M C
30465	Repair nasal stenosis	11.64	NA	9.58	0.97	NA	NA	22.19	$803.26	090	M A+
30520	Repair of nasal septum	5.70	NA	5.93	0.41	NA	NA	12.04	$435.84	090	M A
30540	Repair nasal defect	7.75	NA	6.71	0.53	NA	NA	14.99	$542.63	090	M
30545	Repair nasal defect	11.38	NA	9.19	0.80	NA	NA	21.37	$773.58	090	M
30560	Release of nasal adhesions	1.26	2.37	1.52	0.09	3.72	$134.66	2.87	$103.89	010	M A
30580	Repair upper jaw fistula	6.69	5.00	5.00	0.50	12.19	$441.27	12.19	$441.27	090	M A
30600	Repair mouth/nose fistula	6.02	4.90	4.90	0.70	11.62	$420.63	11.62	$420.63	090	M A+
30620	Intranasal reconstruction	5.97	NA	6.69	0.45	NA	NA	13.11	$474.57	090	M A
30630	Repair nasal septum defect	7.12	NA	7.23	0.51	NA	NA	14.86	$537.92	090	M A+
30801	Cauterization, inner nose	1.09	2.57	2.31	0.08	3.74	$135.39	3.48	$125.97	010	M A
30802	Cauterization, inner nose	2.03	3.14	2.87	0.15	5.32	$192.58	5.05	$182.81	010	M A
30901	Control of nosebleed	1.21	1.43	0.34	0.09	2.73	$98.82	1.64	$59.37	000	M B A
30903	Control of nosebleed	1.54	3.20	0.53	0.12	4.86	$175.93	2.19	$79.28	000	M B A
30905	Control of nosebleed	1.97	3.85	0.80	0.15	5.97	$216.11	2.92	$105.70	000	M A
30906	Repeat control of nosebleed	2.45	4.27	1.27	0.17	6.89	$249.41	3.89	$140.81	000	M A
30915	Ligation, nasal sinus artery	7.20	NA	7.13	0.50	NA	NA	14.83	$536.83	090	M A
30920	Ligation, upper jaw artery	9.83	NA	8.64	0.69	NA	NA	19.16	$693.58	090	M A
30930	Therapy, fracture of nose	1.26	NA	2.17	0.09	NA	NA	3.52	$127.42	010	M B A
30999	Nasal surgery procedure	0.00	0.00	0.00	0.00	0.00	$0.00	0.00	$0.00	YYY	M A+ C+ T+
31000	Irrigation, maxillary sinus	1.15	2.43	0.66	0.08	3.66	$132.49	1.89	$68.42	010	M B A

Code	Description											
31002	Irrigation, sphenoid sinus	1.91	NA	2.07	0.14	NA	NA	4.12	$149.14	010	M	B	A+
31020	Exploration, maxillary sinus	2.94	4.20	3.68	0.20	7.34	$265.70	6.82	$246.88	090	M	B	A
31030	Exploration, maxillary sinus	5.92	4.85	4.68	0.42	11.19	$405.07	11.02	$398.92	090	M	B	A
31032	Explore sinus,remove polyps	6.57	NA	6.16	0.47	NA	NA	13.20	$477.83	090	M	B	A
31040	Exploration behind upper jaw	9.42	NA	7.34	0.71	NA	NA	17.47	$632.40	090	M	B	A	C+
31050	Exploration, sphenoid sinus	5.28	NA	5.12	0.39	NA	NA	10.79	$390.59	090	M	B	A
31051	Sphenoid sinus surgery	7.11	NA	6.66	0.55	NA	NA	14.32	$518.37	090	M	B	A
31070	Exploration of frontal sinus	4.28	NA	5.04	0.30	NA	NA	9.62	$348.24	090	M	B	A
31075	Exploration of frontal sinus	9.16	NA	8.38	0.64	NA	NA	18.18	$658.10	090	M	B		C+
31080	Removal of frontal sinus	11.42	NA	9.13	0.78	NA	NA	21.33	$772.13	090	M	B		
31081	Removal of frontal sinus	12.75	NA	9.97	1.84	NA	NA	24.56	$889.05	090	M	B		C+
31084	Removal of frontal sinus	13.51	NA	10.76	0.96	NA	NA	25.23	$913.31	090	M	B		C+
31085	Removal of frontal sinus	14.20	NA	11.12	1.18	NA	NA	26.50	$959.28	090	M	B		C+
31086	Removal of frontal sinus	12.86	NA	10.50	0.90	NA	NA	24.26	$878.19	090	M	B		
31087	Removal of frontal sinus	13.10	NA	10.32	1.15	NA	NA	24.57	$889.41	090	M	B		C+
31090	Exploration of sinuses	9.53	NA	9.05	0.66	NA	NA	19.24	$696.47	090	M	B	A
31200	Removal of ethmoid sinus	4.97	NA	5.86	0.25	NA	NA	11.08	$401.09	090	M	B	A
31201	Removal of ethmoid sinus	8.37	NA	7.91	0.58	NA	NA	16.86	$610.32	090	M	B	A
31205	Removal of ethmoid sinus	10.24	NA	8.66	0.58	NA	NA	19.48	$705.16	090	M	B		C+
31225	Removal of upper jaw	19.23	NA	15.42	1.38	NA	NA	36.03	$1,304.26	090	M	B		C+
31230	Removal of upper jaw	21.94	NA	17.21	1.57	NA	NA	40.72	$1,474.03	090	M	B		C+
31231	Nasal endoscopy, dx	1.10	2.01	0.61	0.08	3.19	$115.48	1.79	$64.80	000	M	B	A
31233	Nasal/sinus endoscopy, dx	2.18	2.66	1.24	0.16	5.00	$181.00	3.58	$129.59	000	M	B	A
31235	Nasal/sinus endoscopy, dx	2.64	2.93	1.49	0.18	5.75	$208.15	4.31	$156.02	000	M	B	A
31237	Nasal/sinus endoscopy, surg	2.98	3.22	1.66	0.21	6.41	$232.04	4.85	$175.57	000	M	B	A
31238	Nasal/sinus endoscopy, surg	3.26	3.75	1.89	0.23	7.24	$262.08	5.38	$194.75	000	M	B	A+
31239	Nasal/sinus endoscopy, surg	8.70	NA	6.72	0.46	NA	NA	15.88	$574.84	010	M	B	A+
31240	Nasal/sinus endoscopy, surg	2.61	NA	1.62	0.18	NA	NA	4.41	$159.64	000	M	B	A+

* **M** = multiple surgery adjustment applies
Me = multiple endoscopy rules may apply
B = bilateral surgery adjustment applies
A = assistant-at-surgery restriction

A+ = assistant-at-surgery restriction unless medical necessity established with documentation
C = cosurgeons payable
C+ = cosurgeons payable if medical necessity established with documentation

T = team surgeons permitted
T+ = team surgeons payable if medical necessity established with documentation
§ = indicates services that are not covered by Medicare.

199 CPT five-digit codes, two-digit numeric modifiers, and descriptions only are © 2001 American Medical Association

Medicare RBRVS: The Physicians' Guide

Relative value units

CPT Code and Modifier	Description	Work RVU	Non Facility Practice Expense RVU	Facility Practice Expense RVU	PLI RVU	Total Non Facility RVUs	Medicare Payment Non Facility	Total Facility RVUs	Medicare Payment Facility	Global Period	Payment Policy Indicators*			
31254	Revision of ethmoid sinus	4.65	NA	2.79	0.32	NA	NA	7.76	$280.91	000	M	B	A	
31255	Removal of ethmoid sinus	6.96	NA	4.14	0.49	NA	NA	11.59	$419.55	000	M	B	A	
31256	Exploration maxillary sinus	3.29	NA	2.01	0.23	NA	NA	5.53	$200.18	000	M	B	A	
31267	Endoscopy, maxillary sinus	5.46	NA	3.27	0.38	NA	NA	9.11	$329.77	000	M	B	A	
31276	Sinus endoscopy, surgical	8.85	NA	5.24	0.62	NA	NA	14.71	$532.49	000	M	B	A	
31287	Nasal/sinus endoscopy, surg	3.92	NA	2.37	0.27	NA	NA	6.56	$237.47	000	M	B	A+	
31288	Nasal/sinus endoscopy, surg	4.58	NA	2.75	0.32	NA	NA	7.65	$276.92	000	M	B	A+	
31290	Nasal/sinus endoscopy, surg	17.24	NA	11.86	1.20	NA	NA	30.30	$1,096.84	010	M	B	A+	
31291	Nasal/sinus endoscopy, surg	18.19	NA	12.28	1.73	NA	NA	32.20	$1,165.61	010	M	B	A+	
31292	Nasal/sinus endoscopy, surg	14.76	NA	10.36	0.99	NA	NA	26.11	$945.16	010	M	B	A+	
31293	Nasal/sinus endoscopy, surg	16.21	NA	11.16	0.97	NA	NA	28.34	$1,025.89	010	M	B	A+	
31294	Nasal/sinus endoscopy, surg	19.06	NA	12.46	1.04	NA	NA	32.56	$1,178.65	010	M	B	A+	
31299	Sinus surgery procedure	0.00	0.00	0.00	0.00	0.00	$0.00	0.00	$0.00	YYY	M		A+	T+
31300	Removal of larynx lesion	14.29	NA	17.46	0.99	NA	NA	32.74	$1,185.16	090	M			C+
31320	Diagnostic incision, larynx	5.26	NA	12.54	0.40	NA	NA	18.20	$658.83	090	M		A+	
31360	Removal of larynx	17.08	NA	19.24	1.20	NA	NA	37.52	$1,358.19	090	M			C+
31365	Removal of larynx	24.16	NA	23.20	1.72	NA	NA	49.08	$1,776.66	090	M			C+
31367	Partial removal of larynx	21.86	NA	23.92	1.57	NA	NA	47.35	$1,714.03	090	M			C+
31368	Partial removal of larynx	27.09	NA	28.64	1.90	NA	NA	57.63	$2,086.16	090	M			C+
31370	Partial removal of larynx	21.38	NA	23.46	1.51	NA	NA	46.35	$1,677.83	090	M			C+
31375	Partial removal of larynx	20.21	NA	21.16	1.43	NA	NA	42.80	$1,549.33	090	M			C+
31380	Partial removal of larynx	20.21	NA	21.41	1.40	NA	NA	43.02	$1,557.29	090	M			C+
31382	Partial removal of larynx	20.52	NA	23.06	1.44	NA	NA	45.02	$1,629.69	090	M			C+
31390	Removal of larynx & pharynx	27.53	NA	28.90	1.95	NA	NA	58.38	$2,113.31	090	M			C+
31395	Reconstruct larynx & pharynx	31.09	NA	35.02	2.27	NA	NA	68.38	$2,475.30	090	M			C+
31400	Revision of larynx	10.31	NA	15.75	0.72	NA	NA	26.78	$969.41	090	M			
31420	Removal of epiglottis	10.22	NA	15.60	0.71	NA	NA	26.53	$960.36	090	M			C+

Code	Description									
31500	Insert emergency airway	2.33	NA	0.69	0.15	NA	3.17	$114.75	000		A
31502	Change of windpipe airway	0.65	1.97	0.27	0.04	2.66	0.96	$34.75	000	M	A
31505	Diagnostic laryngoscopy	0.61	1.85	0.35	0.04	2.50	1.00	$36.20	000	M	A
31510	Laryngoscopy with biopsy	1.92	2.86	1.04	0.15	4.93	3.11	$112.58	000	Me	A+
31511	Remove foreign body, larynx	2.16	3.15	0.75	0.16	5.47	3.07	$111.13	000	Me	A
31512	Removal of larynx lesion	2.07	3.00	1.10	0.16	5.23	3.33	$120.54	000	Me	A+
31513	Injection into vocal cord	2.10	NA	1.32	0.15	NA	3.57	$129.23	000	Me	A+
31515	Laryngoscopy for aspiration	1.80	2.30	0.90	0.12	4.22	2.82	$102.08	000	M	A
31520	Diagnostic laryngoscopy	2.56	NA	1.41	0.17	NA	4.14	$149.86	000	M	A+
31525	Diagnostic laryngoscopy	2.63	2.94	1.53	0.18	5.75	4.34	$157.10	000	M	A
31526	Diagnostic laryngoscopy	2.57	NA	1.59	0.18	NA	4.34	$157.10	000	M	A
31527	Laryngoscopy for treatment	3.27	NA	1.77	0.21	NA	5.25	$190.05	000	Me	A+
31528	Laryngoscopy and dilation	2.37	NA	1.24	0.16	NA	3.77	$136.47	000	Me	A+
31529	Laryngoscopy and dilation	2.68	NA	1.62	0.18	NA	4.48	$162.17	000	Me	A+
31530	Operative laryngoscopy	3.39	NA	1.89	0.24	NA	5.52	$199.82	000	Me	A
31531	Operative laryngoscopy	3.59	NA	2.18	0.25	NA	6.02	$217.92	000	Me	A+
31535	Operative laryngoscopy	3.16	NA	1.88	0.22	NA	5.26	$190.41	000	Me	A
31536	Operative laryngoscopy	3.56	NA	2.16	0.25	NA	5.97	$216.11	000	Me	A
31540	Operative laryngoscopy	4.13	NA	2.48	0.29	NA	6.90	$249.77	000	Me	A
31541	Operative laryngoscopy	4.53	NA	2.72	0.32	NA	7.57	$274.03	000	Me	A
31560	Operative laryngoscopy	5.46	NA	3.11	0.38	NA	8.95	$323.98	000	Me	A+
31561	Operative laryngoscopy	6.00	NA	2.96	0.42	NA	9.38	$339.55	000	Me	A+
31570	Laryngoscopy with injection	3.87	3.97	2.31	0.24	8.08	6.42	$232.40	000	Me	A
31571	Laryngoscopy with injection	4.27	NA	2.46	0.30	NA	7.03	$254.48	000	Me	A
31575	Diagnostic laryngoscopy	1.10	2.08	0.59	0.08	3.26	1.77	$64.07	000	M	A
31576	Laryngoscopy with biopsy	1.97	2.26	1.08	0.13	4.36	3.18	$115.11	000	Me	A
31577	Remove foreign body, larynx	2.47	2.90	1.31	0.17	5.54	3.95	$142.99	000	Me	A+
31578	Removal of larynx lesion	2.84	3.13	1.62	0.20	6.17	4.66	$168.69	000	Me	A+

* **M** = multiple surgery adjustment applies
Me = multiple endoscopy rules may apply
B = bilateral surgery adjustment applies
A = assistant-at-surgery restriction

A+ = assistant-at-surgery restriction unless medical necessity established with documentation
C = cosurgeons payable
C+ = cosurgeons payable if medical necessity established with documentation

T = team surgeons permitted
T+ = team surgeons payable if medical necessity established with documentation
$ = indicates services that are not covered by Medicare.

CPT five-digit codes, two-digit numeric modifiers, and descriptions only are © 2001 American Medical Association

Medicare RBRVS: The Physicians' Guide

Relative value units

CPT Code and Modifier	Description	Work RVU	Non Facility Practice Expense RVU	Facility Practice Expense RVU	PLI RVU	Total Non Facility RVUs	Medicare Payment Non Facility	Total Facility RVUs	Medicare Payment Facility	Global Period	Payment Policy Indicators*			
31579	Diagnostic laryngoscopy	2.26	2.97	1.27	0.16	5.39	$195.11	3.69	$133.58	000	Me	A		
31580	Revision of larynx	12.38	NA	16.85	0.87	NA	NA	30.10	$1,089.60	090	M		C+	
31582	Revision of larynx	21.62	NA	22.06	1.52	NA	NA	45.20	$1,636.20	090	M	A	C+	
31584	Treat larynx fracture	19.64	NA	19.05	1.42	NA	NA	40.11	$1,451.95	090	M		C+	
31585	Treat larynx fracture	4.64	NA	8.92	0.30	NA	NA	13.86	$501.72	090	M	A+		
31586	Treat larynx fracture	8.03	NA	12.71	0.56	NA	NA	21.30	$771.04	090	M	A+		
31587	Revision of larynx	11.99	NA	14.77	0.88	NA	NA	27.64	$1,000.55	090	M		C+	
31588	Revision of larynx	13.11	NA	17.21	0.92	NA	NA	31.24	$1,130.86	090	M			
31590	Reinnervate larynx	6.97	NA	12.63	0.50	NA	NA	20.10	$727.60	090	M		C+	
31595	Larynx nerve surgery	8.34	NA	11.90	0.62	NA	NA	20.86	$755.12	090	M		C+	
31599	Larynx surgery procedure	0.00	0.00	0.00	0.00	0.00	$0.00	0.00	$0.00	YYY	M	A+	C+	T+
31600	Incision of windpipe	7.18	NA	3.15	0.34	NA	NA	10.67	$386.25	000	M	A		
31601	Incision of windpipe	4.45	NA	2.20	0.39	NA	NA	7.04	$254.84	090	M		C+	
31603	Incision of windpipe	4.15	NA	1.88	0.35	NA	NA	6.38	$230.95	000	M	A		
31605	Incision of windpipe	3.58	NA	1.24	0.33	NA	NA	5.15	$186.43	000	M	A		
31610	Incision of windpipe	8.76	NA	10.98	0.69	NA	NA	20.43	$739.55	090	M	A		
31611	Surgery/speech prosthesis	5.64	NA	10.28	0.40	NA	NA	16.32	$590.77	090	M		C+	
31612	Puncture/clear windpipe	0.91	1.53	0.48	0.06	2.50	$90.50	1.45	$52.49	000	M	A+		
31613	Repair windpipe opening	4.59	NA	8.94	0.37	NA	NA	13.90	$503.17	090	M	A		
31614	Repair windpipe opening	7.12	NA	12.47	0.51	NA	NA	20.10	$727.60	090	M	A		
31615	Visualization of windpipe	2.09	3.76	1.20	0.14	5.99	$216.83	3.43	$124.16	000	M	A		
31622	Dx bronchoscope/wash	2.78	3.69	1.20	0.14	6.61	$239.28	4.12	$149.14	000	M	A		
31623	Dx bronchoscope/brush	2.88	2.97	1.17	0.14	5.99	$216.83	4.19	$151.67	000	Me	A		
31624	Dx bronchoscope/lavage	2.88	2.75	1.17	0.13	5.76	$208.51	4.18	$151.31	000	Me	A		
31625	Bronchoscopy with biopsy	3.37	2.96	1.34	0.16	6.49	$234.93	4.87	$176.29	000	Me	A		
31628	Bronchoscopy with biopsy	3.81	3.38	1.45	0.14	7.33	$265.34	5.40	$195.48	000	Me	A		

Code	Description										
31629	Bronchoscopy with biopsy	3.37	NA	1.32	0.13	NA	NA	4.82	$174.48	000	Me	A
31630	Bronchoscopy with repair	3.82	NA	1.99	0.30	NA	NA	6.11	$221.18	000	Me	A
31631	Bronchoscopy with dilation	4.37	NA	2.04	0.31	NA	NA	6.72	$243.26	000	Me	A
31635	Remove foreign body, airway	3.68	NA	1.70	0.21	NA	NA	5.59	$202.35	000	Me	A
31640	Bronchoscopy & remove lesion	4.94	NA	2.36	0.37	NA	NA	7.67	$277.65	000	Me	A
31641	Bronchoscopy, treat blockage	5.03	NA	2.20	0.30	NA	NA	7.53	$272.58	000	Me	A
31643	Diag bronchoscope/catheter	3.50	1.17	1.17	0.15	4.82	$174.48	4.82	$174.48	000	M	A
31645	Bronchoscopy, clear airways	3.16	NA	1.27	0.13	NA	NA	4.56	$165.07	000	Me	A
31646	Bronchoscopy, reclear airway	2.72	NA	1.12	0.12	NA	NA	3.96	$143.35	000	M	A
31656	Bronchoscopy, inj for xray	2.17	NA	1.05	0.10	NA	NA	3.32	$120.18	000	M	A+
31700	Insertion of airway catheter	1.34	3.44	0.68	0.07	4.85	$175.57	2.09	$75.66	000	M	A+
31708	Instill airway contrast dye	1.41	NA	0.64	0.06	NA	NA	2.11	$76.38	000	M	B A+
31710	Insertion of airway catheter	1.30	NA	0.75	0.06	NA	NA	2.11	$76.38	000	M	B A+
31715	Injection for bronchus x-ray	1.11	NA	0.73	0.06	NA	NA	1.90	$68.78	000	M	B A+
31717	Bronchial brush biopsy	2.12	3.25	0.89	0.09	5.46	$197.65	3.10	$112.22	000	M	A
31720	Clearance of airways	1.06	1.90	0.35	0.06	3.02	$109.32	1.47	$53.21	000	M	A
31725	Clearance of airways	1.96	NA	0.61	0.10	NA	NA	2.67	$96.65	000	M	A
31730	Intro, windpipe wire/tube	2.85	2.54	1.13	0.15	5.54	$200.54	4.13	$149.50	000	M	A
31750	Repair of windpipe	13.02	NA	16.22	1.02	NA	NA	30.26	$1,095.39	090	M	C+
31755	Repair of windpipe	15.93	NA	19.27	1.15	NA	NA	36.35	$1,315.84	090	M	C+
31760	Repair of windpipe	22.35	NA	12.79	1.48	NA	NA	36.62	$1,325.61	090	M	C+
31766	Reconstruction of windpipe	30.43	NA	15.03	3.16	NA	NA	48.62	$1,760.01	090	M	C+
31770	Repair/graft of bronchus	22.51	NA	15.67	2.27	NA	NA	40.45	$1,464.26	090	M	C+
31775	Reconstruct bronchus	23.54	NA	15.14	2.91	NA	NA	41.59	$1,505.52	090	M	C+
31780	Reconstruct windpipe	17.72	NA	12.97	1.55	NA	NA	32.24	$1,167.06	090	M	C+
31781	Reconstruct windpipe	23.53	NA	15.49	2.04	NA	NA	41.06	$1,486.34	090	M	C+
31785	Remove windpipe lesion	17.23	NA	13.05	1.36	NA	NA	31.64	$1,145.34	090	M	C+
31786	Remove windpipe lesion	23.98	NA	14.41	2.20	NA	NA	40.59	$1,469.33	090	M	C+

* **M** = multiple surgery adjustment applies
Me = multiple endoscopy rules may apply
B = bilateral surgery adjustment applies
A = assistant-at-surgery restriction
A+ = assistant-at-surgery restriction unless medical necessity established with documentation
C = cosurgeons payable
C+ = cosurgeons payable if medical necessity established with documentation
T = team surgeons permitted
T+ = team surgeons payable if medical necessity established with documentation
§ = indicates services that are not covered by Medicare.

203   CPT five-digit codes, two-digit numeric modifiers, and descriptions only are © 2001 American Medical Association

Medicare RBRVS: The Physicians' Guide

Relative value units

CPT Code and Modifier	Description	Work RVU	Non Facility Practice Expense RVU	Facility Practice Expense RVU	PLI RVU	Total Non Facility RVUs	Medicare Payment Non Facility	Total Facility RVUs	Medicare Payment Facility	Global Period	Payment Policy Indicators*
31800	Repair of windpipe injury	7.43	NA	6.81	0.67	NA	NA	14.91	$539.73	090	M A+
31805	Repair of windpipe injury	13.13	NA	10.72	1.45	NA	NA	25.30	$915.84	090	M C+
31820	Closure of windpipe lesion	4.49	8.24	8.07	0.35	13.08	$473.49	12.91	$467.33	090	M A+
31825	Repair of windpipe defect	6.81	10.86	10.86	0.50	18.17	$657.74	18.17	$657.74	090	M A+
31830	Revise windpipe scar	4.50	7.82	7.82	0.36	12.68	$459.01	12.68	$459.01	090	M A+
31899	Airways surgical procedure	0.00	0.00	0.00	0.00	0.00	$0.00	0.00	$0.00	YYY	M A+ C+ T+
32000	Drainage of chest	1.54	3.10	0.51	0.07	4.71	$170.50	2.12	$76.74	000	A
32002	Treatment of collapsed lung	2.19	NA	0.87	0.11	NA	NA	3.17	$114.75	000	M A C+
32005	Treat lung lining chemically	2.19	NA	0.88	0.17	NA	NA	3.24	$117.29	000	M A
32020	Insertion of chest tube	3.98	NA	1.48	0.36	NA	NA	5.82	$210.68	000	A
32035	Exploration of chest	8.67	NA	7.83	1.02	NA	NA	17.52	$634.21	090	M C+
32036	Exploration of chest	9.68	NA	8.39	1.20	NA	NA	19.27	$697.56	090	M C+
32095	Biopsy through chest wall	8.36	NA	8.05	0.99	NA	NA	17.40	$629.87	090	M C+
32100	Exploration/biopsy of chest	15.24	NA	10.30	1.45	NA	NA	26.99	$977.02	090	M C+
32110	Explore/repair chest	23.00	NA	12.72	1.63	NA	NA	37.35	$1,352.04	090	M C+
32120	Re-exploration of chest	11.54	NA	9.34	1.42	NA	NA	22.30	$807.24	090	M C+
32124	Explore chest free adhesions	12.72	NA	9.53	1.51	NA	NA	23.76	$860.09	090	M C+
32140	Removal of lung lesion(s)	13.93	NA	9.79	1.68	NA	NA	25.40	$919.46	090	M C+
32141	Remove/treat lung lesions	14.00	NA	9.98	1.72	NA	NA	25.70	$930.32	090	M C+
32150	Removal of lung lesion(s)	14.15	NA	9.70	1.60	NA	NA	25.45	$921.27	090	M C+
32151	Remove lung foreign body	14.21	NA	10.20	1.49	NA	NA	25.90	$937.56	090	M C+
32160	Open chest heart massage	9.30	NA	6.34	1.01	NA	NA	16.65	$602.72	090	M C+
32200	Drain, open, lung lesion	15.29	NA	10.08	1.46	NA	NA	26.83	$971.22	090	M C+
32201	Drain, percut, lung lesion	4.00	NA	5.67	0.18	NA	NA	9.85	$356.56	000	M
32215	Treat chest lining	11.33	NA	9.16	1.34	NA	NA	21.83	$790.23	090	M C+
32220	Release of lung	24.00	NA	13.56	2.39	NA	NA	39.95	$1,446.16	090	M C+
32225	Partial release of lung	13.96	NA	9.95	1.70	NA	NA	25.61	$927.06	090	M C+

Code	Description									
32310	Removal of chest lining	13.44	NA	9.86	1.65	NA	24.95	$903.17	090	M		C+
32320	Free/remove chest lining	24.00	NA	13.21	2.50	NA	39.71	$1,437.47	090	M		C+
32400	Needle biopsy chest lining	1.76	1.89	0.59	0.07	3.72	2.42	$87.60	000	M	A	
32402	Open biopsy chest lining	7.56	NA	7.76	0.91	NA	16.23	$587.51	090	M		C+
32405	Biopsy, lung or mediastinum	1.93	2.33	0.67	0.09	4.35	2.69	$97.38	000	M	A	
32420	Puncture/clear lung	2.18	NA	0.88	0.11	NA	3.17	$114.75	000	M	A	
32440	Removal of lung	25.00	NA	13.57	2.56	NA	41.13	$1,488.87	090	M		C+
32442	Sleeve pneumonectomy	26.24	NA	14.35	3.12	NA	43.71	$1,582.27	090	M		C+
32445	Removal of lung	25.09	NA	13.83	3.11	NA	42.03	$1,521.45	090	M		C+
32480	Partial removal of lung	23.75	NA	12.78	2.24	NA	38.77	$1,403.44	090	M		C+
32482	Bilobectomy	25.00	NA	13.39	2.35	NA	40.74	$1,474.76	090	M		C+
32484	Segmentectomy	20.69	NA	11.97	2.54	NA	35.20	$1,274.21	090	M		C+
32486	Sleeve lobectomy	23.92	NA	13.32	3.00	NA	40.24	$1,456.66	090	M		C+
32488	Completion pneumonectomy	25.71	NA	13.89	3.18	NA	42.78	$1,548.60	090	M		C+
32491	Lung volume reduction	21.25	NA	12.67	2.66	NA	36.58	$1,324.17	090	M	B	C+
32500	Partial removal of lung	22.00	NA	12.70	1.77	NA	36.47	$1,320.18	090	M		C+
32501	Repair bronchus add-on	4.69	NA	1.59	0.56	NA	6.84	$247.60	ZZZ		B	
32520	Remove lung & revise chest	21.68	NA	12.56	2.71	NA	36.95	$1,337.56	090	M		C+
32522	Remove lung & revise chest	24.20	NA	13.63	2.84	NA	40.67	$1,472.22	090	M		C+
32525	Remove lung & revise chest	26.50	NA	14.22	3.25	NA	43.97	$1,591.68	090	M		C+
32540	Removal of lung lesion	14.64	NA	9.99	1.84	NA	26.47	$958.19	090	M		C+
32601	Thoracoscopy, diagnostic	5.46	NA	3.60	0.63	NA	9.69	$350.77	000	M	A+	
32602	Thoracoscopy, diagnostic	5.96	NA	3.72	0.70	NA	10.38	$375.75	000	M	A+	
32603	Thoracoscopy, diagnostic	7.81	NA	4.33	0.76	NA	12.90	$466.97	000	M	A+	
32604	Thoracoscopy, diagnostic	8.78	NA	4.79	0.97	NA	14.54	$526.34	000	M	A+	
32605	Thoracoscopy, diagnostic	6.93	NA	4.19	0.86	NA	11.98	$433.67	000	M	A+	
32606	Thoracoscopy, diagnostic	8.40	NA	4.55	0.99	NA	13.94	$504.62	000	M	A+	
32650	Thoracoscopy, surgical	10.75	NA	8.47	1.25	NA	20.47	$741.00	090	M		C+

* **M** = multiple surgery adjustment applies
   Me = multiple endoscopy rules may apply
   B = bilateral surgery adjustment applies
   A = assistant-at-surgery restriction

A+ = assistant-at-surgery restriction unless medical necessity established with documentation
C = cosurgeons payable
C+ = cosurgeons payable if medical necessity established with documentation

T = team surgeons permitted
T+ = team surgeons payable if medical necessity established with documentation
$ = indicates services that are not covered by Medicare.

205   CPT five-digit codes, two-digit numeric modifiers, and descriptions only are © 2001 American Medical Association

Medicare RBRVS: The Physicians' Guide

Relative value units

CPT Code and Modifier	Description	Work RVU	Non Facility Practice Expense RVU	Facility Practice Expense RVU	PLI RVU	Total Non Facility RVUs	Medicare Payment Non Facility	Total Facility RVUs	Medicare Payment Facility	Global Period	Payment Policy Indicators*
32651	Thoracoscopy, surgical	12.91	NA	8.84	1.50	NA	NA	23.25	$841.63	090	M C+
32652	Thoracoscopy, surgical	18.66	NA	11.16	2.30	NA	NA	32.12	$1,162.72	090	M C+
32653	Thoracoscopy, surgical	12.87	NA	9.15	1.55	NA	NA	23.57	$853.22	090	M C+
32654	Thoracoscopy, surgical	12.44	NA	7.53	1.51	NA	NA	21.48	$777.56	090	M C+
32655	Thoracoscopy, surgical	13.10	NA	8.86	1.53	NA	NA	23.49	$850.32	090	M C+
32656	Thoracoscopy, surgical	12.91	NA	9.53	1.61	NA	NA	24.05	$870.59	090	M C+
32657	Thoracoscopy, surgical	13.65	NA	9.36	1.64	NA	NA	24.65	$892.31	090	M C+
32658	Thoracoscopy, surgical	11.63	NA	9.05	1.47	NA	NA	22.15	$801.81	090	M C+
32659	Thoracoscopy, surgical	11.59	NA	9.10	1.39	NA	NA	22.08	$799.28	090	M C+
32660	Thoracoscopy, surgical	17.43	NA	10.53	2.09	NA	NA	30.05	$1,087.79	090	M C+
32661	Thoracoscopy, surgical	13.25	NA	9.15	1.66	NA	NA	24.06	$870.95	090	M C+
32662	Thoracoscopy, surgical	16.44	NA	10.59	2.01	NA	NA	29.04	$1,051.22	090	M C+
32663	Thoracoscopy, surgical	18.47	NA	11.22	2.28	NA	NA	31.97	$1,157.29	090	M C+
32664	Thoracoscopy, surgical	14.20	NA	9.43	1.70	NA	NA	25.33	$916.93	090	M B C+
32665	Thoracoscopy, surgical	15.54	NA	9.18	1.79	NA	NA	26.51	$959.64	090	M C+
32800	Repair lung hernia	13.69	NA	10.05	1.51	NA	NA	25.25	$914.03	090	M C+
32810	Close chest after drainage	13.05	NA	10.05	1.55	NA	NA	24.65	$892.31	090	M C+
32815	Close bronchial fistula	23.15	NA	13.32	2.84	NA	NA	39.31	$1,422.99	090	M C+
32820	Reconstruct injured chest	21.48	NA	13.99	2.31	NA	NA	37.78	$1,367.61	090	M C+
32851	Lung transplant, single	38.63	NA	19.94	4.90	NA	NA	63.47	$2,297.56	090	M C+ T
32852	Lung transplant with bypass	41.80	NA	21.40	5.17	NA	NA	68.37	$2,474.94	090	M C+ T
32853	Lung transplant, double	47.81	NA	23.49	6.13	NA	NA	77.43	$2,802.90	090	M C+ T
32854	Lung transplant with bypass	50.98	NA	24.35	6.41	NA	NA	81.74	$2,958.92	090	M C+ T
32900	Removal of rib(s)	20.27	NA	12.27	2.42	NA	NA	34.96	$1,265.52	090	M C+
32905	Revise & repair chest wall	20.75	NA	12.77	2.54	NA	NA	36.06	$1,305.34	090	M C+
32906	Revise & repair chest wall	26.77	NA	14.12	3.30	NA	NA	44.19	$1,599.64	090	M C+
32940	Revision of lung	19.43	NA	11.96	2.47	NA	NA	33.86	$1,225.70	090	M C+

Code	Description											
32960	Therapeutic pneumothorax	1.84	2.16	0.70	4.12	$149.14	2.66	$96.29	000	M	A	
32997	Total lung lavage	6.00	NA	2.00	NA	NA	8.55	$309.50	000	M	A	
32999	Chest surgery procedure	0.00	0.00	0.00	0.00	$0.00	0.00	$0.00	YYY	M		C+ T+
33010	Drainage of heart sac	2.24	NA	1.01	NA	NA	3.38	$122.35	000	M	A	
33011	Repeat drainage of heart sac	2.24	NA	1.05	NA	NA	3.42	$123.80	000	M	A+	
33015	Incision of heart sac	6.80	NA	4.41	0.64	NA	11.85	$428.96	090	M	A	
33020	Incision of heart sac	12.61	NA	7.91	1.50	NA	22.02	$797.11	090	M		C+
33025	Incision of heart sac	12.09	NA	7.77	1.50	NA	21.36	$773.21	090	M		C+
33030	Partial removal of heart sac	18.71	NA	12.12	2.40	NA	33.23	$1,202.90	090	M		C+
33031	Partial removal of heart sac	21.79	NA	13.20	2.78	NA	37.77	$1,367.24	090	M		C+
33050	Removal of heart sac lesion	14.36	NA	10.24	1.73	NA	26.33	$953.12	090	M		C+
33120	Removal of heart lesion	24.56	NA	15.68	3.06	NA	43.30	$1,567.43	090	M		C+
33130	Removal of heart lesion	21.39	NA	12.40	2.51	NA	36.30	$1,314.03	090	M		C+
33140	Heart revascularize (tmr)	20.00	NA	10.57	2.27	NA	32.84	$1,188.78	090	M		C+
33141	Heart tmr w/other procedure	4.84	NA	1.63	0.55	NA	7.02	$254.12	ZZZ		B	
33200	Insertion of heart pacemaker	12.48	NA	9.59	1.17	NA	23.24	$841.27	090	M	A	
33201	Insertion of heart pacemaker	10.18	NA	9.39	1.21	NA	20.78	$752.22	090	M	A	
33206	Insertion of heart pacemaker	6.67	NA	5.35	0.50	NA	12.52	$453.21	090	M	A	C
33207	Insertion of heart pacemaker	8.04	NA	6.00	0.57	NA	14.61	$528.87	090	M	A	C
33208	Insertion of heart pacemaker	8.13	NA	6.14	0.54	NA	14.81	$536.11	090	M	A	C
33210	Insertion of heart electrode	3.30	NA	1.34	0.17	NA	4.81	$174.12	000	M	A	
33211	Insertion of heart electrode	3.40	NA	1.41	0.17	NA	4.98	$180.27	000	M	A	
33212	Insertion of pulse generator	5.52	NA	4.44	0.44	NA	10.40	$376.47	090	M	A	
33213	Insertion of pulse generator	6.37	NA	4.85	0.46	NA	11.68	$422.81	090	M	A	
33214	Upgrade of pacemaker system	7.75	NA	5.95	0.52	NA	14.22	$514.75	090	M	A+	C
33216	Revise eltrd pacing-defib	5.39	NA	4.95	0.36	NA	10.70	$387.33	090	M	A	
33217	Revise eltrd pacing-defib	5.75	NA	5.26	0.36	NA	11.37	$411.58	090	M	A	
33218	Revise eltrd pacing-defib	5.44	NA	4.51	0.40	NA	10.35	$374.66	090	M	A	

* **M** = multiple surgery adjustment applies
Me = multiple endoscopy rules may apply
B = bilateral surgery adjustment applies
A = assistant-at-surgery restriction

A+ = assistant-at-surgery restriction unless medical necessity established with documentation
C = cosurgeons payable
C+ = cosurgeons payable if medical necessity established with documentation

T = team surgeons permitted
T+ = team surgeons payable if medical necessity established with documentation
§ = indicates services that are not covered by Medicare.

207 CPT five-digit codes, two-digit numeric modifiers, and descriptions only are © 2001 American Medical Association

Medicare RBRVS: The Physicians' Guide

Relative value units

CPT Code and Modifier	Description	Work RVU	Non Facility Practice Expense RVU	Facility Practice Expense RVU	PLI RVU	Total Non Facility RVUs	Medicare Payment Non Facility	Total Facility RVUs	Medicare Payment Facility	Global Period	Payment Policy Indicators*
33220	Revise eltrd pacing-defib	5.52	NA	4.45	0.39	NA	NA	10.36	$375.02	090	M A
33222	Revise pocket, pacemaker	4.96	NA	3.93	0.39	NA	NA	9.28	$335.93	090	M A
33223	Revise pocket, pacing-defib	6.46	NA	5.06	0.44	NA	NA	11.96	$432.94	090	M A+
33233	Removal of pacemaker system	3.29	NA	3.80	0.22	NA	NA	7.31	$264.62	090	M A
33234	Removal of pacemaker system	7.82	NA	5.03	0.56	NA	NA	13.41	$485.43	090	M A
33235	Removal pacemaker electrode	9.40	NA	6.26	0.68	NA	NA	16.34	$591.49	090	M A
33236	Remove electrode/thoracotomy	12.60	NA	9.35	1.49	NA	NA	23.44	$848.51	090	M A+ C
33237	Remove electrode/thoracotomy	13.71	NA	9.51	1.57	NA	NA	24.79	$897.38	090	M A+ C
33238	Remove electrode/thoracotomy	15.22	NA	9.24	1.56	NA	NA	26.02	$941.90	090	M A+ C
33240	Insert pulse generator	7.60	NA	5.49	0.53	NA	NA	13.62	$493.03	090	M A
33241	Remove pulse generator	3.24	NA	3.39	0.21	NA	NA	6.84	$247.60	090	M A+
33243	Remove eltrd/thoracotomy	22.64	NA	10.88	2.53	NA	NA	36.05	$1,304.98	090	M C+
33244	Remove eltrd, transven	13.76	NA	8.22	1.05	NA	NA	23.03	$833.67	090	M A C+
33245	Insert epic eltrd pace-defib	14.30	NA	10.79	1.28	NA	NA	26.37	$954.57	090	M C+
33246	Insert epic eltrd/generator	20.71	NA	14.16	2.22	NA	NA	37.09	$1,342.63	090	M C+
33249	Eltrd/insert pace-defib	14.23	NA	8.98	0.80	NA	NA	24.01	$869.14	090	M A C+
33250	Ablate heart dysrhythm focus	21.85	NA	13.65	1.01	NA	NA	36.51	$1,321.63	090	M C+
33251	Ablate heart dysrhythm focus	24.88	NA	14.06	2.41	NA	NA	41.35	$1,496.84	090	M C+
33253	Reconstruct atria	31.06	NA	16.58	3.68	NA	NA	51.32	$1,857.74	090	M C+
33261	Ablate heart dysrhythm focus	24.88	NA	14.47	2.82	NA	NA	42.17	$1,526.52	090	M C+
33282	Implant pat-active ht record	4.17	NA	4.42	0.39	NA	NA	8.98	$325.07	090	M A
33284	Remove pat-active ht record	2.50	NA	3.94	0.23	NA	NA	6.67	$241.45	090	M A
33300	Repair of heart wound	17.92	NA	11.56	1.91	NA	NA	31.39	$1,136.29	090	M C+
33305	Repair of heart wound	21.44	NA	13.24	2.68	NA	NA	37.36	$1,352.40	090	M C+
33310	Exploratory heart surgery	18.51	NA	11.85	2.26	NA	NA	32.62	$1,180.82	090	M C+
33315	Exploratory heart surgery	22.37	NA	13.43	2.90	NA	NA	38.70	$1,400.91	090	M C+
33320	Repair major blood vessel(s)	16.79	NA	11.06	1.66	NA	NA	29.51	$1,068.24	090	M C+

Code	Description								
33321	Repair major vessel	20.20	NA	13.15	2.70	NA	36.05	$1,304.98	090	M	C+
33322	Repair major blood vessel(s)	20.62	NA	13.02	2.51	NA	36.15	$1,308.60	090	M	C+
33330	Insert major vessel graft	21.43	NA	12.35	2.49	NA	36.27	$1,312.94	090	M	C+
33332	Insert major vessel graft	23.96	NA	12.94	2.45	NA	39.35	$1,424.44	090	M	C+
33335	Insert major vessel graft	30.01	NA	16.15	3.79	NA	49.95	$1,808.15	090	M	C+
33400	Repair of aortic valve	28.50	NA	17.04	3.09	NA	48.63	$1,760.37	090	M	C+
33401	Valvuloplasty, open	23.91	NA	14.85	2.71	NA	41.47	$1,501.18	090	M	C+
33403	Valvuloplasty, w/cp bypass	24.89	NA	15.99	2.48	NA	43.36	$1,569.60	090	M	C+
33404	Prepare heart-aorta conduit	28.54	NA	17.22	3.31	NA	49.07	$1,776.29	090	M	C+
33405	Replacement of aortic valve	35.00	NA	17.69	3.86	NA	56.55	$2,047.06	090	M	C+
33406	Replacement of aortic valve	37.50	NA	18.53	4.07	NA	60.10	$2,175.57	090	M	C+
33410	Replacement of aortic valve	32.46	NA	16.93	4.11	NA	53.50	$1,936.66	090	M	C+
33411	Replacement of aortic valve	36.25	NA	18.07	4.16	NA	58.48	$2,116.93	090	M	C+
33412	Replacement of aortic valve	42.00	NA	21.90	4.66	NA	68.56	$2,481.82	090	M	C+
33413	Replacement of aortic valve	43.50	NA	23.05	4.26	NA	70.81	$2,563.27	090	M	C+
33414	Repair of aortic valve	30.35	NA	17.67	3.79	NA	51.81	$1,875.48	090	M	C+
33415	Revision, subvalvular tissue	27.15	NA	16.53	3.25	NA	46.93	$1,698.83	090	M	C+
33416	Revise ventricle muscle	30.35	NA	16.06	3.85	NA	50.26	$1,819.37	090	M	C+
33417	Repair of aortic valve	28.53	NA	17.09	3.58	NA	49.20	$1,781.00	090	M	C+
33420	Revision of mitral valve	22.70	NA	11.77	1.48	NA	35.95	$1,301.36	090	M	A C+
33422	Revision of mitral valve	25.94	NA	14.74	3.30	NA	43.98	$1,592.04	090	M	C+
33425	Repair of mitral valve	27.00	NA	14.98	3.00	NA	44.98	$1,628.24	090	M	C+
33426	Repair of mitral valve	33.00	NA	17.14	3.87	NA	54.01	$1,955.12	090	M	C+
33427	Repair of mitral valve	40.00	NA	19.42	4.30	NA	63.72	$2,306.61	090	M	C+
33430	Replacement of mitral valve	33.50	NA	17.26	3.95	NA	54.71	$1,980.46	090	M	C+
33460	Revision of tricuspid valve	23.60	NA	13.83	3.02	NA	40.45	$1,464.26	090	M	C+
33463	Valvuloplasty, tricuspid	25.62	NA	14.60	3.17	NA	43.39	$1,570.68	090	M	C+
33464	Valvuloplasty, tricuspid	27.33	NA	15.22	3.47	NA	46.02	$1,665.89	090	M	C+

* **M** = multiple surgery adjustment applies
   Me = multiple endoscopy rules may apply
   B = bilateral surgery adjustment applies
   A = assistant-at-surgery restriction

A+ = assistant-at-surgery restriction unless medical necessity established with documentation
C = cosurgeons payable
C+ = cosurgeons payable if medical necessity established with documentation

T = team surgeons permitted
T+ = team surgeons payable if medical necessity established with documentation
$ = indicates services that are not covered by Medicare.

CPT five-digit codes, two-digit numeric modifiers, and descriptions only are © 2001 American Medical Association

Medicare RBRVS: The Physicians' Guide

Relative value units

CPT Code and Modifier	Description	Work RVU	Non Facility Practice Expense RVU	Facility Practice Expense RVU	PLI RVU	Total Non Facility RVUs	Medicare Payment Non Facility	Total Facility RVUs	Medicare Payment Facility	Global Period	Payment Policy Indicators*
33465	Replace tricuspid valve	28.79	NA	15.67	3.61	NA	NA	48.07	$1,740.10	090	M C+
33468	Revision of tricuspid valve	30.12	NA	19.06	4.00	NA	NA	53.18	$1,925.07	090	M C+
33470	Revision of pulmonary valve	20.81	NA	14.20	2.81	NA	NA	37.82	$1,369.05	090	M
33471	Valvotomy, pulmonary valve	22.25	NA	13.13	3.00	NA	NA	38.38	$1,389.33	090	M C+
33472	Revision of pulmonary valve	22.25	NA	13.13	2.92	NA	NA	38.30	$1,386.43	090	M
33474	Revision of pulmonary valve	23.04	NA	13.45	2.84	NA	NA	39.33	$1,423.71	090	M C+
33475	Replacement, pulmonary valve	33.00	NA	18.28	2.64	NA	NA	53.92	$1,951.86	090	M
33476	Revision of heart chamber	25.77	NA	14.23	2.40	NA	NA	42.40	$1,534.85	090	M C+
33478	Revision of heart chamber	26.74	NA	14.43	3.56	NA	NA	44.73	$1,619.19	090	M C+
33496	Repair, prosth valve clot	27.25	NA	16.84	3.44	NA	NA	47.53	$1,720.55	090	M C+
33500	Repair heart vessel fistula	25.55	NA	13.99	2.80	NA	NA	42.34	$1,532.67	090	M C+
33501	Repair heart vessel fistula	17.78	NA	10.24	2.05	NA	NA	30.07	$1,088.51	090	M C
33502	Coronary artery correction	21.04	NA	16.64	2.51	NA	NA	40.19	$1,454.85	090	M C+
33503	Coronary artery graft	21.78	NA	13.90	1.42	NA	NA	37.10	$1,342.99	090	M A+ C+
33504	Coronary artery graft	24.66	NA	16.55	3.04	NA	NA	44.25	$1,601.81	090	M C+
33505	Repair artery w/tunnel	26.84	NA	18.16	1.52	NA	NA	46.52	$1,683.99	090	M C+
33506	Repair artery, translocation	35.50	NA	19.27	3.19	NA	NA	57.96	$2,098.11	090	M C+
33510	CABG, vein, single	29.00	NA	15.53	3.13	NA	NA	47.66	$1,725.25	090	M
33511	CABG, vein, two	30.00	NA	16.05	3.34	NA	NA	49.39	$1,787.88	090	M
33512	CABG, vein, three	31.80	NA	16.65	3.70	NA	NA	52.15	$1,887.79	090	M
33513	CABG, vein, four	32.00	NA	16.77	3.99	NA	NA	52.76	$1,909.87	090	M
33514	CABG, vein, five	32.75	NA	17.00	4.37	NA	NA	54.12	$1,959.10	090	M
33516	Cabg, vein, six or more	35.00	NA	17.74	4.62	NA	NA	57.36	$2,076.39	090	M
33517	CABG, artery-vein, single	2.57	NA	0.86	0.32	NA	NA	3.75	$135.75	ZZZ	
33518	CABG, artery-vein, two	4.85	NA	1.62	0.61	NA	NA	7.08	$256.29	ZZZ	
33519	CABG, artery-vein, three	7.12	NA	2.38	0.89	NA	NA	10.39	$376.11	ZZZ	
33521	CABG, artery-vein, four	9.40	NA	3.15	1.18	NA	NA	13.73	$497.02	ZZZ	

Code	Description								
33522	CABG, artery-vein, five	11.67	NA	3.91	1.48	NA	17.06	$617.56	ZZZ
33523	Cabg, art-vein, six or more	13.95	NA	4.63	1.78	NA	20.36	$737.02	ZZZ
33530	Coronary artery, bypass/reop	5.86	NA	1.96	0.73	NA	8.55	$309.50	ZZZ
33533	CABG, arterial, single	30.00	NA	17.24	3.24	NA	50.48	$1,827.34	090	M
33534	CABG, arterial, two	32.20	NA	17.45	3.63	NA	53.28	$1,928.69	090	M
33535	CABG, arterial, three	34.50	NA	17.77	3.97	NA	56.24	$2,035.84	090	M
33536	Cabg, arterial, four or more	37.50	NA	19.27	3.29	NA	60.06	$2,174.12	090	M
33542	Removal of heart lesion	28.85	NA	17.05	3.61	NA	49.51	$1,792.22	090	M	C+
33545	Repair of heart damage	36.78	NA	19.79	4.40	NA	60.97	$2,207.07	090	M	C+
33572	Open coronary endarterectomy	4.45	NA	1.48	0.55	NA	6.48	$234.57	ZZZ
33600	Closure of valve	29.51	NA	17.79	2.30	NA	49.60	$1,795.48	090	M	C+
33602	Closure of valve	28.54	NA	16.65	2.90	NA	48.09	$1,740.82	090	M	C+
33606	Anastomosis/artery-aorta	30.74	NA	17.53	3.59	NA	51.86	$1,877.29	090	M	C+
33608	Repair anomaly w/conduit	31.09	NA	16.38	4.17	NA	51.64	$1,869.33	090	M	C+
33610	Repair by enlargement	30.61	NA	18.89	4.02	NA	53.52	$1,937.38	090	M	C+
33611	Repair double ventricle	34.00	NA	19.08	3.28	NA	56.36	$2,040.19	090	M	C+
33612	Repair double ventricle	35.00	NA	20.17	4.44	NA	59.61	$2,157.83	090	M	C+
33615	Repair, modified fontan	34.00	NA	19.33	3.15	NA	56.48	$2,044.53	090	M	C+
33617	Repair single ventricle	37.00	NA	21.25	4.09	NA	62.34	$2,256.66	090	M	C+
33619	Repair single ventricle	45.00	NA	26.49	4.71	NA	76.20	$2,758.38	090	M	C+
33641	Repair heart septum defect	21.39	NA	11.82	2.67	NA	35.88	$1,298.83	090	M	C+
33645	Revision of heart veins	24.82	NA	13.92	3.27	NA	42.01	$1,520.73	090	M	C+
33647	Repair heart septum defects	28.73	NA	17.08	3.37	NA	49.18	$1,780.28	090	M	C+
33660	Repair of heart defects	30.00	NA	17.09	2.82	NA	49.91	$1,806.70	090	M	C+
33665	Repair of heart defects	28.60	NA	16.87	3.81	NA	49.28	$1,783.90	090	M	C+
33670	Repair of heart chambers	35.00	NA	16.68	2.18	NA	53.86	$1,949.69	090	M	C+
33681	Repair heart septum defect	30.61	NA	17.83	3.53	NA	51.97	$1,881.27	090	M	C+
33684	Repair heart septum defect	29.65	NA	17.82	3.77	NA	51.24	$1,854.85	090	M	C+

*M = multiple surgery adjustment applies
Me = multiple endoscopy rules may apply
B = bilateral surgery adjustment applies
A = assistant-at-surgery restriction

A+ = assistant-at-surgery restriction unless medical necessity established with documentation
C = cosurgeons payable
C+ = cosurgeons payable if medical necessity established with documentation

T = team surgeons permitted
T+ = team surgeons payable if medical necessity established with documentation
$ = indicates services that are not covered by Medicare.

211   CPT five-digit codes, two-digit numeric modifiers, and descriptions only are © 2001 American Medical Association

Medicare RBRVS: The Physicians' Guide

Relative value units

CPT Code and Modifier	Description	Work RVU	Non Facility Practice Expense RVU	Facility Practice Expense RVU	PLI RVU	Total Non Facility RVUs	Medicare Payment Non Facility	Total Facility RVUs	Medicare Payment Facility	Global Period	Payment Policy Indicators*
33688	Repair heart septum defect	30.62	NA	16.70	3.89	NA	NA	51.21	$1,853.76	090	M C+
33690	Reinforce pulmonary artery	19.55	NA	13.55	2.56	NA	NA	35.66	$1,290.86	090	M C+
33692	Repair of heart defects	30.75	NA	17.52	3.77	NA	NA	52.04	$1,883.81	090	M C+
33694	Repair of heart defects	34.00	NA	17.82	4.27	NA	NA	56.09	$2,030.41	090	M C+
33697	Repair of heart defects	36.00	NA	18.62	4.54	NA	NA	59.16	$2,141.54	090	M C+
33702	Repair of heart defects	26.54	NA	16.53	3.45	NA	NA	46.52	$1,683.99	090	M C+
33710	Repair of heart defects	29.71	NA	16.82	3.85	NA	NA	50.38	$1,823.72	090	M
33720	Repair of heart defect	26.56	NA	16.51	3.21	NA	NA	46.28	$1,675.30	090	M C+
33722	Repair of heart defect	28.41	NA	17.05	3.80	NA	NA	49.26	$1,783.17	090	M C+
33730	Repair heart-vein defect(s)	34.25	NA	18.35	2.85	NA	NA	55.45	$2,007.25	090	M C+
33732	Repair heart-vein defect	28.16	NA	17.95	2.78	NA	NA	48.89	$1,769.78	090	M
33735	Revision of heart chamber	21.39	NA	13.00	1.12	NA	NA	35.51	$1,285.43	090	M C+
33736	Revision of heart chamber	23.52	NA	14.06	2.70	NA	NA	40.28	$1,458.10	090	M C+
33737	Revision of heart chamber	21.76	NA	15.22	2.93	NA	NA	39.91	$1,444.71	090	M C+
33750	Major vessel shunt	21.41	NA	12.83	1.74	NA	NA	35.98	$1,302.45	090	M C+
33755	Major vessel shunt	21.79	NA	12.94	2.93	NA	NA	37.66	$1,363.26	090	M C+
33762	Major vessel shunt	21.79	NA	13.32	1.59	NA	NA	36.70	$1,328.51	090	M C+
33764	Major vessel shunt & graft	21.79	NA	14.22	1.93	NA	NA	37.94	$1,373.40	090	M C+
33766	Major vessel shunt	22.76	NA	15.16	3.04	NA	NA	40.96	$1,482.72	090	M C+
33767	Major vessel shunt	24.50	NA	14.92	3.14	NA	NA	42.56	$1,540.64	090	M C+
33770	Repair great vessels defect	37.00	NA	19.01	4.49	NA	NA	60.50	$2,190.05	090	M C+
33771	Repair great vessels defect	34.65	NA	18.08	4.67	NA	NA	57.40	$2,077.83	090	M C+
33774	Repair great vessels defect	30.98	NA	16.61	4.18	NA	NA	51.77	$1,874.03	090	M C+
33775	Repair great vessels defect	32.20	NA	17.10	4.34	NA	NA	53.64	$1,941.73	090	M
33776	Repair great vessels defect	34.04	NA	17.83	4.58	NA	NA	56.45	$2,043.44	090	M C+
33777	Repair great vessels defect	33.46	NA	17.60	4.51	NA	NA	55.57	$2,011.59	090	M
33778	Repair great vessels defect	40.00	NA	20.21	4.83	NA	NA	65.04	$2,354.40	090	M C+

Code	Description								
33779	Repair great vessels defect	36.21	NA	17.93	2.40	NA	56.54	$2,046.70	090	M	C+
33780	Repair great vessels defect	41.75	NA	20.98	5.21	NA	67.94	$2,459.37	090	M	C+
33781	Repair great vessels defect	36.45	NA	18.80	4.91	NA	60.16	$2,177.74	090	M	C+
33786	Repair arterial trunk	39.00	NA	19.81	4.69	NA	63.50	$2,298.65	090	M	C+
33788	Revision of pulmonary artery	26.62	NA	14.87	3.32	NA	44.81	$1,622.09	090	M	C+
33800	Aortic suspension	16.24	NA	13.12	1.11	NA	30.47	$1,102.99	090	M	C
33802	Repair vessel defect	17.66	NA	12.22	1.56	NA	31.44	$1,138.10	090	M	C+
33803	Repair vessel defect	19.60	NA	13.53	2.63	NA	35.76	$1,294.48	090	M	C+
33813	Repair septal defect	20.65	NA	14.12	2.78	NA	37.55	$1,359.28	090	M	C+
33814	Repair septal defect	25.77	NA	15.61	2.52	NA	43.90	$1,589.14	090	M	C+
33820	Revise major vessel	16.29	NA	10.95	2.10	NA	29.34	$1,062.08	090	M	C+
33822	Revise major vessel	17.32	NA	11.16	2.33	NA	30.81	$1,115.30	090	M	
33824	Revise major vessel	19.52	NA	11.97	2.61	NA	34.10	$1,234.39	090	M	C+
33840	Remove aorta constriction	20.63	NA	14.11	2.36	NA	37.10	$1,342.99	090	M	C+
33845	Remove aorta constriction	22.12	NA	14.85	2.90	NA	39.87	$1,443.26	090	M	C+
33851	Remove aorta constriction	21.27	NA	12.98	2.86	NA	37.11	$1,343.35	090	M	C+
33852	Repair septal defect	23.71	NA	14.14	3.19	NA	41.04	$1,485.62	090	M	
33853	Repair septal defect	31.72	NA	18.25	4.23	NA	54.20	$1,962.00	090	M	C+
33860	Ascending aortic graft	38.00	NA	18.74	4.30	NA	61.04	$2,209.60	090	M	C+
33861	Ascending aortic graft	42.00	NA	20.15	4.24	NA	66.39	$2,403.26	090	M	C+
33863	Ascending aortic graft	45.00	NA	21.10	4.60	NA	70.70	$2,559.28	090	M	C+
33870	Transverse aortic arch graft	44.00	NA	20.69	5.09	NA	69.78	$2,525.98	090	M	C+
33875	Thoracic aortic graft	33.06	NA	17.01	4.08	NA	54.15	$1,960.19	090	M	C+
33877	Thoracoabdominal graft	42.60	NA	19.96	5.07	NA	67.63	$2,448.15	090	M	C+
33910	Remove lung artery emboli	24.59	NA	14.16	3.06	NA	41.81	$1,513.49	090	M	C+
33915	Remove lung artery emboli	21.02	NA	12.31	1.20	NA	34.53	$1,249.96	090	M	C+
33916	Surgery of great vessel	25.83	NA	15.49	3.04	NA	44.36	$1,605.80	090	M	C+
33917	Repair pulmonary artery	24.50	NA	15.36	3.17	NA	43.03	$1,557.65	090	M	C+

* **M** = multiple surgery adjustment applies
Me = multiple endoscopy rules may apply
B = bilateral surgery adjustment applies
A = assistant-at-surgery restriction

A+ = assistant-at-surgery restriction unless medical necessity established with documentation
C = cosurgeons payable
C+ = cosurgeons payable if medical necessity established with documentation

T = team surgeons permitted
T+ = team surgeons payable if medical necessity established with documentation
$ = indicates services that are not covered by Medicare.

213 CPT five-digit codes, two-digit numeric modifiers, and descriptions only are © 2001 American Medical Association

Medicare RBRVS: The Physicians' Guide

Relative value units

CPT Code and Modifier	Description	Work RVU	Non Facility Practice Expense RVU	Facility Practice Expense RVU	PLI RVU	Total Non Facility RVUs	Medicare Payment Non Facility	Total Facility RVUs	Medicare Payment Facility	Global Period	Payment Policy Indicators*		
33918	Repair pulmonary atresia	26.45	NA	14.80	3.42	NA	NA	44.67	$1,617.02	090	M	C+	
33919	Repair pulmonary atresia	40.00	NA	21.02	3.48	NA	NA	64.50	$2,334.85	090	M	C+	
33920	Repair pulmonary atresia	31.95	NA	17.28	3.61	NA	NA	52.84	$1,912.77	090	M	C+	
33922	Transect pulmonary artery	23.52	NA	13.79	2.30	NA	NA	39.61	$1,433.85	090	M	C+	
33924	Remove pulmonary shunt	5.50	NA	2.05	0.74	NA	NA	8.29	$300.09	ZZZ	M	C+	
33935	Transplantation, heart/lung	60.96	NA	27.93	8.15	NA	NA	97.04	$3,512.77	090	M	C+	T
33945	Transplantation of heart	42.10	NA	21.67	5.42	NA	NA	69.19	$2,504.62	090	M	C+	T
33960	External circulation assist	19.36	NA	6.06	2.14	NA	NA	27.56	$997.65	000	M	C+	
33961	External circulation assist	10.93	NA	3.79	1.47	NA	NA	16.19	$586.07	ZZZ	M	C+	
33967	Insert ia percut device	4.85	2.01	1.96	0.27	7.13	$258.10	7.08	$256.29	000	M	A+	
33968	Remove aortic assist device	0.64	NA	0.24	0.07	NA	NA	0.95	$34.39	000	M	A	
33970	Aortic circulation assist	6.75	NA	2.37	0.70	NA	NA	9.82	$355.48	000	M	C+	
33971	Aortic circulation assist	9.69	NA	7.82	0.97	NA	NA	18.48	$668.96	090	M	A	
33973	Insert balloon device	9.76	NA	3.44	1.01	NA	NA	14.21	$514.39	000	M	C+	
33974	Remove intra-aortic balloon	14.41	NA	10.69	1.48	NA	NA	26.58	$962.17	090	M	A	
33975	Implant ventricular device	21.00	NA	7.04	1.72	NA	NA	29.76	$1,077.29	XXX	M		
33976	Implant ventricular device	23.00	NA	7.78	2.82	NA	NA	33.60	$1,216.29	XXX	M		
33977	Remove ventricular device	19.29	NA	10.46	2.44	NA	NA	32.19	$1,165.25	090	M		
33978	Remove ventricular device	21.73	NA	11.27	2.66	NA	NA	35.66	$1,290.86	090	M		
33979	Insert intracorporeal device	0.00	0.00	0.00	0.00	0.00	$0.00	0.00	$0.00	XXX	M		
33980	Remove intracorporeal device	0.00	0.00	0.00	0.00	0.00	$0.00	0.00	$0.00	090	M		
33999	Cardiac surgery procedure	0.00	0.00	0.00	0.00	0.00	$0.00	0.00	$0.00	YYY	M	C+	T+
34001	Removal of artery clot	12.91	NA	5.97	1.46	NA	NA	20.34	$736.29	090	M	C+	B
34051	Removal of artery clot	15.21	NA	7.07	1.90	NA	NA	24.18	$875.30	090	M	C+	B
34101	Removal of artery clot	10.00	NA	4.84	1.11	NA	NA	15.95	$577.38	090	M	C+	B
34111	Removal of arm artery clot	10.00	NA	4.88	0.85	NA	NA	15.73	$569.41	090	M	C+	B
34151	Removal of artery clot	25.00	NA	10.54	1.84	NA	NA	37.38	$1,353.13	090	M	C+	B

Code	Description										
34201	Removal of artery clot	10.03	NA	5.12	1.02	NA	16.17	$585.34	090	M	B		C+
34203	Removal of leg artery clot	16.50	NA	7.65	1.37	NA	25.52	$923.80	090	M	B		C+
34401	Removal of vein clot	25.00	NA	10.47	1.20	NA	36.67	$1,327.42	090	M	B		C+
34421	Removal of vein clot	12.00	NA	6.01	0.95	NA	18.96	$686.34	090	M	B		C+
34451	Removal of vein clot	27.00	NA	11.08	1.59	NA	39.67	$1,436.02	090	M	B		C+
34471	Removal of vein clot	10.18	NA	5.18	0.90	NA	16.26	$588.60	090	M	B	A	C+
34490	Removal of vein clot	9.86	NA	6.26	0.73	NA	16.85	$609.96	090	M	B	A	
34501	Repair valve, femoral vein	16.00	NA	8.98	1.37	NA	26.35	$953.85	090	M	B		C+
34502	Reconstruct vena cava	26.95	NA	11.34	2.99	NA	41.28	$1,494.30	090	M			
34510	Transposition of vein valve	18.95	NA	10.23	1.60	NA	30.78	$1,114.21	090	M	B		C+
34520	Cross-over vein graft	17.95	NA	9.59	1.41	NA	28.95	$1,047.97	090	M	B		C+
34530	Leg vein fusion	16.64	NA	8.48	2.06	NA	27.18	$983.89	090	M	B		C+
34800	Endovasc abdo repair w/tube	20.75	NA	9.79	1.49	NA	32.03	$1,159.46	090	M		A+	C
34802	Endovasc abdo repr w/device	23.00	NA	10.69	1.65	NA	35.34	$1,279.28	090	M	B	A+	C
34804	Endovasc abdo repr w/device	23.00	NA	10.69	1.65	NA	35.34	$1,279.28	090	M		A+	C
34808	Endovasc abdo occlud device	4.13	NA	1.65	0.29	NA	6.07	$219.73	ZZZ			A+	C
34812	Xpose for endoprosth, aortic	6.75	NA	2.69	0.49	NA	9.93	$359.46	000	M	B	A+	C
34813	Xpose for endoprosth, femorl	4.80	NA	1.92	0.34	NA	7.06	$255.57	ZZZ			A+	C
34820	Xpose for endoprosth, iliac	9.75	NA	3.89	0.70	NA	14.34	$519.10	000	M	B	A+	C
34825	Endovasc extend prosth, init	12.00	NA	6.30	0.86	NA	19.16	$693.58	090	M		A+	C
34826	Endovasc exten prosth, addl	4.13	NA	1.65	0.29	NA	6.07	$219.73	ZZZ			A+	C
34830	Open aortic tube prosth repr	32.59	NA	14.89	2.34	NA	49.82	$1,803.44	090	M		A+	C
34831	Open aortoiliac prosth repr	35.34	NA	15.99	2.53	NA	53.86	$1,949.69	090	M	B	A+	C
34832	Open aortofemor prosth repr	35.34	NA	15.99	2.53	NA	53.86	$1,949.69	090	M		A+	C
35001	Repair defect of artery	19.64	NA	8.41	2.44	NA	30.49	$1,103.71	090	M	B		C+
35002	Repair artery rupture, neck	21.00	NA	9.12	1.82	NA	31.94	$1,156.20	090	M	B		C+
35005	Repair defect of artery	18.12	NA	8.04	1.35	NA	27.51	$995.84	090	M	B		C+
35011	Repair defect of artery	18.00	NA	7.59	1.30	NA	26.89	$973.40	090	M	B		C+

* **M** = multiple surgery adjustment applies
   Me = multiple endoscopy rules may apply
   B = bilateral surgery adjustment applies
   A = assistant-at-surgery restriction

A+ = assistant-at-surgery restriction unless medical necessity established with documentation
C = cosurgeons payable
C+ = cosurgeons payable if medical necessity established with documentation

T = team surgeons permitted
T+ = team surgeons payable if medical necessity established with documentation
$ = indicates services that are not covered by Medicare.

CPT five-digit codes, two-digit numeric modifiers, and descriptions only are © 2001 American Medical Association

Medicare RBRVS: The Physicians' Guide

Relative value units

CPT Code and Modifier	Description	Work RVU	Non Facility Practice Expense RVU	Facility Practice Expense RVU	PLI RVU	Total Non Facility RVUs	Medicare Payment Non Facility	Total Facility RVUs	Medicare Payment Facility	Global Period	Payment Policy Indicators*
35013	Repair artery rupture, arm	22.00	NA	8.98	1.91	NA	NA	32.89	$1,190.59	090	M B C+
35021	Repair defect of artery	19.65	NA	8.64	1.93	NA	NA	30.22	$1,093.94	090	M B C+
35022	Repair artery rupture, chest	23.18	NA	9.57	1.99	NA	NA	34.74	$1,257.56	090	M B C+
35045	Repair defect of arm artery	17.57	NA	7.99	1.25	NA	NA	26.81	$970.50	090	M B C+
35081	Repair defect of artery	28.01	NA	11.69	3.20	NA	NA	42.90	$1,552.95	090	M C+
35082	Repair artery rupture, aorta	38.50	NA	15.08	4.07	NA	NA	57.65	$2,086.88	090	M C+
35091	Repair defect of artery	35.40	NA	14.22	4.09	NA	NA	53.71	$1,944.26	090	M B C+
35092	Repair artery rupture, aorta	45.00	NA	17.35	4.31	NA	NA	66.66	$2,413.04	090	M B C+
35102	Repair defect of artery	30.76	NA	12.67	3.44	NA	NA	46.87	$1,696.66	090	M B C+
35103	Repair artery rupture, groin	40.50	NA	15.81	3.79	NA	NA	60.10	$2,175.57	090	M B C+
35111	Repair defect of artery	25.00	NA	10.43	1.81	NA	NA	37.24	$1,348.06	090	M B C+
35112	Repair artery rupture, spleen	30.00	NA	12.06	1.95	NA	NA	44.01	$1,593.13	090	M B C+
35121	Repair defect of artery	30.00	NA	12.39	2.93	NA	NA	45.32	$1,640.55	090	M B
35122	Repair artery rupture, belly	35.00	NA	13.73	3.54	NA	NA	52.27	$1,892.13	090	M B C+
35131	Repair defect of artery	25.00	NA	10.64	2.11	NA	NA	37.75	$1,366.52	090	M B C+
35132	Repair artery rupture, groin	30.00	NA	12.14	2.48	NA	NA	44.62	$1,615.21	090	M B C+
35141	Repair defect of artery	20.00	NA	8.66	1.65	NA	NA	30.31	$1,097.20	090	M B C+
35142	Repair artery rupture, thigh	23.30	NA	9.76	1.75	NA	NA	34.81	$1,260.09	090	M B C+
35151	Repair defect of artery	22.64	NA	9.72	1.93	NA	NA	34.29	$1,241.27	090	M B C+
35152	Repair artery rupture, knee	25.62	NA	10.50	1.93	NA	NA	38.05	$1,377.38	090	M B C+
35161	Repair defect of artery	18.76	NA	8.96	2.21	NA	NA	29.93	$1,083.44	090	M B C+
35162	Repair artery rupture	19.78	NA	9.05	2.21	NA	NA	31.04	$1,123.62	090	M B C+
35180	Repair blood vessel lesion	13.62	NA	6.49	1.44	NA	NA	21.55	$780.09	090	M C+
35182	Repair blood vessel lesion	30.00	NA	12.39	1.88	NA	NA	44.27	$1,602.54	090	M C+
35184	Repair blood vessel lesion	18.00	NA	7.92	1.34	NA	NA	27.26	$986.79	090	M C+
35188	Repair blood vessel lesion	14.28	NA	6.70	1.53	NA	NA	22.51	$814.84	090	M C+
35189	Repair blood vessel lesion	28.00	NA	11.71	2.12	NA	NA	41.83	$1,514.21	090	M C+

Code	Description	Col3	Col4	Col5	Col6	Col7	Fee	Global	M1	M2	M3
35190	Repair blood vessel lesion	12.75	NA	6.03	1.33	NA	20.11	$727.97	090	M	C+
35201	Repair blood vessel lesion	16.14	NA	7.18	1.17	NA	24.49	$886.52	090	M B	C+
35206	Repair blood vessel lesion	13.25	NA	7.60	1.04	NA	21.89	$792.40	090	M B	C+
35207	Repair blood vessel lesion	10.15	NA	9.91	1.15	NA	21.21	$767.79	090	M B A	C+
35211	Repair blood vessel lesion	22.12	NA	13.55	2.83	NA	38.50	$1,393.67	090	M B	C+
35216	Repair blood vessel lesion	18.75	NA	11.83	2.17	NA	32.75	$1,185.52	090	M B	C+
35221	Repair blood vessel lesion	24.39	NA	10.31	1.79	NA	36.49	$1,320.91	090	M B	C+
35226	Repair blood vessel lesion	14.50	NA	8.54	0.84	NA	23.88	$864.44	090	M B	C+
35231	Repair blood vessel lesion	20.00	NA	9.45	1.32	NA	30.77	$1,113.85	090	M B	C+
35236	Repair blood vessel lesion	17.11	NA	8.97	1.19	NA	27.27	$987.15	090	M B	C+
35241	Repair blood vessel lesion	23.12	NA	14.09	2.90	NA	40.11	$1,451.95	090	M B	C+
35246	Repair blood vessel lesion	26.45	NA	14.32	2.22	NA	42.99	$1,556.20	090	M B	C+
35251	Repair blood vessel lesion	30.20	NA	12.39	1.87	NA	44.46	$1,609.42	090	M B	C+
35256	Repair blood vessel lesion	18.36	NA	9.63	1.32	NA	29.31	$1,061.00	090	M B	C+
35261	Repair blood vessel lesion	17.80	NA	7.56	1.34	NA	26.70	$966.52	090	M B	C+
35266	Repair blood vessel lesion	14.91	NA	8.12	1.16	NA	24.19	$875.66	090	M B	C+
35271	Repair blood vessel lesion	22.12	NA	13.43	2.77	NA	38.32	$1,387.15	090	M B	C+
35276	Repair blood vessel lesion	24.25	NA	13.56	2.37	NA	40.18	$1,454.48	090	M B	C+
35281	Repair blood vessel lesion	28.00	NA	11.66	1.82	NA	41.48	$1,501.54	090	M B	C+
35286	Repair blood vessel lesion	16.16	NA	8.88	1.36	NA	26.40	$955.66	090	M B	C+
35301	Rechanneling of artery	18.70	NA	8.39	2.23	NA	29.32	$1,061.36	090	M B	C+
35311	Rechanneling of artery	27.00	NA	11.10	2.75	NA	40.85	$1,478.74	090	M B	C+
35321	Rechanneling of artery	16.00	NA	6.87	1.36	NA	24.23	$877.11	090	M B	C+
35331	Rechanneling of artery	26.20	NA	11.11	2.71	NA	40.02	$1,448.69	090	M B	C+
35341	Rechanneling of artery	25.11	NA	10.70	2.87	NA	38.68	$1,400.19	090	M B	C+
35351	Rechanneling of artery	23.00	NA	9.84	2.29	NA	35.13	$1,271.68	090	M B	C+
35355	Rechanneling of artery	18.50	NA	8.33	1.80	NA	28.63	$1,036.38	090	M B	C+
35361	Rechanneling of artery	28.20	NA	11.60	2.66	NA	42.46	$1,537.02	090	M B	C+

* **M** = multiple surgery adjustment applies
Me = multiple endoscopy rules may apply
B = bilateral surgery adjustment applies
A = assistant-at-surgery restriction

A+ = assistant-at-surgery restriction unless medical necessity established with documentation
C = cosurgeons payable
C+ = cosurgeons payable if medical necessity established with documentation

T = team surgeons permitted
T+ = team surgeons payable if medical necessity established with documentation
§ = indicates services that are not covered by Medicare.

217 CPT five-digit codes, two-digit numeric modifiers, and descriptions only are © 2001 American Medical Association

Medicare RBRVS: The Physicians' Guide

Relative value units

CPT Code and Modifier	Description	Work RVU	Non Facility Practice Expense RVU	Facility Practice Expense RVU	PLI RVU	Total Non Facility RVUs	Medicare Payment Non Facility	Total Facility RVUs	Medicare Payment Facility	Global Period	Payment Policy Indicators*
35363	Rechanneling of artery	30.20	NA	12.54	2.77	NA	NA	45.51	$1,647.43	090	M B C+
35371	Rechanneling of artery	14.72	NA	6.75	1.32	NA	NA	22.79	$824.98	090	M B C+
35372	Rechanneling of artery	18.00	NA	7.91	1.53	NA	NA	27.44	$993.31	090	M B C+
35381	Rechanneling of artery	15.81	NA	7.35	1.80	NA	NA	24.96	$903.53	090	M B C+
35390	Reoperation, carotid add-on	3.19	NA	1.11	0.38	NA	NA	4.68	$169.41	ZZZ	M B C+
35400	Angioscopy	3.00	NA	1.05	0.34	NA	NA	4.39	$158.91	ZZZ	A+ C+
35450	Repair arterial blockage	10.07	NA	4.22	0.84	NA	NA	15.13	$547.69	000	M B C+
35452	Repair arterial blockage	6.91	NA	3.11	0.76	NA	NA	10.78	$390.23	000	M B C+
35454	Repair arterial blockage	6.04	NA	2.83	0.67	NA	NA	9.54	$345.34	000	M B C+
35456	Repair arterial blockage	7.35	NA	3.27	0.82	NA	NA	11.44	$414.12	000	M B C+
35458	Repair arterial blockage	9.49	NA	4.03	1.09	NA	NA	14.61	$528.87	000	M B C+
35459	Repair arterial blockage	8.63	NA	3.69	0.96	NA	NA	13.28	$480.73	000	M B C+
35460	Repair venous blockage	6.04	NA	2.70	0.66	NA	NA	9.40	$340.27	000	M B A C+
35470	Repair arterial blockage	8.63	NA	3.98	0.50	NA	NA	13.11	$474.57	000	M B A
35471	Repair arterial blockage	10.07	NA	4.67	0.50	NA	NA	15.24	$551.68	000	M B A
35472	Repair arterial blockage	6.91	NA	3.32	0.39	NA	NA	10.62	$384.44	000	M B A+
35473	Repair arterial blockage	6.04	NA	3.01	0.34	NA	NA	9.39	$339.91	000	M B A C+
35474	Repair arterial blockage	7.36	NA	3.52	0.40	NA	NA	11.28	$408.33	000	M B A
35475	Repair arterial blockage	9.49	NA	4.23	0.47	NA	NA	14.19	$513.67	000	M B A
35476	Repair venous blockage	6.04	NA	2.94	0.27	NA	NA	9.25	$334.84	000	M B A
35480	Atherectomy, open	11.08	NA	4.58	1.13	NA	NA	16.79	$607.78	000	M C
35481	Atherectomy, open	7.61	NA	3.54	0.84	NA	NA	11.99	$434.03	000	M C
35482	Atherectomy, open	6.65	NA	3.16	0.75	NA	NA	10.56	$382.26	000	M C
35483	Atherectomy, open	8.10	NA	3.52	0.81	NA	NA	12.43	$449.96	000	M C
35484	Atherectomy, open	10.44	NA	4.21	1.13	NA	NA	15.78	$571.22	000	M C
35485	Atherectomy, open	9.49	NA	4.05	1.06	NA	NA	14.60	$528.51	000	M C
35490	Atherectomy, percutaneous	11.08	NA	4.83	0.55	NA	NA	16.46	$595.84	000	M

Code	Description										
35491	Atherectomy, percutaneous	7.61	NA	3.59	0.49	NA	11.69	$423.17	000	M	
35492	Atherectomy, percutaneous	6.65	NA	3.22	0.43	NA	10.30	$372.85	000	M	
35493	Atherectomy, percutaneous	8.10	NA	3.90	0.47	NA	12.47	$451.40	000	M	A
35494	Atherectomy, percutaneous	10.44	NA	4.57	0.48	NA	15.49	$560.73	000	M	A
35495	Atherectomy, percutaneous	9.49	NA	4.52	0.51	NA	14.52	$525.61	000	M	A+
35500	Harvest vein for bypass	6.45	NA	2.25	0.63	NA	9.33	$337.74	ZZZ	M	B	C+
35501	Artery bypass graft	19.19	NA	8.14	2.33	NA	29.66	$1,073.67	090	M	B	C+
35506	Artery bypass graft	19.67	NA	8.32	2.33	NA	30.32	$1,097.56	090	M	B	C+
35507	Artery bypass graft	19.67	NA	8.29	2.27	NA	30.23	$1,094.30	090	M	B	C+
35508	Artery bypass graft	18.65	NA	7.91	2.34	NA	28.90	$1,046.16	090	M	B	C+
35509	Artery bypass graft	18.07	NA	7.70	2.12	NA	27.89	$1,009.60	090	M	B	C+
35511	Artery bypass graft	21.20	NA	8.80	1.74	NA	31.74	$1,148.96	090	M	B	C+
35515	Artery bypass graft	18.65	NA	7.80	2.26	NA	28.71	$1,039.28	090	M	B	C+
35516	Artery bypass graft	16.32	NA	4.94	1.88	NA	23.14	$837.65	090	M	B	C+
35518	Artery bypass graft	21.20	NA	8.80	1.78	NA	31.78	$1,150.41	090	M	B	C+
35521	Artery bypass graft	22.20	NA	9.53	1.82	NA	33.55	$1,214.48	090	M	B	C+
35526	Artery bypass graft	29.95	NA	12.19	2.18	NA	44.32	$1,604.35	090	M	B	C+
35531	Artery bypass graft	36.20	NA	14.53	2.91	NA	53.64	$1,941.73	090	M	B	C+
35533	Artery bypass graft	28.00	NA	11.74	2.35	NA	42.09	$1,523.62	090	M	B	C+
35536	Artery bypass graft	31.70	NA	12.85	2.62	NA	47.17	$1,707.52	090	M	B	C+
35541	Artery bypass graft	25.80	NA	10.98	2.74	NA	39.52	$1,430.59	090	M	B	C+
35546	Artery bypass graft	25.54	NA	10.75	2.84	NA	39.13	$1,416.47	090	M		C+
35548	Artery bypass graft	21.57	NA	9.45	2.45	NA	33.47	$1,211.59	090	M	B	C+
35549	Artery bypass graft	23.35	NA	9.88	2.77	NA	36.00	$1,303.17	090	M		C+
35551	Artery bypass graft	26.67	NA	11.20	3.19	NA	41.06	$1,486.34	090	M	B	C+
35556	Artery bypass graft	21.76	NA	9.45	2.48	NA	33.69	$1,219.55	090	M	B	C+
35558	Artery bypass graft	21.20	NA	9.11	1.58	NA	31.89	$1,154.39	090	M	B	C+
35560	Artery bypass graft	32.00	NA	13.12	2.73	NA	47.85	$1,732.13	090	M	B	C+

* **M** = multiple surgery adjustment applies
Me = multiple endoscopy rules may apply
B = bilateral surgery adjustment applies
A = assistant-at-surgery restriction

A+ = assistant-at-surgery restriction unless medical necessity established with documentation
C = cosurgeons payable
C+ = cosurgeons payable if medical necessity established with documentation

T = team surgeons permitted
T+ = team surgeons payable if medical necessity established with documentation
S = indicates services that are not covered by Medicare.

219 CPT five-digit codes, two-digit numeric modifiers, and descriptions only are © 2001 American Medical Association

Medicare RBRVS: The Physicians' Guide

Relative value units

CPT Code and Modifier	Description	Work RVU	Non Facility Practice Expense RVU	Facility Practice Expense RVU	PLI RVU	Total Non Facility RVUs	Medicare Payment Non Facility	Total Facility RVUs	Medicare Payment Facility	Global Period	Payment Policy Indicators*		
35563	Artery bypass graft	24.20	NA	10.42	1.68	NA	NA	36.30	$1,314.03	090	M	B	C+
35565	Artery bypass graft	23.20	NA	9.99	1.71	NA	NA	34.90	$1,263.35	090	M	B	C+
35566	Artery bypass graft	26.92	NA	11.77	3.02	NA	NA	41.71	$1,509.87	090	M	B	C+
35571	Artery bypass graft	24.06	NA	12.13	2.14	NA	NA	38.33	$1,387.52	090	M	B	C+
35582	Vein bypass graft	27.13	NA	11.35	3.11	NA	NA	41.59	$1,505.52	090	M	B	C+
35583	Vein bypass graft	22.37	NA	10.62	2.53	NA	NA	35.52	$1,285.80	090	M	B	C+
35585	Vein bypass graft	28.39	NA	14.53	3.21	NA	NA	46.13	$1,669.87	090	M	B	C+
35587	Vein bypass graft	24.75	NA	12.79	2.17	NA	NA	39.71	$1,437.47	090	M	B	C+
35600	Harvest artery for cabg	4.95	NA	1.98	0.60	NA	NA	7.53	$272.58	ZZZ		B	C+
35601	Artery bypass graft	17.50	NA	7.49	2.08	NA	NA	27.07	$979.91	090	M	B	C+
35606	Artery bypass graft	18.71	NA	7.93	2.17	NA	NA	28.81	$1,042.90	090	M	B	C+
35612	Artery bypass graft	15.76	NA	6.70	1.72	NA	NA	24.18	$875.30	090	M	B	C+
35616	Artery bypass graft	15.70	NA	7.05	1.84	NA	NA	24.59	$890.14	090	M	B	C+
35621	Artery bypass graft	20.00	NA	8.79	1.68	NA	NA	30.47	$1,102.99	090	M	B	C+
35623	Bypass graft, not vein	24.00	NA	10.22	1.91	NA	NA	36.13	$1,307.88	090	M	B	C+
35626	Artery bypass graft	27.75	NA	11.08	2.89	NA	NA	41.72	$1,510.23	090	M	B	C+
35631	Artery bypass graft	34.00	NA	13.74	2.83	NA	NA	50.57	$1,830.59	090	M	B	C+
35636	Artery bypass graft	29.50	NA	12.26	2.37	NA	NA	44.13	$1,597.47	090	M	B	C+
35641	Artery bypass graft	24.57	NA	10.47	2.83	NA	NA	37.87	$1,370.86	090	M	B	C+
35642	Artery bypass graft	17.98	NA	7.92	1.84	NA	NA	27.74	$1,004.17	090	M	B	C+
35645	Artery bypass graft	17.47	NA	8.36	1.91	NA	NA	27.74	$1,004.17	090	M	B	C+
35646	Artery bypass graft	31.00	NA	13.26	2.98	NA	NA	47.24	$1,710.05	090	M	B	C+
35647	Artery bypass graft	28.00	NA	11.97	2.98	NA	NA	42.95	$1,554.76	090	M	B	C+
35650	Artery bypass graft	19.00	NA	7.93	1.64	NA	NA	28.57	$1,034.21	090	M	B	C+
35651	Artery bypass graft	25.04	NA	10.70	2.53	NA	NA	38.27	$1,385.34	090	M	B	C+
35654	Artery bypass graft	25.00	NA	10.60	2.10	NA	NA	37.70	$1,364.71	090	M	B	C+
35656	Artery bypass graft	19.53	NA	8.44	2.21	NA	NA	30.18	$1,092.49	090	M	B	C+

Code	Description										
35661	Artery bypass graft	19.00	NA	8.26	1.50	NA	28.76	$1,041.09	090	M	B	C+
35663	Artery bypass graft	22.00	NA	9.65	1.55	NA	33.20	$1,201.81	090	M	B	C+
35665	Artery bypass graft	21.00	NA	9.18	1.76	NA	31.94	$1,156.20	090	M	B	C+
35666	Artery bypass graft	22.19	NA	11.93	2.19	NA	36.31	$1,314.39	090	M	B	C+
35671	Artery bypass graft	19.33	NA	10.53	1.68	NA	31.54	$1,141.72	090	M	B	C+
35681	Composite bypass graft	1.60	NA	0.56	0.18	NA	2.34	$84.71	ZZZ			C+
35682	Composite bypass graft	7.20	NA	2.51	0.83	NA	10.54	$381.54	ZZZ		A+	C+
35683	Composite bypass graft	8.50	NA	2.99	0.98	NA	12.47	$451.40	ZZZ		A+	C+
35685	Bypass graft patency/patch	4.05	NA	1.50	0.41	NA	5.96	$215.75	ZZZ		B	C+
35686	Bypass graft/av fist patency	3.35	NA	1.24	0.34	NA	4.93	$178.46	ZZZ		B	C+
35691	Arterial transposition	18.05	NA	7.65	2.06	NA	27.76	$1,004.89	090	M	B	C+
35693	Arterial transposition	15.36	NA	6.66	1.80	NA	23.82	$862.26	090	M	B	C+
35694	Arterial transposition	19.16	NA	8.02	2.13	NA	29.31	$1,061.00	090	M	B	C+
35695	Arterial transposition	19.16	NA	7.92	2.19	NA	29.27	$1,059.55	090	M	B	C+
35700	Reoperation, bypass graft	3.08	NA	1.07	0.36	NA	4.51	$163.26	ZZZ		B	C+
35701	Exploration, carotid artery	8.50	NA	4.70	0.64	NA	13.84	$501.00	090	M	B	C+
35721	Exploration, femoral artery	7.18	NA	5.10	0.59	NA	12.87	$465.88	090	M	B	C+
35741	Exploration popliteal artery	8.00	NA	5.47	0.60	NA	14.07	$509.32	090	M	B	C+
35761	Exploration of artery/vein	5.37	NA	4.47	0.60	NA	10.44	$377.92	090	M	B	C+
35800	Explore neck vessels	7.02	NA	3.95	0.79	NA	11.76	$425.70	090	M		C+
35820	Explore chest vessels	12.88	NA	4.32	1.61	NA	18.81	$680.91	090	M	B	C+
35840	Explore abdominal vessels	9.77	NA	5.21	1.06	NA	16.04	$580.64	090	M	B	C+
35860	Explore limb vessels	5.55	NA	3.62	0.63	NA	9.80	$354.75	090	M	B	C+
35870	Repair vessel graft defect	22.17	NA	10.21	2.47	NA	34.85	$1,261.54	090	M	B	C+
35875	Removal of clot in graft	10.13	NA	6.63	0.97	NA	17.73	$641.81	090	M		A	C+
35876	Removal of clot in graft	17.00	NA	9.16	1.88	NA	28.04	$1,015.03	090	M		C+
35879	Revise graft w/vein	16.00	NA	7.77	1.35	NA	25.12	$909.32	090	M	B	C+
35881	Revise graft w/vein	18.00	NA	8.65	1.44	NA	28.09	$1,016.84	090	M	B	C+

* **M** = multiple surgery adjustment applies
Me = multiple endoscopy rules may apply
B = bilateral surgery adjustment applies
A = assistant-at-surgery restriction

A+ = assistant-at-surgery restriction unless medical necessity established with documentation
C = cosurgeons payable
C+ = cosurgeons payable if medical necessity established with documentation

T = team surgeons permitted
T+ = team surgeons payable if medical necessity established with documentation
§ = indicates services that are not covered by Medicare.

221 CPT five-digit codes, two-digit numeric modifiers, and descriptions only are © 2001 American Medical Association

Medicare RBRVS: The Physicians' Guide

Relative value units

CPT Code and Modifier	Description	Work RVU	Non Facility Practice Expense RVU	Facility Practice Expense RVU	PLI RVU	Total Non Facility RVUs	Medicare Payment Non Facility	Total Facility RVUs	Medicare Payment Facility	Global Period	Payment Policy Indicators*		
35901	Excision, graft, neck	8.19	NA	5.85	0.90	NA	NA	14.94	$540.82	090	M		C+
35903	Excision, graft, extremity	9.39	NA	8.20	1.03	NA	NA	18.62	$674.03	090	M		C+
35905	Excision, graft, thorax	31.25	NA	15.39	2.15	NA	NA	48.79	$1,766.16	090	M		C+
35907	Excision, graft, abdomen	35.00	NA	14.97	2.17	NA	NA	52.14	$1,887.43	090	M		C+
36000	Place needle in vein	0.18	0.65	0.05	0.01	0.84	$30.41	0.24	$8.69	XXX	M	B	A
36002	Pseudoaneurysm injection trt	1.96	2.95	1.03	0.08	4.99	$180.63	3.07	$111.13	000	M		A
36005	Injection ext venography	0.95	7.29	0.34	0.04	8.28	$299.73	1.33	$48.14	000	M		A+
36010	Place catheter in vein	2.43	NA	0.84	0.16	NA	NA	3.43	$124.16	XXX	M	B	A
36011	Place catheter in vein	3.14	NA	1.10	0.17	NA	NA	4.41	$159.64	XXX	M	B	A
36012	Place catheter in vein	3.52	NA	1.23	0.17	NA	NA	4.92	$178.10	XXX	M	B	A
36013	Place catheter in artery	2.52	NA	0.61	0.17	NA	NA	3.30	$119.46	XXX	M	B	A
36014	Place catheter in artery	3.02	NA	1.06	0.14	NA	NA	4.22	$152.76	XXX	M	B	A
36015	Place catheter in artery	3.52	NA	1.24	0.16	NA	NA	4.92	$178.10	XXX	M	B	A
36100	Establish access to artery	3.02	NA	1.16	0.18	NA	NA	4.36	$157.83	XXX	M	B	A
36120	Establish access to artery	2.01	NA	0.69	0.11	NA	NA	2.81	$101.72	XXX	M		A
36140	Establish access to artery	2.01	NA	0.69	0.12	NA	NA	2.82	$102.08	XXX	M		A
36145	Artery to vein shunt	2.01	NA	0.70	0.10	NA	NA	2.81	$101.72	XXX	M		A
36160	Establish access to aorta	2.52	NA	0.90	0.20	NA	NA	3.62	$131.04	XXX	M		A
36200	Place catheter in aorta	3.02	NA	1.09	0.15	NA	NA	4.26	$154.21	XXX	M	B	A
36215	Place catheter in artery	4.68	NA	1.68	0.22	NA	NA	6.58	$238.19	XXX	M	B	A
36216	Place catheter in artery	5.28	NA	1.89	0.24	NA	NA	7.41	$268.24	XXX	M	B	A
36217	Place catheter in artery	6.30	NA	2.29	0.32	NA	NA	8.91	$322.53	XXX	M	B	A
36218	Place catheter in artery	1.01	NA	0.37	0.05	NA	NA	1.43	$51.76	ZZZ			A
36245	Place catheter in artery	4.68	NA	1.78	0.23	NA	NA	6.69	$242.17	XXX	M	B	A
36246	Place catheter in artery	5.28	NA	1.91	0.26	NA	NA	7.45	$269.68	XXX	M	B	A
36247	Place catheter in artery	6.30	NA	2.25	0.32	NA	NA	8.87	$321.09	XXX	M	B	A
36248	Place catheter in artery	1.01	NA	0.37	0.06	NA	NA	1.44	$52.13	ZZZ			A

Code	Description										
36260	Insertion of infusion pump	9.71	NA	5.63	1.00	NA	16.34	$591.49	090	M	A
36261	Revision of infusion pump	5.45	NA	3.47	0.50	NA	9.42	$341.00	090	M	A
36262	Removal of infusion pump	4.02	NA	2.59	0.43	NA	7.04	$254.84	090	M	A
36299	Vessel injection procedure	0.00	0.00	0.00	0.00	0.00	0.00	$0.00	YYY	M	A+ C+ T+
36400	Drawing blood	0.38	0.72	0.10	0.01	1.11	0.49	$17.74	XXX	M	A
36405	Drawing blood	0.31	0.58	0.09	0.01	0.90	0.41	$14.84	XXX	M	A
36406	Drawing blood	0.18	0.94	0.06	0.01	1.13	0.25	$9.05	XXX	M	A
36410	Drawing blood	0.18	0.50	0.05	0.01	0.69	0.24	$8.69	XXX	M	A
36420	Establish access to vein	1.01	NA	0.33	0.09	NA	1.43	$51.76	XXX	M	A+
36425	Establish access to vein	0.76	3.44	0.17	0.05	4.25	0.98	$35.48	XXX	M	A
36430	Blood transfusion service	0.00	0.95	0.95	0.05	1.00	1.00	$36.20	XXX	M	A
36440	Blood transfusion service	1.03	NA	0.31	0.08	NA	1.42	$51.40	XXX	M	A+
36450	Exchange transfusion service	2.23	NA	0.71	0.16	NA	3.10	$112.22	XXX	M	A+
36455	Exchange transfusion service	2.43	NA	0.97	0.10	NA	3.50	$126.70	XXX	M	A
36460	Transfusion service, fetal	6.59	NA	2.55	0.56	NA	9.70	$351.13	XXX	M	
36468	Injection(s), spider veins	0.00	0.00	0.00	0.00	0.00	0.00	$0.00	000	M	A+
36469	Injection(s), spider veins	0.00	0.00	0.00	0.00	0.00	0.00	$0.00	000	M	A+
36470	Injection therapy of vein	1.09	2.60	0.40	0.10	3.79	1.59	$57.56	010	M	A
36471	Injection therapy of veins	1.57	2.65	0.58	0.15	4.37	2.30	$83.26	010	M	A
36481	Insertion of catheter; vein	6.99	NA	2.86	0.40	NA	10.25	$371.04	000	M	A
36488	Insertion of catheter; vein	1.35	NA	0.76	0.09	NA	2.20	$79.64	000	M	A
36489	Insertion of catheter; vein	2.50	4.70	1.08	0.08	7.28	3.66	$132.49	000	M	A
36490	Insertion of catheter; vein	1.67	NA	0.86	0.17	NA	2.70	$97.74	000		A
36491	Insertion of catheter; vein	1.43	NA	0.75	0.13	NA	2.31	$83.62	000		A
36493	Repositioning of cvc	1.21	NA	0.88	0.06	NA	2.15	$77.83	000	M	A
36500	Insertion of catheter; vein	3.52	NA	1.31	0.14	NA	4.97	$179.91	000	M	A
36510	Insertion of catheter; vein	1.09	NA	0.73	0.06	NA	1.88	$68.05	000	M	A+
36520	Plasma and/or cell exchange	1.74	NA	1.07	0.06	NA	2.87	$103.89	000	M	A

* **M** = multiple surgery adjustment applies
Me = multiple endoscopy rules may apply
B = bilateral surgery adjustment applies
A = assistant-at-surgery restriction

A+ = assistant-at-surgery restriction unless medical necessity established with documentation
C = cosurgeons payable
C+ = cosurgeons payable if medical necessity established with documentation

T = team surgeons permitted
T+ = team surgeons payable if medical necessity established with documentation
§ = indicates services that are not covered by Medicare.

223 CPT five-digit codes, two-digit numeric modifiers, and descriptions only are © 2001 American Medical Association

Medicare RBRVS: The Physicians' Guide

Relative value units

CPT Code and Modifier	Description	Work RVU	Non Facility Practice Expense RVU	Facility Practice Expense RVU	PLI RVU	Total Non Facility RVUs	Medicare Payment Non Facility	Total Facility RVUs	Medicare Payment Facility	Global Period	Payment Policy Indicators*		
36521	Apheresis w/ adsorp/reinfuse	1.74	NA	1.07	0.06	NA	NA	2.87	$103.89	000	M	A	
36522	Photopheresis	1.67	6.03	1.16	0.07	7.77	$281.27	2.90	$104.98	000	M	A	
36530	Insertion of infusion pump	6.20	NA	4.17	0.56	NA	NA	10.93	$395.66	010	M	A+	
36531	Revision of infusion pump	4.87	NA	3.32	0.44	NA	NA	8.63	$312.40	010	M	A+	
36532	Removal of infusion pump	3.30	NA	1.57	0.34	NA	NA	5.21	$188.60	010	M	A+	
36533	Insertion of access device	5.32	4.67	3.50	0.49	10.48	$379.37	9.31	$337.01	010	M	A+	
36534	Revision of access device	2.80	NA	1.55	0.19	NA	NA	4.54	$164.34	010	M	A+	
36535	Removal of access device	2.27	2.95	1.89	0.21	5.43	$196.56	4.37	$158.19	010	M	A+	
36550	Declot vascular device	0.00	0.38	0.38	0.31	0.69	$24.98	0.69	$24.98	XXX	M	A+	
36600	Withdrawal of arterial blood	0.32	0.43	0.09	0.02	0.77	$27.87	0.43	$15.57	XXX	M	A	
36620	Insertion catheter, artery	1.15	NA	0.25	0.06	NA	NA	1.46	$52.85	000	M	A	
36625	Insertion catheter, artery	2.11	NA	0.61	0.16	NA	NA	2.88	$104.25	000	M	A	
36640	Insertion catheter, artery	2.10	NA	0.75	0.18	NA	NA	3.03	$109.68	000	M	A	
36660	Insertion catheter, artery	1.40	NA	0.38	0.08	NA	NA	1.86	$67.33	000	M	A+	
36680	Insert needle, bone cavity	1.20	NA	0.66	0.08	NA	NA	1.94	$70.23	000	M	A+	
36800	Insertion of cannula	2.43	NA	1.59	0.17	NA	NA	4.19	$151.67	000	M	A	
36810	Insertion of cannula	3.97	NA	2.22	0.40	NA	NA	6.59	$238.55	000	M	A	
36815	Insertion of cannula	2.62	NA	1.28	0.26	NA	NA	4.16	$150.59	000	M	A	
36819	Av fusion/uppr arm vein	14.00	NA	6.56	1.53	NA	NA	22.09	$799.64	090	M		C+
36820	Av fusion/forearm vein	14.00	NA	6.56	1.53	NA	NA	22.09	$799.64	090	M		C+
36821	Av fusion direct any site	8.93	NA	5.03	0.97	NA	NA	14.93	$540.45	090	M		C+
36822	Insertion of cannula(s)	5.42	NA	6.81	0.63	NA	NA	12.86	$465.52	090	M	A	
36823	Insertion of cannula(s)	21.00	NA	10.63	2.18	NA	NA	33.81	$1,223.89	090	M	A	
36825	Artery-vein graft	9.84	NA	5.58	1.09	NA	NA	16.51	$597.65	090	M		C+
36830	Artery-vein graft	12.00	NA	6.14	1.32	NA	NA	19.46	$704.44	090	M		C+
36831	Open thrombect av fistula	8.00	NA	3.99	0.79	NA	NA	12.78	$462.63	090	M		C+
36832	Av fistula revision, open	10.50	NA	5.59	1.13	NA	NA	17.22	$623.35	090	M		C+

Code	Description										
36833	Av fistula revision	11.95	NA	6.11	1.29	NA	19.35	$700.45	090	M	C+
36834	Repair A-V aneurysm	9.93	NA	3.93	1.06	NA	14.92	$540.09	090	M	C+
36835	Artery to vein shunt	7.15	NA	4.50	0.80	NA	12.45	$450.68	090	M	A
36860	External cannula declotting	2.01	2.52	1.33	0.10	$167.60	3.44	$124.53	000	M	A
36861	Cannula declotting	2.52	NA	1.50	0.14	NA	4.16	$150.59	000	M	A
36870	Percut thrombect av fistula	5.16	41.63	2.45	0.23	$1,702.09	7.84	$283.80	090	M	B A C
37140	Revision of circulation	23.60	NA	10.56	1.21	NA	35.37	$1,280.37	090	M	A C+
37145	Revision of circulation	24.61	NA	12.97	2.48	NA	40.06	$1,450.14	090	M	
37160	Revision of circulation	21.60	NA	9.43	2.16	NA	33.19	$1,201.45	090	M	A C+
37180	Revision of circulation	24.61	NA	10.66	2.63	NA	37.90	$1,371.95	090	M	A C+
37181	Splice spleen/kidney veins	26.68	NA	11.02	2.67	NA	40.37	$1,461.36	090	M	A C+
37195	Thrombolytic therapy, stroke	0.00	7.65	7.65	0.38	$290.68	8.03	$290.68	XXX		A+
37200	Transcatheter biopsy	4.56	NA	1.60	0.19	NA	6.35	$229.86	000	M	A
37201	Transcatheter therapy infuse	5.00	NA	2.59	0.24	NA	7.83	$283.44	000	M	A
37202	Transcatheter therapy infuse	5.68	NA	3.33	0.38	NA	9.39	$339.91	000	M	A
37203	Transcatheter retrieval	5.03	NA	2.62	0.23	NA	7.88	$285.25	000	M	A
37204	Transcatheter occlusion	18.14	NA	6.36	0.85	NA	25.35	$917.65	000	M	A
37205	Transcatheter stent	8.28	NA	3.90	0.43	NA	12.61	$456.47	000	M	A+
37206	Transcatheter stent add-on	4.13	NA	1.54	0.22	NA	5.89	$213.21	ZZZ		A+
37207	Transcatheter stent	8.28	NA	3.61	0.89	NA	12.78	$462.63	000	M	B C
37208	Transcatheter stent add-on	4.13	NA	1.45	0.44	NA	6.02	$217.92	ZZZ		C
37209	Exchange arterial catheter	2.27	NA	0.80	0.11	NA	3.18	$115.11	000	M	A
37250	Iv us first vessel add-on	2.10	NA	0.79	0.17	NA	3.06	$110.77	ZZZ		A+ C+
37251	Iv us each add vessel add-on	1.60	NA	0.58	0.14	NA	2.32	$83.98	ZZZ		A+ C+
37565	Ligation of neck vein	10.88	NA	5.34	0.45	NA	16.67	$603.44	090	M	A+ C+
37600	Ligation of neck artery	11.25	NA	6.51	0.40	NA	18.16	$657.38	090	M	C+
37605	Ligation of neck artery	13.11	NA	6.63	0.77	NA	20.51	$742.45	090	M	A+ C+
37606	Ligation of neck artery	6.28	NA	3.85	0.79	NA	10.92	$395.30	090	M	C+

* **M** = multiple surgery adjustment applies
Me = multiple endoscopy rules may apply
B = bilateral surgery adjustment applies
A = assistant-at-surgery restriction

A+ = assistant-at-surgery restriction unless medical necessity established with documentation
C = cosurgeons payable
C+ = cosurgeons payable if medical necessity established with documentation

T = team surgeons permitted
T+ = team surgeons payable if medical necessity established with documentation
§ = indicates services that are not covered by Medicare.

225 CPT five-digit codes, two-digit numeric modifiers, and descriptions only are © 2001 American Medical Association

Medicare RBRVS: The Physicians' Guide

Relative value units

CPT Code and Modifier	Description	Work RVU	Non Facility Practice Expense RVU	Facility Practice Expense RVU	PLI RVU	Total Non Facility RVUs	Medicare Payment Non Facility	Total Facility RVUs	Medicare Payment Facility	Global Period	Payment Policy Indicators*			
37607	Ligation of a-v fistula	6.16	NA	3.71	0.67	NA	NA	10.54	$381.54	090	M		A	C+
37609	Temporal artery procedure	3.00	7.25	2.58	0.21	10.46	$378.64	5.79	$209.59	010	M		A	
37615	Ligation of neck artery	5.73	NA	3.61	0.57	NA	NA	9.91	$358.73	090	M			C+
37616	Ligation of chest artery	16.49	NA	10.54	1.93	NA	NA	28.96	$1,048.33	090	M			C+
37617	Ligation of abdomen artery	22.06	NA	9.81	1.69	NA	NA	33.56	$1,214.85	090	M			C+
37618	Ligation of extremity artery	4.84	NA	3.56	0.54	NA	NA	8.94	$323.62	090	M			C+
37620	Revision of major vein	10.56	NA	5.53	0.75	NA	NA	16.84	$609.59	090	M		A	C+
37650	Revision of major vein	7.80	NA	4.64	0.56	NA	NA	13.00	$470.59	090	M	B	A	C+
37660	Revision of major vein	21.00	NA	9.44	1.17	NA	NA	31.61	$1,144.26	090	M			C+
37700	Revise leg vein	3.73	NA	3.20	0.40	NA	NA	7.33	$265.34	090	M	B	A	
37720	Removal of leg vein	5.66	NA	3.72	0.61	NA	NA	9.99	$361.63	090	M	B	A	C+
37730	Removal of leg veins	7.33	NA	4.59	0.77	NA	NA	12.69	$459.37	090	M	B	A	C+
37735	Removal of leg veins/lesion	10.53	NA	5.94	1.17	NA	NA	17.64	$638.55	090	M	B		C+
37760	Revision of leg veins	10.47	NA	5.78	1.11	NA	NA	17.36	$628.42	090	M			C+
37780	Revision of leg vein	3.84	NA	2.89	0.41	NA	NA	7.14	$258.46	090	M	B	A	C+
37785	Revise secondary varicosity	3.84	7.18	2.91	0.41	11.43	$413.76	7.16	$259.19	090	M	B	A	
37788	Revascularization, penis	22.01	NA	14.08	1.35	NA	NA	37.44	$1,355.30	090	M			C+
37790	Penile venous occlusion	8.34	NA	6.78	0.63	NA	NA	15.75	$570.14	090	M		A+	
37799	Vascular surgery procedure	0.00	0.00	0.00	0.00	0.00	$0.00	0.00	$0.00	YYY	M		A+	T+

Surgery: Hemic and lymphatic system

38100	Removal of spleen, total	14.50	NA	6.73	1.30	NA	NA	22.53	$815.57	090	M			C+
38101	Removal of spleen, partial	15.31	NA	7.27	1.38	NA	NA	23.96	$867.33	090	M			C+
38102	Removal of spleen, total	4.80	NA	1.73	0.49	NA	NA	7.02	$254.12	ZZZ				C+
38115	Repair of ruptured spleen	15.82	NA	7.23	1.40	NA	NA	24.45	$885.07	090	M			C+
38120	Laparoscopy, splenectomy	17.00	NA	7.58	1.73	NA	NA	26.31	$952.40	090	M			C+
38129	Laparoscope proc, spleen	0.00	0.00	0.00	0.00	0.00	$0.00	0.00	$0.00	YYY	M			
38200	Injection for spleen x-ray	2.64	NA	0.93	0.12	NA	NA	3.69	$133.58	000	M		A+	

Code	Description											
38220	Bone marrow aspiration	1.08	4.64	0.44	0.03	5.75	$208.15	1.55	$56.11	XXX	M	A+
38221	Bone marrow biopsy	1.37	4.74	0.56	0.04	6.15	$222.63	1.97	$71.31	XXX	M	A+
38230	Bone marrow collection	4.54	NA	2.45	0.25	NA	NA	7.24	$262.08	010	M	A+
38231	Stem cell collection	1.50	NA	0.61	0.05	NA	NA	2.16	$78.19	000	M	A+
38240	Bone marrow/stem transplant	2.24	NA	0.88	0.08	NA	NA	3.20	$115.84	XXX	M	A+
38241	Bone marrow/stem transplant	2.24	NA	0.86	0.08	NA	NA	3.18	$115.11	XXX	M	A+
38300	Drainage, lymph node lesion	1.99	4.88	2.65	0.15	7.02	$254.12	4.79	$173.39	010	M	A
38305	Drainage, lymph node lesion	6.00	7.99	6.41	0.36	14.35	$519.46	12.77	$462.26	090	M	A
38308	Incision of lymph channels	6.45	NA	5.40	0.51	NA	NA	12.36	$447.42	090	M		C+
38380	Thoracic duct procedure	7.46	NA	7.61	0.68	NA	NA	15.75	$570.14	090	M		C+
38381	Thoracic duct procedure	12.88	NA	9.72	1.58	NA	NA	24.18	$875.30	090	M		C+
38382	Thoracic duct procedure	10.08	NA	8.81	1.08	NA	NA	19.97	$722.90	090	M		C+
38500	Biopsy/removal, lymph nodes	3.75	3.15	2.63	0.28	7.18	$259.91	6.66	$241.09	010	M	B	A
38505	Needle biopsy, lymph nodes	1.14	3.21	1.13	0.09	4.44	$160.72	2.36	$85.43	000	M	B	A
38510	Biopsy/removal, lymph nodes	6.43	NA	5.55	0.38	NA	NA	12.36	$447.42	010	M	B	A
38520	Biopsy/removal, lymph nodes	6.67	NA	5.67	0.52	NA	NA	12.86	$465.52	090	M	B	A
38525	Biopsy/removal, lymph nodes	6.07	NA	4.51	0.48	NA	NA	11.06	$400.36	090	M	B	A
38530	Biopsy/removal, lymph nodes	7.98	NA	5.78	0.63	NA	NA	14.39	$520.91	090	M	B	C+
38542	Explore deep node(s), neck	5.91	NA	6.09	0.50	NA	NA	12.50	$452.49	090	M	B	C+
38550	Removal, neck/armpit lesion	6.92	NA	5.01	0.69	NA	NA	12.62	$456.83	090	M		A+
38555	Removal, neck/armpit lesion	14.14	NA	9.47	1.46	NA	NA	25.07	$907.51	090	M		C+
38562	Removal, pelvic lymph nodes	10.49	NA	6.79	0.97	NA	NA	18.25	$660.64	090	M		C+
38564	Removal, abdomen lymph nodes	10.83	NA	6.54	1.06	NA	NA	18.43	$667.15	090	M		C+
38570	Laparoscopy, lymph node biop	9.25	NA	4.63	0.89	NA	NA	14.77	$534.66	010	Me		C
38571	Laparoscopy, lymphadenectomy	14.68	NA	6.50	0.80	NA	NA	21.98	$795.66	010	M		C
38572	Laparoscopy, lymphadenectomy	16.59	NA	7.71	1.32	NA	NA	25.62	$927.42	010	M		C
38589	Laparoscope proc, lymphatic	0.00	0.00	0.00	0.00	0.00	$0.00	0.00	$0.00	YYY	M	B	
38700	Removal of lymph nodes, neck	8.24	NA	13.61	0.60	NA	NA	22.45	$812.67	090	M	B	C+

* **M** = multiple surgery adjustment applies
Me = multiple endoscopy rules may apply
B = bilateral surgery adjustment applies
A = assistant-at-surgery restriction

A+ = assistant-at-surgery restriction unless medical necessity established with documentation
C = cosurgeons payable
C+ = cosurgeons payable if medical necessity established with documentation

T = team surgeons permitted
T+ = team surgeons payable if medical necessity established with documentation
S = indicates services that are not covered by Medicare.

227 CPT five-digit codes, two-digit numeric modifiers, and descriptions only are © 2001 American Medical Association

Medicare RBRVS: The Physicians' Guide

Relative value units

CPT Code and Modifier	Description	Work RVU	Non Facility Practice Expense RVU	Facility Practice Expense RVU	PLI RVU	Total Non Facility RVUs	Medicare Payment Non Facility	Total Facility RVUs	Medicare Payment Facility	Global Period	Payment Policy Indicators*
38720	Removal of lymph nodes, neck	13.61	NA	16.25	1.03	NA	NA	30.89	$1,118.19	090	M B C+
38724	Removal of lymph nodes, neck	14.54	NA	16.82	1.10	NA	NA	32.46	$1,175.03	090	M B C+
38740	Remove armpit lymph nodes	10.03	NA	5.89	0.69	NA	NA	16.61	$601.27	090	M C+
38745	Remove armpit lymph nodes	13.10	NA	8.47	0.90	NA	NA	22.47	$813.40	090	M C+
38746	Remove thoracic lymph nodes	4.89	NA	1.65	0.55	NA	NA	7.09	$256.65	ZZZ	C+
38747	Remove abdominal lymph nodes	4.89	NA	1.75	0.50	NA	NA	7.14	$258.46	ZZZ	C+
38760	Remove groin lymph nodes	12.95	NA	7.36	0.88	NA	NA	21.19	$767.06	090	M B C+
38765	Remove groin lymph nodes	19.98	NA	11.57	1.50	NA	NA	33.05	$1,196.38	090	M B C+
38770	Remove pelvis lymph nodes	13.23	NA	7.18	0.94	NA	NA	21.35	$772.85	090	M B C+
38780	Remove abdomen lymph nodes	16.59	NA	9.67	1.60	NA	NA	27.86	$1,008.51	090	M C+
38790	Inject for lymphatic x-ray	1.29	14.77	0.46	0.09	16.15	$584.62	1.84	$66.61	000	M B A
38792	Identify sentinel node	0.52	NA	0.19	0.04	NA	NA	0.75	$27.15	000	M B A
38794	Access thoracic lymph duct	4.45	NA	1.57	0.17	NA	NA	6.19	$224.07	090	M A+
38999	Blood/lymph system procedure	0.00	0.00	0.00	0.00	0.00	$0.00	0.00	$0.00	YYY	M C+ T+

Surgery: Mediastinum and diaphragm

CPT Code and Modifier	Description	Work RVU	Non Facility Practice Expense RVU	Facility Practice Expense RVU	PLI RVU	Total Non Facility RVUs	Medicare Payment Non Facility	Total Facility RVUs	Medicare Payment Facility	Global Period	Payment Policy Indicators*
39000	Exploration of chest	6.10	NA	7.41	0.73	NA	NA	14.24	$515.48	090	M C+
39010	Exploration of chest	11.79	NA	9.31	1.46	NA	NA	22.56	$816.65	090	M C+
39200	Removal chest lesion	13.62	NA	10.10	1.65	NA	NA	25.37	$918.37	090	M C+
39220	Removal chest lesion	17.42	NA	11.29	2.10	NA	NA	30.81	$1,115.30	090	M C+
39400	Visualization of chest	5.61	NA	7.01	0.69	NA	NA	13.31	$481.81	010	M A
39499	Chest procedure	0.00	0.00	0.00	0.00	0.00	$0.00	0.00	$0.00	YYY	M C+ T+
39501	Repair diaphragm laceration	13.19	NA	7.82	1.38	NA	NA	22.39	$810.50	090	M C+
39502	Repair paraesophageal hernia	16.33	NA	8.41	1.68	NA	NA	26.42	$956.38	090	M C+
39503	Repair of diaphragm hernia	95.00	NA	37.24	3.52	NA	NA	135.76	$4,914.40	090	M C+
39520	Repair of diaphragm hernia	16.10	NA	9.59	1.83	NA	NA	27.52	$996.20	090	M C+
39530	Repair of diaphragm hernia	15.41	NA	8.69	1.66	NA	NA	25.76	$932.49	090	M C+
39531	Repair of diaphragm hernia	16.42	NA	8.45	1.83	NA	NA	26.70	$966.52	090	M C+

Code	Description										
39540	Repair of diaphragm hernia	13.32	NA	7.79	1.38	NA	22.49	$814.12	090	M	C+
39541	Repair of diaphragm hernia	14.41	NA	7.97	1.52	NA	23.90	$865.16	090	M	C+
39545	Revision of diaphragm	13.37	NA	9.32	1.55	NA	24.24	$877.47	090	M	C+
39560	Resect diaphragm, simple	12.00	NA	7.62	1.35	NA	20.97	$759.10	090	M	C+
39561	Resect diaphragm, complex	17.50	NA	9.84	1.97	NA	29.31	$1,061.00	090	M	C+
39599	Diaphragm surgery procedure	0.00	0.00	0.00	0.00	0.00	0.00	$0.00	YYY	M	C+ T+

Surgery: Digestive system

Code	Description										
40490	Biopsy of lip	1.22	1.63	0.63	0.06	2.91	1.91	$69.14	000	M	A
40500	Partial excision of lip	4.28	5.72	5.72	0.31	10.31	10.31	$373.21	090	M	A
40510	Partial excision of lip	4.70	6.75	6.52	0.38	11.83	11.60	$419.91	090	M	A
40520	Partial excision of lip	4.67	7.97	7.15	0.42	13.06	12.24	$443.08	090	M	A
40525	Reconstruct lip with flap	7.55	NA	8.84	0.68	NA	17.07	$617.92	090	M	A
40527	Reconstruct lip with flap	9.13	NA	9.60	0.82	NA	19.55	$707.69	090	M	A+
40530	Partial removal of lip	5.40	7.35	6.56	0.47	13.22	12.43	$449.96	090	M	A
40650	Repair lip	3.64	5.78	5.18	0.31	9.73	9.13	$330.50	090	M	A+
40652	Repair lip	4.26	7.08	7.04	0.39	11.73	11.69	$423.17	090	M	A+
40654	Repair lip	5.31	7.95	7.95	0.48	13.74	13.74	$497.38	090	M	A
40700	Repair cleft lip/nasal	12.79	NA	10.88	0.93	NA	24.60	$890.50	090	M	A+
40701	Repair cleft lip/nasal	15.85	NA	14.66	1.36	NA	31.87	$1,153.67	090	M	
40702	Repair cleft lip/nasal	13.04	NA	8.99	1.01	NA	23.04	$834.03	090	M	
40720	Repair cleft lip/nasal	13.55	NA	12.89	1.31	NA	27.75	$1,004.53	090	M	B A+
40761	Repair cleft lip/nasal	14.72	NA	12.76	1.41	NA	28.89	$1,045.79	090	M	A
40799	Lip surgery procedure	0.00	0.00	0.00	0.00	$0.00	0.00	$0.00	YYY	M	C+ T+
40800	Drainage of mouth lesion	1.17	2.01	0.48	0.09	3.27	1.74	$62.99	010	M	A
40801	Drainage of mouth lesion	2.53	2.52	1.98	0.18	5.23	4.69	$169.77	010	M	A
40804	Removal, foreign body, mouth	1.24	2.59	2.03	0.09	3.92	3.36	$121.63	010	M	A+
40805	Removal, foreign body, mouth	2.69	3.27	2.85	0.17	6.13	5.71	$206.70	010	M	A+
40806	Incision of lip fold	0.31	0.89	0.89	0.02	1.22	1.22	$44.16	000	M	A+

*M = multiple surgery adjustment applies
Me = multiple endoscopy rules may apply
B = bilateral surgery adjustment applies
A = assistant-at-surgery restriction

A+ = assistant-at-surgery restriction unless medical necessity established with documentation
C = cosurgeons payable
C+ = cosurgeons payable if medical necessity established with documentation

T = team surgeons permitted
T+ = team surgeons payable if medical necessity established with documentation
§ = indicates services that are not covered by Medicare.

CPT five-digit codes, two-digit numeric modifiers, and descriptions only are © 2001 American Medical Association

Medicare RBRVS: The Physicians' Guide

Relative value units

CPT Code and Modifier	Description	Work RVU	Non Facility Practice Expense RVU	Facility Practice Expense RVU	PLI RVU	Total Non Facility RVUs	Medicare Payment Non Facility	Total Facility RVUs	Medicare Payment Facility	Global Period	Payment Policy Indicators*		
40808	Biopsy of mouth lesion	0.96	2.11	2.11	0.07	3.14	$113.67	3.14	$113.67	010	M	A	
40810	Excision of mouth lesion	1.31	2.70	2.47	0.09	4.10	$148.42	3.87	$140.09	010	M	A	
40812	Excise/repair mouth lesion	2.31	2.95	2.93	0.17	5.43	$196.56	5.41	$195.84	010	M	A	
40814	Excise/repair mouth lesion	3.42	4.08	4.08	0.26	7.76	$280.91	7.76	$280.91	090	M	A	
40816	Excision of mouth lesion	3.67	4.32	4.32	0.27	8.26	$299.01	8.26	$299.01	090	M	A	
40818	Excise oral mucosa for graft	2.41	4.05	4.05	0.14	6.60	$238.91	6.60	$238.91	090	M	A+	
40819	Excise lip or cheek fold	2.41	3.67	3.48	0.17	6.25	$226.25	6.06	$219.37	090	M	A+	
40820	Treatment of mouth lesion	1.28	2.38	2.30	0.08	3.74	$135.39	3.66	$132.49	010	M	A	
40830	Repair mouth laceration	1.76	2.48	2.48	0.14	4.38	$158.55	4.38	$158.55	010	M	A+	
40831	Repair mouth laceration	2.46	2.72	2.72	0.21	5.39	$195.11	5.39	$195.11	010	M	A+	
40840	Reconstruction of mouth	8.73	5.93	5.93	0.79	15.45	$559.28	15.45	$559.28	090	M		
40842	Reconstruction of mouth	8.73	5.90	5.90	0.65	15.28	$553.12	15.28	$553.12	090	M	A+	
40843	Reconstruction of mouth	12.10	7.35	7.35	0.84	20.29	$734.48	20.29	$734.48	090	M		
40844	Reconstruction of mouth	16.01	9.01	9.01	1.63	26.65	$964.71	26.65	$964.71	090	M		
40845	Reconstruction of mouth	18.58	12.25	12.25	1.47	32.30	$1,169.23	32.30	$1,169.23	090	M	A+	
40899	Mouth surgery procedure	0.00	0.00	0.00	0.00	0.00	$0.00	0.00	$0.00	YYY	M	A+	C+ T+
41000	Drainage of mouth lesion	1.30	2.40	1.55	0.09	3.79	$137.19	2.94	$106.43	010	M	A	
41005	Drainage of mouth lesion	1.26	2.33	1.62	0.09	3.68	$133.21	2.97	$107.51	010	M	A+	
41006	Drainage of mouth lesion	3.24	3.58	3.28	0.25	7.07	$255.93	6.77	$245.07	090	M	A+	
41007	Drainage of mouth lesion	3.10	3.78	3.33	0.22	7.10	$257.01	6.65	$240.72	090	M	A+	
41008	Drainage of mouth lesion	3.37	3.69	3.22	0.24	7.30	$264.25	6.83	$247.24	090	M	A+	
41009	Drainage of mouth lesion	3.59	3.65	3.42	0.25	7.49	$271.13	7.26	$262.81	090	M	A+	
41010	Incision of tongue fold	1.06	3.57	3.57	0.06	4.69	$169.77	4.69	$169.77	010	M	A+	
41015	Drainage of mouth lesion	3.96	4.05	3.39	0.29	8.30	$300.45	7.64	$276.56	090	M	A+	
41016	Drainage of mouth lesion	4.07	4.31	3.61	0.28	8.66	$313.49	7.96	$288.15	090	M	A+	
41017	Drainage of mouth lesion	4.07	4.26	3.46	0.32	8.65	$313.12	7.85	$284.16	090	M	A+	
41018	Drainage of mouth lesion	5.10	4.39	3.87	0.35	9.84	$356.20	9.32	$337.38	090	M	A+	

Code	Description											
41100	Biopsy of tongue	1.63	2.67	2.64	0.12	4.42	$160.00	4.39	$158.91	010	M	A
41105	Biopsy of tongue	1.42	2.42	2.42	0.10	3.94	$142.62	3.94	$142.62	010	M	A
41108	Biopsy of floor of mouth	1.05	2.38	2.38	0.08	3.51	$127.06	3.51	$127.06	010	M	A
41110	Excision of tongue lesion	1.51	3.19	2.63	0.11	4.81	$174.12	4.25	$153.85	010	M	A
41112	Excision of tongue lesion	2.73	3.56	3.56	0.20	6.49	$234.93	6.49	$234.93	090	M	A
41113	Excision of tongue lesion	3.19	3.50	3.50	0.23	6.92	$250.50	6.92	$250.50	090	M	A
41114	Excision of tongue lesion	8.47	NA	6.59	0.64	NA	NA	15.70	$568.33	090	M	A+
41115	Excision of tongue fold	1.74	2.69	2.53	0.13	4.56	$165.07	4.40	$159.28	010	M	A+
41116	Excision of mouth lesion	2.44	3.37	3.37	0.17	5.98	$216.47	5.98	$216.47	090	M	A
41120	Partial removal of tongue	9.77	NA	9.12	0.70	NA	NA	19.59	$709.14	090	M	C+
41130	Partial removal of tongue	11.15	NA	9.76	0.81	NA	NA	21.72	$786.25	090	M	C+
41135	Tongue and neck surgery	23.09	NA	16.63	1.66	NA	NA	41.38	$1,497.92	090	M	C+
41140	Removal of tongue	25.50	NA	17.39	1.85	NA	NA	44.74	$1,619.55	090	M	C+
41145	Tongue removal, neck surgery	30.06	NA	21.36	2.11	NA	NA	53.53	$1,937.74	090	M	C+
41150	Tongue, mouth, jaw surgery	23.04	NA	17.64	1.67	NA	NA	42.35	$1,533.04	090	M	C+
41153	Tongue, mouth, neck surgery	23.77	NA	18.04	1.71	NA	NA	43.52	$1,575.39	090	M	C+
41155	Tongue, jaw, & neck surgery	27.72	NA	20.44	2.02	NA	NA	50.18	$1,816.48	090	M	C+
41250	Repair tongue laceration	1.91	2.98	1.77	0.15	5.04	$182.44	3.83	$138.64	010	M	A+
41251	Repair tongue laceration	2.27	3.12	1.88	0.18	5.57	$201.63	4.33	$156.74	010	M	A+
41252	Repair tongue laceration	2.97	3.23	2.33	0.23	6.43	$232.76	5.53	$200.18	010	M	A+
41500	Fixation of tongue	3.71	NA	4.43	0.26	NA	NA	8.40	$304.07	090	M	A+
41510	Tongue to lip surgery	3.42	NA	5.39	0.24	NA	NA	9.05	$327.60	090	M	A+
41520	Reconstruction, tongue fold	2.73	3.06	3.06	0.19	5.98	$216.47	5.98	$216.47	090	M	A+
41599	Tongue and mouth surgery	0.00	0.00	0.00	0.00	0.00	$0.00	0.00	$0.00	YYY	M	A+	C+	T+
41800	Drainage of gum lesion	1.17	1.96	1.43	0.09	3.22	$116.56	2.69	$97.38	010	M	A
41805	Removal foreign body, gum	1.24	2.08	2.08	0.09	3.41	$123.44	3.41	$123.44	010	M	A+
41806	Removal foreign body,jawbone	2.69	2.54	2.54	0.22	5.45	$197.29	5.45	$197.29	010	M	A+
41820	Excision, gum, each quadrant	0.00	0.00	0.00	0.00	0.00	$0.00	0.00	$0.00	000	M	A+

* **M** = multiple surgery adjustment applies
Me = multiple endoscopy rules may apply
B = bilateral surgery adjustment applies
A = assistant-at-surgery restriction

A+ = assistant-at-surgery restriction unless medical necessity established with documentation
C = cosurgeons payable
C+ = cosurgeons payable if medical necessity established with documentation

T = team surgeons permitted
T+ = team surgeons payable if medical necessity established with documentation
§ = indicates services that are not covered by Medicare.

CPT five-digit codes, two-digit numeric modifiers, and descriptions only are © 2001 American Medical Association

Medicare RBRVS: The Physicians' Guide

Relative value units

CPT Code and Modifier	Description	Work RVU	Non Facility Practice Expense RVU	Facility Practice Expense RVU	PLI RVU	Total Non Facility RVUs	Medicare Payment Non Facility	Total Facility RVUs	Medicare Payment Facility	Global Period	Payment Policy Indicators*
41821	Excision of gum flap	0.00	0.00	0.00	0.00	0.00	$0.00	0.00	$0.00	000	M A+
41822	Excision of gum lesion	2.31	2.82	0.98	0.24	5.37	$194.39	3.53	$127.78	010	M A+
41823	Excision of gum lesion	3.30	3.54	3.23	0.29	7.13	$258.10	6.82	$246.88	090	M A+
41825	Excision of gum lesion	1.31	2.43	2.41	0.10	3.84	$139.00	3.82	$138.28	010	M A
41826	Excision of gum lesion	2.31	2.66	2.66	0.17	5.14	$186.06	5.14	$186.06	010	M A
41827	Excision of gum lesion	3.42	3.63	3.63	0.25	7.30	$264.25	7.30	$264.25	090	M A
41828	Excision of gum lesion	3.09	3.07	2.47	0.22	6.38	$230.95	5.78	$209.23	010	M A+
41830	Removal of gum tissue	3.35	3.39	2.98	0.23	6.97	$252.31	6.56	$237.47	010	M A+
41850	Treatment of gum lesion	0.00	0.00	0.00	0.00	0.00	$0.00	0.00	$0.00	000	M A+
41870	Gum graft	0.00	0.00	0.00	0.00	0.00	$0.00	0.00	$0.00	000	M A+
41872	Repair gum	2.59	2.93	2.93	0.18	5.70	$206.34	5.70	$206.34	090	M A+
41874	Repair tooth socket	3.09	2.86	2.45	0.23	6.18	$223.71	5.77	$208.87	090	M A+
41899	Dental surgery procedure	0.00	0.00	0.00	0.00	0.00	$0.00	0.00	$0.00	YYY	M A+ C+ T+
42000	Drainage mouth roof lesion	1.23	2.52	1.51	0.10	3.85	$139.37	2.84	$102.81	010	M A+
42100	Biopsy roof of mouth	1.31	2.47	2.47	0.10	3.88	$140.45	3.88	$140.45	010	M A
42104	Excision lesion, mouth roof	1.64	2.58	2.58	0.12	4.34	$157.10	4.34	$157.10	010	M A
42106	Excision lesion, mouth roof	2.10	2.66	2.66	0.16	4.92	$178.10	4.92	$178.10	010	M A
42107	Excision lesion, mouth roof	4.44	4.26	4.26	0.32	9.02	$326.52	9.02	$326.52	090	M A
42120	Remove palate/lesion	6.17	NA	6.19	0.44	NA	NA	12.80	$463.35	090	M C+
42140	Excision of uvula	1.62	3.91	3.36	0.12	5.65	$204.53	5.10	$184.62	090	M A
42145	Repair palate, pharynx/uvula	8.05	NA	7.59	0.56	NA	NA	16.20	$586.43	090	M A
42160	Treatment mouth roof lesion	1.80	3.25	2.72	0.13	5.18	$187.51	4.65	$168.33	010	M A+
42180	Repair palate	2.50	3.29	2.25	0.19	5.98	$216.47	4.94	$178.82	010	M A+
42182	Repair palate	3.83	3.10	3.10	0.27	7.20	$260.63	7.20	$260.63	010	M A+
42200	Reconstruct cleft palate	12.00	NA	9.78	0.97	NA	NA	22.75	$823.53	090	M
42205	Reconstruct cleft palate	13.29	NA	9.76	0.82	NA	NA	23.87	$864.07	090	M
42210	Reconstruct cleft palate	14.50	NA	11.47	1.24	NA	NA	27.21	$984.98	090	M

Code	Description									
42215	Reconstruct cleft palate	8.82	NA	9.72	0.96	NA	19.50	$705.88	090	M
42220	Reconstruct cleft palate	7.02	NA	6.85	0.41	NA	14.28	$516.92	090	M
42225	Reconstruct cleft palate	9.54	NA	9.16	0.75	NA	19.45	$704.07	090	M
42226	Lengthening of palate	10.01	NA	9.96	0.73	NA	20.70	$749.32	090	M
42227	Lengthening of palate	9.52	NA	9.09	0.70	NA	19.31	$699.01	090	M
42235	Repair palate	7.87	NA	5.93	0.49	NA	14.29	$517.29	090	M
42260	Repair nose to lip fistula	9.80	6.43	6.43	0.85	17.08	17.08	$618.28	090	M
42280	Preparation, palate mold	1.54	1.44	0.60	0.12	3.10	2.26	$81.81	010	M	A+
42281	Insertion, palate prosthesis	1.93	1.57	0.92	0.14	3.64	2.99	$108.24	010	M	A+
42299	Palate/uvula surgery	0.00	0.00	0.00	0.00	0.00	0.00	$0.00	YYY	M	C+ T+
42300	Drainage of salivary gland	1.93	2.65	1.98	0.15	4.73	4.06	$146.97	010	M	A
42305	Drainage of salivary gland	6.07	NA	5.38	0.46	NA	11.91	$431.13	090	M	A+
42310	Drainage of salivary gland	1.56	2.32	1.82	0.11	3.99	3.49	$126.34	010	M	A+
42320	Drainage of salivary gland	2.35	2.79	2.15	0.17	5.31	4.67	$169.05	010	M	A+
42325	Create salivary cyst drain	2.75	3.85	1.26	0.17	6.77	4.18	$151.31	090	M	A
42326	Create salivary cyst drain	3.78	3.33	1.51	0.34	7.45	5.63	$203.80	090	M
42330	Removal of salivary stone	2.21	2.81	1.20	0.16	5.18	3.57	$129.23	010	M	A
42335	Removal of salivary stone	3.31	3.71	3.71	0.23	7.25	7.25	$262.44	090	M	A
42340	Removal of salivary stone	4.60	5.07	5.07	0.34	10.01	10.01	$362.35	090	M	A+
42400	Biopsy of salivary gland	0.78	2.52	0.40	0.06	3.36	1.24	$44.89	000	M	A
42405	Biopsy of salivary gland	3.29	3.44	3.44	0.24	6.97	6.97	$252.31	010	M	A
42408	Excision of salivary cyst	4.54	4.71	4.71	0.34	9.59	9.59	$347.15	090	M	A+
42409	Drainage of salivary cyst	2.81	3.34	3.34	0.20	6.35	6.35	$229.86	090	M
42410	Excise parotid gland/lesion	9.34	NA	8.20	0.77	NA	18.31	$662.81	090	M	C+
42415	Excise parotid gland/lesion	16.89	NA	12.82	1.26	NA	30.97	$1,121.09	090	M	C+
42420	Excise parotid gland/lesion	19.59	NA	14.46	1.45	NA	35.50	$1,285.07	090	M	C+
42425	Excise parotid gland/lesion	13.02	NA	10.70	0.98	NA	24.70	$894.12	090	M	C+
42426	Excise parotid gland/lesion	21.26	NA	15.44	1.57	NA	38.27	$1,385.34	090	M	C+

*M = multiple surgery adjustment applies
Me = multiple endoscopy rules may apply
B = bilateral surgery adjustment applies
A = assistant-at-surgery restriction

A+ = assistant-at-surgery restriction unless medical necessity established with documentation
C = cosurgeons payable
C+ = cosurgeons payable if medical necessity established with documentation

T = team surgeons permitted
T+ = team surgeons payable if medical necessity established with documentation
$ = indicates services that are not covered by Medicare.

233 CPT five-digit codes, two-digit numeric modifiers, and descriptions only are © 2001 American Medical Association

Medicare RBRVS: The Physicians' Guide

Relative value units

CPT Code and Modifier	Description	Work RVU	Non Facility Practice Expense RVU	Facility Practice Expense RVU	PLI RVU	Total Non Facility RVUs	Medicare Payment Non Facility	Total Facility RVUs	Medicare Payment Facility	Global Period	Payment Policy Indicators*		
42440	Excise submaxillary gland	6.97	NA	6.13	0.51	NA	NA	13.61	$492.67	090	M	C+	
42450	Excise sublingual gland	4.62	4.38	4.38	0.34	9.34	$338.10	9.34	$338.10	090	M	A+	
42500	Repair salivary duct	4.30	5.14	5.10	0.30	9.74	$352.58	9.70	$351.13	090	M	A+	
42505	Repair salivary duct	6.18	6.02	6.02	0.44	12.64	$457.56	12.64	$457.56	090	M	A	
42507	Parotid duct diversion	6.11	NA	5.44	0.66	NA	NA	12.21	$441.99	090	M		
42508	Parotid duct diversion	9.10	NA	8.40	0.64	NA	NA	18.14	$656.65	090	M		
42509	Parotid duct diversion	11.54	NA	9.25	1.24	NA	NA	22.03	$797.47	090	M	A+	
42510	Parotid duct diversion	8.15	NA	7.27	0.57	NA	NA	15.99	$578.83	090	M	C+	
42550	Injection for salivary x-ray	1.25	12.45	0.44	0.06	13.76	$498.10	1.75	$63.35	000	M	A	
42600	Closure of salivary fistula	4.82	7.89	5.61	0.34	13.05	$472.40	10.77	$389.87	090	M	A+	
42650	Dilation of salivary duct	0.77	1.13	0.41	0.06	1.96	$70.95	1.24	$44.89	000	M	A	
42660	Dilation of salivary duct	1.13	1.15	1.15	0.07	2.35	$85.07	2.35	$85.07	000	M	A+	
42665	Ligation of salivary duct	2.53	3.03	3.03	0.17	5.73	$207.42	5.73	$207.42	090	M	A+	
42699	Salivary surgery procedure	0.00	0.00	0.00	0.00	0.00	$0.00	0.00	$0.00	YYY	M	C+	T+
42700	Drainage of tonsil abscess	1.62	3.30	1.93	0.12	5.04	$182.44	3.67	$132.85	010	M	A	
42720	Drainage of throat abscess	5.42	4.77	4.77	0.39	10.58	$382.99	10.58	$382.99	010	M	A+	
42725	Drainage of throat abscess	10.72	NA	8.70	0.80	NA	NA	20.22	$731.95	090	M	C+	
42800	Biopsy of throat	1.39	3.09	2.63	0.10	4.58	$165.79	4.12	$149.14	010	M	A	
42802	Biopsy of throat	1.54	3.24	2.72	0.11	4.89	$177.01	4.37	$158.19	010	M	A	
42804	Biopsy of upper nose/throat	1.24	3.04	2.56	0.09	4.37	$158.19	3.89	$140.81	010	M	A	
42806	Biopsy of upper nose/throat	1.58	3.53	2.76	0.12	5.23	$189.32	4.46	$161.45	010	M	A	
42808	Excise pharynx lesion	2.30	5.00	3.17	0.17	7.47	$270.41	5.64	$204.16	010	M	A	
42809	Remove pharynx foreign body	1.81	3.48	1.77	0.13	5.42	$196.20	3.71	$134.30	010	M	A	
42810	Excision of neck cyst	3.25	5.66	4.61	0.25	9.16	$331.58	8.11	$293.58	090	M		
42815	Excision of neck cyst	7.07	NA	6.67	0.53	NA	NA	14.27	$516.56	090	M	C+	
42820	Remove tonsils and adenoids	3.91	NA	4.02	0.28	NA	NA	8.21	$297.20	090	M	A+	
42821	Remove tonsils and adenoids	4.29	NA	4.30	0.30	NA	NA	8.89	$321.81	090	M	A+	

Code	Description	Col1	Col2	Col3	Col4	Col5	Col6	Fee	Global	Mult	Asst	Co
42825	Removal of tonsils	3.42	NA	3.74	0.24	NA	7.40	$267.87	090	M	A+	
42826	Removal of tonsils	3.38	NA	3.81	0.23	NA	7.42	$268.60	090	M	A	
42830	Removal of adenoids	2.57	NA	2.51	0.18	NA	5.26	$190.41	090	M	A+	
42831	Removal of adenoids	2.71	NA	2.59	0.19	NA	5.49	$198.73	090	M	A+	
42835	Removal of adenoids	2.30	NA	3.20	0.17	NA	5.67	$205.25	090	M	A+	
42836	Removal of adenoids	3.18	NA	3.69	0.22	NA	7.09	$256.65	090	M	A+	
42842	Extensive surgery of throat	8.76	NA	7.96	0.61	NA	17.33	$627.33	090	M	A+	
42844	Extensive surgery of throat	14.31	NA	11.57	1.04	NA	26.92	$974.48	090	M		C+
42845	Extensive surgery of throat	24.29	NA	18.00	1.76	NA	44.05	$1,594.57	090	M		C+
42860	Excision of tonsil tags	2.22	NA	3.08	0.16	NA	5.46	$197.65	090	M	A+	
42870	Excision of lingual tonsil	5.40	NA	6.18	0.38	NA	11.96	$432.94	090	M	A+	
42890	Partial removal of pharynx	12.94	NA	11.03	0.91	NA	24.88	$900.64	090	M		C+
42892	Revision of pharyngeal walls	15.83	NA	12.68	1.14	NA	29.65	$1,073.31	090	M		C+
42894	Revision of pharyngeal walls	22.88	NA	17.38	1.64	NA	41.90	$1,516.75	090	M		C+
42900	Repair throat wound	5.25	NA	3.93	0.39	NA	9.57	$346.43	010	M	A+	
42950	Reconstruction of throat	8.10	NA	7.60	0.58	NA	16.28	$589.32	090	M		C+
42953	Repair throat, esophagus	8.96	NA	9.14	0.73	NA	18.83	$681.63	090	M		
42955	Surgical opening of throat	7.39	NA	6.55	0.63	NA	14.57	$527.42	090	M		
42960	Control throat bleeding	2.33	NA	2.13	0.17	NA	4.63	$167.60	010	M	A+	
42961	Control throat bleeding	5.59	NA	5.30	0.40	NA	11.29	$408.69	090	M		
42962	Control throat bleeding	7.14	NA	6.35	0.51	NA	14.00	$506.79	090	M		
42970	Control nose/throat bleeding	5.43	NA	3.99	0.37	NA	9.79	$354.39	090	M	A	
42971	Control nose/throat bleeding	6.21	NA	5.99	0.45	NA	12.65	$457.92	090	M		
42972	Control nose/throat bleeding	7.20	NA	5.73	0.54	NA	13.47	$487.60	090	M		
42999	Throat surgery procedure	0.00	0.00	0.00	0.00	$0.00	0.00	$0.00	YYY	M		T+
43020	Incision of esophagus	8.09	NA	6.77	0.70	NA	15.56	$563.26	090	M	A+	C+
43030	Throat muscle surgery	7.69	NA	7.00	0.60	NA	15.29	$553.49	090	M		C+
43045	Incision of esophagus	20.12	NA	11.14	2.15	NA	33.41	$1,209.42	090	M		C+

* **M** = multiple surgery adjustment applies
Me = multiple endoscopy rules may apply
B = bilateral surgery adjustment applies
A = assistant-at-surgery restriction

A+ = assistant-at-surgery restriction unless medical necessity established with documentation
C = cosurgeons payable
C+ = cosurgeons payable if medical necessity established with documentation

T = team surgeons permitted
T+ = team surgeons payable if medical necessity established with documentation
$ = indicates services that are not covered by Medicare.

235 CPT five-digit codes, two-digit numeric modifiers, and descriptions only are © 2001 American Medical Association

Medicare RBRVS: The Physicians' Guide

Relative value units

CPT Code and Modifier	Description	Work RVU	Non Facility Practice Expense RVU	Facility Practice Expense RVU	PLI RVU	Total Non Facility RVUs	Medicare Payment Non Facility	Total Facility RVUs	Medicare Payment Facility	Global Period	Payment Policy Indicators*
43100	Excision of esophagus lesion	9.19	NA	7.58	0.79	NA	NA	17.56	$635.66	090	M C+
43101	Excision of esophagus lesion	16.24	NA	8.84	1.81	NA	NA	26.89	$973.40	090	M C+
43107	Removal of esophagus	40.00	NA	18.49	3.29	NA	NA	61.78	$2,236.39	090	M C+
43108	Removal of esophagus	34.19	NA	16.39	3.78	NA	NA	54.36	$1,967.79	090	M C+
43112	Removal of esophagus	43.50	NA	20.06	3.67	NA	NA	67.23	$2,433.67	090	M C
43113	Removal of esophagus	35.27	NA	16.38	4.33	NA	NA	55.98	$2,026.43	090	M C
43116	Partial removal of esophagus	31.22	NA	18.49	2.62	NA	NA	52.33	$1,894.30	090	M C+
43117	Partial removal of esophagus	40.00	NA	18.51	3.51	NA	NA	62.02	$2,245.07	090	M C
43118	Partial removal of esophagus	33.20	NA	15.76	3.56	NA	NA	52.52	$1,901.18	090	M C
43121	Partial removal of esophagus	29.19	NA	15.08	3.44	NA	NA	47.71	$1,727.06	090	M C
43122	Parital removal of esophagus	40.00	NA	18.05	3.27	NA	NA	61.32	$2,219.73	090	M C+
43123	Partial removal of esophagus	33.20	NA	15.58	3.96	NA	NA	52.74	$1,909.15	090	M C+
43124	Removal of esophagus	27.32	NA	15.15	2.95	NA	NA	45.42	$1,644.17	090	M C+
43130	Removal of esophagus pouch	11.75	NA	9.05	1.06	NA	NA	21.86	$791.31	090	M C+
43135	Removal of esophagus pouch	16.10	NA	10.09	1.85	NA	NA	28.04	$1,015.03	090	M C+
43200	Esophagus endoscopy	1.59	7.92	1.22	0.11	9.62	$348.24	2.92	$105.70	000	M A
43202	Esophagus endoscopy, biopsy	1.89	6.46	1.15	0.12	8.47	$306.61	3.16	$114.39	000	Me A
43204	Esophagus endoscopy & inject	3.77	NA	1.71	0.18	NA	NA	5.66	$204.89	000	Me A
43205	Esophagus endoscopy/ligation	3.79	NA	1.71	0.17	NA	NA	5.67	$205.25	000	Me A+
43215	Esophagus endoscopy	2.60	NA	1.26	0.17	NA	NA	4.03	$145.88	000	Me A
43216	Esophagus endoscopy/lesion	2.40	NA	1.20	0.15	NA	NA	3.75	$135.75	000	Me A+
43217	Esophagus endoscopy	2.90	NA	1.35	0.17	NA	NA	4.42	$160.00	000	Me A
43219	Esophagus endoscopy	2.80	NA	1.43	0.16	NA	NA	4.39	$158.91	000	Me A
43220	Esoph endoscopy, dilation	2.10	NA	1.14	0.12	NA	NA	3.36	$121.63	000	Me A
43226	Esoph endoscopy, dilation	2.34	NA	1.21	0.12	NA	NA	3.67	$132.85	000	Me A
43227	Esoph endoscopy, repair	3.60	NA	1.64	0.18	NA	NA	5.42	$196.20	000	Me A
43228	Esoph endoscopy, ablation	3.77	NA	1.77	0.25	NA	NA	5.79	$209.59	000	Me A

43231	Esoph endoscopy w/us exam	3.19	NA	1.60	0.20	NA	NA	4.99	$180.63	000	Me	A+
43232	Esoph endoscopy w/us fn bx	4.48	NA	2.15	0.26	NA	NA	6.89	$249.41	000	Me	A+ C
43234	Upper GI endoscopy, exam	2.01	4.58	1.06	0.13	6.72	$243.26	3.20	$115.84	000	M	A
43235	Uppr gi endoscopy, diagnosis	2.39	6.38	1.23	0.13	8.90	$322.17	3.75	$135.75	000	M	A
43239	Upper GI endoscopy, biopsy	2.87	6.79	1.27	0.14	9.80	$354.75	4.28	$154.93	000	Me	A
43240	Esoph endoscope w/drain cyst	6.86	NA	2.97	0.36	NA	NA	10.19	$368.87	000	Me	A
43241	Upper GI endoscopy with tube	2.59	NA	1.27	0.14	NA	NA	4.00	$144.80	000	Me	A
43242	Uppr gi endoscopy w/us fn bx	7.31	2.64	2.64	0.29	10.24	$370.68	10.24	$370.68	000	Me	A+
43243	Upper gi endoscopy & inject	4.57	NA	2.00	0.21	NA	NA	6.78	$245.43	000	Me	A
43244	Upper GI endoscopy/ligation	5.05	NA	2.18	0.21	NA	NA	7.44	$269.32	000	Me	A+
43245	Operative upper GI endoscopy	3.39	NA	1.55	0.18	NA	NA	5.12	$185.34	000	Me	A
43246	Place gastrostomy tube	4.33	NA	1.84	0.24	NA	NA	6.41	$232.04	000	Me	A+
43247	Operative upper GI endoscopy	3.39	NA	1.56	0.17	NA	NA	5.12	$185.34	000	Me	A
43248	Uppr gi endoscopy/guide wire	3.15	NA	1.49	0.15	NA	NA	4.79	$173.39	000	M	A
43249	Esoph endoscopy, dilation	2.90	NA	1.39	0.15	NA	NA	4.44	$160.72	000	Me	A
43250	Upper GI endoscopy/tumor	3.20	NA	1.48	0.17	NA	NA	4.85	$175.57	000	Me	A
43251	Operative upper GI endoscopy	3.70	NA	1.67	0.19	NA	NA	5.56	$201.27	000	Me	A
43255	Operative upper GI endoscopy	4.82	NA	1.97	0.20	NA	NA	6.99	$253.03	000	Me	A
43256	Uppr gi endoscopy w stent	4.60	1.66	1.66	0.23	6.49	$234.93	6.49	$234.93	000	Me	A
43258	Operative upper GI endoscopy	4.55	NA	1.99	0.22	NA	NA	6.76	$244.71	000	Me	A
43259	Endoscopic ultrasound exam	4.89	NA	2.22	0.22	NA	NA	7.33	$265.34	000	Me	A+
43260	Endo cholangiopancreatograph	5.96	NA	2.50	0.27	NA	NA	8.73	$316.02	000	M	A
43261	Endo cholangiopancreatograph	6.27	NA	2.62	0.29	NA	NA	9.18	$332.31	000	Me	A
43262	Endo cholangiopancreatograph	7.39	NA	3.03	0.34	NA	NA	10.76	$389.50	000	Me	A
43263	Endo cholangiopancreatograph	7.29	NA	3.00	0.28	NA	NA	10.57	$382.63	000	Me	A
43264	Endo cholangiopancreatograph	8.90	NA	3.58	0.41	NA	NA	12.89	$466.61	000	Me	A
43265	Endo cholangiopancreatograph	10.02	NA	3.99	0.42	NA	NA	14.43	$522.35	000	Me	A
43267	Endo cholangiopancreatograph	7.39	NA	3.04	0.34	NA	NA	10.77	$389.87	000	Me	A

*M = multiple surgery adjustment applies
Me = multiple endoscopy rules may apply
B = bilateral surgery adjustment applies
A = assistant-at-surgery restriction

A+ = assistant-at-surgery restriction unless medical necessity established with documentation
C = cosurgeons payable
C+ = cosurgeons payable if medical necessity established with documentation

T = team surgeons permitted
T+ = team surgeons payable if medical necessity established with documentation
$ = indicates services that are not covered by Medicare.

237 CPT five-digit codes, two-digit numeric modifiers, and descriptions only are © 2001 American Medical Association

Medicare RBRVS: The Physicians' Guide

Relative value units

CPT Code and Modifier	Description	Work RVU	Non Facility Practice Expense RVU	Facility Practice Expense RVU	PLI RVU	Total Non Facility RVUs	Medicare Payment Non Facility	Total Facility RVUs	Medicare Payment Facility	Global Period	Payment Policy Indicators*
43268	Endo cholangiopancreatograph	7.39	NA	3.03	0.34	NA	NA	10.76	$389.50	000	Me A
43269	Endo cholangiopancreatograph	8.21	NA	3.33	0.28	NA	NA	11.82	$427.87	000	Me A
43271	Endo cholangiopancreatograph	7.39	NA	3.02	0.34	NA	NA	10.75	$389.14	000	Me A
43272	Endo cholangiopancreatograph	7.39	NA	3.04	0.34	NA	NA	10.77	$389.87	000	Me A+
43280	Laparoscopy, fundoplasty	17.25	NA	8.43	1.76	NA	NA	27.44	$993.31	090	M C+
43289	Laparoscope proc, esoph	0.00	0.00	0.00	0.00	0.00	$0.00	0.00	$0.00	YYY	M B
43300	Repair of esophagus	9.14	NA	7.31	0.85	NA	NA	17.30	$626.25	090	M C+
43305	Repair esophagus and fistula	17.39	NA	12.84	1.36	NA	NA	31.59	$1,143.53	090	M C+
43310	Repair of esophagus	25.39	NA	14.51	3.18	NA	NA	43.08	$1,559.46	090	M C+
43312	Repair esophagus and fistula	28.42	NA	17.45	3.38	NA	NA	49.25	$1,782.81	090	M C+
43313	Esophagoplasty congential	45.28	NA	22.01	5.43	NA	NA	72.72	$2,632.41	090	M C+
43314	Tracheo-esophagoplasty cong	50.27	NA	24.07	5.53	NA	NA	79.87	$2,891.23	090	M C+
43320	Fuse esophagus & stomach	19.93	NA	10.67	1.59	NA	NA	32.19	$1,165.25	090	M C+
43324	Revise esophagus & stomach	20.57	NA	9.79	1.72	NA	NA	32.08	$1,161.27	090	M C+
43325	Revise esophagus & stomach	20.06	NA	10.08	1.65	NA	NA	31.79	$1,150.77	090	M C+
43326	Revise esophagus & stomach	19.74	NA	10.33	1.84	NA	NA	31.91	$1,155.12	090	M C+
43330	Repair of esophagus	19.77	NA	9.78	1.52	NA	NA	31.07	$1,124.71	090	M C+
43331	Repair of esophagus	20.13	NA	11.41	1.93	NA	NA	33.47	$1,211.59	090	M C+
43340	Fuse esophagus & intestine	19.61	NA	10.31	1.53	NA	NA	31.45	$1,138.46	090	M C+
43341	Fuse esophagus & intestine	20.85	NA	11.17	2.14	NA	NA	34.16	$1,236.56	090	M C+
43350	Surgical opening, esophagus	15.78	NA	10.50	1.15	NA	NA	27.43	$992.94	090	M C+
43351	Surgical opening, esophagus	18.35	NA	10.91	1.51	NA	NA	30.77	$1,113.85	090	M C+
43352	Surgical opening, esophagus	15.26	NA	9.59	1.28	NA	NA	26.13	$945.89	090	M C+
43360	Gastrointestinal repair	35.70	NA	17.43	3.00	NA	NA	56.13	$2,031.86	090	M C+
43361	Gastrointestinal repair	40.50	NA	17.93	3.52	NA	NA	61.95	$2,242.54	090	M C+
43400	Ligate esophagus veins	21.20	NA	10.46	0.99	NA	NA	32.65	$1,181.90	090	M C+
43401	Esophagus surgery for veins	22.09	NA	10.34	1.73	NA	NA	34.16	$1,236.56	090	M C+

43405	Ligate/staple esophagus	20.01	NA	9.45	1.63	NA	31.09	$1,125.43	090	M		C+
43410	Repair esophagus wound	13.47	NA	9.35	1.15	NA	23.97	$867.69	090	M		C+
43415	Repair esophagus wound	25.00	NA	12.50	1.92	NA	39.42	$1,426.97	090	M		C+
43420	Repair esophagus opening	14.35	NA	9.15	0.86	NA	24.36	$881.81	090	M	A+	C+
43425	Repair esophagus opening	21.03	NA	11.00	2.03	NA	34.06	$1,232.94	090	M		C+
43450	Dilate esophagus	1.38	1.47	0.63	0.07	2.92	2.08	$75.29	000	M	A	
43453	Dilate esophagus	1.51	NA	0.68	0.08	NA	2.27	$82.17	000	M	A	
43456	Dilate esophagus	2.57	NA	1.07	0.14	NA	3.78	$136.83	000	M	A	
43458	Dilate esophagus	3.06	NA	1.26	0.17	NA	4.49	$162.53	000	M	A	
43460	Pressure treatment esophagus	3.80	NA	1.54	0.21	NA	5.55	$200.91	000	M	A	
43496	Free jejunum flap, microvasc	0.00	0.00	0.00	0.00	0.00	0.00	$0.00	090	M		C+
43499	Esophagus surgery procedure	0.00	0.00	0.00	0.00	$0.00	0.00	$0.00	YYY	M		C+ T+
43500	Surgical opening of stomach	11.05	NA	5.23	0.84	NA	17.12	$619.73	090	M		C+
43501	Surgical repair of stomach	20.04	NA	8.86	1.55	NA	30.45	$1,102.27	090	M		C+
43502	Surgical repair of stomach	23.13	NA	10.16	1.83	NA	35.12	$1,271.32	090	M		C+
43510	Surgical opening of stomach	13.08	NA	7.50	0.90	NA	21.48	$777.56	090	M		C+
43520	Incision of pyloric muscle	9.99	NA	5.73	0.84	NA	16.56	$599.46	090	M		C+
43600	Biopsy of stomach	1.91	NA	1.05	0.11	NA	3.07	$111.13	000	M	A	
43605	Biopsy of stomach	11.98	NA	5.55	0.93	NA	18.46	$668.24	090	M		C+
43610	Excision of stomach lesion	14.60	NA	6.85	1.14	NA	22.59	$817.74	090	M		C+
43611	Excision of stomach lesion	17.84	NA	8.12	1.38	NA	27.34	$989.69	090	M		C+
43620	Removal of stomach	30.04	NA	12.89	2.29	NA	45.22	$1,636.93	090	M		C+
43621	Removal of stomach	30.73	NA	13.21	2.36	NA	46.30	$1,676.02	090	M		C+
43622	Removal of stomach	32.53	NA	13.79	2.48	NA	48.80	$1,766.52	090	M		C+
43631	Removal of stomach, partial	22.59	NA	9.72	1.99	NA	34.30	$1,241.63	090	M		C+
43632	Removal of stomach, partial	22.59	NA	9.73	2.00	NA	34.32	$1,242.36	090	M		C+
43633	Removal of stomach, partial	23.10	NA	9.87	2.05	NA	35.02	$1,267.70	090	M		C+
43634	Removal of stomach, partial	25.12	NA	10.84	2.18	NA	38.14	$1,380.64	090	M		C+

*M = multiple surgery adjustment applies
Me = multiple endoscopy rules may apply
B = bilateral surgery adjustment applies
A = assistant-at-surgery restriction

A+ = assistant-at-surgery restriction unless medical necessity established with documentation
C = cosurgeons payable
C+ = cosurgeons payable if medical necessity established with documentation

T = team surgeons permitted
T+ = team surgeons payable if medical necessity established with documentation
$ = indicates services that are not covered by Medicare.

239   CPT five-digit codes, two-digit numeric modifiers, and descriptions only are © 2001 American Medical Association

Medicare RBRVS: The Physicians' Guide

Relative value units

CPT Code and Modifier	Description	Work RVU	Non Facility Practice Expense RVU	Facility Practice Expense RVU	PLI RVU	Total Non Facility RVUs	Medicare Payment Non Facility	Total Facility RVUs	Medicare Payment Facility	Global Period	Payment Policy Indicators*	
43635	Removal of stomach, partial	2.06	NA	0.74	0.21	NA	NA	3.01	$108.96	ZZZ		C+
43638	Removal of stomach, partial	29.00	NA	12.13	2.24	NA	NA	43.37	$1,569.96	090	M	C+
43639	Removal of stomach, partial	29.65	NA	12.30	2.31	NA	NA	44.26	$1,602.18	090	M	C+
43640	Vagotomy & pylorus repair	17.02	NA	7.72	1.51	NA	NA	26.25	$950.23	090	M	C+
43641	Vagotomy & pylorus repair	17.27	NA	7.82	1.53	NA	NA	26.62	$963.62	090	M	C+
43651	Laparoscopy, vagus nerve	10.15	NA	4.71	1.03	NA	NA	15.89	$575.21	090	M	C+
43652	Laparoscopy, vagus nerve	12.15	NA	5.53	1.25	NA	NA	18.93	$685.25	090	M	C+
43653	Laparoscopy, gastrostomy	7.73	NA	4.37	0.78	NA	NA	12.88	$466.25	090	M	C+
43659	Laparoscope proc, stom	0.00	0.00	0.00	0.00	0.00	$0.00	0.00	$0.00	YYY	M B	
43750	Place gastrostomy tube	4.49	NA	2.72	0.33	NA	NA	7.54	$272.94	010	M	A
43760	Change gastrostomy tube	1.10	1.47	0.46	0.07	2.64	$95.57	1.63	$59.00	000	M	A
43761	Reposition gastrostomy tube	2.01	NA	0.83	0.10	NA	NA	2.94	$106.43	000	M	A
43800	Reconstruction of pylorus	13.69	NA	6.60	1.07	NA	NA	21.36	$773.21	090	M	C+
43810	Fusion of stomach and bowel	14.65	NA	6.94	1.10	NA	NA	22.69	$821.36	090	M	C+
43820	Fusion of stomach and bowel	15.37	NA	7.15	1.18	NA	NA	23.70	$857.92	090	M	C+
43825	Fusion of stomach and bowel	19.22	NA	8.56	1.50	NA	NA	29.28	$1,059.91	090	M	C+
43830	Place gastrostomy tube	9.53	NA	5.06	0.69	NA	NA	15.28	$553.12	090	M	C+
43831	Place gastrostomy tube	7.84	NA	4.67	0.81	NA	NA	13.32	$482.17	090	M	C+
43832	Place gastrostomy tube	15.60	NA	7.66	1.13	NA	NA	24.39	$882.90	090	M	C+
43840	Repair of stomach lesion	15.56	NA	7.21	1.20	NA	NA	23.97	$867.69	090	M	C+
43842	Gastroplasty for obesity	18.47	NA	11.24	1.51	NA	NA	31.22	$1,130.14	090	M	C
43843	Gastroplasty for obesity	18.65	NA	11.25	1.53	NA	NA	31.43	$1,137.74	090	M	C
43846	Gastric bypass for obesity	24.05	NA	13.68	1.96	NA	NA	39.69	$1,436.75	090	M	C+
43847	Gastric bypass for obesity	26.92	NA	15.28	2.14	NA	NA	44.34	$1,605.07	090	M	C+
43848	Revision gastroplasty	29.39	NA	16.54	2.39	NA	NA	48.32	$1,749.15	090	M	C+
43850	Revise stomach-bowel fusion	24.72	NA	10.42	1.97	NA	NA	37.11	$1,343.35	090	M	C+
43855	Revise stomach-bowel fusion	26.16	NA	11.12	2.01	NA	NA	39.29	$1,422.27	090	M	C+

Code	Description	Col1	Col2	Col3	Col4	Col5	Fee	Days	Mod1	Mod2	Mod3
43860	Revise stomach-bowel fusion	25.00	NA	10.58	2.03	NA	37.61	$1,361.45	090	M		C+
43865	Revise stomach-bowel fusion	26.52	NA	11.21	2.15	NA	39.88	$1,443.62	090	M		C+
43870	Repair stomach opening	9.69	NA	5.22	0.71	NA	15.62	$565.43	090	M		C+
43880	Repair stomach-bowel fistula	24.65	NA	10.87	1.94	NA	37.46	$1,356.02	090	M		C+
43999	Stomach surgery procedure	0.00	0.00	0.00	0.00	$0.00	0.00	$0.00	YYY	M	A+	C+	T+
44005	Freeing of bowel adhesion	16.23	NA	7.40	1.39	NA	25.02	$905.70	090	M		C+
44010	Incision of small bowel	12.52	NA	6.48	1.05	NA	20.05	$725.79	090	M		C+
44015	Insert needle cath bowel	2.62	NA	0.93	0.25	NA	3.80	$137.56	ZZZ			C+
44020	Explore small intestine	13.99	NA	6.56	1.20	NA	21.75	$787.33	090	M		C+
44021	Decompress small bowel	14.08	NA	7.02	1.18	NA	22.28	$806.52	090	M		C+
44025	Incision of large bowel	14.28	NA	6.65	1.21	NA	22.14	$801.45	090	M		C+
44050	Reduce bowel obstruction	14.03	NA	6.60	1.15	NA	21.78	$788.42	090	M		C+
44055	Correct malrotation of bowel	22.00	NA	9.51	1.32	NA	32.83	$1,188.42	090	M		C+
44100	Biopsy of bowel	2.01	NA	1.09	0.12	NA	3.22	$116.56	000	M	A	
44110	Excise intestine lesion(s)	11.81	NA	5.84	1.00	NA	18.65	$675.12	090	M		C+
44111	Excision of bowel lesion(s)	14.29	NA	7.10	1.22	NA	22.61	$818.46	090	M		C+
44120	Removal of small intestine	17.00	NA	7.67	1.46	NA	26.13	$945.89	090	M		C+
44121	Removal of small intestine	4.45	NA	1.60	0.45	NA	6.50	$235.29	ZZZ			C+
44125	Removal of small intestine	17.54	NA	7.86	1.49	NA	26.89	$973.40	090	M		C+
44126	Enterectomy w/o taper, cong	35.50	NA	18.03	0.36	NA	53.89	$1,950.77	090	M		C+
44127	Enterectomy w/taper, cong	41.00	NA	20.56	0.41	NA	61.97	$2,243.26	090	M		C+
44128	Enterectomy cong, add-on	4.45	NA	1.78	0.45	NA	6.68	$241.81	ZZZ			C+
44130	Bowel to bowel fusion	14.49	NA	6.78	1.23	NA	22.50	$814.48	090	M		C+
44132	Enterectomy, cadaver donor	0.00	0.00	0.00	0.00	$0.00	0.00	$0.00	XXX		A+	
44133	Enterectomy, live donor	0.00	0.00	0.00	0.00	$0.00	0.00	$0.00	XXX		A+	
44135	Intestine transplnt, cadaver	0.00	0.00	0.00	0.00	$0.00	0.00	$0.00	XXX		A+	
44136	Intestine transplant, live	0.00	0.00	0.00	0.00	$0.00	0.00	$0.00	XXX		A+	
44139	Mobilization of colon	2.23	NA	0.80	0.21	NA	3.24	$117.29	ZZZ			C+

* **M** = multiple surgery adjustment applies
Me = multiple endoscopy rules may apply
B = bilateral surgery adjustment applies
A = assistant-at-surgery restriction

A+ = assistant-at-surgery restriction unless medical necessity established with documentation
C = cosurgeons payable
C+ = cosurgeons payable if medical necessity established with documentation

T = team surgeons permitted
T+ = team surgeons payable if medical necessity established with documentation
$ = indicates services that are not covered by Medicare.

241 CPT five-digit codes, two-digit numeric modifiers, and descriptions only are © 2001 American Medical Association

Medicare RBRVS: The Physicians' Guide

Relative value units

CPT Code and Modifier	Description	Work RVU	Non Facility Practice Expense RVU	Facility Practice Expense RVU	PLI RVU	Total Non Facility RVUs	Medicare Payment Non Facility	Total Facility RVUs	Medicare Payment Facility	Global Period	Payment Policy Indicators*
44140	Partial removal of colon	21.00	NA	9.53	1.83	NA	NA	32.36	$1,171.41	090	M C+
44141	Partial removal of colon	19.51	NA	11.93	1.95	NA	NA	33.39	$1,208.69	090	M C+
44143	Partial removal of colon	22.99	NA	13.14	2.02	NA	NA	38.15	$1,381.00	090	M C+
44144	Partial removal of colon	21.53	NA	11.75	1.89	NA	NA	35.17	$1,273.13	090	M C+
44145	Partial removal of colon	26.42	NA	11.90	2.22	NA	NA	40.54	$1,467.52	090	M C+
44146	Partial removal of colon	27.54	NA	15.41	2.20	NA	NA	45.15	$1,634.39	090	M C+
44147	Partial removal of colon	20.71	NA	10.15	1.74	NA	NA	32.60	$1,180.09	090	M C+
44150	Removal of colon	23.95	NA	14.08	2.05	NA	NA	40.08	$1,450.86	090	M C+
44151	Removal of colon/ileostomy	26.88	NA	15.74	1.97	NA	NA	44.59	$1,614.12	090	M C+
44152	Removal of colon/ileostomy	27.83	NA	17.01	2.36	NA	NA	47.20	$1,708.60	090	M C+
44153	Removal of colon/ileostomy	30.59	NA	16.64	2.33	NA	NA	49.56	$1,794.03	090	M C+
44155	Removal of colon/ileostomy	27.86	NA	15.28	2.26	NA	NA	45.40	$1,643.44	090	M C+
44156	Removal of colon/ileostomy	30.79	NA	17.86	2.19	NA	NA	50.84	$1,840.37	090	M C+
44160	Removal of colon	18.62	NA	8.65	1.55	NA	NA	28.82	$1,043.26	090	M C+
44200	Laparoscopy, enterolysis	14.44	NA	6.79	1.46	NA	NA	22.69	$821.36	090	M C+
44201	Laparoscopy, jejunostomy	9.78	NA	5.16	0.97	NA	NA	15.91	$575.93	090	M C+
44202	Lap resect s/intestine singl	22.04	NA	9.82	2.16	NA	NA	34.02	$1,231.50	090	M C+
44203	Lap resect s/intestine, addl	4.45	NA	1.60	0.45	NA	NA	6.50	$235.29	ZZZ	C+
44204	Laparo partial colectomy	25.08	NA	10.46	1.83	NA	NA	37.37	$1,352.76	090	M C+
44205	Lap colectomy part w/ileum	22.23	NA	9.31	1.55	NA	NA	33.09	$1,197.83	090	M C+
44209	Laparoscope proc, intestine	0.00	0.00	0.00	0.00	0.00	$0.00	0.00	$0.00	YYY	M B
44300	Open bowel to skin	12.11	NA	6.79	0.88	NA	NA	19.78	$716.02	090	M C+
44310	Ileostomy/jejunostomy	15.95	NA	10.50	1.13	NA	NA	27.58	$998.37	090	M C+
44312	Revision of ileostomy	8.02	NA	5.25	0.54	NA	NA	13.81	$499.91	090	M A+
44314	Revision of ileostomy	15.05	NA	10.37	0.99	NA	NA	26.41	$956.02	090	M C+
44316	Devise bowel pouch	21.09	NA	13.77	1.41	NA	NA	36.27	$1,312.94	090	M C+
44320	Colostomy	17.64	NA	12.13	1.28	NA	NA	31.05	$1,123.99	090	M C+

Code	Description										
44322	Colostomy with biopsies	11.98	NA	10.41	1.18	NA	23.57	$853.22	090	M	C+
44340	Revision of colostomy	7.72	NA	4.86	0.56	NA	13.14	$475.66	090	M	A C+
44345	Revision of colostomy	15.43	NA	8.34	1.11	NA	24.88	$900.64	090	M	C+
44346	Revision of colostomy	16.99	NA	8.91	1.20	NA	27.10	$981.00	090	M	C+
44360	Small bowel endoscopy	2.59	NA	1.39	0.14	NA	4.12	$149.14	000	M	A
44361	Small bowel endoscopy/biopsy	2.87	NA	1.50	0.15	NA	4.52	$163.62	000	Me	A
44363	Small bowel endoscopy	3.50	NA	1.71	0.19	NA	5.40	$195.48	000	Me	A+
44364	Small bowel endoscopy	3.74	NA	1.80	0.21	NA	5.75	$208.15	000	Me	A+
44365	Small bowel endoscopy	3.31	NA	1.68	0.18	NA	5.17	$187.15	000	Me	A+
44366	Small bowel endoscopy	4.41	NA	2.05	0.22	NA	6.68	$241.81	000	Me	A
44369	Small bowel endoscopy	4.52	NA	2.05	0.23	NA	6.80	$246.15	000	Me	A+
44370	Small bowel endoscopy/stent	4.80	1.74	1.74	0.21	6.75	6.75	$244.34	000	Me	A+
44372	Small bowel endoscopy	4.41	NA	2.04	0.27	NA	6.72	$243.26	000	Me	A
44373	Small bowel endoscopy	3.50	NA	1.80	0.19	NA	5.49	$198.73	000	Me	A
44376	Small bowel endoscopy	5.26	NA	2.36	0.29	NA	7.91	$286.34	000	M	A+
44377	Small bowel endoscopy/biopsy	5.53	NA	2.47	0.28	NA	8.28	$299.73	000	Me	A+
44378	Small bowel endoscopy	7.13	NA	3.06	0.37	NA	10.56	$382.26	000	Me	A+
44379	S bowel endoscope w/stent	7.47	2.67	2.67	0.38	10.52	10.52	$380.82	000	Me	A+
44380	Small bowel endoscopy	1.05	NA	0.79	0.08	NA	1.92	$69.50	000	M	A
44382	Small bowel endoscopy	1.27	NA	0.90	0.09	NA	2.26	$81.81	000	M	A
44383	Ileoscopy w/stent	3.26	1.16	1.16	0.13	4.55	4.55	$164.71	000	M	A
44385	Endoscopy of bowel pouch	1.82	5.26	0.95	0.12	7.20	2.89	$104.62	000	M	A
44386	Endoscopy, bowel pouch/biop	2.12	6.98	1.09	0.15	9.25	3.36	$121.63	000	M	A+
44388	Colon endoscopy	2.82	6.91	1.42	0.18	9.91	4.42	$160.00	000	M	A
44389	Colonoscopy with biopsy	3.13	7.62	1.55	0.18	10.93	4.86	$175.93	000	Me	A
44390	Colonoscopy for foreign body	3.83	6.68	1.80	0.22	10.73	5.85	$211.77	000	Me	A+
44391	Colonoscopy for bleeding	4.32	6.04	1.78	0.23	10.59	6.33	$229.14	000	Me	A+
44392	Colonoscopy & polypectomy	3.82	8.21	1.79	0.23	12.26	5.84	$211.40	000	Me	A

* **M** = multiple surgery adjustment applies
Me = multiple endoscopy rules may apply
B = bilateral surgery adjustment applies
A = assistant-at-surgery restriction

A+ = assistant-at-surgery restriction unless medical necessity established with documentation
C = cosurgeons payable
C+ = cosurgeons payable if medical necessity established with documentation

T = team surgeons permitted
T+ = team surgeons payable if medical necessity established with documentation
$ = indicates services that are not covered by Medicare.

243 CPT five-digit codes, two-digit numeric modifiers, and descriptions only are © 2001 American Medical Association

Medicare RBRVS: The Physicians' Guide

Relative value units

CPT Code and Modifier	Description	Work RVU	Non Facility Practice Expense RVU	Facility Practice Expense RVU	PLI RVU	Total Non Facility RVUs	Medicare Payment Non Facility	Total Facility RVUs	Medicare Payment Facility	Global Period	Payment Policy Indicators*		
44393	Colonoscopy, lesion removal	4.84	8.45	2.19	0.27	13.56	$490.86	7.30	$264.25	000	Me	A	
44394	Colonoscopy w/snare	4.43	7.71	2.04	0.26	12.40	$448.87	6.73	$243.62	000	Me	A	
44397	Colonoscopy w stent	4.71	NA	2.10	0.28	NA	NA	7.09	$256.65	000	Me	A	
44500	Intro, gastrointestinal tube	0.49	NA	0.37	0.02	NA	NA	0.88	$31.86	000		A+	
44602	Suture, small intestine	16.03	NA	7.34	1.07	NA	NA	24.44	$884.71	090	M		C+
44603	Suture, small intestine	18.66	NA	8.25	1.39	NA	NA	28.30	$1,024.44	090	M		C+
44604	Suture, large intestine	16.03	NA	7.35	1.42	NA	NA	24.80	$897.74	090	M		C+
44605	Repair of bowel lesion	19.53	NA	8.94	1.54	NA	NA	30.01	$1,086.34	090	M		C+
44615	Intestinal stricturoplasty	15.93	NA	7.32	1.39	NA	NA	24.64	$891.95	090	M		C+
44620	Repair bowel opening	12.20	NA	5.81	1.05	NA	NA	19.06	$689.96	090	M		C+
44625	Repair bowel opening	15.05	NA	6.86	1.30	NA	NA	23.21	$840.18	090	M		C+
44626	Repair bowel opening	25.36	NA	10.60	2.19	NA	NA	38.15	$1,381.00	090	M		C+
44640	Repair bowel-skin fistula	21.65	NA	9.70	1.46	NA	NA	32.81	$1,187.70	090	M		C+
44650	Repair bowel fistula	22.57	NA	10.01	1.49	NA	NA	34.07	$1,233.31	090	M		C+
44660	Repair bowel-bladder fistula	21.36	NA	9.51	1.14	NA	NA	32.01	$1,158.74	090	M		C+
44661	Repair bowel-bladder fistula	24.81	NA	10.73	1.53	NA	NA	37.07	$1,341.90	090	M		C+
44680	Surgical revision, intestine	15.40	NA	7.47	1.37	NA	NA	24.24	$877.47	090	M		C+
44700	Suspend bowel w/prosthesis	16.11	NA	7.57	1.21	NA	NA	24.89	$901.00	090	M		C+
44799	Intestine surgery procedure	0.00	0.00	0.00	0.00	0.00	$0.00	0.00	$0.00	YYY	M		C+ T+
44800	Excision of bowel pouch	11.23	NA	5.61	1.11	NA	NA	17.95	$649.78	090	M		C+
44820	Excision of mesentery lesion	12.09	NA	5.98	1.03	NA	NA	19.10	$691.40	090	M		C+
44850	Repair of mesentery	10.74	NA	5.41	0.99	NA	NA	17.14	$620.45	090	M		C+
44899	Bowel surgery procedure	0.00	NA	0.00	0.00	NA	$0.00	0.00	$0.00	YYY	M		C+ T+
44900	Drain app abscess, open	10.14	NA	5.96	0.84	NA	NA	16.94	$613.21	090	M		C+
44901	Drain app abscess, percut	3.38	NA	5.01	0.17	NA	NA	8.56	$309.87	000	M		
44950	Appendectomy	10.00	NA	5.31	0.88	NA	NA	16.19	$586.07	090	M		C+
44955	Appendectomy add-on	1.53	NA	0.57	0.16	NA	NA	2.26	$81.81	ZZZ			C+

Code	Description										
44960	Appendectomy	12.34	NA	6.50	1.09	NA	19.93	$721.45	090	M	C+
44970	Laparoscopy, appendectomy	8.70	NA	4.21	0.88	NA	13.79	$499.19	090	M	C
44979	Laparoscope proc, app	0.00	0.00	0.00	0.00	0.00	0.00	$0.00	YYY	M	B
45000	Drainage of pelvic abscess	4.52	NA	3.80	0.37	NA	8.69	$314.57	090	M	A
45005	Drainage of rectal abscess	1.99	4.58	1.62	0.18	6.75	3.79	$137.19	010	M	A
45020	Drainage of rectal abscess	4.72	NA	4.21	0.41	NA	9.34	$338.10	090	M	A
45100	Biopsy of rectum	3.68	4.86	2.12	0.33	8.87	6.13	$221.90	090	M	A
45108	Removal of anorectal lesion	4.76	6.40	2.95	0.46	11.62	8.17	$295.75	090	M	A
45110	Removal of rectum	28.00	NA	13.26	2.26	NA	43.52	$1,575.39	090	M	C+
45111	Partial removal of rectum	16.48	NA	8.78	1.60	NA	26.86	$972.31	090	M	C+
45112	Removal of rectum	30.54	NA	13.70	2.35	NA	46.59	$1,686.52	090	M	C+
45113	Partial proctectomy	30.58	NA	13.39	2.13	NA	46.10	$1,668.78	090	M	C+
45114	Partial removal of rectum	27.32	NA	12.61	2.28	NA	42.21	$1,527.97	090	M	C+
45116	Partial removal of rectum	24.58	NA	11.58	2.00	NA	38.16	$1,381.36	090	M	C+
45119	Remove rectum w/reservoir	30.84	NA	13.25	2.13	NA	46.22	$1,673.13	090	M	C+
45120	Removal of rectum	24.60	NA	11.63	2.28	NA	38.51	$1,394.03	090	M	C+
45121	Removal of rectum and colon	27.04	NA	12.53	2.66	NA	42.23	$1,528.69	090	M	C+
45123	Partial proctectomy	16.71	NA	8.21	1.04	NA	25.96	$939.73	090	M	C+
45126	Pelvic exenteration	45.16	NA	19.12	3.23	NA	67.51	$2,443.81	090	M	C+
45130	Excision of rectal prolapse	16.44	NA	7.80	1.12	NA	25.36	$918.01	090	M	C+
45135	Excision of rectal prolapse	19.28	NA	9.10	1.52	NA	29.90	$1,082.36	090	M	C+
45136	Excise ileoanal reservoir	27.30	NA	12.66	2.19	NA	42.15	$1,525.80	090	M	C+
45150	Excision of rectal stricture	5.67	5.89	3.19	0.46	12.02	9.32	$337.38	090	M	A+
45160	Excision of rectal lesion	15.32	NA	7.14	1.07	NA	23.53	$851.77	090	M	C+
45170	Excision of rectal lesion	11.49	NA	5.89	0.89	NA	18.27	$661.36	090	M	C+
45190	Destruction, rectal tumor	9.74	NA	5.33	0.76	NA	15.83	$573.03	090	M	C+
45300	Proctosigmoidoscopy dx	0.38	1.34	0.23	0.05	1.77	0.66	$23.89	000	M	A
45303	Proctosigmoidoscopy dilate	0.44	1.55	0.27	0.06	2.05	0.77	$27.87	000	Me	A

* **M** = multiple surgery adjustment applies
Me = multiple endoscopy rules may apply
B = bilateral surgery adjustment applies
A = assistant-at-surgery restriction

A+ = assistant-at-surgery restriction unless medical necessity established with documentation
C = cosurgeons payable
C+ = cosurgeons payable if medical necessity established with documentation

T = team surgeons permitted
T+ = team surgeons payable if medical necessity established with documentation
$ = indicates services that are not covered by Medicare.

245 CPT five-digit codes, two-digit numeric modifiers, and descriptions only are © 2001 American Medical Association

Medicare RBRVS: The Physicians' Guide

Relative value units

CPT Code and Modifier	Description	Work RVU	Non Facility Practice Expense RVU	Facility Practice Expense RVU	PLI RVU	Total Non Facility RVUs	Medicare Payment Non Facility	Total Facility RVUs	Medicare Payment Facility	Global Period	Payment Policy Indicators*
45305	Protosigmoidoscopy w/bx	1.01	1.64	0.46	0.09	2.74	$99.19	1.56	$56.47	000	Me A
45307	Protosigmoidoscopy fb	0.94	2.68	0.44	0.15	3.77	$136.47	1.53	$55.38	000	Me A+
45308	Protosigmoidoscopy removal	0.83	1.59	0.39	0.13	2.55	$92.31	1.35	$48.87	000	Me A
45309	Protosigmoidoscopy removal	2.01	2.43	0.81	0.17	4.61	$166.88	2.99	$108.24	000	Me A
45315	Protosigmoidoscopy removal	1.40	2.84	0.60	0.20	4.44	$160.72	2.20	$79.64	000	Me A
45317	Protosigmoidoscopy bleed	1.50	1.94	0.63	0.20	3.64	$131.77	2.33	$84.34	000	Me A
45320	Protosigmoidoscopy ablate	1.58	1.88	0.68	0.20	3.66	$132.49	2.46	$89.05	000	Me A
45321	Protosigmoidoscopy volvul	1.17	NA	0.52	0.17	NA	NA	1.86	$67.33	000	Me A
45327	Proctosigmoidoscopy w/stent	1.65	NA	0.89	0.10	NA	NA	2.64	$95.57	000	Me A
45330	Diagnostic sigmoidoscopy	0.96	1.92	0.53	0.05	2.93	$106.06	1.54	$55.75	000	M Me
45331	Sigmoidoscopy and biopsy	1.15	2.38	0.54	0.07	3.60	$130.32	1.76	$63.71	000	Me A
45332	Sigmoidoscopy w/fb removal	1.79	4.36	0.76	0.11	6.26	$226.61	2.66	$96.29	000	Me A
45333	Sigmoidoscopy & polypectomy	1.79	3.93	0.77	0.12	5.84	$211.40	2.68	$97.01	000	Me A
45334	Sigmoidoscopy for bleeding	2.73	NA	1.12	0.16	NA	NA	4.01	$145.16	000	Me A
45337	Sigmoidoscopy & decompress	2.36	NA	0.97	0.15	NA	NA	3.48	$125.97	000	Me A
45338	Sigmoidoscopy w/tumr remove	2.34	4.75	0.97	0.15	7.24	$262.08	3.46	$125.25	000	Me A
45339	Sigmoidoscopy w/ablate tumr	3.14	3.62	1.27	0.17	6.93	$250.86	4.58	$165.79	000	Me A
45341	Sigmoidoscopy w/ultrasound	2.60	NA	1.40	0.20	NA	NA	4.20	$152.04	000	M A
45342	Sigmoidoscopy w/us guide bx	4.06	NA	1.85	0.23	NA	NA	6.14	$222.26	000	M A
45345	Sigmodoscopy w/stent	2.92	NA	1.44	0.15	NA	NA	4.51	$163.26	000	Me A
45355	Surgical colonoscopy	3.52	NA	1.28	0.26	NA	NA	5.06	$183.17	000	M A
45378	Diagnostic colonoscopy	3.70	8.79	1.77	0.20	12.69	$459.37	5.67	$205.25	000	M A
45378-53	Diagnostic colonoscopy	0.96	1.92	0.53	0.05	2.93	$106.06	1.54	$55.75	000	M A
45379	Colonoscopy w/fb removal	4.69	8.25	2.13	0.25	13.19	$477.47	7.07	$255.93	000	Me A
45380	Colonoscopy and biopsy	4.44	9.28	2.05	0.21	13.93	$504.25	6.70	$242.53	000	M A
45382	Colonoscopy/control bleeding	5.69	10.32	2.29	0.27	16.28	$589.32	8.25	$298.64	000	Me A
45383	Lesion removal colonoscopy	5.87	10.01	2.56	0.32	16.20	$586.43	8.75	$316.74	000	Me A

Code	Description										
45384	Lesion remove colonoscopy	4.70	9.74	2.14	0.24	14.68	$531.40	7.08	$256.29	000	Me	A
45385	Lesion removal colonoscopy	5.31	10.19	2.36	0.28	15.78	$571.22	7.95	$287.78	000	Me	A
45387	Colonoscopy w/stent	5.91	NA	2.57	0.33	NA	NA	8.81	$318.91	000	Me	A
45500	Repair of rectum	7.29	NA	4.24	0.56	NA	NA	12.09	$437.65	090	M	A+
45505	Repair of rectum	7.58	NA	3.86	0.50	NA	NA	11.94	$432.22	090	M	A
45520	Treatment of rectal prolapse	0.55	0.77	0.20	0.04	1.36	$49.23	0.79	$28.60	000	M	A
45540	Correct rectal prolapse	16.27	NA	8.18	1.17	NA	NA	25.62	$927.42	090	M		C+
45541	Correct rectal prolapse	13.40	NA	7.03	0.88	NA	NA	21.31	$771.40	000	M		C+
45550	Repair rectum/remove sigmoid	23.00	NA	10.40	1.58	NA	NA	34.98	$1,266.25	000	M		C+
45560	Repair of rectocele	10.58	NA	6.12	0.73	NA	NA	17.43	$630.95	000	M		C+
45562	Exploration/repair of rectum	15.38	NA	7.52	1.15	NA	NA	24.05	$870.59	000	M		C+
45563	Exploration/repair of rectum	23.47	NA	11.34	1.84	NA	NA	36.65	$1,326.70	000	M		C+
45800	Repair rect/bladder fistula	17.77	NA	8.23	1.14	NA	NA	27.14	$982.45	000	M		C+
45805	Repair fistula w/colostomy	20.78	NA	10.72	1.47	NA	NA	32.97	$1,193.49	000	M		C+
45820	Repair rectourethral fistula	18.48	NA	8.55	1.17	NA	NA	28.20	$1,020.82	000	M		C+
45825	Repair fistula w/colostomy	21.25	NA	10.57	0.97	NA	NA	32.79	$1,186.97	000	M		C+
45900	Reduction of rectal prolapse	2.61	NA	1.04	0.17	NA	NA	3.82	$138.28	010	M	A+
45905	Dilation of anal sphincter	2.30	12.19	0.96	0.14	14.63	$529.59	3.40	$123.08	010	M	A
45910	Dilation of rectal narrowing	2.80	17.62	1.15	0.14	20.56	$744.26	4.09	$148.05	010	M	A
45915	Remove rectal obstruction	3.14	4.89	1.16	0.17	8.20	$296.83	4.47	$161.81	010	M	A
45999	Rectum surgery procedure	0.00	0.00	0.00	0.00	0.00	$0.00	0.00	$0.00	YYY	M	A+	C+	T+
46020	Placement of seton	2.90	3.09	2.36	0.22	6.21	$224.80	5.48	$198.37	010	M	A
46030	Removal of rectal marker	1.23	2.90	1.22	0.11	4.24	$153.48	2.56	$92.67	010	M	A+
46040	Incision of rectal abscess	4.96	5.57	3.15	0.48	11.01	$398.55	8.59	$310.95	090	M	A
46045	Incision of rectal abscess	4.32	NA	2.88	0.40	NA	NA	7.60	$275.11	090	M	A
46050	Incision of anal abscess	1.19	3.68	1.37	0.11	4.98	$180.27	2.67	$96.65	010	M	A
46060	Incision of rectal abscess	5.69	NA	3.83	0.52	NA	NA	10.04	$363.44	090	M	A
46070	Incision of anal septum	2.71	NA	2.54	0.27	NA	NA	5.52	$199.82	090	M	A+

* **M** = multiple surgery adjustment applies
Me = multiple endoscopy rules may apply
B = bilateral surgery adjustment applies
A = assistant-at-surgery restriction

A+ = assistant-at-surgery restriction unless medical necessity established with documentation
C = cosurgeons payable
C+ = cosurgeons payable if medical necessity established with documentation

T = team surgeons permitted
T+ = team surgeons payable if medical necessity established with documentation
§ = indicates services that are not covered by Medicare.

247   CPT five-digit codes, two-digit numeric modifiers, and descriptions only are © 2001 American Medical Association

Medicare RBRVS: The Physicians' Guide

Relative value units

CPT Code and Modifier	Description	Work RVU	Non Facility Practice Expense RVU	Facility Practice Expense RVU	PLI RVU	Total Non Facility RVUs	Medicare Payment Non Facility	Total Facility RVUs	Medicare Payment Facility	Global Period	Payment Policy Indicators*
46080	Incision of anal sphincter	2.49	3.81	1.65	0.23	6.53	$236.38	4.37	$158.19	010	M A
46083	Incise external hemorrhoid	1.40	4.78	1.59	0.12	6.30	$228.05	3.11	$112.58	010	M A
46200	Removal of anal fissure	3.42	4.01	2.42	0.30	7.73	$279.82	6.14	$222.26	090	M A
46210	Removal of anal crypt	2.67	5.12	2.17	0.26	8.05	$291.40	5.10	$184.62	090	M A+
46211	Removal of anal crypts	4.25	4.97	3.10	0.37	9.59	$347.15	7.72	$279.46	090	M A+
46220	Removal of anal tab	1.56	1.32	0.56	0.14	3.02	$109.32	2.26	$81.81	010	M A
46221	Ligation of hemorrhoid(s)	2.04	1.80	1.12	0.12	3.96	$143.35	3.28	$118.73	010	M A
46230	Removal of anal tabs	2.57	4.38	1.69	0.22	7.17	$259.55	4.48	$162.17	010	M A
46250	Hemorrhoidectomy	3.89	5.59	2.71	0.43	9.91	$358.73	7.03	$254.48	090	M A
46255	Hemorrhoidectomy	4.60	6.45	2.96	0.51	11.56	$418.46	8.07	$292.13	090	M A
46257	Remove hemorrhoids & fissure	5.40	NA	3.12	0.59	NA	NA	9.11	$329.77	090	M A
46258	Remove hemorrhoids & fistula	5.73	NA	3.30	0.64	NA	NA	9.67	$350.05	090	M A+
46260	Hemorrhoidectomy	6.37	NA	4.04	0.68	NA	NA	11.09	$401.45	090	M A
46261	Remove hemorrhoids & fissure	7.08	NA	4.19	0.70	NA	NA	11.97	$433.30	090	M A
46262	Remove hemorrhoids & fistula	7.50	NA	4.35	0.76	NA	NA	12.61	$456.47	090	M A
46270	Removal of anal fistula	3.72	5.23	2.65	0.36	9.31	$337.01	6.73	$243.62	090	M A
46275	Removal of anal fistula	4.56	4.65	2.85	0.40	9.61	$347.87	7.81	$282.72	090	M A
46280	Removal of anal fistula	5.98	NA	3.83	0.50	NA	NA	10.31	$373.21	090	M A
46285	Removal of anal fistula	4.09	4.28	2.69	0.34	8.71	$315.30	7.12	$257.74	090	M A
46288	Repair anal fistula	7.13	NA	4.25	0.60	NA	NA	11.98	$433.67	090	M A
46320	Removal of hemorrhoid clot	1.61	4.00	1.57	0.14	5.75	$208.15	3.32	$120.18	010	M A
46500	Injection into hemorrhoid(s)	1.61	2.89	0.58	0.12	4.62	$167.24	2.31	$83.62	010	M A
46600	Diagnostic anoscopy	0.50	0.82	0.15	0.04	1.36	$49.23	0.69	$24.98	000	M A
46604	Anoscopy and dilation	1.31	0.99	0.47	0.09	2.39	$86.52	1.87	$67.69	000	Me A
46606	Anoscopy and biopsy	0.81	0.87	0.29	0.07	1.75	$63.35	1.17	$42.35	000	Me A
46608	Anoscopy/ remove for body	1.51	1.81	0.49	0.13	3.45	$124.89	2.13	$77.10	000	Me A+
46610	Anoscopy/remove lesion	1.32	1.46	0.48	0.12	2.90	$104.98	1.92	$69.50	000	Me A

Code	Description										
46611	Anoscopy	1.81	2.07	0.65	0.15	4.03	$145.88	2.61	$94.48	000	Me	A+
46612	Anoscopy/ remove lesions	2.34	2.65	0.85	0.18	5.17	$187.15	3.37	$121.99	000	Me	A+
46614	Anoscopy/control bleeding	2.01	1.90	0.71	0.14	4.05	$146.61	2.86	$103.53	000	Me	A
46615	Anoscopy	2.68	1.76	0.96	0.23	4.67	$169.05	3.87	$140.09	000	Me	A+
46700	Repair of anal stricture	9.13	NA	4.78	0.56	NA	NA	14.47	$523.80	090	M	A
46705	Repair of anal stricture	6.90	NA	4.53	0.73	NA	NA	12.16	$440.18	090	M		C+
46715	Repair of anovaginal fistula	7.20	NA	4.46	0.76	NA	NA	12.42	$449.59	090	M	
46716	Repair of anovaginal fistula	15.07	NA	8.05	1.30	NA	NA	24.42	$883.98	090	M		C+
46730	Construction of absent anus	26.75	NA	12.25	2.03	NA	NA	41.03	$1,485.25	090	M		C+
46735	Construction of absent anus	32.17	NA	15.49	2.64	NA	NA	50.30	$1,820.82	090	M		C+
46740	Construction of absent anus	30.00	NA	14.61	1.99	NA	NA	46.60	$1,686.88	090	M		C+
46742	Repair of imperforated anus	35.80	NA	18.31	2.63	NA	NA	56.74	$2,053.94	090	M		C+
46744	Repair of cloacal anomaly	52.63	NA	22.78	2.27	NA	NA	77.68	$2,811.95	090	M		C+
46746	Repair of cloacal anomaly	58.22	NA	27.19	2.51	NA	NA	87.92	$3,182.63	090	M		C+
46748	Repair of cloacal anomaly	64.21	NA	29.58	2.77	NA	NA	96.56	$3,495.39	090	M		C+
46750	Repair of anal sphincter	10.25	NA	5.79	0.69	NA	NA	16.73	$605.61	090	M		C+
46751	Repair of anal sphincter	8.77	NA	6.14	0.78	NA	NA	15.69	$567.97	090	M		C+
46753	Reconstruction of anus	8.29	NA	4.13	0.58	NA	NA	13.00	$470.59	090	M	A
46754	Removal of suture from anus	2.20	5.36	1.43	0.12	7.68	$278.01	3.75	$135.75	010	M	A+
46760	Repair of anal sphincter	14.43	NA	7.07	0.86	NA	NA	22.36	$809.41	090	M		C+
46761	Repair of anal sphincter	13.84	NA	6.87	0.84	NA	NA	21.55	$780.09	090	M		C+
46762	Implant artificial sphincter	12.71	NA	6.08	0.71	NA	NA	19.50	$705.88	090	M		C+
46900	Destruction, anal lesion(s)	1.91	3.52	0.74	0.13	5.56	$201.27	2.78	$100.63	010	M	A
46910	Destruction, anal lesion(s)	1.86	3.81	1.48	0.14	5.81	$210.32	3.48	$125.97	010	M	A
46916	Cryosurgery, anal lesion(s)	1.86	3.24	1.68	0.09	5.19	$187.87	3.63	$131.40	010	M	A
46917	Laser surgery, anal lesions	1.86	5.32	1.62	0.16	7.34	$265.70	3.64	$131.77	010	M	A
46922	Excision of anal lesion(s)	1.86	3.96	1.46	0.17	5.99	$216.83	3.49	$126.34	010	M	A
46924	Destruction, anal lesion(s)	2.76	4.81	1.77	0.20	7.77	$281.27	4.73	$171.22	010	M	A

* **M** = multiple surgery adjustment applies
Me = multiple endoscopy rules may apply
B = bilateral surgery adjustment applies
A = assistant-at-surgery restriction

A+ = assistant-at-surgery restriction unless medical necessity established with documentation
C = cosurgeons payable
C+ = cosurgeons payable if medical necessity established with documentation

T = team surgeons permitted
T+ = team surgeons payable if medical necessity established with documentation
§ = indicates services that are not covered by Medicare.

249   CPT five-digit codes, two-digit numeric modifiers, and descriptions only are © 2001 American Medical Association

Medicare RBRVS: The Physicians' Guide

Relative value units

CPT Code and Modifier	Description	Work RVU	Non Facility Practice Expense RVU	Facility Practice Expense RVU	PLI RVU	Total Non Facility RVUs	Medicare Payment Non Facility	Total Facility RVUs	Medicare Payment Facility	Global Period	Payment Policy Indicators*		
46934	Destruction of hemorrhoids	3.51	6.62	3.77	0.26	10.39	$376.11	7.54	$272.94	090	M	A	
46935	Destruction of hemorrhoids	2.43	4.60	0.87	0.17	7.20	$260.63	3.47	$125.61	010	M	A	
46936	Destruction of hemorrhoids	3.69	6.67	3.58	0.30	10.66	$385.88	7.57	$274.03	090	M	A	
46937	Cryotherapy of rectal lesion	2.69	4.51	1.72	0.12	7.32	$264.98	4.53	$163.98	010	M	A+	
46938	Cryotherapy of rectal lesion	4.66	6.22	3.27	0.40	11.28	$408.33	8.33	$301.54	090	M	A+	
46940	Treatment of anal fissure	2.32	3.47	0.83	0.17	5.96	$215.75	3.32	$120.18	010	M	A	
46942	Treatment of anal fissure	2.04	2.84	0.71	0.14	5.02	$181.72	2.89	$104.62	010	M	A+	
46945	Ligation of hemorrhoids	1.84	4.04	2.29	0.17	6.05	$219.01	4.30	$155.66	090	M	A	
46946	Ligation of hemorrhoids	2.58	5.40	2.61	0.22	8.20	$296.83	5.41	$195.84	090	M	A	
46999	Anus surgery procedure	0.00	0.00	0.00	0.00	0.00	$0.00	0.00	$0.00	YYY	M	A+	C+ T+
47000	Needle biopsy of liver	1.90	8.36	0.67	0.09	10.35	$374.66	2.66	$96.29	000	M	A	
47001	Needle biopsy, liver add-on	1.90	NA	0.68	0.18	NA	NA	2.76	$99.91	ZZZ	M	A	C+
47010	Open drainage, liver lesion	16.01	NA	9.60	0.65	NA	NA	26.26	$950.59	090	M		C+
47011	Percut drain, liver lesion	3.70	NA	4.61	0.17	NA	NA	8.48	$306.97	000	M		
47015	Inject/aspirate liver cyst	15.11	NA	8.23	0.86	NA	NA	24.20	$876.02	090	M		C+
47100	Wedge biopsy of liver	11.67	NA	6.50	0.75	NA	NA	18.92	$684.89	090	M		C+
47120	Partial removal of liver	35.50	NA	17.02	2.29	NA	NA	54.81	$1,984.08	090	M		C+
47122	Extensive removal of liver	55.13	NA	24.11	3.60	NA	NA	82.84	$2,998.74	090	M		C+
47125	Partial removal of liver	49.19	NA	22.12	3.18	NA	NA	74.49	$2,696.48	090	M		C+
47130	Partial removal of liver	53.35	NA	23.49	3.47	NA	NA	80.31	$2,907.16	090	M		C+
47134	Partial removal, donor liver	39.15	NA	13.91	3.98	NA	NA	57.04	$2,064.80	XXX	M		C+ T
47135	Transplantation of liver	81.52	NA	43.28	8.13	NA	NA	132.93	$4,811.96	090	M		C+ T
47136	Transplantation of liver	68.60	NA	47.00	6.93	NA	NA	122.53	$4,435.49	090	M		C+ T
47300	Surgery for liver lesion	15.08	NA	7.75	0.97	NA	NA	23.80	$861.54	090	M		C+
47350	Repair liver wound	19.56	NA	9.45	1.25	NA	NA	30.26	$1,095.39	090	M		C+
47360	Repair liver wound	26.92	NA	12.96	1.71	NA	NA	41.59	$1,505.52	090	M		C+
47361	Repair liver wound	47.12	NA	19.94	3.11	NA	NA	70.17	$2,540.10	090	M		C+

Code	Description											
47362	Repair liver wound	18.51	NA	9.77	1.22	NA	29.50	$1,067.88	090	M		C+
47370	Laparo ablate liver tumor rf	18.00	7.19	7.19	0.85	$942.63	26.04	$942.63	090	M		C+
47371	Laparo ablate liver cryosug	16.94	6.76	6.76	0.85	$888.69	24.55	$888.69	090	M		C+
47379	Laparoscope procedure, liver	0.00	0.00	0.00	0.00	$0.00	0.00	$0.00	YYY	M		
47380	Open ablate liver tumor rf	21.25	8.48	8.48	0.85	$1,106.97	30.58	$1,106.97	090	M		C+
47381	Open ablate liver tumor cryo	21.00	8.38	8.38	0.85	$1,094.30	30.23	$1,094.30	090	M		C+
47382	Percut ablate liver rf	12.00	NA	5.37	0.85	NA	18.22	$659.55	010	M		
47399	Liver surgery procedure	0.00	0.00	0.00	0.00	$0.00	0.00	$0.00	YYY	M		C+ T+
47400	Incision of liver duct	32.49	NA	14.99	1.82	NA	49.30	$1,784.62	090	M		C+
47420	Incision of bile duct	19.88	NA	9.46	1.70	NA	31.04	$1,123.62	090	M		C+
47425	Incision of bile duct	19.83	NA	9.38	1.60	NA	30.81	$1,115.30	090	M		C+
47460	Incise bile duct sphincter	18.04	NA	9.26	1.24	NA	28.54	$1,033.13	090	M		C+
47480	Incision of gallbladder	10.82	NA	6.80	0.85	NA	18.47	$668.60	090	M		C+
47490	Incision of gallbladder	7.23	NA	7.67	0.33	NA	15.23	$551.31	090	M	A	
47500	Injection for liver x-rays	1.96	NA	0.68	0.09	NA	2.73	$98.82	000	M	A	
47505	Injection for liver x-rays	0.76	2.88	0.26	0.03	$132.85	1.05	$38.01	000	M	A+	
47510	Insert catheter, bile duct	7.83	NA	9.46	0.36	NA	17.65	$638.92	090	M	A	
47511	Insert bile duct drain	10.50	NA	10.57	0.47	NA	21.54	$779.73	090	M	B A	
47525	Change bile duct catheter	5.55	NA	3.34	0.24	NA	9.13	$330.50	010	M	A	
47530	Revise/reinsert bile tube	5.85	NA	5.07	0.29	NA	11.21	$405.79	090	M	A	
47550	Bile duct endoscopy add-on	3.02	NA	1.08	0.30	NA	4.40	$159.28	ZZZ	M		C+
47552	Biliary endoscopy thru skin	6.04	NA	2.52	0.42	NA	8.98	$325.07	000	M	A	C+
47553	Biliary endoscopy thru skin	6.35	NA	2.70	0.30	NA	9.35	$338.46	000	Me	A	
47554	Biliary endoscopy thru skin	9.06	NA	3.55	0.74	NA	13.35	$483.26	000	Me	A	C+
47555	Biliary endoscopy thru skin	7.56	NA	3.15	0.35	NA	11.06	$400.36	000	Me	A	
47556	Biliary endoscopy thru skin	8.56	NA	3.49	0.38	NA	12.43	$449.96	000	M	A	
47560	Laparoscopy w/cholangio	4.89	NA	1.89	0.49	NA	7.27	$263.17	000	M	A+	
47561	Laparo w/cholangio/biopsy	5.18	NA	2.19	0.49	NA	7.86	$284.53	000	M	A+	

* **M** = multiple surgery adjustment applies
   Me = multiple endoscopy rules may apply
   B = bilateral surgery adjustment applies
   A = assistant-at-surgery restriction

A+ = assistant-at-surgery restriction unless medical necessity established with documentation
C = cosurgeons payable
C+ = cosurgeons payable if medical necessity established with documentation

T = team surgeons permitted
T+ = team surgeons payable if medical necessity established with documentation
$ = indicates services that are not covered by Medicare.

251 CPT five-digit codes, two-digit numeric modifiers, and descriptions only are © 2001 American Medical Association

Medicare RBRVS: The Physicians' Guide

Relative value units

CPT Code and Modifier	Description	Work RVU	Non Facility Practice Expense RVU	Facility Practice Expense RVU	PLI RVU	Total Non Facility RVUs	Medicare Payment Non Facility	Total Facility RVUs	Medicare Payment Facility	Global Period	Payment Policy Indicators*
47562	Laparoscopic cholecystectomy	11.09	NA	5.15	1.13	NA	NA	17.37	$628.78	090	M C+
47563	Laparo cholecystectomy/graph	11.94	NA	5.43	1.21	NA	NA	18.58	$672.58	090	M C+
47564	Laparo cholecystectomy/explr	14.23	NA	6.26	1.44	NA	NA	21.93	$793.85	090	M C+
47570	Laparo cholecystoenterostomy	12.58	NA	5.67	1.28	NA	NA	19.53	$706.97	090	M C+
47579	Laparoscope proc, biliary	0.00	0.00	0.00	0.00	0.00	$0.00	0.00	$0.00	YYY	M B
47600	Removal of gallbladder	13.58	NA	6.86	1.16	NA	NA	21.60	$781.90	090	M C+
47605	Removal of gallbladder	14.69	NA	7.23	1.25	NA	NA	23.17	$838.74	090	M C+
47610	Removal of gallbladder	18.82	NA	8.80	1.61	NA	NA	29.23	$1,058.10	090	M C+
47612	Removal of gallbladder	18.78	NA	8.70	1.60	NA	NA	29.08	$1,052.67	090	M C+
47620	Removal of gallbladder	20.64	NA	9.35	1.77	NA	NA	31.76	$1,149.69	090	M C+
47630	Remove bile duct stone	9.11	NA	3.20	0.46	NA	NA	12.77	$462.26	090	M A
47700	Exploration of bile ducts	15.62	NA	8.79	1.40	NA	NA	25.81	$934.30	090	M C+
47701	Bile duct revision	27.81	NA	13.60	3.00	NA	NA	44.41	$1,607.61	090	M A+
47711	Excision of bile duct tumor	23.03	NA	11.34	1.98	NA	NA	36.35	$1,315.84	090	M C+
47712	Excision of bile duct tumor	30.24	NA	14.00	2.67	NA	NA	46.91	$1,698.10	090	M C+
47715	Excision of bile duct cyst	18.80	NA	8.95	1.59	NA	NA	29.34	$1,062.08	090	M C+
47716	Fusion of bile duct cyst	16.44	NA	8.19	1.41	NA	NA	26.04	$942.63	090	M C+
47720	Fuse gallbladder & bowel	15.91	NA	8.66	1.37	NA	NA	25.94	$939.01	090	M C+
47721	Fuse upper gi structures	19.12	NA	9.90	1.63	NA	NA	30.65	$1,109.51	090	M C+
47740	Fuse gallbladder & bowel	18.48	NA	9.64	1.59	NA	NA	29.71	$1,075.48	090	M C+
47741	Fuse gallbladder & bowel	21.34	NA	10.62	1.82	NA	NA	33.78	$1,222.81	090	M C+
47760	Fuse bile ducts and bowel	25.85	NA	12.28	2.21	NA	NA	40.34	$1,460.28	090	M C+
47765	Fuse liver ducts & bowel	24.88	NA	12.73	2.18	NA	NA	39.79	$1,440.37	090	M C+
47780	Fuse bile ducts and bowel	26.50	NA	12.49	2.27	NA	NA	41.26	$1,493.58	090	M C+
47785	Fuse bile ducts and bowel	31.18	NA	14.97	2.69	NA	NA	48.84	$1,767.97	090	M C+
47800	Reconstruction of bile ducts	23.30	NA	11.57	1.95	NA	NA	36.82	$1,332.85	090	M C+
47801	Placement, bile duct support	15.17	NA	10.21	0.69	NA	NA	26.07	$943.71	090	M C+

Code	Description									
47802	Fuse liver duct & intestine	21.55	NA	11.60	1.84	NA	NA	34.99	$1,266.61	090	M		C+
47900	Suture bile duct injury	19.90	NA	10.25	1.65	NA	NA	31.80	$1,151.13	090	M		C+
47999	Bile tract surgery procedure	0.00	0.00	0.00	0.00	NA	$0.00	0.00	$0.00	YYY	M		C+ T+
48000	Drainage of abdomen	28.07	NA	12.59	1.32	NA	NA	41.98	$1,519.64	090	M		C+
48001	Placement of drain, pancreas	35.45	NA	15.04	1.90	NA	NA	52.39	$1,896.48	090	M		C+
48005	Resect/debride pancreas	42.17	NA	17.39	2.26	NA	NA	61.82	$2,237.83	090	M		C+
48020	Removal of pancreatic stone	15.70	NA	7.44	1.36	NA	NA	24.50	$886.88	090	M		C+
48100	Biopsy of pancreas, open	12.23	NA	7.03	1.08	NA	NA	20.34	$736.29	090	M		C+
48102	Needle biopsy, pancreas	4.68	8.96	2.45	0.20	13.84	$501.00	7.33	$265.34	010	M	A	
48120	Removal of pancreas lesion	15.85	NA	7.69	1.35	NA	NA	24.89	$901.00	090	M		C+
48140	Partial removal of pancreas	22.94	NA	10.78	2.12	NA	NA	35.84	$1,297.38	090	M		C+
48145	Partial removal of pancreas	24.02	NA	11.48	2.25	NA	NA	37.75	$1,366.52	090	M		C+
48146	Pancreatectomy	26.40	NA	13.96	2.43	NA	NA	42.79	$1,548.96	090	M		C+
48148	Removal of pancreatic duct	17.34	NA	9.15	1.61	NA	NA	28.10	$1,017.20	090	M		C+
48150	Partial removal of pancreas	48.00	NA	21.29	4.43	NA	NA	73.72	$2,668.61	090	M		C+
48152	Pancreatectomy	43.75	NA	20.74	4.07	NA	NA	68.56	$2,481.82	090	M		C+
48153	Pancreatectomy	47.89	NA	22.18	4.40	NA	NA	74.47	$2,695.75	090	M		C+
48154	Pancreatectomy	44.10	NA	20.82	4.10	NA	NA	69.02	$2,498.47	090	M		C+
48155	Removal of pancreas	24.64	NA	13.89	2.30	NA	NA	40.83	$1,478.01	090	M		C+
48180	Fuse pancreas and bowel	24.72	NA	11.16	2.24	NA	NA	38.12	$1,379.91	090	M		C+
48400	Injection, intraop add-on	1.95	NA	0.69	0.10	NA	NA	2.74	$99.19	ZZZ	M	A+	
48500	Surgery of pancreatic cyst	15.28	NA	7.74	1.35	NA	NA	24.37	$882.17	090	M		C+
48510	Drain pancreatic pseudocyst	14.31	NA	7.45	1.07	NA	NA	22.83	$826.43	090	M		C+
48511	Drain pancreatic pseudocyst	4.00	NA	3.95	0.17	NA	NA	8.12	$293.94	000	M		
48520	Fuse pancreas cyst and bowel	15.59	NA	7.49	1.41	NA	NA	24.49	$886.52	090	M		C+
48540	Fuse pancreas cyst and bowel	19.72	NA	8.84	1.82	NA	NA	30.38	$1,099.73	090	M		C+
48545	Pancreatorrhaphy	18.18	NA	8.88	1.61	NA	NA	28.67	$1,037.83	090	M		C+
48547	Duodenal exclusion	25.83	NA	11.04	2.30	NA	NA	39.17	$1,417.92	090	M		C+

*M = multiple surgery adjustment applies
Me = multiple endoscopy rules may apply
B = bilateral surgery adjustment applies
A = assistant-at-surgery restriction

A+ = assistant-at-surgery restriction unless medical necessity established with documentation
C = cosurgeons payable
C+ = cosurgeons payable if medical necessity established with documentation

T = team surgeons permitted
T+ = team surgeons payable if medical necessity established with documentation
$ = indicates services that are not covered by Medicare.

CPT five-digit codes, two-digit numeric modifiers, and descriptions only are © 2001 American Medical Association

Medicare RBRVS: The Physicians' Guide

Relative value units

CPT Code and Modifier	Description	Work RVU	Non Facility Practice Expense RVU	Facility Practice Expense RVU	PLI RVU	Total Non Facility RVUs	Medicare Payment Non Facility	Total Facility RVUs	Medicare Payment Facility	Global Period	Payment Policy Indicators*			
48554	Transpl allograft pancreas	34.17	NA	12.27	3.30	NA	NA	49.74	$1,800.55	090	M		C	T
48556	Removal, allograft pancreas	15.71	NA	8.71	1.52	NA	NA	25.94	$939.01	090	M		C	T
48999	Pancreas surgery procedure	0.00	0.00	0.00	0.00	0.00	$0.00	0.00	$0.00	YYY	M		C+	T+
49000	Exploration of abdomen	11.68	NA	6.22	1.17	NA	NA	19.07	$690.32	090	M		C+	
49002	Reopening of abdomen	10.49	NA	6.10	1.06	NA	NA	17.65	$638.92	090	M		C+	
49010	Exploration behind abdomen	12.28	NA	7.05	1.22	NA	NA	20.55	$743.89	090	M		C+	
49020	Drain abdominal abscess	22.84	NA	11.41	1.31	NA	NA	35.56	$1,287.24	090	M			
49021	Drain abdominal abscess	3.38	NA	5.84	0.16	NA	NA	9.38	$339.55	000	M	A		
49040	Drain, open, abdom abscess	13.52	NA	8.02	0.84	NA	NA	22.38	$810.14	090	M		C+	
49041	Drain, percut, abdom abscess	4.00	NA	6.07	0.18	NA	NA	10.25	$371.04	000	M			
49060	Drain, open, retrop abscess	15.86	NA	9.62	0.77	NA	NA	26.25	$950.23	090	M	A	C+	
49061	Drain, percut, retroper absc	3.70	NA	5.99	0.17	NA	NA	9.86	$356.92	000	M			
49062	Drain to peritoneal cavity	11.36	NA	7.06	1.08	NA	NA	19.50	$705.88	090	M		C+	
49080	Puncture, peritoneal cavity	1.35	4.56	0.48	0.07	5.98	$216.47	1.90	$68.78	000	M	A		
49081	Removal of abdominal fluid	1.26	3.14	0.60	0.06	4.46	$161.45	1.92	$69.50	000	M	A		
49085	Remove abdomen foreign body	12.14	NA	6.72	0.88	NA	NA	19.74	$714.57	090	M	A	C+	
49180	Biopsy, abdominal mass	1.73	8.50	0.60	0.08	10.31	$373.21	2.41	$87.24	000	M	A		
49200	Removal of abdominal lesion	10.25	NA	6.59	0.89	NA	NA	17.73	$641.81	090	M		C+	
49201	Removal of abdominal lesion	14.84	NA	8.90	1.44	NA	NA	25.18	$911.50	090	M		C+	
49215	Excise sacral spine tumor	33.50	NA	15.52	2.48	NA	NA	51.50	$1,864.26	090	M		C+	
49220	Multiple surgery, abdomen	14.88	NA	7.94	1.51	NA	NA	24.33	$880.73	090	M		C+	
49250	Excision of umbilicus	8.35	NA	5.26	0.84	NA	NA	14.45	$523.08	090	M	A	C+	
49255	Removal of omentum	11.14	NA	6.66	1.12	NA	NA	18.92	$684.89	090	M		C+	
49320	Diag laparo separate proc	5.10	NA	3.08	0.50	NA	NA	8.68	$314.21	010	M			
49321	Laparoscopy, biopsy	5.40	NA	3.07	0.53	NA	NA	9.00	$325.79	010	Me		C	
49322	Laparoscopy, aspiration	5.70	NA	3.53	0.57	NA	NA	9.80	$354.75	010	Me		C	
49323	Laparo drain lymphocele	9.48	NA	4.18	0.88	NA	NA	14.54	$526.34	090	Me		C	

49329	Laparo proc, abdm/per/oment	0.00	0.00	0.00	0.00	0.00	0.00	$0.00	0.00	YYY	M	B
49400	Air injection into abdomen	1.88	NA	0.82	0.11	NA	NA	$101.72	2.81	000	M	A
49420	Insert abdominal drain	2.22	NA	0.98	0.13	NA	NA	$120.54	3.33	000	M	A
49421	Insert abdominal drain	5.54	NA	4.08	0.55	NA	NA	$368.15	10.17	090	M	A
49422	Remove perm cannula/catheter	6.25	NA	3.01	0.63	NA	NA	$358.01	9.89	010	M	A
49423	Exchange drainage catheter	1.46	NA	0.70	0.07	NA	NA	$80.72	2.23	000	M	A+
49424	Assess cyst, contrast inject	0.76	NA	0.45	0.03	NA	NA	$44.89	1.24	000	M	A+
49425	Insert abdomen-venous drain	11.37	NA	6.79	1.21	NA	NA	$701.18	19.37	090	M		C+
49426	Revise abdomen-venous shunt	9.63	NA	6.17	0.93	NA	NA	$605.61	16.73	090	M	A
49427	Injection, abdominal shunt	0.89	NA	0.50	0.05	NA	NA	$52.13	1.44	000	M	A+
49428	Ligation of shunt	6.06	NA	3.19	0.31	NA	NA	$346.06	9.56	100	M	A
49429	Removal of shunt	7.40	NA	3.55	0.81	NA	NA	$425.70	11.76	010	M	A
49491	Repairing hern premie reduc	11.13	NA	5.65	1.00	NA	NA	$643.62	17.78	090	M	B	C+
49492	Rpr ing hern premie, blocked	14.03	NA	6.40	1.42	NA	NA	$790.95	21.85	090	M	B	C+
49495	Rpr ing hernia baby, reduc	5.89	NA	3.72	0.55	NA	NA	$367.78	10.16	090	M	B	C+
49496	Rerepair ing hernia baby, blocked	8.79	NA	5.94	0.89	NA	NA	$565.43	15.62	090	M	B	C+
49500	Rpr ing hernia, init, reduce	5.48	NA	3.48	0.46	NA	NA	$341.00	9.42	090	M	B	C+
49501	Rpr ing hernia, init blocked	8.88	NA	4.62	0.76	NA	NA	$516.20	14.26	090	M	B	C+
49505	Rpr i/hern init reduc>5 yr	7.60	4.58	4.13	0.65	12.83	$464.44	$448.15	12.38	090	M	B	C+
49507	Rpr i/hern init block>5 yr	9.57	NA	6.17	0.83	NA	NA	$599.82	16.57	090	M	B	C+
49520	Rerepair ing hernia, reduce	9.63	NA	5.49	0.84	NA	NA	$577.74	15.96	090	M	B	C+
49521	Rerepair ing hernia, blocked	11.97	NA	5.85	1.04	NA	NA	$682.72	18.86	090	M	B	C+
49525	Repair ing hernia, sliding	8.57	NA	4.97	0.74	NA	NA	$516.92	14.28	090	M	B	C+
49540	Repair lumbar hernia	10.39	NA	5.65	0.90	NA	NA	$613.21	16.94	090	M	B	C+
49550	Rpr fem hernia, init, reduce	8.63	NA	4.55	0.75	NA	NA	$504.25	13.93	090	M	B	C+
49553	Rpr fem hernia, init blocked	9.44	NA	4.95	0.83	NA	NA	$550.95	15.22	090	M	B	C+
49555	Rerepair fem hernia, reduce	9.03	NA	5.30	0.79	NA	NA	$547.33	15.12	090	M	B	C+
49557	Rerepair fem hernia, blocked	11.15	NA	5.59	0.97	NA	NA	$641.09	17.71	090	M	B	C+

* **M** = multiple surgery adjustment applies
Me = multiple endoscopy rules may apply
B = bilateral surgery adjustment applies
A = assistant-at-surgery restriction

A+ = assistant-at-surgery restriction unless medical necessity established with documentation
C = cosurgeons payable
C+ = cosurgeons payable if medical necessity established with documentation

T = team surgeons permitted
T+ = team surgeons payable if medical necessity established with documentation
$ = indicates services that are not covered by Medicare.

255 CPT five-digit codes, two-digit numeric modifiers, and descriptions only are © 2001 American Medical Association

Medicare RBRVS: The Physicians' Guide

Relative value units

CPT Code and Modifier	Description	Work RVU	Non Facility Practice Expense RVU	Facility Practice Expense RVU	PLI RVU	Total Non Facility RVUs	Medicare Payment Non Facility	Total Facility RVUs	Medicare Payment Facility	Global Period	Payment Policy Indicators*		
49560	Rpr ventral hern init, reduc	11.57	NA	6.11	1.00	NA	NA	18.68	$676.20	090	M	B	C+
49561	Rpr ventral hern init, block	14.25	NA	6.71	1.23	NA	NA	22.19	$803.26	090	M	B	C+
49565	Rerepair ventrl hern, reduce	11.57	NA	6.27	1.00	NA	NA	18.84	$681.99	090	M	B	C+
49566	Rerepair ventrl hern, block	14.40	NA	6.79	1.24	NA	NA	22.43	$811.95	090	M	B	C+
49568	Hernia repair w/mesh	4.89	NA	1.76	0.50	NA	NA	7.15	$258.82	ZZZ		B	C+
49570	Rpr epigastric hern, reduce	5.69	NA	3.54	0.50	NA	NA	9.73	$352.22	090	M		C+
49572	Rpr epigastric hern, blocked	6.73	NA	4.00	0.58	NA	NA	11.31	$409.41	090	M	B	C+
49580	Rpr umbil hern, reduc <5 yr	4.11	NA	3.03	0.34	NA	NA	7.48	$270.77	090	M		C+
49582	Rpr umbil hern, block < 5 yr	6.65	NA	5.02	0.57	NA	NA	12.24	$443.08	090	M		C+
49585	Rpr umbil hern, reduc > 5 yr	6.23	NA	4.15	0.53	NA	NA	10.91	$394.93	090	M		C+
49587	Rpr umbil hern, block > 5 yr	7.56	NA	4.27	0.65	NA	NA	12.48	$451.77	090	M		C+
49590	Repair spigelian hernia	8.54	NA	4.96	0.74	NA	NA	14.24	$515.48	090	M	B	C+
49600	Repair umbilical lesion	10.96	NA	6.30	1.13	NA	NA	18.39	$665.70	090	M		C+
49605	Repair umbilical lesion	76.00	NA	30.79	2.57	NA	NA	109.36	$3,958.74	090	M		C+
49606	Repair umbilical lesion	18.60	NA	9.61	2.22	NA	NA	30.43	$1,101.54	090	M		C+
49610	Repair umbilical lesion	10.50	NA	6.87	0.77	NA	NA	18.14	$656.65	090	M		C+
49611	Repair umbilical lesion	8.92	NA	6.56	0.65	NA	NA	16.13	$583.89	090	M		C+
49650	Laparo hernia repair initial	6.27	NA	3.33	0.64	NA	NA	10.24	$370.68	090	M	B	C+
49651	Laparo hernia repair recur	8.24	NA	4.40	0.84	NA	NA	13.48	$487.97	090	M	B	C+
49659	Laparo proc, hernia repair	0.00	0.00	0.00	0.00	0.00	$0.00	0.00	$0.00	YYY	M	B	
49900	Repair of abdominal wall	12.28	NA	6.80	1.23	NA	NA	20.31	$735.21	090	M		C+
49905	Omental flap	6.55	NA	2.44	0.61	NA	NA	9.60	$347.51	ZZZ			C
49906	Free omental flap, microvasc	0.00	0.00	0.00	0.00	0.00	$0.00	0.00	$0.00	090	M	A	C+
49999	Abdomen surgery procedure	0.00	0.00	0.00	0.00	0.00	$0.00	0.00	$0.00	YYY	M		C+ T+

Surgery: Urinary system

| 50010 | Exploration of kidney | 10.98 | NA | 7.07 | 0.79 | NA | NA | 18.84 | $681.99 | 090 | M | | C+ |
| 50020 | Renal abscess, open drain | 14.66 | NA | 13.72 | 0.80 | NA | NA | 29.18 | $1,056.29 | 090 | M | A | C+ |

Code	Description									
50021	Renal abscess, percut drain	3.38	NA	10.46	0.15	NA	13.99	$506.43	000	M
50040	Drainage of kidney	14.94	NA	11.56	0.82	NA	27.32	$988.96	090	M	A	C+
50045	Exploration of kidney	15.46	NA	8.55	1.06	NA	25.07	$907.51	090	M		C+
50060	Removal of kidney stone	19.30	NA	10.03	1.14	NA	30.47	$1,102.99	090	M		C+
50065	Incision of kidney	20.79	NA	10.56	1.13	NA	32.48	$1,175.75	090	M		
50070	Incision of kidney	20.32	NA	10.70	1.20	NA	32.22	$1,166.34	090	M		C+
50075	Removal of kidney stone	25.34	NA	12.65	1.51	NA	39.50	$1,429.87	090	M		C+
50080	Removal of kidney stone	14.71	NA	11.03	0.86	NA	26.60	$962.90	090	M	A	
50081	Removal of kidney stone	21.80	NA	13.27	1.30	NA	36.37	$1,316.56	090	M		C+
50100	Revise kidney blood vessels	16.09	NA	9.34	1.64	NA	27.07	$979.91	090	M		C+
50120	Exploration of kidney	15.91	NA	8.93	1.04	NA	25.88	$936.84	090	M		C+
50125	Explore and drain kidney	16.52	NA	9.48	1.07	NA	27.07	$979.91	090	M		C+
50130	Removal of kidney stone	17.29	NA	9.24	1.04	NA	27.57	$998.01	090	M		C+
50135	Exploration of kidney	19.18	NA	9.93	1.18	NA	30.29	$1,096.47	090	M		C+
50200	Biopsy of kidney	2.63	NA	0.96	0.12	NA	3.71	$134.30	000	M	A	
50205	Biopsy of kidney	11.31	NA	6.52	0.94	NA	18.77	$679.46	090	M		C+
50220	Remove kidney, open	17.15	NA	9.29	1.16	NA	27.60	$999.10	090	M		C+
50225	Removal kidney open, complex	20.23	NA	10.30	1.26	NA	31.79	$1,150.77	090	M		C+
50230	Removal kidney open, radical	22.07	NA	10.92	1.35	NA	34.34	$1,243.08	090	M		C
50234	Removal of kidney & ureter	22.40	NA	11.05	1.37	NA	34.82	$1,260.46	090	M		C+
50236	Removal of kidney & ureter	24.86	NA	14.27	1.50	NA	40.63	$1,470.77	090	M		C+
50240	Partial removal of kidney	22.00	NA	13.32	1.36	NA	36.68	$1,327.79	090	M		C+
50280	Removal of kidney lesion	15.67	NA	8.69	0.99	NA	25.35	$917.65	090	M		C+
50290	Removal of kidney lesion	14.73	NA	8.49	1.11	NA	24.33	$880.73	090	M		C+
50320	Removal of donor kidney	22.21	NA	10.98	1.78	NA	34.97	$1,265.89	090	M	B	C+
50340	Removal of kidney	12.15	NA	9.31	1.15	NA	22.61	$818.46	090	M	B	C+
50360	Transplantation of kidney	31.53	NA	17.87	2.97	NA	52.37	$1,895.75	090	M		C	T
50365	Transplantation of kidney	36.81	NA	21.29	3.51	NA	61.61	$2,230.23	090	M	B	C	T

* **M** = multiple surgery adjustment applies
Me = multiple endoscopy rules may apply
B = bilateral surgery adjustment applies
A = assistant-at-surgery restriction

A+ = assistant-at-surgery restriction unless medical necessity established with documentation
C = cosurgeons payable
C+ = cosurgeons payable if medical necessity established with documentation

T = team surgeons permitted
T+ = team surgeons payable if medical necessity established with documentation
$ = indicates services that are not covered by Medicare.

257 CPT five-digit codes, two-digit numeric modifiers, and descriptions only are © 2001 American Medical Association

Medicare RBRVS: The Physicians' Guide

Relative value units

CPT Code and Modifier	Description	Work RVU	Non Facility Practice Expense RVU	Facility Practice Expense RVU	PLI RVU	Total Non Facility RVUs	Medicare Payment Non Facility	Total Facility RVUs	Medicare Payment Facility	Global Period	Payment Policy Indicators*			
50370	Remove transplanted kidney	13.72	NA	9.88	1.26	NA	NA	24.86	$899.91	090	M			C+
50380	Reimplantation of kidney	20.76	NA	13.52	1.80	NA	NA	36.08	$1,306.07	090	M			C+
50390	Drainage of kidney lesion	1.96	NA	0.68	0.09	NA	NA	2.73	$98.82	000	M	B	A	
50392	Insert kidney drain	3.38	NA	1.18	0.15	NA	NA	4.71	$170.50	000	M	B	A	
50393	Insert ureteral tube	4.16	NA	1.44	0.18	NA	NA	5.78	$209.23	000	M	B	A	
50394	Injection for kidney x-ray	0.76	2.60	0.26	0.04	3.40	$123.08	1.06	$38.37	000	M	B	A	
50395	Create passage to kidney	3.38	NA	1.17	0.16	NA	NA	4.71	$170.50	000	M	B	A	
50396	Measure kidney pressure	2.09	NA	0.89	0.10	NA	NA	3.08	$111.49	000	M	B	A+	
50398	Change kidney tube	1.46	1.06	0.51	0.07	2.59	$93.76	2.04	$73.85	000	M	B	A	
50400	Revision of kidney/ureter	19.50	NA	10.06	1.21	NA	NA	30.77	$1,113.85	090	M			C+
50405	Revision of kidney/ureter	23.93	NA	11.84	1.45	NA	NA	37.22	$1,347.33	090	M			C+
50500	Repair of kidney wound	19.57	NA	11.37	1.45	NA	NA	32.39	$1,172.49	090	M			C+
50520	Close kidney-skin fistula	17.23	NA	11.80	1.26	NA	NA	30.29	$1,096.47	090	M			C+
50525	Repair renal-abdomen fistula	22.27	NA	13.30	1.51	NA	NA	37.08	$1,342.27	090	M			C+
50526	Repair renal-abdomen fistula	24.02	NA	14.86	1.62	NA	NA	40.50	$1,466.07	090	M			C+
50540	Revision of horseshoe kidney	19.93	NA	10.42	1.28	NA	NA	31.63	$1,144.98	090	M			C+
50541	Laparo ablate renal cyst	16.00	NA	6.79	0.99	NA	NA	23.78	$860.82	090	M			C+
50544	Laparoscopy, pyeloplasty	22.40	NA	9.04	1.41	NA	NA	32.85	$1,189.14	090	M			C+
50545	Laparo radical nephrectomy	24.00	NA	9.65	1.53	NA	NA	35.18	$1,273.49	090	M	B		C+
50546	Laparoscopic nephrectomy	20.48	NA	8.40	1.37	NA	NA	30.25	$1,095.03	090	M			C+
50547	Laparo removal donor kidney	25.50	NA	11.27	2.04	NA	NA	38.81	$1,404.89	090	M	B		C+
50548	Laparo remove k/ureter	24.40	NA	9.70	1.49	NA	NA	35.59	$1,288.33	090	M			C+
50549	Laparoscope proc, renal	0.00	0.00	0.00	0.00	0.00	$0.00	0.00	$0.00	YYY	M	B		
50551	Kidney endoscopy	5.60	4.93	1.90	0.33	10.86	$393.12	7.83	$283.44	000	M	B	A+	
50553	Kidney endoscopy	5.99	16.25	2.05	0.35	22.59	$817.74	8.39	$303.71	000	M	B	A	
50555	Kidney endoscopy & biopsy	6.53	20.11	2.25	0.38	27.02	$978.10	9.16	$331.58	000	Me	B	A+	
50557	Kidney endoscopy & treatment	6.62	20.23	2.25	0.39	27.24	$986.07	9.26	$335.20	000	Me	B	A+	

Code	Description											
50559	Renal endoscopy/radiotracer	6.78	NA	2.42	0.27	NA	NA	9.47	$342.81	000	Me	B	A+
50561	Kidney endoscopy & treatment	7.59	18.31	2.58	0.44	26.34	$953.49	10.61	$384.07	000	Me	B	A+
50570	Kidney endoscopy	9.54	NA	3.24	0.56	NA	NA	13.34	$482.90	000	M	B	A+
50572	Kidney endoscopy	10.35	NA	3.52	0.64	NA	NA	14.51	$525.25	000	Me	B	A+
50574	Kidney endoscopy & biopsy	11.02	NA	3.87	0.65	NA	NA	15.54	$562.54	000	Me	B	A+
50575	Kidney endoscopy	13.98	NA	4.73	0.84	NA	NA	19.55	$707.69	000	Me	B	A
50576	Kidney endoscopy & treatment	10.99	NA	3.74	0.66	NA	NA	15.39	$557.11	000	Me	B	A+
50578	Renal endoscopy/radiotracer	11.35	NA	4.01	0.67	NA	NA	16.03	$580.27	000	Me	B	A+
50580	Kidney endoscopy & treatment	11.86	NA	4.03	0.70	NA	NA	16.59	$600.54	000	Me	B	A+
50590	Fragmenting of kidney stone	9.09	10.78	5.35	0.54	20.41	$738.83	14.98	$542.26	090	M	B	A
50600	Exploration of ureter	15.84	NA	9.07	0.99	NA	NA	25.90	$937.56	090	M	B	C+
50605	Insert ureteral support	15.46	NA	8.88	1.13	NA	NA	25.47	$921.99	090	M	B	C+
50610	Removal of ureter stone	15.92	NA	9.09	1.08	NA	NA	26.09	$944.44	090	M	B	C+
50620	Removal of ureter stone	15.16	NA	8.55	0.91	NA	NA	24.62	$891.22	090	M	B	C+
50630	Removal of ureter stone	14.94	NA	8.48	0.90	NA	NA	24.32	$880.36	090	M	B	C+
50650	Removal of ureter	17.41	NA	9.71	1.07	NA	NA	28.19	$1,020.46	090	M		C+
50660	Removal of ureter	19.55	NA	10.43	1.19	NA	NA	31.17	$1,128.33	090	M		C+
50684	Injection for ureter x-ray	0.76	15.02	0.26	0.04	15.82	$572.67	1.06	$38.37	000	M	B	A
50686	Measure ureter pressure	1.51	5.08	0.65	0.09	6.68	$241.81	2.25	$81.45	000	M		A+
50688	Change of ureter tube	1.17	NA	1.76	0.06	NA	NA	2.99	$108.24	010	M		A
50690	Injection for ureter x-ray	1.16	15.40	0.40	0.06	16.62	$601.63	1.62	$58.64	000	M		A
50700	Revision of ureter	15.21	NA	9.09	0.86	NA	NA	25.16	$910.77	090	M		C+
50715	Release of ureter	18.90	NA	12.37	1.68	NA	NA	32.95	$1,192.76	090	M	B	C+
50722	Release of ureter	16.35	NA	10.42	1.41	NA	NA	28.18	$1,020.09	090	M		C+
50725	Release/revise ureter	18.49	NA	10.61	1.44	NA	NA	30.54	$1,105.52	090	M		C+
50727	Revise ureter	8.18	NA	6.54	0.51	NA	NA	15.23	$551.31	090	M		C
50728	Revise ureter	12.02	NA	8.18	0.88	NA	NA	21.08	$763.08	090	M		C
50740	Fusion of ureter & kidney	18.42	NA	9.66	1.49	NA	NA	29.57	$1,070.41	090	M		C+

* **M** = multiple surgery adjustment applies
   Me = multiple endoscopy rules may apply
   B = bilateral surgery adjustment applies
   A = assistant-at-surgery restriction

A+ = assistant-at-surgery restriction unless medical necessity established with documentation
C = cosurgeons payable
C+ = cosurgeons payable if medical necessity established with documentation

T = team surgeons permitted
T+ = team surgeons payable if medical necessity established with documentation
$ = indicates services that are not covered by Medicare.

259 CPT five-digit codes, two-digit numeric modifiers, and descriptions only are © 2001 American Medical Association

Medicare RBRVS: The Physicians' Guide

Relative value units

CPT Code and Modifier	Description	Work RVU	Non Facility Practice Expense RVU	Facility Practice Expense RVU	PLI RVU	Total Non Facility RVUs	Medicare Payment Non Facility	Total Facility RVUs	Medicare Payment Facility	Global Period	Payment Policy Indicators*
50750	Fusion of ureter & kidney	19.51	NA	10.48	1.24	NA	NA	31.23	$1,130.50	090	M C+
50760	Fusion of ureters	18.42	NA	10.11	1.25	NA	NA	29.78	$1,078.01	090	M C+
50770	Splicing of ureters	19.51	NA	10.43	1.25	NA	NA	31.19	$1,129.05	090	M C+
50780	Reimplant ureter in bladder	18.36	NA	10.01	1.20	NA	NA	29.57	$1,070.41	090	M B C+
50782	Reimplant ureter in bladder	19.54	NA	11.91	1.13	NA	NA	32.58	$1,179.37	090	M B C
50783	Reimplant ureter in bladder	20.55	NA	11.22	1.35	NA	NA	33.12	$1,198.92	090	M B C
50785	Reimplant ureter in bladder	20.52	NA	10.83	1.30	NA	NA	32.65	$1,181.90	090	M B C+
50800	Implant ureter in bowel	14.52	NA	10.02	0.92	NA	NA	25.46	$921.63	090	M C+
50810	Fusion of ureter & bowel	20.05	NA	12.23	1.78	NA	NA	34.06	$1,232.94	090	M B C+
50815	Urine shunt to intestine	19.93	NA	11.71	1.31	NA	NA	32.95	$1,192.76	090	M B C+
50820	Construct bowel bladder	21.89	NA	12.38	1.38	NA	NA	35.65	$1,290.50	090	M B C+
50825	Construct bowel bladder	28.18	NA	15.30	1.81	NA	NA	45.29	$1,639.46	090	M C+
50830	Revise urine flow	31.28	NA	15.96	2.20	NA	NA	49.44	$1,789.69	090	M C+
50840	Replace ureter by bowel	20.00	NA	11.83	1.26	NA	NA	33.09	$1,197.83	090	M B C+
50845	Appendico-vesicostomy	20.89	NA	10.20	1.26	NA	NA	32.35	$1,171.04	090	M C+
50860	Transplant ureter to skin	15.36	NA	8.93	1.01	NA	NA	25.30	$915.84	090	M B C+
50900	Repair of ureter	13.62	NA	8.08	0.98	NA	NA	22.68	$821.00	090	M C+
50920	Closure ureter/skin fistula	14.33	NA	8.37	0.84	NA	NA	23.54	$852.13	090	M C+
50930	Closure ureter/bowel fistula	18.72	NA	10.80	1.57	NA	NA	31.09	$1,125.43	090	M C+
50940	Release of ureter	14.51	NA	8.44	1.04	NA	NA	23.99	$868.42	090	M B C+
50945	Laparoscopy ureterolithotomy	17.00	NA	7.42	1.15	NA	NA	25.57	$925.61	090	M B C+
50947	Laparo new ureter/bladder	24.50	NA	11.74	1.99	NA	NA	38.23	$1,383.90	090	M B C+
50948	Laparo new ureter/bladder	22.50	NA	10.61	1.83	NA	NA	34.94	$1,264.80	090	M B C+
50949	Laparoscope proc, ureter	0.00	0.00	0.00	0.00	0.00	$0.00	0.00	$0.00	YYY	M B C+
50951	Endoscopy of ureter	5.84	5.28	1.98	0.35	11.47	$415.20	8.17	$295.75	000	M B A+
50953	Endoscopy of ureter	6.24	16.55	2.12	0.37	23.16	$838.37	8.73	$316.02	000	Me B A+
50955	Ureter endoscopy & biopsy	6.75	21.11	2.38	0.38	28.24	$1,022.27	9.51	$344.25	000	Me B A+

Code	Description										
50957	Ureter endoscopy & treatment	6.79	19.64	2.28	0.40	26.83	$971.22	9.47	$342.81	000	Me B A+
50959	Ureter endoscopy & tracer	4.40	NA	1.58	0.18	NA	NA	6.16	$222.99	000	Me B A+
50961	Ureter endoscopy & treatment	6.05	23.38	2.04	0.35	29.78	$1,078.01	8.44	$305.52	000	Me B A+
50970	Ureter endoscopy	7.14	NA	2.43	0.43	NA	NA	10.00	$361.99	000	M B A+
50972	Ureter endoscopy & catheter	6.89	NA	2.52	0.39	NA	NA	9.80	$354.75	000	M B A+
50974	Ureter endoscopy & biopsy	9.17	NA	3.16	0.53	NA	NA	12.86	$465.52	000	Me B A+
50976	Ureter endoscopy & treatment	9.04	NA	3.09	0.53	NA	NA	12.66	$458.28	000	Me B A+
50978	Ureter endoscopy & tracer	5.10	NA	1.88	0.30	NA	NA	7.28	$263.53	000	M B A+
50980	Ureter endoscopy & treatment	6.85	NA	2.34	0.41	NA	NA	9.60	$347.51	000	M B A+
51000	Drainage of bladder	0.78	2.03	0.25	0.05	2.86	$103.53	1.08	$39.10	000	M A
51005	Drainage of bladder	1.02	3.37	0.35	0.08	4.47	$161.81	1.45	$52.49	000	M A
51010	Drainage of bladder	3.53	4.42	2.37	0.23	8.18	$296.11	6.13	$221.90	010	M A
51020	Incise & treat bladder	6.71	NA	5.72	0.42	NA	NA	12.85	$465.16	090	M C+
51030	Incise & treat bladder	6.77	NA	6.01	0.42	NA	NA	13.20	$477.83	090	M A+
51040	Incise & drain bladder	4.40	NA	4.47	0.27	NA	NA	9.14	$330.86	090	M C+
51045	Incise bladder/drain ureter	6.77	NA	6.01	0.47	NA	NA	13.25	$479.64	090	M
51050	Removal of bladder stone	6.92	NA	5.27	0.42	NA	NA	12.61	$456.47	090	M C+
51060	Removal of ureter stone	8.85	NA	6.53	0.54	NA	NA	15.92	$576.29	090	M C+
51065	Remove ureter calculus	8.85	NA	6.06	0.53	NA	NA	15.44	$558.92	090	M A+
51080	Drainage of bladder abscess	5.96	NA	5.67	0.35	NA	NA	11.98	$433.67	090	M C+
51500	Removal of bladder cyst	10.14	NA	6.13	0.88	NA	NA	17.15	$620.82	090	M C+
51520	Removal of bladder lesion	9.29	NA	6.66	0.58	NA	NA	16.53	$598.37	090	M C+
51525	Removal of bladder lesion	13.97	NA	8.15	0.85	NA	NA	22.97	$831.50	090	M C+
51530	Removal of bladder lesion	12.38	NA	7.81	0.82	NA	NA	21.01	$760.55	090	M C+
51535	Repair of ureter lesion	12.57	NA	8.23	0.90	NA	NA	21.70	$785.52	090	M B C+
51550	Partial removal of bladder	15.66	NA	8.68	1.05	NA	NA	25.39	$919.10	090	M C+
51555	Partial removal of bladder	21.23	NA	11.00	1.37	NA	NA	33.60	$1,216.29	090	M C+
51565	Revise bladder & ureter(s)	21.62	NA	11.62	1.40	NA	NA	34.64	$1,253.94	090	M C+

* **M** = multiple surgery adjustment applies
Me = multiple endoscopy rules may apply
B = bilateral surgery adjustment applies
A = assistant-at-surgery restriction

A+ = assistant-at-surgery restriction unless medical necessity established with documentation
C = cosurgeons payable
C+ = cosurgeons payable if medical necessity established with documentation

T = team surgeons permitted
T+ = team surgeons payable if medical necessity established with documentation
S = indicates services that are not covered by Medicare.

CPT five-digit codes, two-digit numeric modifiers, and descriptions only are © 2001 American Medical Association

Medicare RBRVS: The Physicians' Guide

Relative value units

CPT Code and Modifier	Description	Work RVU	Non Facility Practice Expense RVU	Facility Practice Expense RVU	PLI RVU	Total Non Facility RVUs	Medicare Payment Non Facility	Total Facility RVUs	Medicare Payment Facility	Global Period	Payment Policy Indicators*	
51570	Removal of bladder	24.24	NA	12.60	1.59	NA	NA	38.43	$1,391.14	090	M	C+
51575	Removal of bladder & nodes	30.45	NA	15.35	1.88	NA	NA	47.68	$1,725.98	090	M	C+
51580	Remove bladder/revise tract	31.08	NA	16.01	1.94	NA	NA	49.03	$1,774.85	090	M	C+
51585	Removal of bladder & nodes	35.23	NA	17.34	2.18	NA	NA	54.75	$1,981.91	090	M	C+
51590	Remove bladder/revise tract	32.66	NA	16.01	2.01	NA	NA	50.68	$1,834.58	090	M	C+
51595	Remove bladder/revise tract	37.14	NA	17.55	2.23	NA	NA	56.92	$2,060.46	090	M	C+
51596	Remove bladder/create pouch	39.52	NA	18.94	2.39	NA	NA	60.85	$2,202.72	090	M	C+
51597	Removal of pelvic structures	38.35	NA	18.06	2.49	NA	NA	58.90	$2,132.13	090	M	C+
51600	Injection for bladder x-ray	0.88	5.51	0.30	0.04	6.43	$232.76	1.22	$44.16	000	M	A
51605	Preparation for bladder xray	0.64	16.73	0.22	0.04	17.41	$630.23	0.90	$32.58	000	M	A
51610	Injection for bladder x-ray	1.05	16.20	0.36	0.05	17.30	$626.25	1.46	$52.85	000	M	A
51700	Irrigation of bladder	0.88	1.32	0.30	0.05	2.25	$81.45	1.23	$44.53	000	M	A
51705	Change of bladder tube	1.02	2.15	0.65	0.06	3.23	$116.92	1.73	$62.62	010	M	A
51710	Change of bladder tube	1.49	5.11	1.47	0.09	6.69	$242.17	3.05	$110.41	010	M	A
51715	Endoscopic injection/implant	3.74	4.44	1.29	0.24	8.42	$304.80	5.27	$190.77	000	M	A+
51720	Treatment of bladder lesion	1.96	1.68	0.74	0.12	3.76	$136.11	2.82	$102.08	000	M	A
51725	Simple cystometrogram	1.51	5.92	5.92	0.13	7.56	$273.67	7.56	$273.67	000	M	A+
51725-26	Simple cystometrogram	1.51	0.52	0.52	0.10	2.13	$77.10	2.13	$77.10	000	M	A+
51725-TC	Simple cystometrogram	0.00	5.40	5.40	0.03	5.43	$196.56	5.43	$196.56	000		A+
51726	Complex cystometrogram	1.71	4.65	4.65	0.15	6.51	$235.66	6.51	$235.66	000	M	A
51726-26	Complex cystometrogram	1.71	0.59	0.59	0.11	2.41	$87.24	2.41	$87.24	000	M	A
51726-TC	Complex cystometrogram	0.00	4.06	4.06	0.04	4.10	$148.42	4.10	$148.42	000		A
51736	Urine flow measurement	0.61	1.07	1.07	0.05	1.73	$62.62	1.73	$62.62	000	M	A+
51736-26	Urine flow measurement	0.61	0.21	0.21	0.04	0.86	$31.13	0.86	$31.13	000	M	A
51736-TC	Urine flow measurement	0.00	0.86	0.86	0.01	0.87	$31.49	0.87	$31.49	000		A+
51741	Electro-uroflowmetry, first	1.14	1.93	1.93	0.09	3.16	$114.39	3.16	$114.39	000	M	A
51741-26	Electro-uroflowmetry, first	1.14	0.40	0.40	0.07	1.61	$58.28	1.61	$58.28	000	M	A

Code	Description	col1	col2	col3	col4	col5	col6	col7	col8	col9	col10
51741-TC	Electro-uroflowmetry, first	0.00	1.53	1.53	0.02	1.55	$56.11	1.55	$56.11	000	A
51772	Urethra pressure profile	1.61	4.73	4.73	0.16	6.50	$235.29	6.50	$235.29	000	M	A+
51772-26	Urethra pressure profile	1.61	0.59	0.59	0.12	2.32	$83.98	2.32	$83.98	000	M	A+
51772-TC	Urethra pressure profile	0.00	4.14	4.14	0.04	4.18	$151.31	4.18	$151.31	000		A+
51784	Anal/urinary muscle study	1.53	3.36	3.36	0.13	5.02	$181.72	5.02	$181.72	000	M	A
51784-26	Anal/urinary muscle study	1.53	0.53	0.53	0.10	2.16	$78.19	2.16	$78.19	000	M	A
51784-TC	Anal/urinary muscle study	0.00	2.83	2.83	0.03	2.86	$103.53	2.86	$103.53	000		A
51785	Anal/urinary muscle study	1.53	3.46	3.46	0.12	5.11	$184.98	5.11	$184.98	000	M	A+
51785-26	Anal/urinary muscle study	1.53	0.53	0.53	0.09	2.15	$77.83	2.15	$77.83	000	M	A+
51785-TC	Anal/urinary muscle study	0.00	2.93	2.93	0.03	2.96	$107.15	2.96	$107.15	000		A+
51792	Urinary reflex study	1.10	3.33	3.33	0.20	4.63	$167.60	4.63	$167.60	000	M	A+
51792-26	Urinary reflex study	1.10	0.43	0.43	0.09	1.62	$58.64	1.62	$58.64	000	M	A+
51792-TC	Urinary reflex study	0.00	2.90	2.90	0.11	3.01	$108.96	3.01	$108.96	000		A+
51795	Urine voiding pressure study	1.53	4.84	4.84	0.18	6.55	$237.10	6.55	$237.10	000	M	A+
51795-26	Urine voiding pressure study	1.53	0.53	0.53	0.10	2.16	$78.19	2.16	$78.19	000	M	A+
51795-TC	Urine voiding pressure study	0.00	4.31	4.31	0.08	4.39	$158.91	4.39	$158.91	000		A+
51797	Intraabdominal pressure test	1.60	4.87	4.87	0.14	6.61	$239.28	6.61	$239.28	000	M	A+
51797-26	Intraabdominal pressure test	1.60	0.56	0.56	0.10	2.26	$81.81	2.26	$81.81	000	M	A+
51797-TC	Intraabdominal pressure test	0.00	4.31	4.31	0.04	4.35	$157.47	4.35	$157.47	000		A+
51800	Revision of bladder/urethra	17.42	NA	9.59	1.17	28.18	$1,020.09	NA	NA	090	M	C+
51820	Revision of urinary tract	17.89	NA	10.91	1.45	30.25	$1,095.03	NA	NA	090	M	C+
51840	Attach bladder/urethra	10.71	NA	6.88	0.87	18.46	$668.24	NA	NA	090	M	C+
51841	Attach bladder/urethra	13.03	NA	8.57	1.04	22.64	$819.55	NA	NA	090	M	C+
51845	Repair bladder neck	9.73	NA	6.90	0.62	17.25	$624.44	NA	NA	090	M	C+
51860	Repair of bladder wound	12.02	NA	7.90	0.89	20.81	$753.31	NA	NA	090	M	C+
51865	Repair of bladder wound	15.04	NA	8.93	1.01	24.98	$904.26	NA	NA	090	M	C+
51880	Repair of bladder opening	7.66	NA	5.98	0.54	14.18	$513.30	NA	NA	090	M	C+
51900	Repair bladder/vagina lesion	12.97	NA	8.29	0.87	22.13	$801.09	NA	NA	090	M	C+

* **M** = multiple surgery adjustment applies
Me = multiple endoscopy rules may apply
B = bilateral surgery adjustment applies
A = assistant-at-surgery restriction

A+ = assistant-at-surgery restriction unless medical necessity established with documentation
C = cosurgeons payable
C+ = cosurgeons payable if medical necessity established with documentation

T = team surgeons permitted
T+ = team surgeons payable if medical necessity established with documentation
$ = indicates services that are not covered by Medicare.

263 CPT five-digit codes, two-digit numeric modifiers, and descriptions only are © 2001 American Medical Association

Medicare RBRVS: The Physicians' Guide

Relative value units

CPT Code and Modifier	Description	Work RVU	Non Facility Practice Expense RVU	Facility Practice Expense RVU	PLI RVU	Total Non Facility RVUs	Medicare Payment Non Facility	Total Facility RVUs	Medicare Payment Facility	Global Period	Payment Policy Indicators*		
51920	Close bladder-uterus fistula	11.81	NA	7.65	0.86	NA	NA	20.32	$735.57	090	M	C+	
51925	Hysterectomy/bladder repair	15.58	NA	9.65	1.48	NA	NA	26.71	$966.88	090	M	C+	
51940	Correction of bladder defect	28.43	NA	16.41	1.97	NA	NA	46.81	$1,694.48	090	M	C+	
51960	Revision of bladder & bowel	23.01	NA	13.39	1.41	NA	NA	37.81	$1,368.69	090	M	C+	
51980	Construct bladder opening	11.36	NA	7.30	0.74	NA	NA	19.40	$702.26	090	M	C+	
51990	Laparo urethral suspension	12.50	NA	6.79	1.02	NA	NA	20.31	$735.21	090	M	C+	
51992	Laparo sling operation	14.01	NA	6.81	0.93	NA	NA	21.75	$787.33	090	M	C+	
52000	Cystoscopy	2.01	3.45	0.69	0.12	5.58	$201.99	2.82	$102.08	000	M	A	
52001	Cystoscopy, removal of clots	2.37	NA	0.98	0.32	NA	NA	3.67	$132.85	000	M	A	
52005	Cystoscopy & ureter catheter	2.37	13.40	0.91	0.15	15.92	$576.29	3.43	$124.16	000	M	A	
52007	Cystoscopy and biopsy	3.02	NA	1.02	0.18	NA	NA	4.22	$152.76	000	Me	A	B
52010	Cystoscopy & duct catheter	3.02	5.91	1.02	0.18	9.11	$329.77	4.22	$152.76	000	Me	A	
52204	Cystoscopy	2.37	6.17	0.80	0.15	8.69	$314.57	3.32	$120.18	000	Me	A	
52214	Cystoscopy and treatment	3.71	6.53	1.26	0.22	10.46	$378.64	5.19	$187.87	000	Me	A	
52224	Cystoscopy and treatment	3.14	6.41	1.07	0.18	9.73	$352.22	4.39	$158.91	000	Me	A	
52234	Cystoscopy and treatment	4.63	NA	1.68	0.27	NA	NA	6.58	$238.19	000	M	A	
52235	Cystoscopy and treatment	5.45	NA	1.97	0.32	NA	NA	7.74	$280.18	000	M	A	
52240	Cystoscopy and treatment	9.72	NA	3.43	0.58	NA	NA	13.73	$497.02	000	M	A	
52250	Cystoscopy and radiotracer	4.50	NA	1.53	0.27	NA	NA	6.30	$228.05	000	Me	A	
52260	Cystoscopy and treatment	3.92	NA	1.34	0.23	NA	NA	5.49	$198.73	000	Me	A	
52265	Cystoscopy and treatment	2.94	3.77	1.00	0.18	6.89	$249.41	4.12	$149.14	000	Me	A	
52270	Cystoscopy & revise urethra	3.37	6.88	1.14	0.20	10.45	$378.28	4.71	$170.50	000	Me	A	
52275	Cystoscopy & revise urethra	4.70	7.42	1.59	0.28	12.40	$448.87	6.57	$237.83	000	Me	A	
52276	Cystoscopy and treatment	5.00	7.55	1.70	0.30	12.85	$465.16	7.00	$253.39	000	Me	A	
52277	Cystoscopy and treatment	6.17	NA	2.12	0.38	NA	NA	8.67	$313.85	000	Me	A+	
52281	Cystoscopy and treatment	2.80	14.54	1.08	0.17	17.51	$633.85	4.05	$146.61	000	Me	A	
52282	Cystoscopy, implant stent	6.40	15.36	2.18	0.38	22.14	$801.45	8.96	$324.34	000	Me	A	

Code	Description										
52283	Cystoscopy and treatment	3.74	6.58	1.27	0.22	10.54	$381.54	5.23	$189.32	000	Me	A
52285	Cystoscopy and treatment	3.61	7.06	1.23	0.22	10.89	$394.21	5.06	$183.17	000	Me	A
52290	Cystoscopy and treatment	4.59	NA	1.56	0.27	NA	NA	6.42	$232.40	000	Me	A
52300	Cystoscopy and treatment	5.31	NA	1.80	0.32	NA	NA	7.43	$268.96	000	Me	A+
52301	Cystoscopy and treatment	5.51	NA	1.82	0.39	NA	NA	7.72	$279.46	000	Me	A+
52305	Cystoscopy and treatment	5.31	NA	1.80	0.31	NA	NA	7.42	$268.60	000	Me	A
52310	Cystoscopy and treatment	2.81	3.85	1.02	0.17	6.83	$247.24	4.00	$144.80	000	Me	A
52315	Cystoscopy and treatment	5.21	16.43	1.76	0.31	21.95	$794.57	7.28	$263.53	000	Me	A
52317	Remove bladder stone	6.72	26.09	2.28	0.40	33.21	$1,202.18	9.40	$340.27	000	Me	A
52318	Remove bladder stone	9.19	NA	3.11	0.54	NA	NA	12.84	$464.80	000	Me	A
52320	Cystoscopy and treatment	4.70	NA	1.59	0.28	NA	NA	6.57	$237.83	000	Me	B	A
52325	Cystoscopy, stone removal	6.16	NA	2.08	0.37	NA	NA	8.61	$311.68	000	Me	B	A
52327	Cystoscopy, inject material	5.19	NA	1.77	0.32	NA	NA	7.28	$263.53	000	Me	B	A
52330	Cystoscopy and treatment	5.04	20.79	1.71	0.30	26.13	$945.89	7.05	$255.20	000	Me	B	A
52332	Cystoscopy and treatment	2.83	18.84	1.07	0.17	21.84	$790.59	4.07	$147.33	000	Me	B	A
52334	Create passage to kidney	4.83	NA	1.63	0.28	NA	NA	6.74	$243.98	000	Me	B	A
52341	Cysto w/ureter stricture tx	6.00	NA	2.40	0.37	NA	NA	8.77	$317.47	000	Me	B	A
52342	Cysto w/up stricture tx	6.50	NA	2.59	0.40	NA	NA	9.49	$343.53	000	Me	B	A
52343	Cysto w/renal stricture tx	7.20	NA	2.87	0.44	NA	NA	10.51	$380.45	000	Me	B	A
52344	Cysto/uretero, stone remove	7.70	NA	3.07	0.47	NA	NA	11.24	$406.88	000	Me	B	A
52345	Cysto/uretero w/up stricture	8.20	NA	3.27	0.50	NA	NA	11.97	$433.30	000	Me	B	A+
52346	Cystouretero w/renal strict	9.23	NA	3.68	0.57	NA	NA	13.48	$487.97	000	Me	A+
52347	Cystoscopy, resect ducts	5.28	NA	2.14	0.33	NA	NA	7.75	$280.54	000	Me	A+
52351	Cystouretero & or pyeloscope	5.86	NA	1.99	0.36	NA	NA	8.21	$297.20	000	M	A
52352	Cystouretero w/stone remove	6.88	NA	2.33	0.42	NA	NA	9.63	$348.60	000	Me	B	A
52353	Cystouretero w/lithotripsy	7.97	NA	2.69	0.49	NA	NA	11.15	$403.62	000	Me	B	A
52354	Cystouretero w/biopsy	7.34	NA	2.49	0.45	NA	NA	10.28	$372.13	000	Me	B	A
52355	Cystouretero w/excise tumor	8.82	NA	2.99	0.55	NA	NA	12.36	$447.42	000	Me	B	A

* **M** = multiple surgery adjustment applies
Me = multiple endoscopy rules may apply
B = bilateral surgery adjustment applies
A = assistant-at-surgery restriction

A+ = assistant-at-surgery restriction unless medical necessity established with documentation
C = cosurgeons payable
C+ = cosurgeons payable if medical necessity established with documentation

T = team surgeons permitted
T+ = team surgeons payable if medical necessity established with documentation
$ = indicates services that are not covered by Medicare.

CPT five-digit codes, two-digit numeric modifiers, and descriptions only are © 2001 American Medical Association

Medicare RBRVS: The Physicians' Guide

Relative value units

CPT Code and Modifier	Description	Work RVU	Non Facility Practice Expense RVU	Facility Practice Expense RVU	PLI RVU	Total Non Facility RVUs	Medicare Payment Non Facility	Total Facility RVUs	Medicare Payment Facility	Global Period	Payment Policy Indicators*
52400	Cystouretero w/congen repr	9.68	NA	5.75	0.60	NA	NA	16.03	$580.27	090	M A
52450	Incision of prostate	7.64	NA	6.56	0.46	NA	NA	14.66	$530.68	090	M A
52500	Revision of bladder neck	8.47	NA	6.81	0.50	NA	NA	15.78	$571.22	090	M A
52510	Dilation prostatic urethra	6.72	NA	5.80	0.40	NA	NA	12.92	$467.69	090	M A
52601	Prostatectomy (TURP)	12.37	NA	8.16	0.74	NA	NA	21.27	$769.96	090	M A
52606	Control postop bleeding	8.13	NA	6.27	0.49	NA	NA	14.89	$539.01	090	M A
52612	Prostatectomy, first stage	7.98	NA	6.72	0.48	NA	NA	15.18	$549.50	090	M A
52614	Prostatectomy, second stage	6.84	NA	6.30	0.41	NA	NA	13.55	$490.50	090	M A
52620	Remove residual prostate	6.61	NA	6.22	0.39	NA	NA	13.22	$478.55	090	M A
52630	Remove prostate regrowth	7.26	NA	6.44	0.43	NA	NA	14.13	$511.49	090	M A
52640	Relieve bladder contracture	6.62	NA	5.73	0.39	NA	NA	12.74	$461.18	090	M A
52647	Laser surgery of prostate	10.36	59.33	4.85	0.61	70.30	$2,544.80	15.82	$572.67	090	M A
52648	Laser surgery of prostate	11.21	NA	7.63	0.66	NA	NA	19.50	$705.88	090	M A
52700	Drainage of prostate abscess	6.80	NA	6.32	0.41	NA	NA	13.53	$489.78	090	M A+
53000	Incision of urethra	2.28	7.47	2.63	0.13	9.88	$357.65	5.04	$182.44	010	M A
53010	Incision of urethra	3.64	NA	4.12	0.20	NA	NA	7.96	$288.15	090	M A
53020	Incision of urethra	1.77	4.43	0.67	0.11	6.31	$228.42	2.55	$92.31	000	M A
53025	Incision of urethra	1.13	4.81	0.45	0.07	6.01	$217.56	1.65	$59.73	000	M A+
53040	Drainage of urethra abscess	6.40	14.74	8.33	0.41	21.55	$780.09	15.14	$548.06	090	M A+
53060	Drainage of urethra abscess	2.63	6.21	2.91	0.23	9.07	$328.33	5.77	$208.87	010	M A
53080	Drainage of urinary leakage	6.29	NA	8.37	0.42	NA	NA	15.08	$545.88	090	M A
53085	Drainage of urinary leakage	10.27	NA	10.29	0.67	NA	NA	21.23	$768.51	090	M C+
53200	Biopsy of urethra	2.59	5.63	0.97	0.17	8.39	$303.71	3.73	$135.02	000	M A
53210	Removal of urethra	12.57	NA	8.00	0.81	NA	NA	21.38	$773.94	090	M C+
53215	Removal of urethra	15.58	NA	8.81	0.93	NA	NA	25.32	$916.56	090	M C+
53220	Treatment of urethra lesion	7.00	NA	5.71	0.44	NA	NA	13.15	$476.02	090	M A+
53230	Removal of urethra lesion	9.58	NA	6.36	0.60	NA	NA	16.54	$598.73	090	M C+

Code	Description									
53235	Removal of urethra lesion	10.14	NA	6.49	0.60	NA	17.23	$623.71	090	M	C+
53240	Surgery for urethra pouch	6.45	NA	5.32	0.42	NA	12.19	$441.27	090	M	A
53250	Removal of urethra gland	5.89	NA	4.74	0.35	NA	10.98	$397.47	090	M	A
53260	Treatment of urethra lesion	2.98	6.11	2.44	0.23	9.32	5.65	$204.53	010	M	A
53265	Treatment of urethra lesion	3.12	6.60	2.42	0.20	9.92	5.74	$207.78	010	M	A
53270	Removal of urethra gland	3.09	7.03	2.83	0.21	10.33	6.13	$221.90	010	M	A
53275	Repair of urethra defect	4.53	NA	3.43	0.28	NA	8.24	$298.28	010	M	A
53400	Revise urethra, stage 1	12.77	NA	8.31	0.85	NA	21.93	$793.85	090	M	C+
53405	Revise urethra, stage 2	14.48	NA	8.61	0.91	NA	24.00	$868.78	090	M	C+
53410	Reconstruction of urethra	16.44	NA	9.21	0.99	NA	26.64	$964.35	090	M	C+
53415	Reconstruction of urethra	19.41	NA	10.16	1.16	NA	30.73	$1,112.40	090	M	C+
53420	Reconstruct urethra, stage 1	14.08	NA	8.82	0.90	NA	23.80	$861.54	090	M	A
53425	Reconstruct urethra, stage 2	15.98	NA	9.02	0.97	NA	25.97	$940.09	090	M	C+
53430	Reconstruction of urethra	16.34	NA	9.34	1.01	NA	26.69	$966.16	090	M	C+
53431	Reconstruct urethra/bladder	19.89	7.94	7.94	1.25	29.08	29.08	$1,052.67	090	M	C+
53440	Correct bladder function	12.34	NA	8.09	0.73	NA	21.16	$765.98	090	M	C+
53442	Remove perineal prosthesis	8.27	NA	6.08	0.55	NA	14.90	$539.37	090	M	
53444	Insert tandem cuff	13.40	NA	6.66	0.79	NA	20.85	$754.75	090	M	C+
53445	Insert uro/ves nck sphincter	14.06	NA	8.72	0.84	NA	23.62	$855.03	090	M	C+
53446	Remove uro sphincter	10.23	NA	8.46	0.61	NA	19.30	$698.64	090	M	C+
53447	Remove/replace ur sphincter	13.49	NA	7.90	0.79	NA	22.18	$802.90	090	M	C+
53448	Remov/replc ur sphinctr comp	21.15	NA	12.35	1.27	NA	34.77	$1,258.65	090	M	C+
53449	Repair uro sphincter	9.70	NA	6.73	0.57	NA	17.00	$615.39	090	M	C+
53450	Revision of urethra	6.14	NA	5.16	0.37	NA	11.67	$422.44	090	M	A
53460	Revision of urethra	7.12	NA	5.50	0.43	NA	13.05	$472.40	090	M	A+
53502	Repair of urethra injury	7.63	NA	5.80	0.50	NA	13.93	$504.25	090	M	A
53505	Repair of urethra injury	7.63	NA	5.62	0.46	NA	13.71	$496.29	090	M	
53510	Repair of urethra injury	10.11	NA	6.58	0.60	NA	17.29	$625.88	090	M	C+

*   **M** = multiple surgery adjustment applies
    Me = multiple endoscopy rules may apply
    B = bilateral surgery adjustment applies
    A = assistant-at-surgery restriction

    A+ = assistant-at-surgery restriction unless medical necessity established with documentation
    C = cosurgeons payable
    C+ = cosurgeons payable if medical necessity established with documentation

    T = team surgeons permitted
    T+ = team surgeons payable if medical necessity established with documentation
    $ = indicates services that are not covered by Medicare.

CPT five-digit codes, two-digit numeric modifiers, and descriptions only are © 2001 American Medical Association

Medicare RBRVS: The Physicians' Guide

Relative value units

CPT Code and Modifier	Description	Work RVU	Non Facility Practice Expense RVU	Facility Practice Expense RVU	PLI RVU	Total Non Facility RVUs	Medicare Payment Non Facility	Total Facility RVUs	Medicare Payment Facility	Global Period	Payment Policy Indicators*
53515	Repair of urethra injury	13.31	NA	7.81	0.83	NA	NA	21.95	$794.57	090	M C+
53520	Repair of urethra defect	8.68	NA	6.12	0.53	NA	NA	15.33	$554.93	090	M A
53600	Dilate urethra stricture	1.21	1.19	0.46	0.07	2.47	$89.41	1.74	$62.99	000	M A
53601	Dilate urethra stricture	0.98	1.31	0.40	0.06	2.35	$85.07	1.44	$52.13	000	M A
53605	Dilate urethra stricture	1.28	NA	0.44	0.08	NA	NA	1.80	$65.16	000	M A
53620	Dilate urethra stricture	1.62	1.91	0.63	0.10	3.63	$131.40	2.35	$85.07	000	M A
53621	Dilate urethra stricture	1.35	2.00	0.52	0.08	3.43	$124.16	1.95	$70.59	000	M A
53660	Dilation of urethra	0.71	1.22	0.33	0.04	1.97	$71.31	1.08	$39.10	000	M A
53661	Dilation of urethra	0.72	1.21	0.31	0.04	1.97	$71.31	1.07	$38.73	000	M A
53665	Dilation of urethra	0.76	NA	0.27	0.05	NA	NA	1.08	$39.10	000	M A
53670	Insert urinary catheter	0.50	1.74	0.18	0.03	2.27	$82.17	0.71	$25.70	000	M A
53675	Insert urinary catheter	1.47	2.63	0.58	0.09	4.19	$151.67	2.14	$77.47	000	M A
53850	Prostatic microwave thermotx	9.45	87.54	4.50	0.56	97.55	$3,531.23	14.51	$525.25	090	M A
53852	Prostatic rf thermotx	9.88	75.53	4.68	0.58	85.99	$3,112.77	15.14	$548.06	090	M A
53853	Prostatic water thermother	4.14	52.75	2.55	0.38	57.27	$2,073.13	7.07	$255.93	090	M A
53899	Urology surgery procedure	0.00	0.00	0.00	0.00	0.00	$0.00	0.00	$0.00	YYY	M A+ C+ T+
54000	Slitting of prepuce	1.54	5.66	1.51	0.10	7.30	$264.25	3.15	$114.03	010	M A+
54001	Slitting of prepuce	2.19	6.56	2.15	0.14	8.89	$321.81	4.48	$162.17	010	M A
54015	Drain penis lesion	5.32	7.95	3.21	0.33	13.60	$492.31	8.86	$320.72	010	M A+
54050	Destruction, penis lesion(s)	1.24	2.85	0.47	0.07	4.16	$150.59	1.78	$64.43	010	M A
54055	Destruction, penis lesion(s)	1.22	6.64	1.42	0.07	7.93	$287.06	2.71	$98.10	010	M A
54056	Cryosurgery, penis lesion(s)	1.24	2.96	0.58	0.06	4.26	$154.21	1.88	$68.05	010	M A
54057	Laser surg, penis lesion(s)	1.24	2.97	1.41	0.08	4.29	$155.29	2.73	$98.82	010	M A
54060	Excision of penis lesion(s)	1.93	5.65	1.66	0.12	7.70	$278.73	3.71	$134.30	010	M A
54065	Destruction, penis lesion(s)	2.42	5.38	2.24	0.13	7.93	$287.06	4.79	$173.39	010	M A
54100	Biopsy of penis	1.90	3.54	0.77	0.10	5.54	$200.54	2.77	$100.27	000	M A
54105	Biopsy of penis	3.50	6.75	2.19	0.21	10.46	$378.64	5.90	$213.58	010	M A

Code	Description										
54110	Treatment of penis lesion	10.13	NA	8.20	0.60	NA	NA	18.93	$685.25	090	M	
54111	Treat penis lesion, graft	13.57	NA	9.37	0.79	NA	NA	23.73	$859.01	090	M	C+
54112	Treat penis lesion, graft	15.86	NA	10.08	0.94	NA	NA	26.88	$973.03	090	M	C+
54115	Treatment of penis lesion	6.15	11.63	6.77	0.39	18.17	$657.74	13.31	$481.81	090	M	
54120	Partial removal of penis	9.97	NA	8.14	0.60	NA	NA	18.71	$677.29	090	M	C+
54125	Removal of penis	13.53	NA	9.37	0.81	NA	NA	23.71	$858.28	090	M	C+
54130	Remove penis & nodes	20.14	NA	12.00	1.19	NA	NA	33.33	$1,206.52	090	M	C+
54135	Remove penis & nodes	26.36	NA	14.68	1.58	NA	NA	42.62	$1,542.81	090	M	
54150	Circumcision	1.81	6.04	1.87	0.17	8.02	$290.32	3.85	$139.37	010	M	A+
54152	Circumcision	2.31	NA	1.76	0.16	NA	NA	4.23	$153.12	010	M	A
54160	Circumcision	2.48	5.04	1.82	0.16	7.68	$278.01	4.46	$161.45	010	M	A
54161	Circumcision	3.27	NA	2.10	0.20	NA	NA	5.57	$201.63	010	M	A
54162	Lysis penil circumcis lesion	3.00	NA	2.91	0.18	NA	NA	6.09	$220.45	010	M	A
54163	Repair of circumcision	3.00	NA	2.54	0.18	NA	NA	5.72	$207.06	010	M	A
54164	Frenulotomy of penis	2.50	NA	2.37	0.15	NA	NA	5.02	$181.72	010	M	A
54200	Treatment of penis lesion	1.06	2.87	0.38	0.06	3.99	$144.43	1.50	$54.30	010	M	A
54205	Treatment of penis lesion	7.93	NA	7.50	0.47	NA	NA	15.90	$575.57	090	M	A
54220	Treatment of penis lesion	2.42	2.08	1.04	0.15	4.65	$168.33	3.61	$130.68	000	M	A
54230	Prepare penis study	1.34	NA	0.46	0.08	NA	NA	1.88	$68.05	000	M	A
54231	Dynamic cavernosometry	2.04	2.26	0.83	0.14	4.44	$160.72	3.01	$108.96	000	M	A
54235	Penile injection	1.19	1.19	0.41	0.07	2.45	$88.69	1.67	$60.45	000	M	A
54240	Penis study	1.31	1.59	1.59	0.13	3.03	$109.68	3.03	$109.68	000	M	A+
54240-26	Penis study	1.31	0.45	0.45	0.08	1.84	$66.61	1.84	$66.61	000	M	A+
54240-TC	Penis study	0.00	1.14	1.14	0.05	1.19	$43.08	1.19	$43.08	000		A+
54250	Penis study	2.22	2.90	2.90	0.16	5.28	$191.13	5.28	$191.13	000	M	A+
54250-26	Penis study	2.22	0.75	0.75	0.14	3.11	$112.58	3.11	$112.58	000	M	A+
54250-TC	Penis study	0.00	2.15	2.15	0.02	2.17	$78.55	2.17	$78.55	000		A+
54300	Revision of penis	10.41	NA	8.89	0.64	NA	NA	19.94	$721.81	090	M	C+

* **M** = multiple surgery adjustment applies
Me = multiple endoscopy rules may apply
B = bilateral surgery adjustment applies
A = assistant-at-surgery restriction

A+ = assistant-at-surgery restriction unless medical necessity established with documentation
C = cosurgeons payable
C+ = cosurgeons payable if medical necessity established with documentation

T = team surgeons permitted
T+ = team surgeons payable if medical necessity established with documentation
$ = indicates services that are not covered by Medicare.

269 CPT five-digit codes, two-digit numeric modifiers, and descriptions only are © 2001 American Medical Association

Medicare RBRVS: The Physicians' Guide

Relative value units

CPT Code and Modifier	Description	Work RVU	Non Facility Practice Expense RVU	Facility Practice Expense RVU	PLI RVU	Total Non Facility RVUs	Medicare Payment Non Facility	Total Facility RVUs	Medicare Payment Facility	Global Period	Payment Policy Indicators*
54304	Revision of penis	12.49	NA	10.04	0.74	NA	NA	23.27	$842.36	090	M
54308	Reconstruction of urethra	11.83	NA	9.94	0.70	NA	NA	22.47	$813.40	090	M C+
54312	Reconstruction of urethra	13.57	NA	10.73	0.81	NA	NA	25.11	$908.96	090	M C+
54316	Reconstruction of urethra	16.82	NA	11.67	1.00	NA	NA	29.49	$1,067.51	090	M C+
54318	Reconstruction of urethra	11.25	NA	10.06	1.15	NA	NA	22.46	$813.03	090	M C+
54322	Reconstruction of urethra	13.01	NA	9.56	0.77	NA	NA	23.34	$844.89	090	M
54324	Reconstruction of urethra	16.31	NA	12.02	1.03	NA	NA	29.36	$1,062.81	090	M C+
54326	Reconstruction of urethra	15.72	NA	11.17	0.93	NA	NA	27.82	$1,007.06	090	M C+
54328	Revise penis/urethra	15.65	NA	11.59	0.92	NA	NA	28.16	$1,019.37	090	M C+
54332	Revise penis/urethra	17.08	NA	11.87	1.01	NA	NA	29.96	$1,084.53	090	M C+
54336	Revise penis/urethra	20.04	NA	13.59	1.90	NA	NA	35.53	$1,286.16	090	M C+
54340	Secondary urethral surgery	8.91	NA	9.80	0.72	NA	NA	19.43	$703.35	090	M C+
54344	Secondary urethral surgery	15.94	NA	10.91	1.10	NA	NA	27.95	$1,011.77	090	M C+
54348	Secondary urethral surgery	17.15	NA	12.10	1.02	NA	NA	30.27	$1,095.75	090	M C+
54352	Reconstruct urethra/penis	24.74	NA	16.53	1.62	NA	NA	42.89	$1,552.58	090	M C+
54360	Penis plastic surgery	11.93	NA	8.82	0.72	NA	NA	21.47	$777.20	090	M C+
54380	Repair penis	13.18	NA	10.79	1.16	NA	NA	25.13	$909.69	090	M C+
54385	Repair penis	15.39	NA	12.20	0.71	NA	NA	28.30	$1,024.44	090	M C+
54390	Repair penis and bladder	21.61	NA	14.69	1.28	NA	NA	37.58	$1,360.37	090	M C+
54400	Insert semi-rigid prosthesis	8.99	NA	6.53	0.53	NA	NA	16.05	$581.00	090	M A C+
54401	Insert self-contd prosthesis	10.28	NA	7.37	0.61	NA	NA	18.26	$661.00	090	M A C+
54405	Insert multi-comp penis pros	13.43	NA	8.45	0.80	NA	NA	22.68	$821.00	090	M C+
54406	Remove multi-comp penis pros	12.10	NA	6.09	0.80	NA	NA	18.99	$687.42	090	M C+
54408	Repair multi-comp penis pros	12.75	NA	6.46	0.80	NA	NA	20.01	$724.35	090	M C+
54410	Remove/replace penis prosth	15.50	NA	7.36	0.80	NA	NA	23.66	$856.47	090	M C+
54411	Remv/replc penis pros, comp	16.00	NA	8.98	0.80	NA	NA	25.78	$933.22	090	M C+
54415	Remove self-contd penis pros	8.20	NA	5.35	0.55	NA	NA	14.10	$510.41	090	M C+

Code	Description										
54416	Remv/repl penis contain pros	10.87	NA	6.94	NA	NA	18.36	$664.62	090	M		C+
54417	Remv/replc penis pros, compl	14.19	NA	7.89	0.55	NA	22.63	$819.19	090	M		C+
54420	Revision of penis	11.42	NA	8.70	0.72	NA	20.84	$754.39	090	M		
54430	Revision of penis	10.15	NA	8.17	0.60	NA	18.92	$684.89	090	M		
54435	Revision of penis	6.12	NA	6.30	0.36	NA	12.78	$462.63	090	M		A
54440	Repair of penis	0.00	0.00	0.00	0.00	$0.00	0.00	$0.00	090	M		C+
54450	Preputial stretching	1.12	1.10	0.49	0.07	$82.90	1.68	$60.81	000	M		A
54500	Biopsy of testis	1.31	6.26	0.45	0.08	$276.92	1.84	$66.61	000	M	B	A+
54505	Biopsy of testis	3.46	NA	2.75	0.21	NA	6.42	$232.40	010	M	B	A+
54512	Excise lesion testis	8.58	NA	5.19	0.56	NA	14.33	$518.73	090	M	B	C+
54520	Removal of testis	5.23	NA	3.75	0.33	NA	9.31	$337.01	090	M	B	A
54522	Orchiectomy, partial	9.50	NA	6.15	0.62	NA	16.27	$588.96	090	M	B	C+
54530	Removal of testis	8.58	NA	5.46	0.53	NA	14.57	$527.42	090	M	B	C+
54535	Extensive testis surgery	12.16	NA	7.62	0.83	NA	20.61	$746.07	090	M	B	
54550	Exploration for testis	7.78	NA	4.97	0.49	NA	13.24	$479.28	090	M	B	
54560	Exploration for testis	11.13	NA	7.10	0.79	NA	19.02	$688.51	090	M	B	C+
54600	Reduce testis torsion	7.01	NA	4.38	0.45	NA	11.84	$428.60	090	M	B	A
54620	Suspension of testis	4.90	NA	3.26	0.31	NA	8.47	$306.61	010	M	B	A
54640	Suspension of testis	6.90	NA	4.40	0.49	NA	11.79	$426.79	090	M	B	A
54650	Orchiopexy (Fowler-Stephens)	11.45	NA	7.29	0.81	NA	19.55	$707.69	090	M	B	
54660	Revision of testis	5.11	NA	3.65	0.35	NA	9.11	$329.77	090	M	B	A+
54670	Repair testis injury	6.41	NA	4.30	0.41	NA	11.12	$402.54	090	M	B	A+
54680	Relocation of testis(es)	12.65	NA	7.65	0.94	NA	21.24	$768.87	090	M	B	C+
54690	Laparoscopy, orchiectomy	10.96	NA	7.08	0.99	NA	19.03	$688.87	090	M	B	C+
54692	Laparoscopy, orchiopexy	12.88	NA	5.84	0.87	NA	19.59	$709.14	090	M	B	A
54699	Laparoscope proc, testis	0.00	0.00	0.00	0.00	$0.00	0.00	$0.00	YYY	M	B	
54700	Drainage of scrotum	3.43	8.80	3.53	0.23	$451.04	7.19	$260.27	010	M		A

* **M** = multiple surgery adjustment applies
   Me = multiple endoscopy rules may apply
   B = bilateral surgery adjustment applies
   A = assistant-at-surgery restriction

A+ = assistant-at-surgery restriction unless medical necessity established with documentation
C = cosurgeons payable
C+ = cosurgeons payable if medical necessity established with documentation

T = team surgeons permitted
T+ = team surgeons payable if medical necessity established with documentation
$ = indicates services that are not covered by Medicare.

Medicare RBRVS: The Physicians' Guide

Relative value units

CPT Code and Modifier	Description	Work RVU	Non Facility Practice Expense RVU	Facility Practice Expense RVU	PLI RVU	Total Non Facility RVUs	Medicare Payment Non Facility	Total Facility RVUs	Medicare Payment Facility	Global Period	Payment Policy Indicators*		
54800	Biopsy of epididymis	2.33	6.45	0.79	0.14	8.92	$322.90	3.26	$118.01	000	M		A+
54820	Exploration of epididymis	5.14	NA	3.61	0.33	NA	NA	9.08	$328.69	090	M		A+
54830	Remove epididymis lesion	5.38	NA	3.85	0.34	NA	NA	9.57	$346.43	090	M		A+
54840	Remove epididymis lesion	5.20	NA	3.79	0.31	NA	NA	9.30	$336.65	090	M		A
54860	Removal of epididymis	6.32	NA	4.40	0.38	NA	NA	11.10	$401.81	090	M		A
54861	Removal of epididymis	8.90	NA	5.28	0.52	NA	NA	14.70	$532.13	090	M		A+
54900	Fusion of spermatic ducts	13.20	NA	6.99	1.34	NA	NA	21.53	$779.37	090	M		A+
54901	Fusion of spermatic ducts	17.94	NA	9.27	1.83	NA	NA	29.04	$1,051.22	090	M		A+
55000	Drainage of hydrocele	1.43	2.24	0.49	0.10	3.77	$136.47	2.02	$73.12	000	M		A
55040	Removal of hydrocele	5.36	NA	3.56	0.35	NA	NA	9.27	$335.57	090	M		A
55041	Removal of hydroceles	7.74	NA	4.63	0.50	NA	NA	12.87	$465.88	090	M		A
55060	Repair of hydrocele	5.52	NA	3.64	0.37	NA	NA	9.53	$344.98	090	M	B	A+
55100	Drainage of scrotum abscess	2.13	10.06	3.63	0.15	12.34	$446.70	5.91	$213.94	010	M		A
55110	Explore scrotum	5.70	NA	3.71	0.36	NA	NA	9.77	$353.67	090	M		A
55120	Removal of scrotum lesion	5.09	NA	3.52	0.33	NA	NA	8.94	$323.62	090	M		A+
55150	Removal of scrotum	7.22	NA	4.76	0.47	NA	NA	12.45	$450.68	090	M		C+
55175	Revision of scrotum	5.24	NA	3.88	0.33	NA	NA	9.45	$342.08	090	M		A+
55180	Revision of scrotum	10.72	NA	6.38	0.72	NA	NA	17.82	$645.07	090	M		A+
55200	Incision of sperm duct	4.24	NA	3.10	0.25	NA	NA	7.59	$274.75	090	M		A+
55250	Removal of sperm duct(s)	3.29	9.72	3.28	0.21	13.22	$478.55	6.78	$245.43	090	M		A
55300	Prepare, sperm duct x-ray	3.51	NA	1.56	0.20	NA	NA	5.27	$190.77	000	M		A+
55400	Repair of sperm duct	8.49	NA	5.32	0.50	NA	NA	14.31	$518.01	090	M	B	C+
55450	Ligation of sperm duct	4.12	8.08	2.62	0.24	12.44	$450.32	6.98	$252.67	010	M		A+
55500	Removal of hydrocele	5.59	NA	3.76	0.43	NA	NA	9.78	$354.03	090	M		A+
55520	Removal of sperm cord lesion	6.03	NA	3.82	0.56	NA	NA	10.41	$376.83	090	M		C+
55530	Revise spermatic cord veins	5.66	NA	3.92	0.36	NA	NA	9.94	$359.82	090	M	B	A	C+

Code	Description											
55535	Revise spermatic cord veins	6.56	NA	4.23	0.42	NA	11.21	$405.79	090	M	B		C+
55540	Revise hernia & sperm veins	7.67	NA	4.37	0.74	NA	12.78	$462.63	090	M	B		C+
55550	Laparo ligate spermatic vein	6.57	NA	3.67	0.47	NA	10.71	$387.69	090	M	B		C+
55559	Laparo proc, spermatic cord	0.00	0.00	0.00	0.00	$0.00	0.00	$0.00	YYY	M	B		
55600	Incise sperm duct pouch	6.38	NA	4.41	0.38	NA	11.17	$404.35	090	M	B	A+	C+
55605	Incise sperm duct pouch	7.96	NA	5.39	0.54	NA	13.89	$502.81	090	M	B	A+	
55650	Remove sperm duct pouch	11.80	NA	6.44	0.72	NA	18.96	$686.34	090	M	B		C+
55680	Remove sperm pouch lesion	5.19	NA	3.77	0.31	NA	9.27	$335.57	090	M		A+	
55700	Biopsy of prostate	1.57	4.68	0.73	0.10	6.35	2.40	$86.88	000	M		A	
55705	Biopsy of prostate	4.57	NA	3.92	0.26	NA	8.75	$316.74	000	M		A	C+
55720	Drainage of prostate abscess	7.64	NA	5.88	0.44	NA	13.96	$505.34	010	M			C+
55725	Drainage of prostate abscess	8.68	NA	6.58	0.51	NA	15.77	$570.86	090	M			C+
55801	Removal of prostate	17.80	NA	9.78	1.08	NA	28.66	$1,037.47	090	M			C+
55810	Extensive prostate surgery	22.58	NA	11.85	1.35	NA	35.78	$1,295.21	090	M			C+
55812	Extensive prostate surgery	27.51	NA	13.91	1.69	NA	43.11	$1,560.55	090	M			C+
55815	Extensive prostate surgery	30.46	NA	15.01	1.84	NA	47.31	$1,712.58	090	M			C+
55821	Removal of prostate	14.25	NA	8.20	0.85	NA	23.30	$843.44	090	M			C+
55831	Removal of prostate	15.62	NA	8.67	0.94	NA	25.23	$913.31	090	M			C+
55840	Extensive prostate surgery	22.69	NA	12.32	1.37	NA	36.38	$1,316.93	090	M			C+
55842	Extensive prostate surgery	24.38	NA	12.86	1.48	NA	38.72	$1,401.63	090	M			C+
55845	Extensive prostate surgery	28.55	NA	14.26	1.71	NA	44.52	$1,611.59	090	M			C+
55859	Percut/needle insert, pros	12.52	NA	7.71	0.74	NA	20.97	$759.10	090	M		A+	
55860	Surgical exposure, prostate	14.45	NA	7.93	0.82	NA	23.20	$839.82	090	M		A	C+
55862	Extensive prostate surgery	18.39	NA	9.69	1.14	NA	29.22	$1,057.74	090	M			C+
55865	Extensive prostate surgery	22.87	NA	11.49	1.37	NA	35.73	$1,293.40	090	M			C+
55870	Electroejaculation	2.58	1.96	0.98	0.14	$169.41	3.70	$133.94	000	M		A	C+
55873	Cryoablate prostate	19.47	NA	10.65	1.02	NA	31.14	$1,127.24	090	M		A	
55899	Genital surgery procedure	0.00	0.00	0.00	0.00	$0.00	0.00	$0.00	YYY	M		A	C+ T+

* **M** = multiple surgery adjustment applies
Me = multiple endoscopy rules may apply
B = bilateral surgery adjustment applies
A = assistant-at-surgery restriction

A+ = assistant-at-surgery restriction unless medical necessity established with documentation
C = cosurgeons payable
C+ = cosurgeons payable if medical necessity established with documentation

T = team surgeons permitted
T+ = team surgeons payable if medical necessity established with documentation
§ = indicates services that are not covered by Medicare.

273 CPT five-digit codes, two-digit numeric modifiers, and descriptions only are © 2001 American Medical Association

Medicare RBRVS: The Physicians' Guide

Relative value units

CPT Code and Modifier	Description	Work RVU	Non Facility Practice Expense RVU	Facility Practice Expense RVU	PLI RVU	Total Non Facility RVUs	Medicare Payment Non Facility	Total Facility RVUs	Medicare Payment Facility	Global Period	Payment Policy Indicators*		
Surgery: Female genital system													
56405	I & D of vulva/perineum	1.44	2.50	1.33	0.14	4.08	$147.69	2.91	$105.34	010	M	A	C
56420	Drainage of gland abscess	1.39	2.48	1.33	0.13	4.00	$144.80	2.85	$103.17	010	M	A	
56440	Surgery for vulva lesion	2.84	3.83	2.40	0.28	6.95	$251.58	5.52	$199.82	010	M	A	
56441	Lysis of labial lesion(s)	1.97	2.74	2.11	0.17	4.88	$176.65	4.25	$153.85	010	M	A+	
56501	Destroy, vulva lesions, simp	1.53	2.42	1.42	0.15	4.10	$148.42	3.10	$112.22	010	M	A	
56515	Destroy vulva lesion/s compl	2.76	3.20	2.46	0.18	6.14	$222.26	5.40	$195.48	010	M	A	
56605	Biopsy of vulva/perineum	1.10	1.90	0.50	0.11	3.11	$112.58	1.71	$61.90	000	M	A	C
56606	Biopsy of vulva/perineum	0.55	1.69	0.23	0.06	2.30	$83.26	0.84	$30.41	ZZZ	M	A	C
56620	Partial removal of vulva	7.47	NA	5.13	0.76	NA	NA	13.36	$483.62	090	M		C+
56625	Complete removal of vulva	8.40	NA	6.20	0.84	NA	NA	15.44	$558.92	090	M		C+
56630	Extensive vulva surgery	12.36	NA	7.93	1.23	NA	NA	21.52	$779.01	090	M		C+
56631	Extensive vulva surgery	16.20	NA	10.80	1.63	NA	NA	28.63	$1,036.38	090	M		C
56632	Extensive vulva surgery	20.29	NA	12.42	2.03	NA	NA	34.74	$1,257.56	090	M		C
56633	Extensive vulva surgery	16.47	NA	9.70	1.66	NA	NA	27.83	$1,007.42	090	M		C
56634	Extensive vulva surgery	17.88	NA	11.25	1.78	NA	NA	30.91	$1,118.92	090	M		C
56637	Extensive vulva surgery	21.97	NA	13.16	2.18	NA	NA	37.31	$1,350.59	090	M		C
56640	Extensive vulva surgery	22.17	NA	12.58	2.26	NA	NA	37.01	$1,339.73	090	M	B	C+
56700	Partial removal of hymen	2.52	3.18	2.16	0.24	5.94	$215.02	4.92	$178.10	010	M		C+
56720	Incision of hymen	0.68	1.79	0.57	0.07	2.54	$91.95	1.32	$47.78	000	M	A+	
56740	Remove vagina gland lesion	4.57	4.08	3.08	0.37	9.02	$326.52	8.02	$290.32	010	M	A	
56800	Repair of vagina	3.89	NA	2.86	0.37	NA	NA	7.12	$257.74	010	M		C+
56805	Repair clitoris	18.86	NA	9.69	1.82	NA	NA	30.37	$1,099.37	090	M		C+
56810	Repair of perineum	4.13	NA	2.91	0.41	NA	NA	7.45	$269.68	010	M		C
57000	Exploration of vagina	2.97	NA	2.49	0.28	NA	NA	5.74	$207.78	010	M	A+	
57010	Drainage of pelvic abscess	6.03	NA	4.08	0.57	NA	NA	10.68	$386.61	090	M	A+	

Code	Description										
57020	Drainage of pelvic fluid	1.50	1.63	0.66	0.15	3.28	$118.73	2.31	$83.62	000	M	A+
57022	I & d vaginal hematoma, pp	2.56	NA	2.14	0.24	NA	NA	4.94	$178.82	010	M	A+
57023	I & d vag hematoma, non-ob	4.75	NA	3.01	0.24	NA	NA	8.00	$289.59	010	M	A+
57061	Destroy vag lesions, simple	1.25	2.37	1.33	0.13	3.75	$135.75	2.71	$98.10	010	M	A
57065	Destroy vag lesions, complex	2.61	3.09	2.41	0.26	5.96	$215.75	5.28	$191.13	010	M	A
57100	Biopsy of vagina	1.20	1.64	0.53	0.10	2.94	$106.43	1.83	$66.24	000	M	A
57105	Biopsy of vagina	1.69	2.35	2.34	0.17	4.21	$152.40	4.20	$152.04	010	M	A
57106	Remove vagina wall, partial	6.36	2.67	2.67	0.58	9.61	$347.87	9.61	$347.87	090	M		C+
57107	Remove vagina tissue, part	23.00	NA	10.65	2.17	NA	NA	35.82	$1,296.66	090	M		C+
57109	Vaginectomy partial w/nodes	27.00	NA	13.89	1.97	NA	NA	42.86	$1,551.50	090	M		C+
57110	Remove vagina wall, complete	14.29	NA	7.56	1.43	NA	NA	23.28	$842.72	090	M		C+
57111	Remove vagina tissue, compl	27.00	NA	12.85	2.71	NA	NA	42.56	$1,540.64	090	M		C+
57112	Vaginectomy w/nodes, compl	29.00	NA	14.38	2.19	NA	NA	45.57	$1,649.60	090	M		C+
57120	Closure of vagina	7.41	NA	4.85	0.75	NA	NA	13.01	$470.95	090	M		C+
57130	Remove vagina lesion	2.43	NA	2.25	0.23	NA	NA	4.91	$177.74	010	M		C+
57135	Remove vagina lesion	2.67	3.09	2.35	0.26	6.02	$217.92	5.28	$191.13	010	M	A
57150	Treat vagina infection	0.55	1.04	0.22	0.06	1.65	$59.73	0.83	$30.05	000	M	A
57155	Insert uteri tandems/ovoids	6.27	NA	3.67	0.63	NA	NA	10.57	$382.63	090	M	A
57160	Insert pessary/other device	0.89	1.12	0.41	0.09	2.10	$76.02	1.39	$50.32	000	M	A
57170	Fitting of diaphragm/cap	0.91	1.46	0.36	0.09	2.46	$89.05	1.36	$49.23	000	M	A+
57180	Treat vaginal bleeding	1.58	2.37	1.55	0.16	4.11	$148.78	3.29	$119.10	010	M	A
57200	Repair of vagina	3.94	NA	3.14	0.38	NA	NA	7.46	$270.05	090	M		C+
57210	Repair vagina/perineum	5.17	NA	3.69	0.50	NA	NA	9.36	$338.82	090	M		C+
57220	Revision of urethra	4.31	NA	3.52	0.42	NA	NA	8.25	$298.64	090	M		C+
57230	Repair of urethral lesion	5.64	NA	4.49	0.50	NA	NA	10.63	$384.80	090	M		C+
57240	Repair bladder & vagina	6.07	NA	4.62	0.53	NA	NA	11.22	$406.16	090	M		C+
57250	Repair rectum & vagina	5.53	NA	4.01	0.54	NA	NA	10.08	$364.89	090	M		C+
57260	Repair of vagina	8.27	NA	5.17	0.83	NA	NA	14.27	$516.56	090	M		C+

* **M** = multiple surgery adjustment applies
Me = multiple endoscopy rules may apply
B = bilateral surgery adjustment applies
A = assistant-at-surgery restriction

A+ = assistant-at-surgery restriction unless medical necessity established with documentation
C = cosurgeons payable
C+ = cosurgeons payable if medical necessity established with documentation

T = team surgeons permitted
T+ = team surgeons payable if medical necessity established with documentation
$ = indicates services that are not covered by Medicare.

275 CPT five-digit codes, two-digit numeric modifiers, and descriptions only are © 2001 American Medical Association

Medicare RBRVS: The Physicians' Guide

Relative value units

CPT Code and Modifier	Description	Work RVU	Non Facility Practice Expense RVU	Facility Practice Expense RVU	PLI RVU	Total Non Facility RVUs	Medicare Payment Non Facility	Total Facility RVUs	Medicare Payment Facility	Global Period	Payment Policy Indicators*	
57265	Extensive repair of vagina	11.34	NA	7.22	1.14	NA	NA	19.70	$713.12	090	M	C+
57268	Repair of bowel bulge	6.76	NA	4.54	0.66	NA	NA	11.96	$432.94	090	M	C+
57270	Repair of bowel pouch	12.11	NA	6.58	1.17	NA	NA	19.86	$718.92	090	M	C+
57280	Suspension of vagina	15.04	NA	7.74	1.44	NA	NA	24.22	$876.74	090	M	C+
57282	Repair of vaginal prolapse	8.86	NA	5.44	0.86	NA	NA	15.16	$548.78	090	M	C+
57284	Repair paravaginal defect	12.70	NA	7.45	1.17	NA	NA	21.32	$771.77	090	M	C
57287	Revise/remove sling repair	10.71	NA	7.47	0.74	NA	NA	18.92	$684.89	090	M	C+
57288	Repair bladder defect	13.02	NA	7.24	0.86	NA	NA	21.12	$764.53	090	M	C+
57289	Repair bladder & vagina	11.58	NA	7.12	0.95	NA	NA	19.65	$711.31	090	M	C+
57291	Construction of vagina	7.95	NA	5.93	0.78	NA	NA	14.66	$530.68	090	M	
57292	Construct vagina with graft	13.09	NA	7.20	1.29	NA	NA	21.58	$781.18	090	M	C+
57300	Repair rectum-vagina fistula	7.61	NA	4.82	0.70	NA	NA	13.13	$475.30	090	M	C+
57305	Repair rectum-vagina fistula	13.77	NA	7.00	1.33	NA	NA	22.10	$800.00	090	M	C+
57307	Fistula repair & colostomy	15.93	NA	7.72	1.59	NA	NA	25.24	$913.67	090	M	C+
57308	Fistula repair, transperine	9.94	NA	5.96	0.91	NA	NA	16.81	$608.51	090	M	C+
57310	Repair urethrovaginal lesion	6.78	NA	4.95	0.45	NA	NA	12.18	$440.91	090	M	C+
57311	Repair urethrovaginal lesion	7.98	NA	5.45	0.51	NA	NA	13.94	$504.62	090	M	C+
57320	Repair bladder-vagina lesion	8.01	NA	5.68	0.60	NA	NA	14.29	$517.29	090	M	C+
57330	Repair bladder-vagina lesion	12.35	NA	6.96	0.86	NA	NA	20.17	$730.14	090	M	C+
57335	Repair vagina	18.73	NA	9.84	1.66	NA	NA	30.23	$1,094.30	090	M	C+
57400	Dilation of vagina	2.27	NA	1.18	0.22	NA	NA	3.67	$132.85	000	M	A+
57410	Pelvic examination	1.75	2.75	1.12	0.14	4.64	$167.96	3.01	$108.96	000	M	A
57415	Remove vaginal foreign body	2.17	3.71	2.18	0.19	6.07	$219.73	4.54	$164.34	010	M	A+
57452	Examination of vagina	0.99	1.69	0.46	0.10	2.78	$100.63	1.55	$56.11	000	M	A
57454	Vagina examination & biopsy	1.27	1.88	0.62	0.13	3.28	$118.73	2.02	$73.12	000	Me	A
57460	Cervix excision	2.83	2.17	1.19	0.28	5.28	$191.13	4.30	$155.66	000	Me	A
57500	Biopsy of cervix	0.97	2.29	0.50	0.10	3.36	$121.63	1.57	$56.83	000	M	A

Code	Description										
57505	Endocervical curettage	1.14	2.05	1.36	0.12	3.31	$119.82	2.62	$94.84	010	M	A
57510	Cauterization of cervix	1.90	3.39	1.66	0.18	5.47	$198.01	3.74	$135.39	010	M	A
57511	Cryocautery of cervix	1.90	2.54	0.77	0.18	4.62	$167.24	2.85	$103.17	010	M	A
57513	Laser surgery of cervix	1.90	2.72	1.66	0.19	4.81	$174.12	3.75	$135.75	010	M	A
57520	Conization of cervix	4.04	4.43	2.93	0.41	8.88	$321.45	7.38	$267.15	090	M	A
57522	Conization of cervix	3.36	4.02	2.68	0.34	7.72	$279.46	6.38	$230.95	090	M	A
57530	Removal of cervix	4.79	NA	3.78	0.48	NA	NA	9.05	$327.60	090	M	C+
57531	Removal of cervix, radical	28.00	NA	14.44	2.46	NA	NA	44.90	$1,625.34	090	M	C+
57540	Removal of residual cervix	12.22	NA	6.49	1.21	NA	NA	19.92	$721.09	090	M	C+
57545	Remove cervix/repair pelvis	13.03	NA	6.95	1.30	NA	NA	21.28	$770.32	090	M	C+
57550	Removal of residual cervix	5.53	NA	3.98	0.55	NA	NA	10.06	$364.16	090	M	C+
57555	Remove cervix/repair vagina	8.95	NA	5.90	0.89	NA	NA	15.74	$569.78	090	M	C+
57556	Remove cervix, repair bowel	8.37	NA	5.14	0.80	NA	NA	14.31	$518.01	090	M	C+
57700	Revision of cervix	3.55	NA	2.71	0.33	NA	NA	6.59	$238.55	090	M	A+
57720	Revision of cervix	4.13	NA	3.41	0.41	NA	NA	7.95	$287.78	090	M	
57800	Dilation of cervical canal	0.77	1.22	0.36	0.08	2.07	$74.93	1.21	$43.80	000	M	A
57820	D & c of residual cervix	1.67	2.70	2.40	0.17	4.54	$164.34	4.24	$153.48	010	M	A
58100	Biopsy of uterus lining	1.53	1.56	0.76	0.07	3.16	$114.39	2.36	$85.43	000	M	A
58120	Dilation and curettage	3.27	4.01	2.55	0.33	7.61	$275.48	6.15	$222.63	010	M	A
58140	Removal of uterus lesion	14.60	NA	7.38	1.46	NA	NA	23.44	$848.51	090	M	C+
58145	Removal of uterus lesion	8.04	NA	5.11	0.80	NA	NA	13.95	$504.98	090	M	C+
58150	Total hysterectomy	15.24	NA	7.90	1.53	NA	NA	24.67	$893.03	090	M	C+
58152	Total hysterectomy	20.60	NA	10.17	1.52	NA	NA	32.29	$1,168.87	090	M	C+
58180	Partial hysterectomy	15.29	NA	7.90	1.54	NA	NA	24.73	$895.21	090	M	C+
58200	Extensive hysterectomy	21.59	NA	11.62	2.15	NA	NA	35.36	$1,280.00	090	M	C+
58210	Extensive hysterectomy	28.85	NA	14.67	2.91	NA	NA	46.43	$1,680.73	090	M	C+
58240	Removal of pelvis contents	38.39	NA	19.71	3.76	NA	NA	61.86	$2,239.28	090	M	C+
58260	Vaginal hysterectomy	12.98	NA	6.90	1.23	NA	NA	21.11	$764.17	090	M	C+

* **M** = multiple surgery adjustment applies
Me = multiple endoscopy rules may apply
B = bilateral surgery adjustment applies
A = assistant-at-surgery restriction

A+ = assistant-at-surgery restriction unless medical necessity established with documentation
C = cosurgeons payable
C+ = cosurgeons payable if medical necessity established with documentation

T = team surgeons permitted
T+ = team surgeons payable if medical necessity established with documentation
§ = indicates services that are not covered by Medicare.

CPT five-digit codes, two-digit numeric modifiers, and descriptions only are © 2001 American Medical Association

Medicare RBRVS: The Physicians' Guide

Relative value units

CPT Code and Modifier	Description	Work RVU	Non Facility Practice Expense RVU	Facility Practice Expense RVU	PLI RVU	Total Non Facility RVUs	Medicare Payment Non Facility	Total Facility RVUs	Medicare Payment Facility	Global Period	Payment Policy Indicators*		
58262	Vaginal hysterectomy	14.77	NA	7.66	1.42	NA	NA	23.85	$863.35	090	M		C
58263	Vaginal hysterectomy	16.06	NA	8.22	1.55	NA	NA	25.83	$935.03	090	M		C
58267	Hysterectomy & vagina repair	17.04	NA	8.81	1.51	NA	NA	27.36	$990.41	090	M		C+
58270	Hysterectomy & vagina repair	14.26	NA	7.43	1.37	NA	NA	23.06	$834.75	090	M		C+
58275	Hysterectomy/revise vagina	15.76	NA	7.94	1.51	NA	NA	25.21	$912.58	090	M		C+
58280	Hysterectomy/revise vagina	17.01	NA	8.46	1.54	NA	NA	27.01	$977.74	090	M		C+
58285	Extensive hysterectomy	22.26	NA	11.15	1.88	NA	NA	35.29	$1,277.47	090	M		C+
58300 §	Insert intrauterine device	1.01	1.42	0.40	0.10	2.53	$91.58	1.51	$54.66	XXX			
58301	Remove intrauterine device	1.27	1.62	0.51	0.13	3.02	$109.32	1.91	$69.14	000	M		A+
58321	Artificial insemination	0.92	1.03	0.37	0.10	2.05	$74.21	1.39	$50.32	000	M		A+
58322	Artificial insemination	1.10	1.05	0.42	0.11	2.26	$81.81	1.63	$59.00	000	M		A+
58323	Sperm washing	0.23	0.53	0.10	0.02	0.78	$28.24	0.35	$12.67	000	M		A+
58340	Catheter for hysterography	0.88	12.42	0.33	0.08	13.38	$484.35	1.29	$46.70	000	M		A
58345	Reopen fallopian tube	4.66	NA	1.73	0.36	NA	NA	6.75	$244.34	010	M	B	C
58346	Insert heyman uteri capsule	6.75	NA	3.84	0.68	NA	NA	11.27	$407.96	090	M		A
58350	Reopen fallopian tube	1.01	2.15	1.17	0.10	3.26	$118.01	2.28	$82.53	010	M		A
58353	Endometr ablate, thermal	3.56	NA	2.28	0.37	NA	NA	6.21	$224.80	010	M	B	C
58400	Suspension of uterus	6.36	NA	4.17	0.62	NA	NA	11.15	$403.62	090	M		C+
58410	Suspension of uterus	12.73	NA	6.84	1.09	NA	NA	20.66	$747.88	090	M		C+
58520	Repair of ruptured uterus	11.92	NA	6.24	1.17	NA	NA	19.33	$699.73	090	M		C+
58540	Revision of uterus	14.64	NA	6.96	1.28	NA	NA	22.88	$828.24	090	M		C
58550	Laparo-asst vag hysterectomy	14.19	NA	7.11	1.44	NA	NA	22.74	$823.17	010	Me		C
58551	Laparoscopy, remove myoma	14.21	NA	7.09	1.45	NA	NA	22.75	$823.53	010	Me		C
58555	Hysteroscopy, dx, sep proc	3.33	2.95	1.49	0.34	6.62	$239.64	5.16	$186.79	000	M		A+ C
58558	Hysteroscopy, biopsy	4.75	3.55	2.13	0.49	8.79	$318.19	7.37	$266.79	000	Me		A C
58559	Hysteroscopy, lysis	6.17	2.59	2.59	0.62	9.38	$339.55	9.38	$339.55	000	Me		A C
58560	Hysteroscopy, resect septum	7.00	3.01	3.01	0.71	10.72	$388.06	10.72	$388.06	000	Me		C

58561	Hysteroscopy, remove myoma	10.00	3.78	3.78	1.02	14.80	$535.75	000	Me	A+	C
58562	Hysteroscopy, remove fb	5.21	NA	2.34	0.52	NA	$292.13	000	Me	A	C
58563	Hysteroscopy, ablation	6.17	2.62	2.62	0.62	9.41	$340.63	000	Me	A+	C
58578	Laparo proc, uterus	0.00	0.00	0.00	0.00	0.00	$0.00	YYY	M		B
58579	Hysteroscope procedure	0.00	0.00	0.00	0.00	0.00	$0.00	YYY	M		B
58600	Division of fallopian tube	5.60	NA	3.51	0.39	NA	$343.89	090	M		C+
58605	Division of fallopian tube	5.00	NA	3.32	0.33	NA	$313.12	090	M		
58611	Ligate oviduct(s) add-on	1.45	NA	0.61	0.07	NA	$77.10	ZZZ			
58615	Occlude fallopian tube(s)	3.90	NA	3.35	0.40	NA	$276.92	010	M		C
58660	Laparoscopy, lysis	11.29	NA	5.78	1.14	NA	$659.19	090	Me		C
58661	Laparoscopy, remove adnexa	11.05	NA	5.47	1.12	NA	$638.55	010	Me		C
58662	Laparoscopy, excise lesions	11.79	NA	5.75	1.18	NA	$677.65	090	Me		C
58670	Laparoscopy, tubal cautery	5.60	NA	3.73	0.55	NA	$357.65	090	Me	A	C
58671	Laparoscopy, tubal block	5.60	NA	3.74	0.56	NA	$358.37	090	Me	A	C
58672	Laparoscopy, fimbrioplasty	12.88	NA	6.81	1.22	NA	$756.93	090	Me	B	
58673	Laparoscopy, salpingostomy	13.74	NA	7.16	1.40	NA	$807.24	090	Me	B	
58679	Laparo proc, oviduct-ovary	0.00	0.00	0.00	0.00	0.00	$0.00	YYY	M	B	
58700	Removal of fallopian tube	12.05	NA	6.05	0.64	NA	$678.37	090	M		C+
58720	Removal of ovary/tube(s)	11.36	NA	6.05	1.14	NA	$671.50	090	M		C+
58740	Revise fallopian tube(s)	14.00	NA	7.34	0.59	NA	$793.85	090	M		C+
58750	Repair oviduct	14.84	NA	7.60	1.52	NA	$867.33	090	M		C+
58752	Revise ovarian tube(s)	14.84	NA	7.92	1.51	NA	$878.55	090	M		
58760	Remove tubal obstruction	13.13	NA	7.00	1.34	NA	$777.20	090	M	B	C+
58770	Create new tubal opening	13.97	NA	7.24	1.42	NA	$819.19	090	M	B	
58800	Drainage of ovarian cyst(s)	4.14	4.43	4.36	0.36	8.93	$320.72	090	M	A	
58805	Drainage of ovarian cyst(s)	5.88	NA	3.66	0.56	NA	$365.61	090	M		C+
58820	Drain ovary abscess, open	4.22	NA	3.38	0.29	NA	$285.61	090	M		
58822	Drain ovary abscess, percut	10.13	NA	5.20	0.92	NA	$588.24	090	M		C+

* **M** = multiple surgery adjustment applies
Me = multiple endoscopy rules may apply
B = bilateral surgery adjustment applies
A = assistant-at-surgery restriction

A+ = assistant-at-surgery restriction unless medical necessity established with documentation
C = cosurgeons payable
C+ = cosurgeons payable if medical necessity established with documentation

T = team surgeons permitted
T+ = team surgeons payable if medical necessity established with documentation
$ = indicates services that are not covered by Medicare.

279   CPT five-digit codes, two-digit numeric modifiers, and descriptions only are © 2001 American Medical Association

Medicare RBRVS: The Physicians' Guide

Relative value units

CPT Code and Modifier	Description	Work RVU	Non Facility Practice Expense RVU	Facility Practice Expense RVU	PLI RVU	Total Non Facility RVUs	Medicare Payment Non Facility	Total Facility RVUs	Medicare Payment Facility	Global Period	Payment Policy Indicators*	
58823	Drain pelvic abscess, percut	3.38	NA	2.38	0.18	NA	NA	5.94	$215.02	000	M	
58825	Transposition, ovary(s)	10.98	NA	5.95	0.62	NA	NA	17.55	$635.30	090	M	C+
58900	Biopsy of ovary(s)	5.99	NA	3.64	0.56	NA	NA	10.19	$368.87	090	M	C+
58920	Partial removal of ovary(s)	11.36	NA	5.85	0.68	NA	NA	17.89	$647.60	090	M	C+
58925	Removal of ovarian cyst(s)	11.36	NA	5.79	1.14	NA	NA	18.29	$662.08	090	M	C+
58940	Removal of ovary(s)	7.29	NA	4.18	0.73	NA	NA	12.20	$441.63	090	M	C+
58943	Removal of ovary(s)	18.43	NA	9.92	1.86	NA	NA	30.21	$1,093.58	090	M	C+
58950	Resect ovarian malignancy	16.93	NA	9.41	1.55	NA	NA	27.89	$1,009.60	090	M	C+
58951	Resect ovarian malignancy	22.38	NA	11.81	2.20	NA	NA	36.39	$1,317.29	090	M	C+
58952	Resect ovarian malignancy	25.01	NA	12.99	2.50	NA	NA	40.50	$1,466.07	090	M	C+
58953	Tah, rad dissect for debulk	32.00	NA	15.59	3.20	NA	NA	50.79	$1,838.56	090	M	C+
58954	Tah rad debulk/lymph remove	35.00	NA	16.71	3.50	NA	NA	55.21	$1,998.56	090	M	C+
58960	Exploration of abdomen	14.65	NA	8.52	1.47	NA	NA	24.64	$891.95	090	M	C+
58970	Retrieval of oocyte	3.53	8.56	1.92	0.36	12.45	$450.68	5.81	$210.32	000	M	A+
58974	Transfer of embryo	0.00	0.00	0.00	0.00	0.00	$0.00	0.00	$0.00	000	M	C+
58976	Transfer of embryo	3.83	2.30	1.53	0.39	6.52	$236.02	5.75	$208.15	000	M	C+
58999	Genital surgery procedure	0.00	0.00	0.00	0.00	0.00	$0.00	0.00	$0.00	YYY	M	C+ T+

Surgery: Maternity care and delivery

CPT Code and Modifier	Description	Work RVU	Non Facility Practice Expense RVU	Facility Practice Expense RVU	PLI RVU	Total Non Facility RVUs	Medicare Payment Non Facility	Total Facility RVUs	Medicare Payment Facility	Global Period	Payment Policy Indicators*
59000	Amniocentesis, diagnostic	1.30	2.05	0.72	0.23	3.58	$129.59	2.25	$81.45	000	M	A
59001	Amniocentesis, therapeutic	3.00	NA	1.37	0.23	NA	NA	4.60	$166.52	000	M	A
59012	Fetal cord puncture,prenatal	3.45	NA	1.71	0.62	NA	NA	5.78	$209.23	000	M	A+
59015	Chorion biopsy	2.20	1.64	1.11	0.40	4.24	$153.48	3.71	$134.30	000	M	A+
59020	Fetal contract stress test	0.66	0.78	0.78	0.20	1.64	$59.37	1.64	$59.37	000	M	A+
59020-26	Fetal contract stress test	0.66	0.28	0.28	0.12	1.06	$38.37	1.06	$38.37	000	M	A+
59020-TC	Fetal contract stress test	0.00	0.50	0.50	0.08	0.58	$21.00	0.58	$21.00	000		A+
59025	Fetal non-stress test	0.53	0.44	0.44	0.12	1.09	$39.46	1.09	$39.46	000	M	A+
59025-26	Fetal non-stress test	0.53	0.22	0.22	0.10	0.85	$30.77	0.85	$30.77	000	M	A+

Code	Description										
59025-TC	Fetal non-stress test	0.00	0.22	0.22	0.02	0.24	$8.69	0.24	$8.69	000		A+
59030	Fetal scalp blood sample	1.99	NA	1.14	0.36	NA	NA	3.49	$126.34	000	M	A+
59050	Fetal monitor w/report	0.89	NA	0.38	0.16	NA	NA	1.43	$51.76	XXX		A+
59051	Fetal monitor/interpret only	0.74	NA	0.31	0.14	NA	NA	1.19	$43.08	XXX		A+
59100	Remove uterus lesion	12.35	NA	6.61	2.21	NA	NA	21.17	$766.34	090	M	C+
59120	Treat ectopic pregnancy	11.49	NA	6.35	2.06	NA	NA	19.90	$720.36	090	M	C+
59121	Treat ectopic pregnancy	11.67	NA	6.39	2.09	NA	NA	20.15	$729.41	090	M	C+
59130	Treat ectopic pregnancy	14.22	NA	7.16	2.54	NA	NA	23.92	$865.88	090	M	A+
59135	Treat ectopic pregnancy	13.88	NA	7.27	2.49	NA	NA	23.64	$855.75	090	M	A+
59136	Treat ectopic pregnancy	13.18	NA	6.36	2.36	NA	NA	21.90	$792.76	090	M	
59140	Treat ectopic pregnancy	5.46	NA	3.70	0.98	NA	NA	10.14	$367.06	090	M	
59150	Treat ectopic pregnancy	11.67	NA	6.69	1.23	NA	NA	19.59	$709.14	090	M	
59151	Treat ectopic pregnancy	11.49	NA	6.12	1.41	NA	NA	19.02	$688.51	090	M	
59160	D & c after delivery	2.71	3.73	2.29	0.49	6.93	$250.86	5.49	$198.73	010	M	A+
59200	Insert cervical dilator	0.79	1.41	0.32	0.15	2.35	$85.07	1.26	$45.61	000	M	A
59300	Episiotomy or vaginal repair	2.41	2.01	1.01	0.43	4.85	$175.57	3.85	$139.37	000	M	A+
59320	Revision of cervix	2.48	NA	1.31	0.45	NA	NA	4.24	$153.48	000	M	A+
59325	Revision of cervix	4.07	NA	1.97	0.73	NA	NA	6.77	$245.07	000	M	A+
59350	Repair of uterus	4.95	NA	2.19	0.88	NA	NA	8.02	$290.32	000	M	
59400	Obstetrical care	23.06	NA	15.41	4.14	NA	NA	42.61	$1,542.45	MMM	M	A
59409	Obstetrical care	13.50	NA	5.57	2.42	NA	NA	21.49	$777.92	MMM	M	A+
59410	Obstetrical care	14.78	NA	6.98	2.65	NA	NA	24.41	$883.62	MMM	M	A
59412	Antepartum manipulation	1.71	1.38	0.72	0.31	3.40	$123.08	2.74	$99.19	MMM	M	A+
59414	Deliver placenta	1.61	NA	1.34	0.29	NA	NA	3.24	$117.29	MMM	M	A+
59425	Antepartum care only	4.81	5.36	5.32	0.86	11.03	$399.28	10.99	$397.83	MMM	M	A+
59426	Antepartum care only	8.28	9.14	9.14	1.49	18.91	$684.53	18.91	$684.53	MMM	M	A+
59430	Care after delivery	2.13	1.29	1.29	0.38	3.80	$137.56	3.80	$137.56	MMM	M	A

* **M** = multiple surgery adjustment applies
Me = multiple endoscopy rules may apply
B = bilateral surgery adjustment applies
A = assistant-at-surgery restriction

A+ = assistant-at-surgery restriction unless medical necessity established with documentation
C = cosurgeons payable
C+ = cosurgeons payable if medical necessity established with documentation

T = team surgeons permitted
T+ = team surgeons payable if medical necessity established with documentation
$ = indicates services that are not covered by Medicare.

CPT five-digit codes, two-digit numeric modifiers, and descriptions only are © 2001 American Medical Association

Medicare RBRVS: The Physicians' Guide

Relative value units

CPT Code and Modifier	Description	Work RVU	Non Facility Practice Expense RVU	Facility Practice Expense RVU	PLI RVU	Total Non Facility RVUs	Medicare Payment Non Facility	Total Facility RVUs	Medicare Payment Facility	Global Period	Payment Policy Indicators*		
59510	Cesarean delivery	26.22	NA	17.61	4.70	NA	NA	48.53	$1,756.75	MMM	M	A	
59514	Cesarean delivery only	15.97	NA	6.57	2.86	NA	NA	25.40	$919.46	MMM	M		C+
59515	Cesarean delivery	17.37	NA	8.52	3.12	NA	NA	29.01	$1,050.14	MMM	M	A	
59525	Remove uterus after cesarean	8.54	NA	3.52	1.53	NA	NA	13.59	$491.95	ZZZ	M		C+
59610	Vbac delivery	24.62	NA	16.29	4.41	NA	NA	45.32	$1,640.55	MMM	M	A+	
59612	Vbac delivery only	15.06	NA	6.43	2.70	NA	NA	24.19	$875.66	MMM	M	A+	
59614	Vbac care after delivery	16.34	NA	7.70	2.93	NA	NA	26.97	$976.29	MMM	M	A+	
59618	Attempted vbac delivery	27.78	NA	18.38	4.98	NA	NA	51.14	$1,851.23	MMM	M		
59620	Attempted vbac delivery only	17.53	NA	6.87	3.15	NA	NA	27.55	$997.29	MMM	M	A+	
59622	Attempted vbac after care	18.93	NA	8.91	3.39	NA	NA	31.23	$1,130.50	MMM	M	A+	
59812	Treatment of miscarriage	4.01	3.75	2.51	0.58	8.34	$301.90	7.10	$257.01	090	M	A	
59820	Care of miscarriage	4.01	3.79	2.85	0.72	8.52	$308.42	7.58	$274.39	090	M	A	
59821	Treatment of miscarriage	4.47	3.79	3.01	0.80	9.06	$327.96	8.28	$299.73	090	M	A+	
59830	Treat uterus infection	6.11	NA	3.85	1.10	NA	NA	11.06	$400.36	090	M	A+	
59840	Abortion	3.01	4.01	2.47	0.54	7.56	$273.67	6.02	$217.92	010	M	A+	
59841	Abortion	5.24	5.78	3.72	0.94	11.96	$432.94	9.90	$358.37	010	M	A+	
59850	Abortion	5.91	NA	2.75	1.06	NA	NA	9.72	$351.86	090	M	A+	
59851	Abortion	5.93	NA	3.22	1.06	NA	NA	10.21	$369.59	090	M	A+	
59852	Abortion	8.24	NA	4.58	1.48	NA	NA	14.30	$517.65	090	M	A+	
59855	Abortion	6.12	NA	3.38	1.10	NA	NA	10.60	$383.71	090	M	A+	
59856	Abortion	7.48	NA	3.74	1.34	NA	NA	12.56	$454.66	090	M	A+	
59857	Abortion	9.29	NA	4.46	1.66	NA	NA	15.41	$557.83	090	M	A+	
59866	Abortion (mpr)	4.00	NA	1.60	0.72	NA	NA	6.32	$228.78	000	M		C+
59870	Evacuate mole of uterus	6.01	NA	3.83	0.77	NA	NA	10.61	$384.07	090	M		
59871	Remove cerclage suture	2.13	2.19	0.93	0.38	4.70	$170.14	3.44	$124.53	000	M	A+	
59898	Laparo proc, ob care/deliver	0.00	0.00	0.00	0.00	0.00	$0.00	0.00	$0.00	YYY	M	B	
59899	Maternity care procedure	0.00	0.00	0.00	0.00	0.00	$0.00	0.00	$0.00	YYY	M		C+ T+

Surgery: Endocrine system

Code	Description										
60000	Drain thyroid/tongue cyst	1.76	2.40	2.22	0.14	4.30	$155.66	4.12	$149.14	010	M	A+
60001	Aspirate/inject thyroid cyst	0.97	1.77	0.35	0.06	2.80	$101.36	1.38	$49.95	000	M	A
60100	Biopsy of thyroid	1.56	2.70	0.56	0.05	4.31	$156.02	2.17	$78.55	000	M	A
60200	Remove thyroid lesion	9.55	NA	6.88	0.84	NA	NA	17.27	$625.16	090	M	C+
60210	Partial thyroid excision	10.88	NA	6.63	1.01	NA	NA	18.52	$670.41	090	M	C+
60212	Partial thyroid excision	16.03	NA	8.62	1.51	NA	NA	26.16	$946.97	090	M	C+
60220	Partial removal of thyroid	11.90	NA	7.27	0.97	NA	NA	20.14	$729.05	090	M	C+
60225	Partial removal of thyroid	14.19	NA	8.05	1.31	NA	NA	23.55	$852.49	090	M	C+
60240	Removal of thyroid	16.06	NA	9.32	1.50	NA	NA	26.88	$973.03	090	M	C+
60252	Removal of thyroid	20.57	NA	11.64	1.63	NA	NA	33.84	$1,224.98	090	M	C+
60254	Extensive thyroid surgery	26.99	NA	16.39	1.96	NA	NA	45.34	$1,641.27	090	M	C+
60260	Repeat thyroid surgery	17.47	NA	10.66	1.39	NA	NA	29.52	$1,068.60	090	M	C+
60270	Removal of thyroid	20.27	NA	11.54	1.78	NA	NA	33.59	$1,215.93	090	M	C+
60271	Removal of thyroid	16.83	NA	10.20	1.35	NA	NA	28.38	$1,027.33	090	M	C+
60280	Remove thyroid duct lesion	5.87	NA	5.29	0.45	NA	NA	11.61	$420.27	090	M	C+
60281	Remove thyroid duct lesion	8.53	NA	6.27	0.67	NA	NA	15.47	$560.00	090	M	C+
60500	Explore parathyroid glands	16.23	NA	7.99	1.61	NA	NA	25.83	$935.03	090	M	C+
60502	Re-explore parathyroids	20.35	NA	9.97	2.00	NA	NA	32.32	$1,169.96	090	M	C+
60505	Explore parathyroid glands	21.49	NA	11.53	2.14	NA	NA	35.16	$1,272.76	090	M	C+
60512	Autotransplant parathyroid	4.45	NA	1.72	0.44	NA	NA	6.61	$239.28	ZZZ		C+
60520	Removal of thymus gland	16.81	NA	9.55	1.84	NA	NA	28.20	$1,020.82	090	M	C+
60521	Removal of thymus gland	18.87	NA	11.57	2.34	NA	NA	32.78	$1,186.61	090	M	C+
60522	Removal of thymus gland	23.09	NA	12.88	2.83	NA	NA	38.80	$1,404.53	090	M	C+
60540	Explore adrenal gland	17.03	NA	8.09	1.42	NA	NA	26.54	$960.73	090	M	C+ B
60545	Explore adrenal gland	19.88	NA	9.73	1.75	NA	NA	31.36	$1,135.21	090	M	C+
60600	Remove carotid body lesion	17.93	NA	13.43	1.87	NA	NA	33.23	$1,202.90	090	M	C+
60605	Remove carotid body lesion	20.24	NA	18.12	2.28	NA	NA	40.64	$1,471.14	090	M	C+

* **M** = multiple surgery adjustment applies
Me = multiple endoscopy rules may apply
B = bilateral surgery adjustment applies
A = assistant-at-surgery restriction

A+ = assistant-at-surgery restriction unless medical necessity established with documentation
C = cosurgeons payable
C+ = cosurgeons payable if medical necessity established with documentation

T = team surgeons permitted
T+ = team surgeons payable if medical necessity established with documentation
§ = indicates services that are not covered by Medicare.

283 CPT five-digit codes, two-digit numeric modifiers, and descriptions only are © 2001 American Medical Association

Medicare RBRVS: The Physicians' Guide

Relative value units

CPT Code and Modifier	Description	Work RVU	Non Facility Practice Expense RVU	Facility Practice Expense RVU	PLI RVU	Total Non Facility RVUs	Medicare Payment Non Facility	Total Facility RVUs	Medicare Payment Facility	Global Period	Payment Policy Indicators*			
60650	Laparoscopy adrenalectomy	20.00	NA	8.34	1.98	NA	NA	30.32	$1,097.56	090	M	B		C+
60659	Laparo proc, endocrine	0.00	0.00	0.00	0.00	0.00	$0.00	0.00	$0.00	YYY	M	B		
60699	Endocrine surgery procedure	0.00	0.00	0.00	0.00	0.00	$0.00	0.00	$0.00	YYY	M		C+	T+

Surgery: Nervous system

61000	Remove cranial cavity fluid	1.58	1.79	1.53	0.13	3.50	$126.70	3.24	$117.29	000	M		A	
61001	Remove cranial cavity fluid	1.49	2.08	1.47	0.15	3.72	$134.66	3.11	$112.58	000	M		A	
61020	Remove brain cavity fluid	1.51	2.52	1.51	0.26	4.29	$155.29	3.28	$118.73	000	M		A	
61026	Injection into brain canal	1.69	2.28	1.73	0.21	4.18	$151.31	3.63	$131.40	000	M		A	
61050	Remove brain canal fluid	1.51	NA	1.56	0.13	NA	NA	3.20	$115.84	000	M		A+	
61055	Injection into brain canal	2.10	NA	1.80	0.13	NA	NA	4.03	$145.88	000	M		A	
61070	Brain canal shunt procedure	0.89	7.33	1.22	0.09	8.31	$300.82	2.20	$79.64	000	M		A	
61105	Twist drill hole	5.14	NA	3.67	1.05	NA	NA	9.86	$356.92	090	M		A+	
61107	Drill skull for implantation	5.00	NA	3.12	1.02	NA	NA	9.14	$330.86	000	M		A	
61108	Drill skull for drainage	10.19	NA	7.09	2.04	NA	NA	19.32	$699.37	090	M		A	
61120	Burr hole for puncture	8.76	NA	5.88	1.81	NA	NA	16.45	$595.48	090	M		A+	
61140	Pierce skull for biopsy	15.90	NA	10.00	3.15	NA	NA	29.05	$1,051.59	090	M			
61150	Pierce skull for drainage	17.57	NA	10.74	3.52	NA	NA	31.83	$1,152.22	090	M		A	C+
61151	Pierce skull for drainage	12.42	NA	8.16	2.45	NA	NA	23.03	$833.67	090	M		A	
61154	Pierce skull & remove clot	14.99	NA	9.43	3.05	NA	NA	27.47	$994.39	090	M	B		C+
61156	Pierce skull for drainage	16.32	NA	10.30	3.42	NA	NA	30.04	$1,087.42	090	M			C+
61210	Pierce skull, implant device	5.84	NA	3.53	1.16	NA	NA	10.53	$381.18	000	M		A	
61215	Insert brain-fluid device	4.89	NA	4.24	0.99	NA	NA	10.12	$366.34	090	M		A	C+
61250	Pierce skull & explore	10.42	NA	6.73	2.02	NA	NA	19.17	$693.94	090	M	B		C+
61253	Pierce skull & explore	12.36	NA	7.65	2.26	NA	NA	22.27	$806.16	090	M			
61304	Open skull for exploration	21.96	NA	12.85	4.33	NA	NA	39.14	$1,416.84	090	M			C+
61305	Open skull for exploration	26.61	NA	15.31	5.25	NA	NA	47.17	$1,707.52	090	M			C+
61312	Open skull for drainage	24.57	NA	14.57	4.99	NA	NA	44.13	$1,597.47	090	M			C+

Code	Description									
61313	Open skull for drainage	24.93	NA	14.76	5.07	NA	44.76	$1,620.28	090	M		C+
61314	Open skull for drainage	24.23	NA	11.55	4.00	NA	39.78	$1,440.00	090	M		C+
61315	Open skull for drainage	27.68	NA	16.22	5.62	NA	49.52	$1,792.58	090	M		C+
61320	Open skull for drainage	25.62	NA	15.20	5.20	NA	46.02	$1,665.89	090	M		C+
61321	Open skull for drainage	28.50	NA	16.09	5.35	NA	49.94	$1,807.79	090	M		C+
61330	Decompress eye socket	23.32	NA	19.43	2.58	NA	45.33	$1,640.91	090	M	B	C+
61332	Explore/biopsy eye socket	27.28	NA	20.43	4.15	NA	51.86	$1,877.29	090	M		C+
61333	Explore orbit/remove lesion	27.95	NA	16.45	2.24	NA	46.64	$1,688.33	090	M		C+
61334	Explore orbit/remove object	18.27	NA	10.08	3.02	NA	31.37	$1,135.57	090	M		C+
61340	Relieve cranial pressure	18.66	NA	11.75	3.66	NA	34.07	$1,233.31	090	M	B	C+
61343	Incise skull (press relief)	29.77	NA	17.96	6.04	NA	53.77	$1,946.43	090	M		C+
61345	Relieve cranial pressure	27.20	NA	16.17	5.23	NA	48.60	$1,759.28	090	M		C+
61440	Incise skull for surgery	26.63	NA	12.14	5.57	NA	44.34	$1,605.07	090	M		C+
61450	Incise skull for surgery	25.95	NA	14.46	5.11	NA	45.52	$1,647.79	090	M		C
61458	Incise skull for brain wound	27.29	NA	15.89	5.28	NA	48.46	$1,754.21	090	M		C+
61460	Incise skull for surgery	28.39	NA	16.77	5.13	NA	50.29	$1,820.46	090	M		C+
61470	Incise skull for surgery	26.06	NA	13.74	4.65	NA	44.45	$1,609.05	090	M		C+
61480	Incise skull for surgery	26.49	NA	12.34	5.54	NA	44.37	$1,606.16	090	M		C+
61490	Incise skull for surgery	25.66	NA	15.18	5.37	NA	46.21	$1,672.77	090	M	B	C+
61500	Removal of skull lesion	17.92	NA	11.03	3.26	NA	32.21	$1,165.98	090	M		C+
61501	Remove infected skull bone	14.84	NA	9.62	2.63	NA	27.09	$980.64	090	M		C+
61510	Removal of brain lesion	28.45	NA	16.60	5.77	NA	50.82	$1,839.64	090	M		C+
61512	Remove brain lining lesion	35.09	NA	20.18	7.14	NA	62.41	$2,259.19	090	M		C+
61514	Removal of brain abscess	25.26	NA	14.91	5.12	NA	45.29	$1,639.46	090	M		C+
61516	Removal of brain lesion	24.61	NA	15.01	4.94	NA	44.56	$1,613.04	090	M		C+
61518	Removal of brain lesion	37.32	NA	22.34	7.53	NA	67.19	$2,432.22	090	M		C+
61519	Remove brain lining lesion	41.39	NA	24.42	8.15	NA	73.96	$2,677.29	090	M		C+
61520	Removal of brain lesion	54.84	NA	31.93	10.10	NA	96.87	$3,506.62	090	M		C

* **M** = multiple surgery adjustment applies
Me = multiple endoscopy rules may apply
B = bilateral surgery adjustment applies
A = assistant-at-surgery restriction

A+ = assistant-at-surgery restriction unless medical necessity established with documentation
C = cosurgeons payable
C+ = cosurgeons payable if medical necessity established with documentation

T = team surgeons permitted
T+ = team surgeons payable if medical necessity established with documentation
$ = indicates services that are not covered by Medicare.

CPT five-digit codes, two-digit numeric modifiers, and descriptions only are © 2001 American Medical Association

Medicare RBRVS: The Physicians' Guide

Relative value units

CPT Code and Modifier	Description	Work RVU	Non Facility Practice Expense RVU	Facility Practice Expense RVU	PLI RVU	Total Non Facility RVUs	Medicare Payment Non Facility	Total Facility RVUs	Medicare Payment Facility	Global Period	Payment Policy Indicators*
61521	Removal of brain lesion	44.48	NA	26.22	8.85	NA	NA	79.55	$2,879.65	090	M C+
61522	Removal of brain abscess	29.45	NA	17.20	5.30	NA	NA	51.95	$1,880.55	090	M C+
61524	Removal of brain lesion	27.86	NA	16.83	5.01	NA	NA	49.70	$1,799.10	090	M C+
61526	Removal of brain lesion	52.17	NA	31.55	6.72	NA	NA	90.44	$3,273.86	090	M A C
61530	Removal of brain lesion	43.86	NA	27.43	6.17	NA	NA	77.46	$2,803.99	090	M A C
61531	Implant brain electrodes	14.63	NA	9.56	2.84	NA	NA	27.03	$978.46	090	M C
61533	Implant brain electrodes	19.71	NA	12.21	3.80	NA	NA	35.72	$1,293.04	090	M C+
61534	Removal of brain lesion	20.97	NA	13.30	4.15	NA	NA	38.42	$1,390.77	090	M C+
61535	Remove brain electrodes	11.63	NA	8.16	2.29	NA	NA	22.08	$799.28	090	M C+
61536	Removal of brain lesion	35.52	NA	21.18	6.68	NA	NA	63.38	$2,294.31	090	M C+
61538	Removal of brain tissue	26.81	NA	16.30	5.38	NA	NA	48.49	$1,755.30	090	M C+
61539	Removal of brain tissue	32.08	NA	18.91	6.62	NA	NA	57.61	$2,085.44	090	M C+
61541	Incision of brain tissue	28.85	NA	16.89	5.50	NA	NA	51.24	$1,854.85	090	M C+
61542	Removal of brain tissue	31.02	NA	18.00	6.49	NA	NA	55.51	$2,009.42	090	M C+
61543	Removal of brain tissue	29.22	NA	17.42	6.11	NA	NA	52.75	$1,909.51	090	M C+
61544	Remove & treat brain lesion	25.50	NA	15.21	4.91	NA	NA	45.62	$1,651.41	090	M
61545	Excision of brain tumor	43.80	NA	25.09	8.88	NA	NA	77.77	$2,815.21	090	M C+
61546	Removal of pituitary gland	31.30	NA	18.74	6.06	NA	NA	56.10	$2,030.78	090	M C+
61548	Removal of pituitary gland	21.53	NA	13.74	3.63	NA	NA	38.90	$1,408.15	090	M C
61550	Release of skull seams	14.65	NA	4.89	1.14	NA	NA	20.68	$748.60	090	M C+
61552	Release of skull seams	19.56	NA	9.87	0.88	NA	NA	30.31	$1,097.20	090	M C+
61556	Incise skull/sutures	22.26	NA	11.74	3.57	NA	NA	37.57	$1,360.00	090	M
61557	Incise skull/sutures	22.38	NA	13.41	4.68	NA	NA	40.47	$1,464.98	090	M
61558	Excision of skull/sutures	25.58	NA	12.67	2.61	NA	NA	40.86	$1,479.10	090	M
61559	Excision of skull/sutures	32.79	NA	18.89	6.86	NA	NA	58.54	$2,119.10	090	M C+
61563	Excision of skull tumor	26.83	NA	16.25	4.46	NA	NA	47.54	$1,720.91	090	M C+
61564	Excision of skull tumor	33.83	NA	18.73	7.08	NA	NA	59.64	$2,158.92	090	M C+

Code	Description	Col3	Col4	Col5	Col6	Fee	Global	Col9	Col10	Col11	Col12
61570	Remove foreign body, brain	24.60	NA	13.80	4.60	43.00	$1,556.57	090	M		C+
61571	Incise skull for brain wound	26.39	NA	15.43	5.23	47.05	$1,703.17	090	M		C+
61575	Skull base/brainstem surgery	34.36	NA	21.38	5.02	60.76	$2,199.46	090	M		C+
61576	Skull base/brainstem surgery	52.43	NA	28.89	4.68	86.00	$3,113.13	090	M		C+
61580	Craniofacial approach, skull	30.35	NA	19.96	2.75	53.06	$1,920.73	090	M	B	C+	T
61581	Craniofacial approach, skull	34.60	NA	22.57	3.37	60.54	$2,191.50	090	M	B A	C	T
61582	Craniofacial approach, skull	31.66	NA	19.56	6.30	57.52	$2,082.18	090	M		C+	T
61583	Craniofacial approach, skull	36.21	NA	22.71	6.94	65.86	$2,384.08	090	M	B	C+	T
61584	Orbitocranial approach/skull	34.65	NA	20.99	6.53	62.17	$2,250.50	090	M	B	C+	T
61585	Orbitocranial approach/skull	38.61	NA	22.21	6.19	67.01	$2,425.71	090	M	B	C+	T
61586	Resect nasopharynx, skull	25.10	NA	16.39	3.52	45.01	$1,629.33	090	M		C+	T
61590	Infratemporal approach/skull	41.78	NA	26.12	4.28	72.18	$2,612.86	090	M	B	C+	T
61591	Infratemporal approach/skull	43.68	NA	26.89	5.26	75.83	$2,744.99	090	M	B	C+	T
61592	Orbitocranial approach/skull	39.64	NA	23.59	7.55	70.78	$2,562.18	090	M	B	C+	T
61595	Transtemporal approach/skull	29.57	NA	19.74	3.05	52.36	$1,895.39	090	M	B	C+	T
61596	Transcochlear approach/skull	35.63	NA	21.88	4.25	61.76	$2,235.66	090	M	B	C+	T
61597	Transcondylar approach/skull	37.96	NA	22.41	6.65	67.02	$2,426.07	090	M	B	C+	T
61598	Transpetrosal approach/skull	33.41	NA	20.92	4.60	58.93	$2,133.22	090	M		C+	T
61600	Resect/excise cranial lesion	25.85	NA	15.01	3.12	43.98	$1,592.04	090	M		C+	T
61601	Resect/excise cranial lesion	27.89	NA	17.34	5.29	50.52	$1,828.78	090	M		C+	T
61605	Resect/excise cranial lesion	29.33	NA	18.97	2.51	50.81	$1,839.28	090	M		C+	T
61606	Resect/excise cranial lesion	38.83	NA	23.17	6.81	68.81	$2,490.87	090	M		C+	T
61607	Resect/excise cranial lesion	36.27	NA	22.17	5.69	64.13	$2,321.45	090	M		C+	T
61608	Resect/excise cranial lesion	42.10	NA	24.89	8.31	75.30	$2,725.80	090	M		C+	T
61609	Transect artery, sinus	9.89	NA	5.11	2.07	17.07	$617.92	ZZZ		B	C+	T
61610	Transect artery, sinus	29.67	NA	14.38	3.52	47.57	$1,722.00	ZZZ		B	C+	T
61611	Transect artery, sinus	7.42	NA	2.96	1.55	11.93	$431.86	ZZZ		B	C+	T
61612	Transect artery, sinus	27.88	NA	14.30	3.55	45.73	$1,655.39	ZZZ		B	C+	T

* **M** = multiple surgery adjustment applies
   Me = multiple endoscopy rules may apply
   B = bilateral surgery adjustment applies
   A = assistant-at-surgery restriction

A+ = assistant-at-surgery restriction unless medical necessity established with documentation
C = cosurgeons payable
C+ = cosurgeons payable if medical necessity established with documentation

T = team surgeons permitted
T+ = team surgeons payable if medical necessity established with documentation
$ = indicates services that are not covered by Medicare.

287 CPT five-digit codes, two-digit numeric modifiers, and descriptions only are © 2001 American Medical Association

Medicare RBRVS: The Physicians' Guide

Relative value units

CPT Code and Modifier	Description	Work RVU	Non Facility Practice Expense RVU	Facility Practice Expense RVU	PLI RVU	Total Non Facility RVUs	Medicare Payment Non Facility	Total Facility RVUs	Medicare Payment Facility	Global Period	Payment Policy Indicators*
61613	Remove aneurysm, sinus	40.86	NA	23.34	8.32	NA	NA	72.52	$2,625.17	090	M B C+ T
61615	Resect/excise lesion, skull	32.07	NA	20.81	4.64	NA	NA	57.52	$2,082.18	090	M C+ T
61616	Resect/excise lesion, skull	43.33	NA	26.97	7.02	NA	NA	77.32	$2,798.92	090	M C+ T
61618	Repair dura	16.99	NA	11.43	2.92	NA	NA	31.34	$1,134.48	090	M C+ T
61619	Repair dura	20.71	NA	13.67	3.42	NA	NA	37.80	$1,368.33	090	M C+ T
61624	Occlusion/embolization cath	20.15	NA	7.46	1.15	NA	NA	28.76	$1,041.09	000	M A
61626	Occlusion/embolization cath	16.62	NA	5.88	0.84	NA	NA	23.34	$844.89	000	M A
61680	Intracranial vessel surgery	30.71	NA	18.38	6.04	NA	NA	55.13	$1,995.66	090	M C+
61682	Intracranial vessel surgery	61.57	NA	34.65	12.69	NA	NA	108.91	$3,942.45	090	M C+
61684	Intracranial vessel surgery	39.81	NA	22.60	7.87	NA	NA	70.28	$2,544.08	090	M C+
61686	Intracranial vessel surgery	64.49	NA	36.70	13.20	NA	NA	114.39	$4,140.83	090	M C+
61690	Intracranial vessel surgery	29.31	NA	17.64	5.51	NA	NA	52.46	$1,899.01	090	M C+
61692	Intracranial vessel surgery	51.87	NA	29.51	10.17	NA	NA	91.55	$3,314.04	090	M C+
61697	Brain aneurysm repr, complx	50.52	NA	28.42	10.31	NA	NA	89.25	$3,230.78	090	M C+
61698	Brain aneurysm repr, complx	48.41	NA	27.31	9.99	NA	NA	85.71	$3,102.63	090	M C+
61700	Brain aneurysm repr , simple	50.52	NA	28.42	10.18	NA	NA	89.12	$3,226.07	090	M C+
61702	Inner skull vessel surgery	48.41	NA	27.31	9.75	NA	NA	85.47	$3,093.95	090	M C+
61703	Clamp neck artery	17.47	NA	11.13	3.62	NA	NA	32.22	$1,166.34	090	M C+
61705	Revise circulation to head	36.20	NA	19.89	6.67	NA	NA	62.76	$2,271.86	090	M C+
61708	Revise circulation to head	35.30	NA	16.52	2.18	NA	NA	54.00	$1,954.76	090	M
61710	Revise circulation to head	29.67	NA	14.68	2.42	NA	NA	46.77	$1,693.04	090	M A+
61711	Fusion of skull arteries	36.33	NA	20.68	7.39	NA	NA	64.40	$2,331.23	090	M C+
61720	Incise skull/brain surgery	16.77	NA	10.90	3.51	NA	NA	31.18	$1,128.69	090	M A
61735	Incise skull/brain surgery	20.43	NA	12.77	4.16	NA	NA	37.36	$1,352.40	090	M A
61750	Incise skull/brain biopsy	18.20	NA	11.08	3.71	NA	NA	32.99	$1,194.21	090	M A
61751	Brain biopsy w/ ct/mr guide	17.62	NA	10.92	3.57	NA	NA	32.11	$1,162.36	090	M A
61760	Implant brain electrodes	22.27	NA	12.85	4.59	NA	NA	39.71	$1,437.47	090	M C

Code	Description	Col3	Col4	Col5	Col6	Col7	Fee	Global	*M	A	C
61770	Incise skull for treatment	21.44	NA	13.26	4.09	NA	38.79	$1,404.17	090	M	A	C+
61790	Treat trigeminal nerve	10.86	NA	6.92	1.82	NA	19.60	$709.50	090	M	A	
61791	Treat trigeminal tract	14.61	NA	9.39	3.03	NA	27.03	$978.46	090	M	A+	
61793	Focus radiation beam	17.24	NA	11.07	3.51	NA	31.82	$1,151.86	090	M	A	
61795	Brain surgery using computer	4.04	NA	2.14	0.81	NA	6.99	$253.03	ZZZ		A	
61850	Implant neuroelectrodes	12.39	NA	8.13	2.23	NA	22.75	$823.53	090	M		
61860	Implant neuroelectrodes	20.87	NA	12.59	4.04	NA	37.50	$1,357.47	090	M		
61862	Implant neurostimul, subcort	19.34	NA	12.16	3.97	NA	35.47	$1,283.99	090	M		C+
61870	Implant neuroelectrodes	14.94	NA	9.97	1.70	NA	26.61	$963.26	090	M		C+
61875	Implant neuroelectrodes	15.06	NA	7.39	2.42	NA	24.87	$900.27	090	M		
61880	Revise/remove neuroelectrode	6.29	NA	5.26	1.31	NA	12.86	$465.52	090	M		C+
61885	Implant neurostim one array	5.85	NA	4.36	1.22	NA	11.43	$413.76	090	M	A+	
61886	Implant neurostim arrays	8.00	NA	6.13	1.64	NA	15.77	$570.86	090	M	A+	
61888	Revise/remove neuroreceiver	5.07	NA	3.90	1.04	NA	10.01	$362.35	010	M	A	
62000	Treat skull fracture	12.53	NA	6.19	0.87	NA	19.59	$709.14	090	M	A	
62005	Treat skull fracture	16.17	NA	9.35	2.33	NA	27.85	$1,008.15	090	M		C+
62010	Treatment of head injury	19.81	NA	11.83	4.05	NA	35.69	$1,291.95	090	M		C+
62100	Repair brain fluid leakage	22.03	NA	13.97	4.07	NA	40.07	$1,450.50	090	M		C+
62115	Reduction of skull defect	21.66	NA	11.03	4.53	NA	37.22	$1,347.33	090	M		C+
62116	Reduction of skull defect	23.59	NA	14.04	4.85	NA	42.48	$1,537.74	090	M		C+
62117	Reduction of skull defect	26.60	NA	12.68	5.56	NA	44.84	$1,623.17	090	M		C+
62120	Repair skull cavity lesion	23.35	NA	15.14	3.07	NA	41.56	$1,504.44	090	M		C+
62121	Incise skull repair	21.58	NA	13.52	2.47	NA	37.57	$1,360.00	090	M		
62140	Repair of skull defect	13.51	NA	8.72	2.60	NA	24.83	$898.83	090	M		C+
62141	Repair of skull defect	14.91	NA	9.89	2.85	NA	27.65	$1,000.91	090	M		C+
62142	Remove skull plate/flap	10.79	NA	7.31	2.10	NA	20.20	$731.22	090	M		
62143	Replace skull plate/flap	13.05	NA	8.81	2.55	NA	24.41	$883.62	090	M		C+
62145	Repair of skull & brain	18.82	NA	11.77	3.81	NA	34.40	$1,245.25	090	M		C+

*M = multiple surgery adjustment applies
Me = multiple endoscopy rules may apply
B = bilateral surgery adjustment applies
A = assistant-at-surgery restriction

A+ = assistant-at-surgery restriction unless medical necessity established with documentation
C = cosurgeons payable
C+ = cosurgeons payable if medical necessity established with documentation

T = team surgeons permitted
T+ = team surgeons payable if medical necessity established with documentation
$ = indicates services that are not covered by Medicare.

289   CPT five-digit codes, two-digit numeric modifiers, and descriptions only are © 2001 American Medical Association

Medicare RBRVS: The Physicians' Guide

Relative value units

CPT Code and Modifier	Description	Work RVU	Non Facility Practice Expense RVU	Facility Practice Expense RVU	PLI RVU	Total Non Facility RVUs	Medicare Payment Non Facility	Total Facility RVUs	Medicare Payment Facility	Global Period	Payment Policy Indicators*
62146	Repair of skull with graft	16.12	NA	10.63	2.94	NA	NA	29.69	$1,074.75	090	M C+
62147	Repair of skull with graft	19.34	NA	12.38	3.64	NA	NA	35.36	$1,280.00	090	M C+
62180	Establish brain cavity shunt	21.06	NA	13.08	4.32	NA	NA	38.46	$1,392.22	090	M
62190	Establish brain cavity shunt	11.07	NA	7.77	2.18	NA	NA	21.02	$760.91	090	M C+ A
62192	Establish brain cavity shunt	12.25	NA	8.25	2.46	NA	NA	22.96	$831.13	090	M C+
62194	Replace/irrigate catheter	5.03	NA	2.25	0.50	NA	NA	7.78	$281.63	010	M A+
62200	Establish brain cavity shunt	18.32	NA	11.72	3.70	NA	NA	33.74	$1,221.36	090	M C+
62201	Establish brain cavity shunt	14.86	NA	9.76	2.52	NA	NA	27.14	$982.45	090	M A
62220	Establish brain cavity shunt	13.00	NA	8.60	2.53	NA	NA	24.13	$873.49	090	M C+
62223	Establish brain cavity shunt	12.87	NA	8.54	2.58	NA	NA	23.99	$868.42	090	M C+
62225	Replace/irrigate catheter	5.41	NA	4.11	1.09	NA	NA	10.61	$384.07	090	M A
62230	Replace/revise brain shunt	10.54	NA	6.42	2.10	NA	NA	19.06	$689.96	090	M C+
62252	Csf shunt reprogram	0.74	1.35	1.35	0.18	2.27	$82.17	2.27	$82.17	XXX	A+
62252-26	Csf shunt reprogram	0.74	0.30	0.30	0.16	1.20	$43.44	1.20	$43.44	XXX	A+
62252-TC	Csf shunt reprogram	0.00	1.05	1.05	0.02	1.07	$38.73	1.07	$38.73	XXX	A+
62256	Remove brain cavity shunt	6.60	NA	5.40	1.34	NA	NA	13.34	$482.90	090	M A
62258	Replace brain cavity shunt	14.54	NA	8.82	2.91	NA	NA	26.27	$950.95	090	M C+
62263	Lysis epidural adhesions	6.14	5.15	2.07	0.42	11.71	$423.89	8.63	$312.40	010	M A
62268	Drain spinal cord cyst	4.74	NA	2.74	0.29	NA	NA	7.77	$281.27	010	M A
62269	Needle biopsy, spinal cord	5.02	NA	2.40	0.29	NA	NA	7.71	$279.10	000	M A+
62270	Spinal fluid tap, diagnostic	1.13	4.08	0.48	0.06	5.27	$190.77	1.67	$60.45	000	M A
62272	Drain cerebro spinal fluid	1.35	3.38	0.62	0.13	4.86	$175.93	2.10	$76.02	000	M A
62273	Treat epidural spine lesion	2.15	1.57	1.27	0.14	3.86	$139.73	3.56	$128.87	010	M A
62280	Treat spinal cord lesion	2.63	3.79	0.70	0.17	6.59	$238.55	3.50	$126.70	010	M A
62281	Treat spinal cord lesion	2.66	4.50	0.62	0.16	7.32	$264.98	3.44	$124.53	010	M A
62282	Treat spinal canal lesion	2.33	5.57	0.62	0.14	8.04	$291.04	3.09	$111.86	010	M A
62284	Injection for myelogram	1.54	5.53	0.55	0.10	7.17	$259.55	2.19	$79.28	000	A

Code	Description											
62287	Percutaneous diskectomy	8.08	NA	5.05	0.66	NA	13.79	$499.19	090	M	A	
62290	Inject for spine disk x-ray	3.00	5.68	1.30	0.20	8.88	4.50	$162.90	000	M	A	
62291	Inject for spine disk x-ray	2.91	6.24	1.20	0.17	9.32	4.28	$154.93	000	M	A	
62292	Injection into disk lesion	7.86	NA	5.34	0.65	NA	13.85	$501.36	090	M	A+	
62294	Injection into spinal artery	11.83	NA	7.37	0.85	NA	20.05	$725.79	090	M	A	
62310	Inject spine c/t	1.91	3.71	0.43	0.11	5.73	2.45	$88.69	000	M	A	
62311	Inject spine l/s (cd)	1.54	4.22	0.37	0.09	5.85	2.00	$72.40	000	M	A	
62318	Inject spine w/cath, c/t	2.04	3.83	0.44	0.12	5.99	2.60	$94.12	000	M	A	
62319	Inject spine w/cath l/s (cd)	1.87	3.67	0.40	0.11	5.65	2.38	$86.15	000	M	A	
62350	Implant spinal canal cath	6.87	NA	3.79	0.64	NA	11.30	$409.05	090	M	A	C+
62351	Implant spinal canal cath	10.00	NA	6.90	1.79	NA	18.69	$676.56	090	M		C
62355	Remove spinal canal catheter	5.45	NA	3.02	0.47	NA	8.94	$323.62	090	M	A+	
62360	Insert spine infusion device	2.62	NA	2.46	0.21	NA	5.29	$191.49	090	M	A+	C+
62361	Implant spine infusion pump	5.42	NA	3.67	0.50	NA	9.59	$347.15	090	M	A+	C+
62362	Implant spine infusion pump	7.04	NA	4.06	0.86	NA	11.96	$432.94	090	M	A+	C+
62365	Remove spine infusion device	5.42	NA	3.99	0.58	NA	9.99	$361.63	090	M	A+	
62367	Analyze spine infusion pump	0.00	0.00	0.00	0.00	0.00	0.00	$0.00	XXX		A+	
62367-26	Analyze spine infusion pump	0.48	0.14	0.14	0.03	0.65	0.65	$23.53	XXX	M	A+	
62367-TC	Analyze spine infusion pump	0.00	0.00	0.00	0.00	0.00	0.00	$0.00	XXX	M	A+	
62368	Analyze spine infusion pump	0.00	0.00	0.00	0.00	0.00	0.00	$0.00	XXX	M	A+	
62368-26	Analyze spine infusion pump	0.75	0.20	0.20	0.05	1.00	1.00	$36.20	XXX	M	A+	
62368-TC	Analyze spine infusion pump	0.00	0.00	0.00	0.00	0.00	0.00	$0.00	XXX	M	A+	
63001	Removal of spinal lamina	15.82	NA	11.68	3.03	NA	30.53	$1,105.16	090	M		C
63003	Removal of spinal lamina	15.95	NA	11.95	2.98	NA	30.88	$1,117.83	090	M		C
63005	Removal of spinal lamina	14.92	NA	11.49	2.62	NA	29.03	$1,050.86	090	M		C
63011	Removal of spinal lamina	14.52	NA	11.29	1.43	NA	27.24	$986.07	090	M		C
63012	Removal of spinal lamina	15.40	NA	10.34	2.71	NA	28.45	$1,029.87	090	M		C
63015	Removal of spinal lamina	19.35	NA	13.68	3.84	NA	36.87	$1,334.66	090	M		C

* **M** = multiple surgery adjustment applies
Me = multiple endoscopy rules may apply
B = bilateral surgery adjustment applies
A = assistant-at-surgery restriction

A+ = assistant-at-surgery restriction unless medical necessity established with documentation
C = cosurgeons payable
C+ = cosurgeons payable if medical necessity established with documentation

T = team surgeons permitted
T+ = team surgeons payable if medical necessity established with documentation
§ = indicates services that are not covered by Medicare.

CPT five-digit codes, two-digit numeric modifiers, and descriptions only are © 2001 American Medical Association

Medicare RBRVS: The Physicians' Guide

Relative value units

CPT Code and Modifier	Description	Work RVU	Non Facility Practice Expense RVU	Facility Practice Expense RVU	PLI RVU	Total Non Facility RVUs	Medicare Payment Non Facility	Total Facility RVUs	Medicare Payment Facility	Global Period	Payment Policy Indicators*		
63016	Removal of spinal lamina	19.20	NA	13.66	3.62	NA	NA	36.48	$1,320.55	090	M		C
63017	Removal of spinal lamina	15.94	NA	12.00	2.91	NA	NA	30.85	$1,116.75	090	M		C
63020	Neck spine disk surgery	14.81	NA	11.33	2.89	NA	NA	29.03	$1,050.86	090	M	B	C
63030	Low back disk surgery	12.00	NA	9.92	2.21	NA	NA	24.13	$873.49	090	M		C
63035	Spinal disk surgery add-on	3.15	NA	1.67	0.57	NA	NA	5.39	$195.11	ZZZ		B	C
63040	Laminotomy, single cervical	18.81	NA	13.39	3.36	NA	NA	35.56	$1,287.24	090	M	B	C
63042	Laminotomy, single lumbar	17.47	NA	12.95	3.11	NA	NA	33.53	$1,213.76	090	M	B	C
63043	Laminotomy, addl cervical	0.00	0.00	0.00	0.00	0.00	$0.00	0.00	$0.00	ZZZ			C
63044	Laminotomy, addl lumbar	0.00	0.00	0.00	0.00	0.00	$0.00	0.00	$0.00	ZZZ			C
63045	Removal of spinal lamina	16.50	NA	12.22	3.19	NA	NA	31.91	$1,155.12	090	M		C
63046	Removal of spinal lamina	15.80	NA	12.02	2.89	NA	NA	30.71	$1,111.68	090	M		C
63047	Removal of spinal lamina	14.61	NA	11.42	2.61	NA	NA	28.64	$1,036.75	090	M		C
63048	Remove spinal lamina add-on	3.26	NA	1.75	0.58	NA	NA	5.59	$202.35	ZZZ			C+
63055	Decompress spinal cord	21.99	NA	15.11	4.09	NA	NA	41.19	$1,491.05	090	M		C+
63056	Decompress spinal cord	20.36	NA	14.44	3.34	NA	NA	38.14	$1,380.64	090	M		C+
63057	Decompress spine cord add-on	5.26	NA	2.82	0.81	NA	NA	8.89	$321.81	ZZZ			C+
63064	Decompress spinal cord	24.61	NA	17.12	4.72	NA	NA	46.45	$1,681.45	090	M		C+
63066	Decompress spine cord add-on	3.26	NA	1.76	0.63	NA	NA	5.65	$204.53	ZZZ			C+
63075	Neck spine disk surgery	19.41	NA	13.83	3.73	NA	NA	36.97	$1,338.28	090	M		C
63076	Neck spine disk surgery	4.05	NA	2.16	0.78	NA	NA	6.99	$253.03	ZZZ			C
63077	Spine disk surgery, thorax	21.44	NA	15.47	3.44	NA	NA	40.35	$1,460.64	090	M		C
63078	Spine disk surgery, thorax	3.28	NA	1.72	0.50	NA	NA	5.50	$199.10	ZZZ			C
63081	Removal of vertebral body	23.73	NA	16.68	4.46	NA	NA	44.87	$1,624.26	090	M		C+	T
63082	Remove vertebral body add-on	4.37	NA	2.34	0.82	NA	NA	7.53	$272.58	ZZZ			C+	T
63085	Removal of vertebral body	26.92	NA	17.89	4.70	NA	NA	49.51	$1,792.22	090	M		C	T
63086	Remove vertebral body add-on	3.19	NA	1.66	0.55	NA	NA	5.40	$195.48	ZZZ			C
63087	Removal of vertebral body	35.57	NA	22.45	5.87	NA	NA	63.89	$2,312.77	090	M		C	T

Code	Description										
63088	Remove vertebral body add-on	4.33	NA	2.30	0.77	NA	7.40	$267.87	ZZZ		C	T
63090	Removal of vertebral body	28.16	NA	18.12	4.27	NA	50.55	$1,829.87	090	M	C	T
63091	Remove vertebral body add-on	3.03	NA	1.48	0.45	NA	4.96	$179.55	ZZZ		C	T
63170	Incise spinal cord tract(s)	19.83	NA	13.54	3.89	NA	37.26	$1,348.78	090	M	C+	
63172	Drainage of spinal cyst	17.66	NA	13.37	3.46	NA	34.49	$1,248.51	090	M	C+	
63173	Drainage of spinal cyst	21.99	NA	15.54	4.14	NA	41.67	$1,508.42	090	M	C+	
63180	Revise spinal cord ligaments	18.27	NA	13.04	3.83	NA	35.14	$1,272.04	090	M	C+	
63182	Revise spinal cord ligaments	20.50	NA	13.61	3.48	NA	37.59	$1,360.73	090	M	C+	
63185	Incise spinal column/nerves	15.04	NA	9.70	2.08	NA	26.82	$970.86	090	M	C+	
63190	Incise spinal column/nerves	17.45	NA	11.68	2.88	NA	32.01	$1,158.74	090	M	C+	
63191	Incise spinal column/nerves	17.54	NA	10.65	3.50	NA	31.69	$1,147.15	090	M B	C+	
63194	Incise spinal column & cord	19.19	NA	13.48	4.01	NA	36.68	$1,327.79	090	M	C+	
63195	Incise spinal column & cord	18.84	NA	13.02	3.44	NA	35.30	$1,277.83	090	M	C+	
63196	Incise spinal column & cord	22.30	NA	14.03	4.66	NA	40.99	$1,483.81	090	M	C+	
63197	Incise spinal column & cord	21.11	NA	13.49	4.42	NA	39.02	$1,412.49	090	M	C+	
63198	Incise spinal column & cord	25.38	NA	12.70	5.31	NA	43.39	$1,570.68	090	M	C+	
63199	Incise spinal column & cord	26.89	NA	14.38	5.62	NA	46.89	$1,697.38	090	M	C+	
63200	Release of spinal cord	19.18	NA	13.42	3.61	NA	36.21	$1,310.77	090	M		
63250	Revise spinal cord vessels	40.76	NA	23.15	7.65	NA	71.56	$2,590.41	090	M	C+	
63251	Revise spinal cord vessels	41.20	NA	23.51	7.98	NA	72.69	$2,631.32	090	M	C+	
63252	Revise spinal cord vessels	41.19	NA	23.36	7.75	NA	72.30	$2,617.20	090	M	C+	
63265	Excise intraspinal lesion	21.56	NA	13.21	4.29	NA	39.06	$1,413.94	090	M	C+	
63266	Excise intraspinal lesion	22.30	NA	13.70	4.47	NA	40.47	$1,464.98	090	M	C+	
63267	Excise intraspinal lesion	17.95	NA	11.48	3.50	NA	32.93	$1,192.04	090	M	C+	
63268	Excise intraspinal lesion	18.52	NA	10.97	3.18	NA	32.67	$1,182.63	090	M	C+	
63270	Excise intraspinal lesion	26.80	NA	16.10	5.41	NA	48.31	$1,748.78	090	M	C+	
63271	Excise intraspinal lesion	26.92	NA	16.17	5.56	NA	48.65	$1,761.09	090	M	C+	
63272	Excise intraspinal lesion	25.32	NA	15.31	5.07	NA	45.70	$1,654.30	090	M	C+	

* **M** = multiple surgery adjustment applies
Me = multiple endoscopy rules may apply
B = bilateral surgery adjustment applies
A = assistant-at-surgery restriction

A+ = assistant-at-surgery restriction unless medical necessity established with documentation
C = cosurgeons payable
C+ = cosurgeons payable if medical necessity established with documentation

T = team surgeons permitted
T+ = team surgeons payable if medical necessity established with documentation
§ = indicates services that are not covered by Medicare.

CPT five-digit codes, two-digit numeric modifiers, and descriptions only are © 2001 American Medical Association

Medicare RBRVS: The Physicians' Guide

Relative value units

CPT Code and Modifier	Description	Work RVU	Non Facility Practice Expense RVU	Facility Practice Expense RVU	PLI RVU	Total Non Facility RVUs	Medicare Payment Non Facility	Total Facility RVUs	Medicare Payment Facility	Global Period	Payment Policy Indicators*
63273	Excise intraspinal lesion	24.29	NA	14.84	5.08	NA	NA	44.21	$1,600.37	090	M
63275	Biopsy/excise spinal tumor	23.68	NA	14.47	4.68	NA	NA	42.83	$1,550.41	090	M C+
63276	Biopsy/excise spinal tumor	23.45	NA	14.27	4.63	NA	NA	42.35	$1,533.04	090	M C+
63277	Biopsy/excise spinal tumor	20.83	NA	12.99	4.03	NA	NA	37.85	$1,370.14	090	M C+
63278	Biopsy/excise spinal tumor	20.56	NA	13.08	4.02	NA	NA	37.66	$1,363.26	090	M C+
63280	Biopsy/excise spinal tumor	28.35	NA	16.76	5.80	NA	NA	50.91	$1,842.90	090	M C+
63281	Biopsy/excise spinal tumor	28.05	NA	16.73	5.67	NA	NA	50.45	$1,826.25	090	M C+
63282	Biopsy/excise spinal tumor	26.39	NA	15.79	5.33	NA	NA	47.51	$1,719.82	090	M C+
63283	Biopsy/excise spinal tumor	25.00	NA	15.07	5.12	NA	NA	45.19	$1,635.84	090	M C+
63285	Biopsy/excise spinal tumor	36.00	NA	20.82	7.31	NA	NA	64.13	$2,321.45	090	M C+
63286	Biopsy/excise spinal tumor	35.63	NA	20.51	7.07	NA	NA	63.21	$2,288.15	090	M C+
63287	Biopsy/excise spinal tumor	36.70	NA	21.03	7.48	NA	NA	65.21	$2,360.55	090	M C+
63290	Biopsy/excise spinal tumor	37.38	NA	21.58	7.65	NA	NA	66.61	$2,411.23	090	M C+
63300	Removal of vertebral body	24.43	NA	14.63	4.78	NA	NA	43.84	$1,586.97	090	M C+
63301	Removal of vertebral body	27.60	NA	15.65	5.03	NA	NA	48.28	$1,747.70	090	M C+
63302	Removal of vertebral body	27.81	NA	16.45	5.25	NA	NA	49.51	$1,792.22	090	M C+
63303	Removal of vertebral body	30.50	NA	17.71	5.21	NA	NA	53.42	$1,933.76	090	M C+
63304	Removal of vertebral body	30.33	NA	17.80	4.72	NA	NA	52.85	$1,913.13	090	M
63305	Removal of vertebral body	32.03	NA	19.24	5.39	NA	NA	56.66	$2,051.05	090	M C+
63306	Removal of vertebral body	32.22	NA	18.19	2.39	NA	NA	52.80	$1,911.32	090	M C+
63307	Removal of vertebral body	31.63	NA	17.29	4.23	NA	NA	53.15	$1,923.99	090	M C+
63308	Remove vertebral body add-on	5.25	NA	2.74	1.01	NA	NA	9.00	$325.79	ZZZ	
63600	Remove spinal cord lesion	14.02	NA	6.38	1.22	NA	NA	21.62	$782.63	090	M A+
63610	Stimulation of spinal cord	8.73	NA	3.90	0.43	NA	NA	13.06	$472.76	000	M A+
63615	Remove lesion of spinal cord	16.28	NA	9.50	2.85	NA	NA	28.63	$1,036.38	090	M A C+
63650	Implant neuroelectrodes	6.74	NA	2.97	0.48	NA	NA	10.19	$368.87	090	M A
63655	Implant neuroelectrodes	10.29	NA	7.26	1.85	NA	NA	19.40	$702.26	090	M C+

Code	Description										
63660	Revise/remove neuroelectrode	6.16	NA	3.67	0.65	NA	10.48	$379.37	090	M	A	C+
63685	Implant neuroreceiver	7.04	NA	4.15	0.96	NA	12.15	$439.82	090	M		C+
63688	Revise/remove neuroreceiver	5.39	NA	3.69	0.70	NA	9.78	$354.03	090	M	A	
63700	Repair of spinal herniation	16.53	NA	10.47	2.69	NA	29.69	$1,074.75	090	M		C+
63702	Repair of spinal herniation	18.48	NA	9.90	1.36	NA	29.74	$1,076.56	090	M		C+
63704	Repair of spinal herniation	21.18	NA	12.37	3.84	NA	37.39	$1,353.49	090	M		C+
63706	Repair of spinal herniation	24.11	NA	13.60	4.73	NA	42.44	$1,536.29	090	M		C+
63707	Repair spinal fluid leakage	11.26	NA	8.06	1.96	NA	21.28	$770.32	090	M		C+
63709	Repair spinal fluid leakage	14.32	NA	9.79	2.49	NA	26.60	$962.90	090	M		C+
63710	Graft repair of spine defect	14.07	NA	9.54	2.61	NA	26.22	$949.14	090	M		C+
63740	Install spinal shunt	11.36	NA	7.79	2.15	NA	21.30	$771.04	090	M		C+
63741	Install spinal shunt	8.25	NA	4.72	1.05	NA	14.02	$507.51	090	M		C+
63744	Revision of spinal shunt	8.10	NA	5.72	1.51	NA	15.33	$554.93	090	M		C+
63746	Removal of spinal shunt	6.43	NA	4.96	1.15	NA	12.54	$453.94	090	M	A+	
64400	Injection for nerve block	1.11	2.70	0.29	0.06	3.87	1.46	$52.85	000	M	A	
64402	Injection for nerve block	1.25	4.38	0.45	0.07	5.70	1.77	$64.07	000	M	A	
64405	Injection for nerve block	1.32	1.34	0.37	0.08	2.74	1.77	$64.07	000	M	A	
64408	Injection for nerve block	1.41	2.95	0.62	0.09	4.45	2.12	$76.74	000	M	A+	
64410	Injection for nerve block	1.43	3.27	0.35	0.08	4.78	1.86	$67.33	000	M	A+	
64412	Injection for nerve block	1.18	2.49	0.37	0.08	3.75	1.63	$59.00	000	M	A	
64413	Injection for nerve block	1.40	2.81	0.34	0.09	4.30	1.83	$66.24	000	M	A	
64415	Injection for nerve block	1.48	2.65	0.32	0.08	4.21	1.88	$68.05	000	M	A	
64417	Injection for nerve block	1.44	3.21	0.38	0.09	4.74	1.91	$69.14	000	M	A	
64418	Injection for nerve block	1.32	2.49	0.29	0.07	3.88	1.68	$60.81	000	M	A	
64420	Injection for nerve block	1.18	2.37	0.27	0.07	3.62	1.52	$55.02	000	M	A	
64421	Injection for nerve block	1.68	2.91	0.38	0.10	4.69	2.16	$78.19	000	M	A	
64425	Injection for nerve block	1.75	2.33	0.41	0.11	4.19	2.27	$82.17	000	M	A	
64430	Injection for nerve block	1.46	2.89	0.47	0.11	4.46	2.04	$73.85	000	M	A	

*M = multiple surgery adjustment applies
Me = multiple endoscopy rules may apply
B = bilateral surgery adjustment applies
A = assistant-at-surgery restriction

A+ = assistant-at-surgery restriction unless medical necessity established with documentation
C = cosurgeons payable
C+ = cosurgeons payable if medical necessity established with documentation

T = team surgeons permitted
T+ = team surgeons payable if medical necessity established with documentation
§ = indicates services that are not covered by Medicare.

295 CPT five-digit codes, two-digit numeric modifiers, and descriptions only are © 2001 American Medical Association

Medicare RBRVS: The Physicians' Guide

Relative value units

CPT Code and Modifier	Description	Work RVU	Non Facility Practice Expense RVU	Facility Practice Expense RVU	PLI RVU	Total Non Facility RVUs	Medicare Payment Non Facility	Total Facility RVUs	Medicare Payment Facility	Global Period	Payment Policy Indicators*
64435	Injection for nerve block	1.45	2.96	0.60	0.15	4.56	$165.07	2.20	$79.64	000	M A
64445	Injection for nerve block	1.48	1.60	0.42	0.08	3.16	$114.39	1.98	$71.67	000	M A
64450	Injection for nerve block	1.27	1.79	0.33	0.08	3.14	$113.67	1.68	$60.81	000	M A
64470	Inj paravertebral c/t	1.85	4.02	0.48	0.12	5.99	$216.83	2.45	$88.69	000	M B A
64472	Inj paravertebral c/t add-on	1.29	3.90	0.33	0.09	5.28	$191.13	1.71	$61.90	ZZZ	M B A
64475	Inj paravertebral l/s	1.41	3.82	0.39	0.09	5.32	$192.58	1.89	$68.42	000	M B A
64476	Inj paravertebral l/s add-on	0.98	3.86	0.26	0.06	4.90	$177.38	1.30	$47.06	ZZZ	M B A
64479	Inj foramen epidural c/t	2.20	4.40	0.64	0.14	6.74	$243.98	2.98	$107.87	000	M B A
64480	Inj foramen epidural add-on	1.54	4.07	0.50	0.09	5.70	$206.34	2.13	$77.10	ZZZ	M B A
64483	Inj foramen epidural l/s	1.90	4.44	0.56	0.12	6.46	$233.85	2.58	$93.39	000	M B A
64484	Inj foramen epidural add-on	1.33	4.05	0.40	0.08	5.46	$197.65	1.81	$65.52	ZZZ	M B A
64505	Injection for nerve block	1.36	2.41	0.35	0.08	3.85	$139.37	1.79	$64.80	000	M A
64508	Injection for nerve block	1.12	2.32	0.48	0.06	3.50	$126.70	1.66	$60.09	000	M A+
64510	Injection for nerve block	1.22	2.53	0.26	0.07	3.82	$138.28	1.55	$56.11	000	M A
64520	Injection for nerve block	1.35	3.49	0.31	0.08	4.92	$178.10	1.74	$62.99	000	M A+
64530	Injection for nerve block	1.58	3.07	0.37	0.09	4.74	$171.58	2.04	$73.85	000	M A
64550	Apply neurostimulator	0.18	0.56	0.07	0.01	0.75	$27.15	0.26	$9.41	000	M A
64553	Implant neuroelectrodes	2.31	4.25	1.33	0.17	6.73	$243.62	3.81	$137.92	010	M A+
64555	Implant neuroelectrodes	2.27	2.38	0.77	0.11	4.76	$172.31	3.15	$114.03	010	M A
64560	Implant neuroelectrodes	2.36	2.30	0.94	0.17	4.83	$174.84	3.47	$125.61	010	M A+
64561	Implant neuroelectrodes	6.74	15.28	3.83	0.11	22.13	$801.09	10.68	$386.61	010	M A
64565	Implant neuroelectrodes	1.76	3.41	0.69	0.08	5.25	$190.05	2.53	$91.58	010	M A
64573	Implant neuroelectrodes	7.50	NA	5.40	1.48	NA	NA	14.38	$520.54	090	M A+
64575	Implant neuroelectrodes	4.35	NA	3.03	0.37	NA	NA	7.75	$280.54	090	M A
64577	Implant neuroelectrodes	4.62	NA	3.44	0.50	NA	NA	8.56	$309.87	090	M A
64580	Implant neuroelectrodes	4.12	NA	3.94	0.21	NA	NA	8.27	$299.37	090	M
64581	Implant neuroelectrodes	13.50	NA	6.72	0.37	NA	NA	20.59	$745.34	090	M A

Code	Description											
64585	Revise/remove neuroelectrode	2.06	2.82	2.20	0.29	5.17	$187.15	4.55	$164.71	010	M		
64590	Implant neuroreceiver	2.40	NA	2.17	0.40	NA	NA	4.97	$179.91	010	M		C+
64595	Revise/remove neuroreceiver	1.73	NA	2.08	0.22	NA	NA	4.03	$145.88	010	M		A
64600	Injection treatment of nerve	3.45	2.98	2.06	0.28	6.71	$242.90	5.79	$209.59	010	M		A
64605	Injection treatment of nerve	5.61	3.62	2.90	0.53	9.76	$353.30	9.04	$327.24	010	M		A+
64610	Injection treatment of nerve	7.16	NA	4.18	1.12	NA	NA	12.46	$451.04	010	M		A
64612	Destroy nerve, face muscle	1.96	3.00	1.65	0.09	5.05	$182.81	3.70	$133.94	010	M	B	A
64613	Destroy nerve, spine muscle	1.96	1.82	1.48	0.10	3.88	$140.45	3.54	$128.15	010	M		A
64614	Destroy nerve, extrem musc	2.20	3.23	0.82	0.09	5.52	$199.82	3.11	$112.58	010	M	B	A
64620	Injection treatment of nerve	2.84	2.98	0.67	0.17	5.99	$216.83	3.68	$133.21	010	M		A
64622	Destr paravertebrl nerve l/s	3.00	4.77	0.74	0.17	7.94	$287.42	3.91	$141.54	010	M	B	A
64623	Destr paravertebral n add-on	0.99	3.85	0.24	0.06	4.90	$177.38	1.29	$46.70	ZZZ		B	A
64626	Destr paravertebrl nerve c/t	3.28	4.34	0.80	0.22	7.84	$283.80	4.30	$155.66	010	M	B	A
64627	Destr paravertebral n add-on	1.16	3.74	0.29	0.08	4.98	$180.27	1.53	$55.38	ZZZ		B	A
64630	Injection treatment of nerve	3.00	3.66	0.88	0.16	6.82	$246.88	4.04	$146.24	010	M		A+
64640	Injection treatment of nerve	2.76	3.67	1.72	0.11	6.54	$236.74	4.59	$166.15	010	M		A
64680	Injection treatment of nerve	2.62	2.89	0.76	0.15	5.66	$204.89	3.53	$127.78	010	M		A
64702	Revise finger/toe nerve	4.23	NA	4.05	0.51	NA	NA	8.79	$318.19	090	M		A
64704	Revise hand/foot nerve	4.57	NA	3.23	0.59	NA	NA	8.39	$303.71	090	M		C+
64708	Revise arm/leg nerve	6.12	NA	5.19	0.82	NA	NA	12.13	$439.10	090	M		C+
64712	Revision of sciatic nerve	7.75	NA	5.61	0.54	NA	NA	13.90	$503.17	090	M		C+
64713	Revision of arm nerve(s)	11.00	NA	6.66	1.01	NA	NA	18.67	$675.84	090	M		C+
64714	Revise low back nerve(s)	10.33	NA	4.25	0.64	NA	NA	15.22	$550.95	090	M		C+
64716	Revision of cranial nerve	6.31	NA	5.18	0.59	NA	NA	12.08	$437.29	090	M		C+
64718	Revise ulnar nerve at elbow	5.99	NA	5.29	0.87	NA	NA	12.15	$439.82	090	M		A+
64719	Revise ulnar nerve at wrist	4.85	NA	4.78	0.63	NA	NA	10.26	$371.40	090	M		A
64721	Carpal tunnel surgery	4.29	6.59	6.14	0.59	11.47	$415.20	11.02	$398.92	090	M	B	A
64722	Relieve pressure on nerve(s)	4.70	NA	3.49	0.32	NA	NA	8.51	$308.06	090	M		C+

* **M** = multiple surgery adjustment applies
   Me = multiple endoscopy rules may apply
   B = bilateral surgery adjustment applies
   A = assistant-at-surgery restriction

A+ = assistant-at-surgery restriction unless medical necessity established with documentation
C = cosurgeons payable
C+ = cosurgeons payable if medical necessity established with documentation

T = team surgeons permitted
T+ = team surgeons payable if medical necessity established with documentation
S = indicates services that are not covered by Medicare.

297   CPT five-digit codes, two-digit numeric modifiers, and descriptions only are © 2001 American Medical Association

Medicare RBRVS: The Physicians' Guide

Relative value units

CPT Code and Modifier	Description	Work RVU	Non Facility Practice Expense RVU	Facility Practice Expense RVU	PLI RVU	Total Non Facility RVUs	Medicare Payment Non Facility	Total Facility RVUs	Medicare Payment Facility	Global Period	Payment Policy Indicators*
64726	Release foot/toe nerve	4.18	NA	3.14	0.57	NA	NA	7.89	$285.61	090	M A
64727	Internal nerve revision	3.10	NA	1.68	0.40	NA	NA	5.18	$187.51	ZZZ	A
64732	Incision of brow nerve	4.41	NA	3.69	0.77	NA	NA	8.87	$321.09	090	M
64734	Incision of cheek nerve	4.92	NA	3.80	0.83	NA	NA	9.55	$345.70	090	M A+
64736	Incision of chin nerve	4.60	NA	2.98	0.71	NA	NA	8.29	$300.09	090	M
64738	Incision of jaw nerve	5.73	NA	3.92	0.84	NA	NA	10.49	$379.73	090	M
64740	Incision of tongue nerve	5.59	NA	4.11	0.43	NA	NA	10.13	$366.70	090	M
64742	Incision of facial nerve	6.22	NA	4.96	0.69	NA	NA	11.87	$429.68	090	M
64744	Incise nerve, back of head	5.24	NA	3.94	0.98	NA	NA	10.16	$367.78	090	M B A+
64746	Incise diaphragm nerve	5.93	NA	4.58	0.75	NA	NA	11.26	$407.60	090	M C+
64752	Incision of vagus nerve	7.06	NA	4.96	0.83	NA	NA	12.85	$465.16	090	M C+
64755	Incision of stomach nerves	13.52	NA	6.40	1.16	NA	NA	21.08	$763.08	090	M C+
64760	Incision of vagus nerve	6.96	NA	4.05	0.51	NA	NA	11.52	$417.01	090	M C+
64761	Incision of pelvis nerve	6.41	NA	3.48	0.26	NA	NA	10.15	$367.42	090	M B
64763	Incise hip/thigh nerve	6.93	NA	6.21	0.77	NA	NA	13.91	$503.53	090	M B C+
64766	Incise hip/thigh nerve	8.67	NA	4.73	0.99	NA	NA	14.39	$520.91	090	M B
64771	Sever cranial nerve	7.35	NA	5.44	1.32	NA	NA	14.11	$510.77	090	M
64772	Incision of spinal nerve	7.21	NA	4.88	1.20	NA	NA	13.29	$481.09	090	M C+
64774	Remove skin nerve lesion	5.17	NA	3.92	0.60	NA	NA	9.69	$350.77	090	M A
64776	Remove digit nerve lesion	5.12	NA	3.89	0.63	NA	NA	9.64	$348.96	090	M A+
64778	Digit nerve surgery add-on	3.11	NA	1.64	0.38	NA	NA	5.13	$185.70	ZZZ	M A
64782	Remove limb nerve lesion	6.23	NA	3.93	0.79	NA	NA	10.95	$396.38	090	M A C+
64783	Limb nerve surgery add-on	3.72	NA	1.95	0.48	NA	NA	6.15	$222.63	ZZZ	M A
64784	Remove nerve lesion	9.82	NA	6.99	1.17	NA	NA	17.98	$650.86	090	M A+
64786	Remove sciatic nerve lesion	15.46	NA	10.41	2.22	NA	NA	28.09	$1,016.84	090	M
64787	Implant nerve end	4.30	NA	2.28	0.56	NA	NA	7.14	$258.46	ZZZ	A+
64788	Remove skin nerve lesion	4.61	NA	3.50	0.54	NA	NA	8.65	$313.12	090	M A

Code	Description										
64790	Removal of nerve lesion	11.31	NA	7.53	1.68	NA	20.52	$742.81	090	M		A+
64792	Removal of nerve lesion	14.92	NA	9.13	1.88	NA	25.93	$938.65	090	M			C+
64795	Biopsy of nerve	3.01	NA	1.81	0.40	NA	5.22	$188.96	000	M		A	
64802	Remove sympathetic nerves	9.15	NA	5.17	0.87	NA	15.19	$549.87	090	M	B		C+
64804	Remove sympathetic nerves	14.64	NA	6.83	1.79	NA	23.26	$841.99	090	M	B		C+
64809	Remove sympathetic nerves	13.67	NA	6.04	0.96	NA	20.67	$748.24	090	M	B		C+
64818	Remove sympathetic nerves	10.30	NA	5.76	1.08	NA	17.14	$620.45	090	M	B		C+
64820	Remove sympathetic nerves	10.37	NA	6.48	1.17	NA	18.02	$652.31	090	M		A	
64821	Remove sympathetic nerves	8.75	NA	7.09	0.99	NA	16.83	$609.23	090	M		A	
64822	Remove sympathetic nerves	8.75	NA	7.09	0.99	NA	16.83	$609.23	090	M		A	
64823	Remove sympathetic nerves	10.37	NA	7.89	1.17	NA	19.43	$703.35	090	M		A	
64831	Repair of digit nerve	9.44	NA	7.44	1.14	NA	18.02	$652.31	090	M		A	
64832	Repair nerve add-on	5.66	NA	3.11	0.68	NA	9.45	$342.08	ZZZ			A+	
64834	Repair of hand or foot nerve	10.19	NA	7.40	1.23	NA	18.82	$681.27	090	M		A+	
64835	Repair of hand or foot nerve	10.94	NA	8.06	1.36	NA	20.36	$737.02	090	M			C+
64836	Repair of hand or foot nerve	10.94	NA	7.94	1.32	NA	20.20	$731.22	090	M			C+
64837	Repair nerve add-on	6.26	NA	3.47	0.80	NA	10.53	$381.18	ZZZ				C+
64840	Repair of leg nerve	13.02	NA	7.79	0.86	NA	21.67	$784.44	090	M			
64856	Repair/transpose nerve	13.80	NA	9.66	1.71	NA	25.17	$911.13	090	M		A	C+
64857	Repair arm/leg nerve	14.49	NA	10.21	1.76	NA	26.46	$957.83	090	M			C+
64858	Repair sciatic nerve	16.49	NA	11.04	2.78	NA	30.31	$1,097.20	090	M			C+
64859	Nerve surgery	4.26	NA	2.24	0.50	NA	7.00	$253.39	ZZZ				C+
64861	Repair of arm nerves	19.24	NA	13.02	2.45	NA	34.71	$1,256.47	090	M			C+
64862	Repair of low back nerves	19.44	NA	12.29	2.47	NA	34.20	$1,238.01	090	M			
64864	Repair of facial nerve	12.55	NA	8.63	1.13	NA	22.31	$807.60	090	M			C+
64865	Repair of facial nerve	15.24	NA	10.46	1.37	NA	27.07	$979.91	090	M			C+
64866	Fusion of facial/other nerve	15.74	NA	9.84	1.06	NA	26.64	$964.35	090	M			C+
64868	Fusion of facial/other nerve	14.04	NA	9.57	1.40	NA	25.01	$905.34	090	M			C+

* **M** = multiple surgery adjustment applies
   Me = multiple endoscopy rules may apply
   B = bilateral surgery adjustment applies
   A = assistant-at-surgery restriction

A+ = assistant-at-surgery restriction unless medical necessity established with documentation
C = cosurgeons payable
C+ = cosurgeons payable if medical necessity established with documentation

T = team surgeons permitted
T+ = team surgeons payable if medical necessity established with documentation
§ = indicates services that are not covered by Medicare.

CPT five-digit codes, two-digit numeric modifiers, and descriptions only are © 2001 American Medical Association

Medicare RBRVS: The Physicians' Guide

Relative value units

CPT Code and Modifier	Description	Work RVU	Non Facility Practice Expense RVU	Facility Practice Expense RVU	PLI RVU	Total Non Facility RVUs	Medicare Payment Non Facility	Total Facility RVUs	Medicare Payment Facility	Global Period	Payment Policy Indicators*		
64870	Fusion of facial/other nerve	15.99	NA	9.65	1.08	NA	NA	26.72	$967.24	090	M		C+
64872	Subsequent repair of nerve	1.99	NA	1.08	0.24	NA	NA	3.31	$119.82	ZZZ			C+
64874	Repair & revise nerve add-on	2.98	NA	1.64	0.34	NA	NA	4.96	$179.55	ZZZ			C+
64876	Repair nerve/shorten bone	3.38	NA	1.35	0.39	NA	NA	5.12	$185.34	ZZZ			C+
64885	Nerve graft, head or neck	17.53	NA	11.66	1.51	NA	NA	30.70	$1,111.32	090	M		C+
64886	Nerve graft, head or neck	20.75	NA	13.60	1.73	NA	NA	36.08	$1,306.07	090	M		C+
64890	Nerve graft, hand or foot	15.15	NA	10.27	1.74	NA	NA	27.16	$983.17	090	M		
64891	Nerve graft, hand or foot	16.14	NA	5.75	1.38	NA	NA	23.27	$842.36	090	M		C+
64892	Nerve graft, arm or leg	14.65	NA	8.96	1.65	NA	NA	25.26	$914.39	090	M		
64893	Nerve graft, arm or leg	15.60	NA	10.75	1.77	NA	NA	28.12	$1,017.92	090	M		C+
64895	Nerve graft, hand or foot	19.25	NA	8.62	2.04	NA	NA	29.91	$1,082.72	090	M		C+
64896	Nerve graft, hand or foot	20.49	NA	11.75	1.85	NA	NA	34.09	$1,234.03	090	M		
64897	Nerve graft, arm or leg	18.24	NA	10.92	2.64	NA	NA	31.80	$1,151.13	090	M		C+
64898	Nerve graft, arm or leg	19.50	NA	10.75	2.71	NA	NA	32.96	$1,193.13	090	M		C+
64901	Nerve graft add-on	10.22	NA	5.75	0.99	NA	NA	16.96	$613.94	ZZZ			
64902	Nerve graft add-on	11.83	NA	6.32	1.10	NA	NA	19.25	$696.83	ZZZ			C+
64905	Nerve pedicle transfer	14.02	NA	8.93	1.52	NA	NA	24.47	$885.79	090	M		C+
64907	Nerve pedicle transfer	18.83	NA	12.07	1.79	NA	NA	32.69	$1,183.35	090	M		C+
64999	Nervous system surgery	0.00	0.00	0.00	0.00	0.00	$0.00	0.00	$0.00	YYY	M	A+	T+

Surgery: Eye and ocular adnexa

CPT Code and Modifier	Description	Work RVU	Non Facility Practice Expense RVU	Facility Practice Expense RVU	PLI RVU	Total Non Facility RVUs	Medicare Payment Non Facility	Total Facility RVUs	Medicare Payment Facility	Global Period	Payment Policy Indicators*		
65091	Revise eye	6.46	NA	11.59	0.26	NA	NA	18.31	$662.81	090	M	B	A+
65093	Revise eye with implant	6.87	NA	11.83	0.28	NA	NA	18.98	$687.06	090	M	B	A
65101	Removal of eye	7.03	NA	12.04	0.28	NA	NA	19.35	$700.45	090	M	B	A
65103	Remove eye/insert implant	7.57	NA	12.17	0.30	NA	NA	20.04	$725.43	090	M	B	A
65105	Remove eye/attach implant	8.49	NA	12.67	0.34	NA	NA	21.50	$778.28	090	M	B	C+
65110	Removal of eye	13.95	NA	15.90	0.68	NA	NA	30.53	$1,105.16	090	M	B	C+
65112	Remove eye/revise socket	16.38	NA	17.26	0.96	NA	NA	34.60	$1,252.49	090	M	B	C+

Code	Description											
65114	Remove eye/revise socket	17.53	NA	18.54	0.94	NA	NA	37.01	$1,339.73	090	M	B	C+
65125	Revise ocular implant	3.12	6.23	1.48	0.15	9.50	$343.89	4.75	$171.95	090	M	B	A	C+
65130	Insert ocular implant	7.15	NA	11.46	0.28	NA	NA	18.89	$683.80	090	M	B	A	C+
65135	Insert ocular implant	7.33	NA	12.37	0.29	NA	NA	19.99	$723.62	090	M	B	A
65140	Attach ocular implant	8.02	NA	12.36	0.31	NA	NA	20.69	$748.96	090	M	B	A
65150	Revise ocular implant	6.26	NA	10.94	0.25	NA	NA	17.45	$631.68	090	M	B	A+
65155	Reinsert ocular implant	8.66	NA	12.59	0.40	NA	NA	21.65	$783.71	090	M	B	A
65175	Removal of ocular implant	6.28	NA	11.35	0.26	NA	NA	17.89	$647.60	090	M	B	A	C+
65205	Remove foreign body from eye	0.71	0.63	0.20	0.03	1.37	$49.59	0.94	$34.03	000	M	B	A
65210	Remove foreign body from eye	0.84	0.78	0.32	0.03	1.65	$59.73	1.19	$43.08	000	M	B	A
65220	Remove foreign body from eye	0.71	8.23	0.19	0.05	8.99	$325.43	0.95	$34.39	000	M	B	A
65222	Remove foreign body from eye	0.93	0.80	0.29	0.04	1.77	$64.07	1.26	$45.61	000	M	B	A
65235	Remove foreign body from eye	7.57	NA	7.04	0.30	NA	NA	14.91	$539.73	090	M	B	A+
65260	Remove foreign body from eye	10.96	NA	12.66	0.43	NA	NA	24.05	$870.59	090	M	B
65265	Remove foreign body from eye	12.59	NA	14.38	0.50	NA	NA	27.47	$994.39	090	M	B		C+
65270	Repair of eye wound	1.90	4.07	2.44	0.08	6.05	$219.01	4.42	$160.00	010	M	B	A+
65272	Repair of eye wound	3.82	5.76	4.75	0.16	9.74	$352.58	8.73	$316.02	090	M	B	A
65273	Repair of eye wound	4.36	NA	5.15	0.17	NA	NA	9.68	$350.41	090	M	B	A	C+
65275	Repair of eye wound	5.34	5.50	5.32	0.27	11.11	$402.17	10.93	$395.66	090	M	B	A+
65280	Repair of eye wound	7.66	NA	7.88	0.30	NA	NA	15.84	$573.40	090	M	B	A+
65285	Repair of eye wound	12.90	NA	13.86	0.51	NA	NA	27.27	$987.15	090	M	B
65286	Repair of eye wound	5.51	9.12	7.85	0.21	14.84	$537.20	13.57	$491.22	090	M	B	A
65290	Repair of eye socket wound	5.41	NA	6.60	0.26	NA	NA	12.27	$444.16	090	M	B	A	C+
65400	Removal of eye lesion	6.06	8.61	7.13	0.24	14.91	$539.73	13.43	$486.16	090	M	B	A
65410	Biopsy of cornea	1.47	1.76	0.71	0.06	3.29	$119.10	2.24	$81.09	000	M	B	A+
65420	Removal of eye lesion	4.17	8.36	7.22	0.17	12.70	$459.73	11.56	$418.46	090	M	B	A
65426	Removal of eye lesion	5.25	8.01	6.75	0.20	13.46	$487.24	12.20	$441.63	090	M	B	A
65430	Corneal smear	1.47	8.68	0.71	0.06	10.21	$369.59	2.24	$81.09	000	M	B	A

* **M** = multiple surgery adjustment applies
Me = multiple endoscopy rules may apply
B = bilateral surgery adjustment applies
A = assistant-at-surgery restriction

A+ = assistant-at-surgery restriction unless medical necessity established with documentation
C = cosurgeons payable
C+ = cosurgeons payable if medical necessity established with documentation

T = team surgeons permitted
T+ = team surgeons payable if medical necessity established with documentation
§ = indicates services that are not covered by Medicare.

301 CPT five-digit codes, two-digit numeric modifiers, and descriptions only are © 2001 American Medical Association

Medicare RBRVS: The Physicians' Guide

Relative value units

CPT Code and Modifier	Description	Work RVU	Non Facility Practice Expense RVU	Facility Practice Expense RVU	PLI RVU	Total Non Facility RVUs	Medicare Payment Non Facility	Total Facility RVUs	Medicare Payment Facility	Global Period	Payment Policy Indicators*			
65435	Curette/treat cornea	0.92	1.37	0.41	0.04	2.33	$84.34	1.37	$49.59	000	M	B	A	
65436	Curette/treat cornea	4.19	6.02	5.03	0.17	10.38	$375.75	9.39	$339.91	090	M	B	A	
65450	Treatment of corneal lesion	3.27	7.97	6.80	0.13	11.37	$411.58	10.20	$369.23	090	M	B	A	
65600	Revision of cornea	3.40	5.54	1.54	0.14	9.08	$328.69	5.08	$183.89	090	M	B	A	
65710	Corneal transplant	12.35	NA	13.25	0.49	NA	NA	26.09	$944.44	090	M	B	A	C+
65730	Corneal transplant	14.25	NA	12.16	0.56	NA	NA	26.97	$976.29	090	M	B	A	C+
65750	Corneal transplant	15.00	NA	14.54	0.59	NA	NA	30.13	$1,090.68	090	M	B	A	C+
65755	Corneal transplant	14.89	NA	14.48	0.58	NA	NA	29.95	$1,084.17	090	M	B	A	C+
65770	Revise cornea with implant	17.56	NA	15.48	0.69	NA	NA	33.73	$1,221.00	090	M	B		
65772	Correction of astigmatism	4.29	7.51	6.47	0.17	11.97	$433.30	10.93	$395.66	090	M	B	A	
65775	Correction of astigmatism	5.79	NA	8.63	0.22	NA	NA	14.64	$529.96	090	M	B	A	
65800	Drainage of eye	1.91	2.33	1.45	0.08	4.32	$156.38	3.44	$124.53	000	M	B	A	
65805	Drainage of eye	1.91	2.34	1.46	0.08	4.33	$156.74	3.45	$124.89	000	M	B	A	
65810	Drainage of eye	4.87	NA	8.95	0.19	NA	NA	14.01	$507.15	090	M	B	A	
65815	Drainage of eye	5.05	9.40	8.16	0.20	14.65	$530.32	13.41	$485.43	090	M	B	A	
65820	Relieve inner eye pressure	8.13	NA	10.99	0.32	NA	NA	19.44	$703.71	090	M	B	A+	
65850	Incision of eye	10.52	NA	10.35	0.41	NA	NA	21.28	$770.32	090	M	B	A	C+
65855	Laser surgery of eye	3.85	5.17	3.70	0.17	9.19	$332.67	7.72	$279.46	010	M	B	A	
65860	Incise inner eye adhesions	3.55	4.15	3.18	0.14	7.84	$283.80	6.87	$248.69	090	M	B	A+	
65865	Incise inner eye adhesions	5.60	NA	6.92	0.22	NA	NA	12.74	$461.18	090	M	B	A	C+
65870	Incise inner eye adhesions	6.27	NA	7.25	0.24	NA	NA	13.76	$498.10	090	M	B	A	C+
65875	Incise inner eye adhesions	6.54	NA	7.37	0.25	NA	NA	14.16	$512.58	090	M	B	A	C+
65880	Incise inner eye adhesions	7.09	NA	7.64	0.28	NA	NA	15.01	$543.35	090	M	B	A	
65900	Remove eye lesion	10.93	NA	12.75	0.46	NA	NA	24.14	$873.85	090	M	B		
65920	Remove implant of eye	8.40	NA	8.26	0.33	NA	NA	16.99	$615.02	090	M	B	A	C+
65930	Remove blood clot from eye	7.44	NA	8.83	0.29	NA	NA	16.56	$599.46	090	M	B	A	C+
66020	Injection treatment of eye	1.59	2.43	1.57	0.07	4.09	$148.05	3.23	$116.92	010	M	B	A	

Code	Description												
66030	Injection treatment of eye	1.25	2.25	1.40	0.05	3.55	$128.51	2.70	$97.74	010	M	B	A
66130	Remove eye lesion	7.69	7.63	6.71	0.31	15.63	$565.79	14.71	$532.49	090	M	B	A+
66150	Glaucoma surgery	8.30	NA	10.98	0.33	NA	NA	19.61	$709.87	090	M	B	A	C+
66155	Glaucoma surgery	8.29	NA	10.94	0.32	NA	NA	19.55	$707.69	090	M	B	A
66160	Glaucoma surgery	10.17	NA	11.84	0.41	NA	NA	22.42	$811.59	090	M	B	A	C+
66165	Glaucoma surgery	8.01	NA	10.72	0.31	NA	NA	19.04	$689.23	090	M	B	
66170	Glaucoma surgery	12.16	NA	17.11	0.48	NA	NA	29.75	$1,076.93	090	M	B	A	C+
66172	Incision of eye	15.04	NA	15.67	0.59	NA	NA	31.30	$1,133.03	090	M	B	A	C+
66180	Implant eye shunt	14.55	NA	12.44	0.57	NA	NA	27.56	$997.65	090	M	B	A	C+
66185	Revise eye shunt	8.14	NA	8.47	0.32	NA	NA	16.93	$612.85	090	M	B	
66220	Repair eye lesion	7.77	NA	9.99	0.32	NA	NA	18.08	$654.48	090	M	B	A	C+
66225	Repair/graft eye lesion	11.05	NA	9.65	0.44	NA	NA	21.14	$765.25	090	M	B	A	C+
66250	Follow-up surgery of eye	5.98	8.08	6.48	0.23	14.29	$517.29	12.69	$459.37	090	M	B	A
66500	Incision of iris	3.71	NA	4.82	0.15	NA	NA	8.68	$314.21	090	M	B	A	C+
66505	Incision of iris	4.08	NA	5.01	0.17	NA	NA	9.26	$335.20	090	M	B	A
66600	Remove iris and lesion	8.68	NA	8.90	0.34	NA	NA	17.92	$648.69	090	M	B	A
66605	Removal of iris	12.79	NA	12.54	0.61	NA	NA	25.94	$939.01	090	M	B	A
66625	Removal of iris	5.13	7.90	6.81	0.20	13.23	$478.92	12.14	$439.46	090	M	B	A
66630	Removal of iris	6.16	NA	7.76	0.24	NA	NA	14.16	$512.58	090	M	B	A
66635	Removal of iris	6.25	NA	6.65	0.24	NA	NA	13.14	$475.66	090	M	B	A
66680	Repair iris & ciliary body	5.44	NA	6.30	0.21	NA	NA	11.95	$432.58	090	M	B	A	C+
66682	Repair iris & ciliary body	6.21	NA	7.75	0.24	NA	NA	14.20	$514.03	090	M	B	A
66700	Destruction, ciliary body	4.78	7.17	7.17	0.19	12.14	$439.46	12.14	$439.46	090	M	B	A+
66710	Destruction, ciliary body	4.78	8.92	7.53	0.18	13.88	$502.44	12.49	$452.13	090	M	B	A
66720	Destruction, ciliary body	4.78	8.40	7.53	0.19	13.37	$483.98	12.50	$452.49	090	M	B	A
66740	Destruction, ciliary body	4.78	NA	6.53	0.18	NA	NA	11.49	$415.93	090	M	B	A
66761	Revision of iris	4.07	5.66	4.38	0.16	9.89	$358.01	8.61	$311.68	090	M	B	A
66762	Revision of iris	4.58	5.65	4.45	0.18	10.41	$376.83	9.21	$333.39	090	M	B	A

* **M** = multiple surgery adjustment applies
Me = multiple endoscopy rules may apply
B = bilateral surgery adjustment applies
A = assistant-at-surgery restriction

A+ = assistant-at-surgery restriction unless medical necessity established with documentation
C = cosurgeons payable
C+ = cosurgeons payable if medical necessity established with documentation

T = team surgeons permitted
T+ = team surgeons payable if medical necessity established with documentation
$ = indicates services that are not covered by Medicare.

303 CPT five-digit codes, two-digit numeric modifiers, and descriptions only are © 2001 American Medical Association

Medicare RBRVS: The Physicians' Guide

Relative value units

CPT Code and Modifier	Description	Work RVU	Non Facility Practice Expense RVU	Facility Practice Expense RVU	PLI RVU	Total Non Facility RVUs	Medicare Payment Non Facility	Total Facility RVUs	Medicare Payment Facility	Global Period	Payment Policy Indicators*
66770	Removal of inner eye lesion	5.18	5.94	4.68	0.20	11.32	$409.77	10.06	$364.16	090	M B A
66820	Incision, secondary cataract	3.89	NA	8.50	0.16	NA	NA	12.55	$454.30	090	M B A
66821	After cataract laser surgery	2.35	3.89	3.46	0.10	6.34	$229.50	5.91	$213.94	090	M B A
66825	Reposition intraocular lens	8.23	NA	10.56	0.32	NA	NA	19.11	$691.77	090	M B A+
66830	Removal of lens lesion	8.20	NA	7.06	0.32	NA	NA	15.58	$563.98	090	M B A
66840	Removal of lens material	7.91	NA	6.92	0.31	NA	NA	15.14	$548.06	090	M B A
66850	Removal of lens material	9.11	NA	7.52	0.36	NA	NA	16.99	$615.02	090	M B A
66852	Removal of lens material	9.97	NA	7.99	0.39	NA	NA	18.35	$664.26	090	M B A+ C+
66920	Extraction of lens	8.86	NA	7.42	0.35	NA	NA	16.63	$601.99	090	M B A+ C+
66930	Extraction of lens	10.18	NA	8.94	0.41	NA	NA	19.53	$706.97	090	M B A+
66940	Extraction of lens	8.93	NA	8.39	0.35	NA	NA	17.67	$639.64	090	M B A+ C+
66982	Cataract surgery, complex	13.50	NA	9.31	0.56	NA	NA	23.37	$845.98	090	M B A
66983	Cataract surg w/iol, 1 stage	8.99	NA	6.34	0.37	NA	NA	15.70	$568.33	090	M B A
66984	Cataract surg w/iol, i stage	10.23	NA	7.85	0.41	NA	NA	18.49	$669.32	090	M B A
66985	Insert lens prosthesis	8.39	NA	7.05	0.33	NA	NA	15.77	$570.86	090	M B A C+
66986	Exchange lens prosthesis	12.28	NA	8.86	0.49	NA	NA	21.63	$782.99	090	M B A C+
66999	Eye surgery procedure	0.00	0.00	0.00	0.00	0.00	$0.00	0.00	$0.00	YYY	M B A+ C+ T+
67005	Partial removal of eye fluid	5.70	NA	2.75	0.22	NA	NA	8.67	$313.85	090	M B A C+
67010	Partial removal of eye fluid	6.87	NA	3.32	0.27	NA	NA	10.46	$378.64	090	M B A C+
67015	Release of eye fluid	6.92	NA	8.38	0.27	NA	NA	15.57	$563.62	090	M B A C+
67025	Replace eye fluid	6.84	18.23	7.77	0.27	25.34	$917.29	14.88	$538.64	090	M B A C+
67027	Implant eye drug system	10.85	15.12	9.26	0.46	26.43	$956.74	20.57	$744.62	090	M B A C+
67028	Injection eye drug	2.52	11.92	1.21	0.11	14.55	$526.70	3.84	$139.00	000	M B A
67030	Incise inner eye strands	4.84	NA	6.96	0.19	NA	NA	11.99	$434.03	090	M B C+
67031	Laser surgery, eye strands	3.67	4.22	3.24	0.15	8.04	$291.04	7.06	$255.57	090	M B A
67036	Removal of inner eye fluid	11.89	NA	9.30	0.47	NA	NA	21.66	$784.07	090	M B C+
67038	Strip retinal membrane	21.24	NA	16.01	0.84	NA	NA	38.09	$1,378.83	090	M B C+

Code	Description												
67039	Laser treatment of retina	14.52	NA	12.74	0.57	NA	27.83	$1,007.42	090	M	B		C+
67040	Laser treatment of retina	17.23	NA	14.08	0.68	NA	31.99	$1,158.01	090	M	B		C+
67101	Repair detached retina	7.53	11.29	9.12	0.29	19.11	16.94	$613.21	090	M	B	A	
67105	Repair detached retina	7.41	7.80	5.70	0.29	15.50	13.40	$485.07	090	M	B	A	
67107	Repair detached retina	14.84	NA	13.63	0.58	NA	29.05	$1,051.59	090	M	B		C+
67108	Repair detached retina	20.82	NA	18.30	0.82	NA	39.94	$1,445.80	090	M	B		C+
67110	Repair detached retina	8.81	21.74	10.56	0.35	30.90	19.72	$713.85	090	M	B	A	
67112	Rerepair detached retina	16.86	NA	15.66	0.66	NA	33.18	$1,201.09	090	M	B		C+
67115	Release encircling material	4.99	NA	7.02	0.19	NA	12.20	$441.63	090	M	B	A	
67120	Remove eye implant material	5.98	17.57	7.36	0.23	23.78	13.57	$491.22	090	M	B	A	
67121	Remove eye implant material	10.67	NA	12.47	0.42	NA	23.56	$852.85	090	M	B		C+
67141	Treatment of retina	5.20	8.29	7.16	0.20	13.69	12.56	$454.66	090	M	B	A	
67145	Treatment of retina	5.37	5.43	4.28	0.21	11.01	9.86	$356.92	090	M	B	A	
67208	Treatment of retinal lesion	6.70	8.62	7.26	0.26	15.58	14.22	$514.75	090	M	B	A	
67210	Treatment of retinal lesion	8.82	7.49	5.93	0.35	16.66	15.10	$546.61	090	M	B	A	
67218	Treatment of retinal lesion	18.53	NA	16.36	0.53	NA	35.42	$1,282.18	090	M	B	A	
67220	Treatment of choroid lesion	13.13	11.18	9.94	0.51	24.82	23.58	$853.58	090	M	B	A	
67221	Ocular photodynamic ther	4.01	4.80	1.95	0.16	8.97	6.12	$221.54	000	M		A	
67225	Eye photodynamic ther add-on	0.47	0.24	0.19	0.50	1.21	1.16	$41.99	ZZZ				
67227	Treatment of retinal lesion	6.58	9.29	7.40	0.26	16.13	14.24	$515.48	090	M	B	A	
67228	Treatment of retinal lesion	12.74	10.17	7.47	0.50	23.41	20.71	$749.69	090	M	B	A	
67250	Reinforce eye wall	8.66	NA	12.10	0.36	NA	21.12	$764.53	090	M	B		C+
67255	Reinforce/graft eye wall	8.90	NA	12.11	0.35	NA	21.36	$773.21	090	M	B		C+
67299	Eye surgery procedure	0.00	0.00	0.00	0.00	0.00	0.00	$0.00	YYY	M	B	A+	C+ T+
67311	Revise eye muscle	6.65	NA	6.36	0.27	NA	13.28	$480.73	090	M	B	A	
67312	Revise two eye muscles	8.54	NA	7.46	0.35	NA	16.35	$591.86	090	M	B	A	
67314	Revise eye muscle	7.52	NA	6.94	0.30	NA	14.76	$534.30	090	M	B	A	
67316	Revise two eye muscles	9.66	NA	7.99	0.40	NA	18.05	$653.40	090	M	B	A+	

* **M** = multiple surgery adjustment applies
   Me = multiple endoscopy rules may apply
   B = bilateral surgery adjustment applies
   A = assistant-at-surgery restriction

A+ = assistant-at-surgery restriction unless medical necessity established with documentation
C = cosurgeons payable
C+ = cosurgeons payable if medical necessity established with documentation

T = team surgeons permitted
T+ = team surgeons payable if medical necessity established with documentation
S = indicates services that are not covered by Medicare.

CPT five-digit codes, two-digit numeric modifiers, and descriptions only are © 2001 American Medical Association

Medicare RBRVS: The Physicians' Guide

Relative value units

CPT Code and Modifier	Description	Work RVU	Non Facility Practice Expense RVU	Facility Practice Expense RVU	PLI RVU	Total Non Facility RVUs	Medicare Payment Non Facility	Total Facility RVUs	Medicare Payment Facility	Global Period	Payment Policy Indicators*			
67318	Revise eye muscle(s)	7.85	NA	7.37	0.31	NA	NA	15.53	$562.17	090	M	B	A	C+
67320	Revise eye muscle(s) add-on	4.33	NA	2.09	0.17	NA	NA	6.59	$238.55	ZZZ	M	B	A	C+
67331	Eye surgery follow-up add-on	4.06	NA	2.02	0.17	NA	NA	6.25	$226.25	ZZZ	M	B	A	C+
67332	Rerevise eye muscles add-on	4.49	NA	2.16	0.18	NA	NA	6.83	$247.24	ZZZ	M	B		C+
67334	Revise eye muscle w/suture	3.98	NA	1.90	0.16	NA	NA	6.04	$218.64	ZZZ	M	B	A	C+
67335	Eye suture during surgery	2.49	NA	1.20	0.10	NA	NA	3.79	$137.19	ZZZ	M	B	A	C+
67340	Revise eye muscle add-on	4.93	NA	2.41	0.19	NA	NA	7.53	$272.58	ZZZ	M	B		
67343	Release eye tissue	7.35	NA	7.26	0.30	NA	NA	14.91	$539.73	090	M	B	A	C+
67345	Destroy nerve of eye muscle	2.96	4.46	1.36	0.13	7.55	$273.30	4.45	$161.09	010	M	B	A	
67350	Biopsy eye muscle	2.87	NA	1.99	0.13	NA	NA	4.99	$180.63	000	M	B	A+	
67399	Eye muscle surgery procedure	0.00	0.00	0.00	0.00	0.00	$0.00	0.00	$0.00	YYY	M	B		C+ T+
67400	Explore/biopsy eye socket	9.76	NA	13.85	0.43	NA	NA	24.04	$870.23	090	M	B		C+
67405	Explore/drain eye socket	7.93	NA	12.56	0.36	NA	NA	20.85	$754.75	090	M	B		
67412	Explore/treat eye socket	9.50	NA	16.02	0.41	NA	NA	25.93	$938.65	090	M	B		C+
67413	Explore/treat eye socket	10.00	NA	13.80	0.43	NA	NA	24.23	$877.11	090	M	B		
67414	Explr/decompress eye socket	11.13	NA	16.90	0.48	NA	NA	28.51	$1,032.04	090	M	B		C+
67415	Aspiration, orbital contents	1.76	NA	0.80	0.09	NA	NA	2.65	$95.93	000	M	B	A+	
67420	Explore/treat eye socket	20.06	NA	20.79	0.84	NA	NA	41.69	$1,509.14	090	M	B		C+
67430	Explore/treat eye socket	13.39	NA	18.38	0.97	NA	NA	32.74	$1,185.16	090	M	B		
67440	Explore/drain eye socket	13.09	NA	18.43	0.58	NA	NA	32.10	$1,161.99	090	M	B		C+
67445	Explr/decompress eye socket	14.42	NA	18.19	0.63	NA	NA	33.24	$1,203.26	090	M	B		C+
67450	Explore/biopsy eye socket	13.51	NA	17.51	0.56	NA	NA	31.58	$1,143.17	090	M	B		C+
67500	Inject/treat eye socket	0.79	0.95	0.20	0.04	1.78	$64.43	1.03	$37.29	000	M	B	A	
67505	Inject/treat eye socket	0.82	0.95	0.21	0.04	1.81	$65.52	1.07	$38.73	000	M	B	A	
67515	Inject/treat eye socket	0.61	0.86	0.29	0.02	1.49	$53.94	0.92	$33.30	000	M	B	A	
67550	Insert eye socket implant	10.19	NA	13.57	0.50	NA	NA	24.26	$878.19	090	M	B	A	C+
67560	Revise eye socket implant	10.60	NA	13.50	0.47	NA	NA	24.57	$889.41	090	M	B	A+	

Code	Description													
67570	Decompress optic nerve	13.58	NA	17.66	0.69	NA	NA	31.93	$1,155.84	090	M	B	A	C+
67599	Orbit surgery procedure	0.00	0.00	0.00	0.00	0.00	0.00	0.00	$0.00	YYY	M	B	A	C+ T+
67700	Drainage of eyelid abscess	1.35	7.80	0.60	0.06	9.21	$333.39	2.01	$72.76	010	M	B	A	
67710	Incision of eyelid	1.02	7.92	0.49	0.04	8.98	$325.07	1.55	$56.11	010	M	B	A	
67715	Incision of eyelid fold	1.22	NA	0.59	0.05	NA	NA	1.86	$67.33	010	M	B	A	
67800	Remove eyelid lesion	1.38	2.67	0.66	0.06	4.11	$148.78	2.10	$76.02	010	M	B	A	
67801	Remove eyelid lesions	1.88	8.23	0.91	0.08	10.19	$368.87	2.87	$103.89	010	M	B	A	
67805	Remove eyelid lesions	2.22	8.41	1.06	0.09	10.72	$388.06	3.37	$121.99	010	M	B	A	
67808	Remove eyelid lesion(s)	3.80	NA	4.34	0.17	NA	NA	8.31	$300.82	090	M	B	A	
67810	Biopsy of eyelid	1.48	5.26	0.72	0.06	6.80	$246.15	2.26	$81.81	000	M	B	A	
67820	Revise eyelashes	0.89	2.02	0.39	0.04	2.95	$106.79	1.32	$47.78	000	M	B	A	
67825	Revise eyelashes	1.38	5.70	1.07	0.06	7.14	$258.46	2.51	$90.86	010	M	B	A	
67830	Revise eyelashes	1.70	11.55	2.20	0.07	13.32	$482.17	3.97	$143.71	010	M	B	A	
67835	Revise eyelashes	5.56	NA	4.90	0.22	NA	NA	10.68	$386.61	090	M	B	A+	
67840	Remove eyelid lesion	2.04	8.19	0.99	0.08	10.31	$373.21	3.11	$112.58	010	M	B	A	
67850	Treat eyelid lesion	1.69	8.79	2.07	0.07	10.55	$381.90	3.83	$138.64	010	M	B	A	
67875	Closure of eyelid by suture	1.35	11.62	2.16	0.06	13.03	$471.68	3.57	$129.23	000	M	B	A	
67880	Revision of eyelid	3.80	12.77	3.24	0.16	16.73	$605.61	7.20	$260.63	090	M	B	A	
67882	Revision of eyelid	5.07	15.42	4.84	0.21	20.70	$749.32	10.12	$366.34	090	M	B	A	
67900	Repair brow defect	6.14	11.29	6.69	0.30	17.73	$641.81	13.13	$475.30	090	M	B	A	
67901	Repair eyelid defect	6.97	NA	7.22	0.32	NA	NA	14.51	$525.25	090	M	B	A	
67902	Repair eyelid defect	7.03	NA	7.17	0.34	NA	NA	14.54	$526.34	090	M	B	A	C+
67903	Repair eyelid defect	6.37	10.72	6.80	0.39	17.48	$632.76	13.56	$490.86	090	M	B	A	C+
67904	Repair eyelid defect	6.26	14.97	8.57	0.26	21.49	$777.92	15.09	$546.25	090	M	B	A	C+
67906	Repair eyelid defect	6.79	9.91	6.30	0.42	17.12	$619.73	13.51	$489.05	090	M	B	A	
67908	Repair eyelid defect	5.13	9.65	6.36	0.20	14.98	$542.26	11.69	$423.17	090	M	B	A	
67909	Revise eyelid defect	5.40	10.20	6.87	0.25	15.85	$573.76	12.52	$453.21	090	M	B	A	
67911	Revise eyelid defect	5.27	NA	6.92	0.23	NA	NA	12.42	$449.59	090	M	B	A	

* **M** = multiple surgery adjustment applies
Me = multiple endoscopy rules may apply
B = bilateral surgery adjustment applies
A = assistant-at-surgery restriction

A+ = assistant-at-surgery restriction unless medical necessity established with documentation
C = cosurgeons payable
C+ = cosurgeons payable if medical necessity established with documentation

T = team surgeons permitted
T+ = team surgeons payable if medical necessity established with documentation
S = indicates services that are not covered by Medicare.

307   CPT five-digit codes, two-digit numeric modifiers, and descriptions only are © 2001 American Medical Association

Medicare RBRVS: The Physicians' Guide

Relative value units

CPT Code and Modifier	Description	Work RVU	Non Facility Practice Expense RVU	Facility Practice Expense RVU	PLI RVU	Total Non Facility RVUs	Medicare Payment Non Facility	Total Facility RVUs	Medicare Payment Facility	Global Period	Payment Policy Indicators*
67914	Repair eyelid defect	3.68	13.22	3.70	0.16	17.06	$617.56	7.54	$272.94	090	M B A
67915	Repair eyelid defect	3.18	11.73	1.52	0.13	15.04	$544.44	4.83	$174.84	090	M B A
67916	Repair eyelid defect	5.31	17.26	5.52	0.22	22.79	$824.98	11.05	$400.00	090	M B A
67917	Repair eyelid defect	6.02	10.63	6.86	0.25	16.90	$611.77	13.13	$475.30	090	M B A
67921	Repair eyelid defect	3.40	12.94	3.47	0.14	16.48	$596.56	7.01	$253.76	090	M B A
67922	Repair eyelid defect	3.06	11.73	3.31	0.13	14.92	$540.09	6.50	$235.29	090	M B A
67923	Repair eyelid defect	5.88	16.33	5.62	0.24	22.45	$812.67	11.74	$424.98	090	M B A
67924	Repair eyelid defect	5.79	9.97	6.20	0.23	15.99	$578.83	12.22	$442.35	090	M B A
67930	Repair eyelid wound	3.61	12.50	3.15	0.17	16.28	$589.32	6.93	$250.86	010	M A
67935	Repair eyelid wound	6.22	16.12	5.60	0.29	22.63	$819.19	12.11	$438.37	090	M A
67938	Remove eyelid foreign body	1.33	9.65	0.53	0.06	11.04	$399.64	1.92	$69.50	010	M A
67950	Revision of eyelid	5.82	9.01	7.67	0.30	15.13	$547.69	13.79	$499.19	090	M A C+
67961	Revision of eyelid	5.69	9.39	6.03	0.26	15.34	$555.30	11.98	$433.67	090	M A+
67966	Revision of eyelid	6.57	9.01	6.25	0.33	15.91	$575.93	13.15	$476.02	090	M A
67971	Reconstruction of eyelid	9.79	NA	7.85	0.42	NA	NA	18.06	$653.76	090	M C+
67973	Reconstruction of eyelid	12.87	NA	9.95	0.59	NA	NA	23.41	$847.42	090	M C+
67974	Reconstruction of eyelid	12.84	NA	9.87	0.54	NA	NA	23.25	$841.63	090	M C+
67975	Reconstruction of eyelid	9.13	NA	7.51	0.38	NA	NA	17.02	$616.11	090	M A
67999	Revision of eyelid	0.00	0.00	0.00	0.00	0.00	$0.00	0.00	$0.00	YYY	M A+ C+ T+
68020	Incise/drain eyelid lining	1.37	7.79	0.65	0.06	9.22	$333.76	2.08	$75.29	010	M A
68040	Treatment of eyelid lesions	0.85	7.68	0.41	0.03	8.56	$309.87	1.29	$46.70	000	M A
68100	Biopsy of eyelid lining	1.35	7.93	0.65	0.06	9.34	$338.10	2.06	$74.57	000	M A
68110	Remove eyelid lining lesion	1.77	8.98	1.41	0.07	10.82	$391.68	3.25	$117.65	010	M A
68115	Remove eyelid lining lesion	2.36	8.47	1.14	0.10	10.93	$395.66	3.60	$130.32	010	M A
68130	Remove eyelid lining lesion	4.93	NA	2.38	0.19	NA	NA	7.50	$271.49	090	M A
68135	Remove eyelid lining lesion	1.84	8.23	0.89	0.07	10.14	$367.06	2.80	$101.36	010	M A
68200	Treat eyelid by injection	0.49	0.76	0.24	0.02	1.27	$45.97	0.75	$27.15	000	M B A

Code	Description										
68320	Revise/graft eyelid lining	5.37	5.75	5.34	0.21	11.33	$410.14	10.92	$395.30	090	M	A	C+
68325	Revise/graft eyelid lining	7.36	NA	6.33	0.30	NA	NA	13.99	$506.43	090	M	A	C+
68326	Revise/graft eyelid lining	7.15	NA	6.26	0.30	NA	NA	13.71	$496.29	090	M	A	
68328	Revise/graft eyelid lining	8.18	NA	7.07	0.40	NA	NA	15.65	$566.52	090	M	A+	
68330	Revise eyelid lining	4.83	7.34	5.82	0.19	12.36	$447.42	10.84	$392.40	090	M	A+	
68335	Revise/graft eyelid lining	7.19	NA	5.68	0.29	NA	NA	13.16	$476.38	090	M	A	C+
68340	Separate eyelid adhesions	4.17	15.87	4.33	0.17	20.21	$731.59	8.67	$313.85	090	M	A+	
68360	Revise eyelid lining	4.37	6.77	5.42	0.17	11.31	$409.41	9.96	$360.54	090	M	A	
68362	Revise eyelid lining	7.34	NA	8.02	0.29	NA	NA	15.65	$566.52	090	M	A	C+
68399	Eyelid lining surgery	0.00	0.00	0.00	0.00	0.00	$0.00	0.00	$0.00	YYY	M	A+	C+ T+
68400	Incise/drain tear gland	1.69	11.48	2.18	0.07	13.24	$479.28	3.94	$142.62	010	M	A	
68420	Incise/drain tear sac	2.30	11.89	2.52	0.10	14.29	$517.29	4.92	$178.10	010	M	A	
68440	Incise tear duct opening	0.94	7.86	0.45	0.04	8.84	$320.00	1.43	$51.76	010	M	A	
68500	Removal of tear gland	11.02	NA	9.13	0.60	NA	NA	20.75	$751.13	090	M	A	
68505	Partial removal, tear gland	10.94	NA	10.31	0.57	NA	NA	21.82	$789.87	090	M	A	
68510	Biopsy of tear gland	4.61	13.09	2.22	0.19	17.89	$647.60	7.02	$254.12	000	M	A+	
68520	Removal of tear sac	7.51	NA	7.47	0.33	NA	NA	15.31	$554.21	090	M	A+	
68525	Biopsy of tear sac	4.43	NA	2.15	0.18	NA	NA	6.76	$244.71	000	M	A	C+
68530	Clearance of tear duct	3.66	15.33	3.18	0.16	19.15	$693.21	7.00	$253.39	010	M	A	
68540	Remove tear gland lesion	10.60	NA	9.73	0.46	NA	NA	20.79	$752.58	090	M	A	C+
68550	Remove tear gland lesion	13.26	NA	10.50	0.66	NA	NA	24.42	$883.98	090	M	A	
68700	Repair tear ducts	6.60	NA	6.87	0.27	NA	NA	13.74	$497.38	090	M	A	
68705	Revise tear duct opening	2.06	8.33	1.00	0.08	10.47	$379.01	3.14	$113.67	010	M	A	
68720	Create tear sac drain	8.96	NA	8.04	0.38	NA	NA	17.38	$629.14	090	M		C+
68745	Create tear duct drain	8.63	NA	7.82	0.38	NA	NA	16.83	$609.23	090	M		C+
68750	Create tear duct drain	8.66	NA	8.46	0.37	NA	NA	17.49	$633.12	090	M		C+
68760	Close tear duct opening	1.73	6.77	1.25	0.07	8.57	$310.23	3.05	$110.41	010	M	B	A
68761	Close tear duct opening	1.36	3.09	1.03	0.06	4.51	$163.26	2.45	$88.69	010	M	B	A+

*M = multiple surgery adjustment applies
Me = multiple endoscopy rules may apply
B = bilateral surgery adjustment applies
A = assistant-at-surgery restriction

A+ = assistant-at-surgery restriction unless medical necessity established with documentation
C = cosurgeons payable
C+ = cosurgeons payable if medical necessity established with documentation

T = team surgeons permitted
T+ = team surgeons payable if medical necessity established with documentation
$ = indicates services that are not covered by Medicare.

309   CPT five-digit codes, two-digit numeric modifiers, and descriptions only are © 2001 American Medical Association

Medicare RBRVS: The Physicians' Guide

Relative value units

CPT Code and Modifier	Description	Work RVU	Non Facility Practice Expense RVU	Facility Practice Expense RVU	PLI RVU	Total Non Facility RVUs	Medicare Payment Non Facility	Total Facility RVUs	Medicare Payment Facility	Global Period	Payment Policy Indicators*
68770	Close tear system fistula	7.02	17.74	6.15	0.28	25.04	$906.43	13.45	$486.88	090	M A+
68801	Dilate tear duct opening	0.94	0.88	0.57	0.04	1.86	$67.33	1.55	$56.11	010	M B A
68810	Probe nasolacrimal duct	1.90	2.48	0.91	0.08	4.46	$161.45	2.89	$104.62	010	M B A
68811	Probe nasolacrimal duct	2.35	NA	2.46	0.10	NA	NA	4.91	$177.74	010	M B A
68815	Probe nasolacrimal duct	3.20	14.08	2.92	0.14	17.42	$630.59	6.26	$226.61	010	M B A
68840	Explore/irrigate tear ducts	1.25	1.62	1.00	0.05	2.92	$105.70	2.30	$83.26	010	M A
68850	Injection for tear sac x-ray	0.80	15.29	0.32	0.03	16.12	$583.53	1.15	$41.63	000	M A
68899	Tear duct system surgery	0.00	0.00	0.00	0.00	0.00	$0.00	0.00	$0.00	YYY	M A+ C+ T+
69000	Drain external ear lesion	1.45	2.14	0.59	0.10	3.69	$133.58	2.14	$77.47	010	M A
69005	Drain external ear lesion	2.11	2.55	2.11	0.16	4.82	$174.48	4.38	$158.55	010	M A
69020	Drain outer ear canal lesion	1.48	2.25	0.71	0.11	3.84	$139.00	2.30	$83.26	010	M A
69100	Biopsy of external ear	0.81	1.44	0.41	0.04	2.29	$82.90	1.26	$45.61	000	M A
69105	Biopsy of external ear canal	0.85	1.51	1.02	0.06	2.42	$87.60	1.93	$69.86	000	M A
69110	Remove external ear, partial	3.44	3.48	2.85	0.24	7.16	$259.19	6.53	$236.38	090	M A
69120	Removal of external ear	4.05	NA	4.68	0.31	NA	NA	9.04	$327.24	090	M A
69140	Remove ear canal lesion(s)	7.97	NA	8.24	0.56	NA	NA	16.77	$607.06	090	M A+
69145	Remove ear canal lesion(s)	2.62	3.41	2.54	0.18	6.21	$224.80	5.34	$193.30	090	M A
69150	Extensive ear canal surgery	13.43	NA	11.38	1.07	NA	NA	25.88	$936.84	090	M A C+
69155	Extensive ear/neck surgery	20.80	NA	16.26	1.51	NA	NA	38.57	$1,396.20	090	M A C+
69200	Clear outer ear canal	0.77	1.45	0.77	0.05	2.27	$82.17	1.59	$57.56	000	M A
69205	Clear outer ear canal	1.20	NA	1.58	0.09	NA	NA	2.87	$103.89	010	M A
69210	Remove impacted ear wax	0.61	0.59	0.25	0.04	1.24	$44.89	0.90	$32.58	000	M A
69220	Clean out mastoid cavity	0.83	1.53	0.44	0.06	2.42	$87.60	1.33	$48.14	000	M B A
69222	Clean out mastoid cavity	1.40	2.24	1.71	0.10	3.74	$135.39	3.21	$116.20	010	M B A
69300	Revise external ear	6.36	NA	4.38	0.43	NA	NA	11.17	$404.35	YYY	M A+
69310	Rebuild outer ear canal	10.79	NA	9.86	0.77	NA	NA	21.42	$775.39	090	M A
69320	Rebuild outer ear canal	16.96	NA	13.77	1.17	NA	NA	31.90	$1,154.75	090	M

Code	Description								YYY				
69399	Outer ear surgery procedure	0.00	0.00	0.00	0.00	0.00	$0.00	0.00		M		A+	
69400	Inflate middle ear canal	0.83	1.51	0.49	0.06	2.40	$86.88	1.38	$49.95	000	M	A	
69401	Inflate middle ear canal	0.63	1.41	0.34	0.04	2.08	$75.29	1.01	$36.56	000	M	A	
69405	Catheterize middle ear canal	2.63	3.09	1.50	0.18	5.90	$213.58	4.31	$156.02	010	M	A+	
69410	Inset middle ear (baffle)	0.33	1.39	0.17	0.02	1.74	$62.99	0.52	$18.82	000	M	A+	
69420	Incision of eardrum	1.33	2.35	0.75	0.10	3.78	$136.83	2.18	$78.91	010	M	B	A
69421	Incision of eardrum	1.73	2.58	1.92	0.13	4.44	$160.72	3.78	$136.83	010	M	B	A
69424	Remove ventilating tube	0.85	1.68	0.94	0.06	2.59	$93.76	1.85	$66.97	000	M		A
69433	Create eardrum opening	1.52	2.32	0.88	0.11	3.95	$142.99	2.51	$90.86	010	M	B	A
69436	Create eardrum opening	1.96	NA	2.05	0.14	NA	NA	4.15	$150.23	010	M	B	A
69440	Exploration of middle ear	7.57	NA	7.41	0.53	NA	NA	15.51	$561.45	090	M		A
69450	Eardrum revision	5.57	NA	6.18	0.39	NA	NA	12.14	$439.46	090	M		A+
69501	Mastoidectomy	9.07	NA	8.22	0.65	NA	NA	17.94	$649.41	090	M		A
69502	Mastoidectomy	12.38	NA	10.80	0.86	NA	NA	24.04	$870.23	090	M		A+
69505	Remove mastoid structures	12.99	NA	10.94	0.92	NA	NA	24.85	$899.55	090	M		A+
69511	Extensive mastoid surgery	13.52	NA	11.45	0.96	NA	NA	25.93	$938.65	090	M		A+
69530	Extensive mastoid surgery	19.19	NA	15.06	1.32	NA	NA	35.57	$1,287.61	090	M		
69535	Remove part of temporal bone	36.14	NA	25.13	2.59	NA	NA	63.86	$2,311.68	090	M		A C+
69540	Remove ear lesion	1.20	2.27	1.61	0.09	3.56	$128.87	2.90	$104.98	010	M		A
69550	Remove ear lesion	10.99	NA	9.97	0.80	NA	NA	21.76	$787.69	090	M		
69552	Remove ear lesion	19.46	NA	14.81	1.36	NA	NA	35.63	$1,289.78	090	M		A+
69554	Remove ear lesion	33.16	NA	21.79	2.32	NA	NA	57.27	$2,073.13	090	M		C+
69601	Mastoid surgery revision	13.24	NA	11.97	0.92	NA	NA	26.13	$945.89	090	M		A+
69602	Mastoid surgery revision	13.58	NA	11.55	0.94	NA	NA	26.07	$943.71	090	M		A+
69603	Mastoid surgery revision	14.02	NA	11.80	1.00	NA	NA	26.82	$970.86	090	M		A+
69604	Mastoid surgery revision	14.02	NA	11.76	0.98	NA	NA	26.76	$968.69	090	M		A
69605	Mastoid surgery revision	18.49	NA	14.37	1.29	NA	NA	34.15	$1,236.20	090	M		
69610	Repair of eardrum	4.43	4.27	3.47	0.31	9.01	$326.15	8.21	$297.20	010	M		A

*M = multiple surgery adjustment applies
Me = multiple endoscopy rules may apply
B = bilateral surgery adjustment applies
A = assistant-at-surgery restriction

A+ = assistant-at-surgery restriction unless medical necessity established with documentation
C = cosurgeons payable
C+ = cosurgeons payable if medical necessity established with documentation

T = team surgeons permitted
T+ = team surgeons payable if medical necessity established with documentation
§ = indicates services that are not covered by Medicare.

CPT five-digit codes, two-digit numeric modifiers, and descriptions only are © 2001 American Medical Association

Medicare RBRVS: The Physicians' Guide

Relative value units

CPT Code and Modifier	Description	Work RVU	Non Facility Practice Expense RVU	Facility Practice Expense RVU	PLI RVU	Total Non Facility RVUs	Medicare Payment Non Facility	Total Facility RVUs	Medicare Payment Facility	Global Period	Payment Policy Indicators*	
69620	Repair of eardrum	5.89	6.90	3.40	0.40	13.19	$477.47	9.69	$350.77	090	M	A
69631	Repair eardrum structures	9.86	NA	9.38	0.69	NA	NA	19.93	$721.45	090	M	A
69632	Rebuild eardrum structures	12.75	NA	11.73	0.89	NA	NA	25.37	$918.37	090	M	A
69633	Rebuild eardrum structures	12.10	NA	11.36	0.84	NA	NA	24.30	$879.64	090	M	A
69635	Repair eardrum structures	13.33	NA	11.41	0.87	NA	NA	25.61	$927.06	090	M	A
69636	Rebuild eardrum structures	15.22	NA	13.23	1.07	NA	NA	29.52	$1,068.60	090	M	A+
69637	Rebuild eardrum structures	15.11	NA	13.16	1.06	NA	NA	29.33	$1,061.72	090	M	A+
69641	Revise middle ear & mastoid	12.71	NA	11.06	0.89	NA	NA	24.66	$892.67	090	M	A
69642	Revise middle ear & mastoid	16.84	NA	14.16	1.18	NA	NA	32.18	$1,164.89	090	M	A
69643	Revise middle ear & mastoid	15.32	NA	13.24	1.08	NA	NA	29.64	$1,072.94	090	M	A
69644	Revise middle ear & mastoid	16.97	NA	14.22	1.19	NA	NA	32.38	$1,172.13	090	M	A
69645	Revise middle ear & mastoid	16.38	NA	13.77	1.16	NA	NA	31.31	$1,133.40	090	M	A
69646	Revise middle ear & mastoid	17.99	NA	14.83	1.26	NA	NA	34.08	$1,233.67	090	M	A+
69650	Release middle ear bone	9.66	NA	8.53	0.68	NA	NA	18.87	$683.08	090	M	A
69660	Revise middle ear bone	11.90	NA	9.86	0.84	NA	NA	22.60	$818.10	090	M	A
69661	Revise middle ear bone	15.74	NA	12.63	1.10	NA	NA	29.47	$1,066.79	090	M	A+
69662	Revise middle ear bone	15.44	NA	12.56	1.08	NA	NA	29.08	$1,052.67	090	M	A
69666	Repair middle ear structures	9.75	NA	8.65	0.68	NA	NA	19.08	$690.68	090	M	A+
69667	Repair middle ear structures	9.76	NA	8.58	0.72	NA	NA	19.06	$689.96	090	M	A+
69670	Remove mastoid air cells	11.51	NA	10.36	0.78	NA	NA	22.65	$819.91	090	M	
69676	Remove middle ear nerve	9.52	NA	9.14	0.69	NA	NA	19.35	$700.45	090	M	B A
69700	Close mastoid fistula	8.23	NA	5.77	0.55	NA	NA	14.55	$526.70	090	M	A
69711	Remove/repair hearing aid	10.44	NA	9.62	0.62	NA	NA	20.68	$748.60	090	M	
69714	Implant temple bone w/stimul	14.00	NA	11.53	1.01	NA	NA	26.54	$960.73	090	M	A
69715	Temple bne implnt w/stimulat	18.25	NA	14.05	1.32	NA	NA	33.62	$1,217.02	090	M	A
69717	Temple bone implant revision	14.98	NA	11.46	1.08	NA	NA	27.52	$996.20	090	M	A
69718	Revise temple bone implant	18.50	NA	14.20	1.34	NA	NA	34.04	$1,232.22	090	M	A

Code	Description									
69720	Release facial nerve	14.38	NA	12.85	1.03	NA	NA	28.26	$1,022.99	090	M	A+	C+
69725	Release facial nerve	25.38	NA	17.97	1.78	NA	NA	45.13	$1,633.67	090	M		T+
69740	Repair facial nerve	15.96	NA	10.90	1.13	NA	NA	27.99	$1,013.22	090	M		
69745	Repair facial nerve	16.69	NA	12.80	1.00	NA	NA	30.49	$1,103.71	090	M		
69799	Middle ear surgery procedure	0.00	0.00	0.00	0.00	0.00	$0.00	0.00	$0.00	YYY	M	A+	C+	T+
69801	Incise inner ear	8.56	NA	7.96	0.60	NA	NA	17.12	$619.73	090	M	A+	
69802	Incise inner ear	13.10	NA	11.37	0.91	NA	NA	25.38	$918.74	090	M		
69805	Explore inner ear	13.82	NA	10.91	0.97	NA	NA	25.70	$930.32	090	M	A	
69806	Explore inner ear	12.35	NA	10.82	0.86	NA	NA	24.03	$869.87	090	M		
69820	Establish inner ear window	10.34	NA	8.78	0.66	NA	NA	19.78	$716.02	090	M	A+	
69840	Revise inner ear window	10.26	NA	9.00	0.64	NA	NA	19.90	$720.36	090	M		
69905	Remove inner ear	11.10	NA	9.94	0.77	NA	NA	21.81	$789.50	090	M	A	
69910	Remove inner ear & mastoid	13.63	NA	11.42	0.94	NA	NA	25.99	$940.82	090	M	A+	
69915	Incise inner ear nerve	21.23	NA	15.88	1.54	NA	NA	38.65	$1,399.10	090	M		C+
69930	Implant cochlear device	16.81	NA	12.94	1.19	NA	NA	30.94	$1,120.00	090	M	A+	
69949	Inner ear surgery procedure	0.00	0.00	0.00	0.00	0.00	$0.00	0.00	$0.00	YYY	M	A+	C+	T+
69950	Incise inner ear nerve	25.64	NA	16.71	2.90	NA	NA	45.25	$1,638.01	090	M	C+	
69955	Release facial nerve	27.04	NA	18.39	1.89	NA	NA	47.32	$1,712.95	090	M	A+	C+
69960	Release inner ear canal	27.04	NA	18.40	2.43	NA	NA	47.87	$1,732.86	090	M	A+	C+
69970	Remove inner ear lesion	30.04	NA	19.12	2.34	NA	NA	51.50	$1,864.26	090	M	A+	C+
69979	Temporal bone surgery	0.00	0.00	0.00	0.00	0.00	$0.00	0.00	$0.00	YYY	M	A+	C+	T+
69990	Microsurgery add-on	3.47	NA	1.87	0.56	NA	NA	5.90	$213.58	ZZZ			

Radiology: Diagnostic radiology (diagnostic imaging)

Code	Description									
70010	Contrast x-ray of brain	1.19	4.53	4.53	0.24	5.96	$215.75	5.96	$215.75	XXX		A+	
70010-26	Contrast x-ray of brain	1.19	0.42	0.42	0.06	1.67	$60.45	1.67	$60.45	XXX		A+	
70010-TC	Contrast x-ray of brain	0.00	4.11	4.11	0.18	4.29	$155.29	4.29	$155.29	XXX		A+	
70015	Contrast x-ray of brain	1.19	1.71	1.71	0.12	3.02	$109.32	3.02	$109.32	XXX		A+	

* **M** = multiple surgery adjustment applies
Me = multiple endoscopy rules may apply
B = bilateral surgery adjustment applies
A = assistant-at-surgery restriction

A+ = assistant-at-surgery restriction unless medical necessity established with documentation
C = cosurgeons payable
C+ = cosurgeons payable if medical necessity established with documentation

T = team surgeons permitted
T+ = team surgeons payable if medical necessity established with documentation
§ = indicates services that are not covered by Medicare.

313 CPT five-digit codes, two-digit numeric modifiers, and descriptions only are © 2001 American Medical Association

Medicare RBRVS: The Physicians' Guide

Relative value units

CPT Code and Modifier	Description	Work RVU	Non Facility Practice Expense RVU	Facility Practice Expense RVU	PLI RVU	Total Non Facility RVUs	Medicare Payment Non Facility	Total Facility RVUs	Medicare Payment Facility	Global Period	Payment Policy Indicators*
70015-26	Contrast x-ray of brain	1.19	0.42	0.42	0.05	1.66	$60.09	1.66	$60.09	XXX	A+
70015-TC	Contrast x-ray of brain	0.00	1.29	1.29	0.07	1.36	$49.23	1.36	$49.23	XXX	A+
70030	X-ray eye for foreign body	0.17	0.45	0.45	0.03	0.65	$23.53	0.65	$23.53	XXX	A+
70030-26	X-ray eye for foreign body	0.17	0.06	0.06	0.01	0.24	$8.69	0.24	$8.69	XXX	A+
70030-TC	X-ray eye for foreign body	0.00	0.39	0.39	0.02	0.41	$14.84	0.41	$14.84	XXX	A+
70100	X-ray exam of jaw	0.18	0.56	0.56	0.03	0.77	$27.87	0.77	$27.87	XXX	A+
70100-26	X-ray exam of jaw	0.18	0.06	0.06	0.01	0.25	$9.05	0.25	$9.05	XXX	A+
70100-TC	X-ray exam of jaw	0.00	0.50	0.50	0.02	0.52	$18.82	0.52	$18.82	XXX	A+
70110	X-ray exam of jaw	0.25	0.68	0.68	0.04	0.97	$35.11	0.97	$35.11	XXX	A+
70110-26	X-ray exam of jaw	0.25	0.09	0.09	0.01	0.35	$12.67	0.35	$12.67	XXX	A+
70110-TC	X-ray exam of jaw	0.00	0.59	0.59	0.03	0.62	$22.44	0.62	$22.44	XXX	A+
70120	X-ray exam of mastoids	0.18	0.65	0.65	0.04	0.87	$31.49	0.87	$31.49	XXX	A+
70120-26	X-ray exam of mastoids	0.18	0.06	0.06	0.01	0.25	$9.05	0.25	$9.05	XXX	A+
70120-TC	X-ray exam of mastoids	0.00	0.59	0.59	0.03	0.62	$22.44	0.62	$22.44	XXX	A+
70130	X-ray exam of mastoids	0.34	0.86	0.86	0.05	1.25	$45.25	1.25	$45.25	XXX	A+
70130-26	X-ray exam of mastoids	0.34	0.12	0.12	0.01	0.47	$17.01	0.47	$17.01	XXX	A+
70130-TC	X-ray exam of mastoids	0.00	0.74	0.74	0.04	0.78	$28.24	0.78	$28.24	XXX	A+
70134	X-ray exam of middle ear	0.34	0.82	0.82	0.05	1.21	$43.80	1.21	$43.80	XXX	A+
70134-26	X-ray exam of middle ear	0.34	0.12	0.12	0.01	0.47	$17.01	0.47	$17.01	XXX	A+
70134-TC	X-ray exam of middle ear	0.00	0.70	0.70	0.04	0.74	$26.79	0.74	$26.79	XXX	A+
70140	X-ray exam of facial bones	0.19	0.66	0.66	0.04	0.89	$32.22	0.89	$32.22	XXX	A+
70140-26	X-ray exam of facial bones	0.19	0.07	0.07	0.01	0.27	$9.77	0.27	$9.77	XXX	A+
70140-TC	X-ray exam of facial bones	0.00	0.59	0.59	0.03	0.62	$22.44	0.62	$22.44	XXX	A+
70150	X-ray exam of facial bones	0.26	0.83	0.83	0.05	1.14	$41.27	1.14	$41.27	XXX	A+
70150-26	X-ray exam of facial bones	0.26	0.09	0.09	0.01	0.36	$13.03	0.36	$13.03	XXX	A+
70150-TC	X-ray exam of facial bones	0.00	0.74	0.74	0.04	0.78	$28.24	0.78	$28.24	XXX	A+
70160	X-ray exam of nasal bones	0.17	0.56	0.56	0.03	0.76	$27.51	0.76	$27.51	XXX	A+

Code	Description								
70160-26	X-ray exam of nasal bones	0.17	0.06	0.06	0.01	0.24	$8.69	XXX	A+
70160-TC	X-ray exam of nasal bones	0.00	0.50	0.50	0.02	0.52	$18.82	XXX	A+
70170	X-ray exam of tear duct	0.30	1.01	1.01	0.06	1.37	$49.59	XXX	A+
70170-26	X-ray exam of tear duct	0.30	0.11	0.11	0.01	0.42	$15.20	XXX	A+
70170-TC	X-ray exam of tear duct	0.00	0.90	0.90	0.05	0.95	$34.39	XXX	A+
70190	X-ray exam of eye sockets	0.21	0.66	0.66	0.04	0.91	$32.94	XXX	A+
70190-26	X-ray exam of eye sockets	0.21	0.07	0.07	0.01	0.29	$10.50	XXX	A+
70190-TC	X-ray exam of eye sockets	0.00	0.59	0.59	0.03	0.62	$22.44	XXX	A+
70200	X-ray exam of eye sockets	0.28	0.84	0.84	0.05	1.17	$42.35	XXX	A+
70200-26	X-ray exam of eye sockets	0.28	0.10	0.10	0.01	0.39	$14.12	XXX	A+
70200-TC	X-ray exam of eye sockets	0.00	0.74	0.74	0.04	0.78	$28.24	XXX	A+
70210	X-ray exam of sinuses	0.17	0.65	0.65	0.04	0.86	$31.13	XXX	A+
70210-26	X-ray exam of sinuses	0.17	0.06	0.06	0.01	0.24	$8.69	XXX	A+
70210-TC	X-ray exam of sinuses	0.00	0.59	0.59	0.03	0.62	$22.44	XXX	A+
70220	X-ray exam of sinuses	0.25	0.83	0.83	0.05	1.13	$40.91	XXX	A+
70220-26	X-ray exam of sinuses	0.25	0.09	0.09	0.01	0.35	$12.67	XXX	A+
70220-TC	X-ray exam of sinuses	0.00	0.74	0.74	0.04	0.78	$28.24	XXX	A+
70240	X-ray exam, pituitary saddle	0.19	0.46	0.46	0.03	0.68	$24.62	XXX	A+
70240-26	X-ray exam, pituitary saddle	0.19	0.07	0.07	0.01	0.27	$9.77	XXX	A+
70240-TC	X-ray exam, pituitary saddle	0.00	0.39	0.39	0.02	0.41	$14.84	XXX	A+
70250	X-ray exam of skull	0.24	0.67	0.67	0.04	0.95	$34.39	XXX	A+
70250-26	X-ray exam of skull	0.24	0.08	0.08	0.01	0.33	$11.95	XXX	A+
70250-TC	X-ray exam of skull	0.00	0.59	0.59	0.03	0.62	$22.44	XXX	A+
70260	X-ray exam of skull	0.34	0.96	0.96	0.06	1.36	$49.23	XXX	A+
70260-26	X-ray exam of skull	0.34	0.12	0.12	0.01	0.47	$17.01	XXX	A+
70260-TC	X-ray exam of skull	0.00	0.84	0.84	0.05	0.89	$32.22	XXX	A+
70300	X-ray exam of teeth	0.10	0.29	0.29	0.03	0.42	$15.20	XXX	A+
70300-26	X-ray exam of teeth	0.10	0.04	0.04	0.01	0.15	$5.43	XXX	A+

* **M** = multiple surgery adjustment applies
Me = multiple endoscopy rules may apply
B = bilateral surgery adjustment applies
A = assistant-at-surgery restriction

A+ = assistant-at-surgery restriction unless medical necessity established with documentation
C = cosurgeons payable
C+ = cosurgeons payable if medical necessity established with documentation

T = team surgeons permitted
T+ = team surgeons payable if medical necessity established with documentation
§ = indicates services that are not covered by Medicare.

CPT five-digit codes, two-digit numeric modifiers, and descriptions only are © 2001 American Medical Association

Medicare RBRVS: The Physicians' Guide

Relative value units

CPT Code and Modifier	Description	Work RVU	Non Facility Practice Expense RVU	Facility Practice Expense RVU	PLI RVU	Total Non Facility RVUs	Medicare Payment Non Facility	Total Facility RVUs	Medicare Payment Facility	Global Period	Payment Policy Indicators*
70300-TC	X-ray exam of teeth	0.00	0.25	0.25	0.02	0.27	$9.77	0.27	$9.77	XXX	A+
70310	X-ray exam of teeth	0.16	0.46	0.46	0.03	0.65	$23.53	0.65	$23.53	XXX	A+
70310-26	X-ray exam of teeth	0.16	0.07	0.07	0.01	0.24	$8.69	0.24	$8.69	XXX	A+
70310-TC	X-ray exam of teeth	0.00	0.39	0.39	0.02	0.41	$14.84	0.41	$14.84	XXX	A+
70320	Full mouth x-ray of teeth	0.22	0.82	0.82	0.05	1.09	$39.46	1.09	$39.46	XXX	A+
70320-26	Full mouth x-ray of teeth	0.22	0.08	0.08	0.01	0.31	$11.22	0.31	$11.22	XXX	A+
70320-TC	Full mouth x-ray of teeth	0.00	0.74	0.74	0.04	0.78	$28.24	0.78	$28.24	XXX	A+
70328	X-ray exam of jaw joint	0.18	0.53	0.53	0.03	0.74	$26.79	0.74	$26.79	XXX	A+
70328-26	X-ray exam of jaw joint	0.18	0.06	0.06	0.01	0.25	$9.05	0.25	$9.05	XXX	A+
70328-TC	X-ray exam of jaw joint	0.00	0.47	0.47	0.02	0.49	$17.74	0.49	$17.74	XXX	A+
70330	X-ray exam of jaw joints	0.24	0.88	0.88	0.05	1.17	$42.35	1.17	$42.35	XXX	A+
70330-26	X-ray exam of jaw joints	0.24	0.08	0.08	0.01	0.33	$11.95	0.33	$11.95	XXX	A+
70330-TC	X-ray exam of jaw joints	0.00	0.80	0.80	0.04	0.84	$30.41	0.84	$30.41	XXX	A+
70332	X-ray exam of jaw joint	0.54	2.18	2.18	0.12	2.84	$102.81	2.84	$102.81	XXX	A+
70332-26	X-ray exam of jaw joint	0.54	0.19	0.19	0.02	0.75	$27.15	0.75	$27.15	XXX	A+
70332-TC	X-ray exam of jaw joint	0.00	1.99	1.99	0.10	2.09	$75.66	2.09	$75.66	XXX	A+
70336	Magnetic image, jaw joint	1.48	11.16	11.16	0.56	13.20	$477.83	13.20	$477.83	XXX	A+
70336-26	Magnetic image, jaw joint	1.48	0.52	0.52	0.07	2.07	$74.93	2.07	$74.93	XXX	A+
70336-TC	Magnetic image, jaw joint	0.00	10.64	10.64	0.49	11.13	$402.90	11.13	$402.90	XXX	A+
70350	X-ray head for orthodontia	0.17	0.42	0.42	0.03	0.62	$22.44	0.62	$22.44	XXX	A+
70350-26	X-ray head for orthodontia	0.17	0.06	0.06	0.01	0.24	$8.69	0.24	$8.69	XXX	A+
70350-TC	X-ray head for orthodontia	0.00	0.36	0.36	0.02	0.38	$13.76	0.38	$13.76	XXX	A+
70355	Panoramic x-ray of jaws	0.20	0.61	0.61	0.04	0.85	$30.77	0.85	$30.77	XXX	A+
70355-26	Panoramic x-ray of jaws	0.20	0.07	0.07	0.01	0.28	$10.14	0.28	$10.14	XXX	A+
70355-TC	Panoramic x-ray of jaws	0.00	0.54	0.54	0.03	0.57	$20.63	0.57	$20.63	XXX	A+
70360	X-ray exam of neck	0.17	0.45	0.45	0.03	0.65	$23.53	0.65	$23.53	XXX	A+
70360-26	X-ray exam of neck	0.17	0.06	0.06	0.01	0.24	$8.69	0.24	$8.69	XXX	A+

Code	Description						
70360-TC	X-ray exam of neck	0.00	0.39	0.02	0.41	$14.84	XXX	A+
70370	Throat x-ray & fluoroscopy	0.32	1.35	0.07	1.74	$62.99	XXX	A+
70370-26	Throat x-ray & fluoroscopy	0.32	0.11	0.01	0.44	$15.93	XXX	A+
70370-TC	Throat x-ray & fluoroscopy	0.00	1.24	0.06	1.30	$47.06	XXX	A+
70371	Speech evaluation, complex	0.84	2.29	0.14	3.27	$118.37	XXX	A+
70371-26	Speech evaluation, complex	0.84	0.30	0.04	1.18	$42.72	XXX	A+
70371-TC	Speech evaluation, complex	0.00	1.99	0.10	2.09	$75.66	XXX	A+
70373	Contrast x-ray of larynx	0.44	1.84	0.11	2.39	$86.52	XXX	A+
70373-26	Contrast x-ray of larynx	0.44	0.15	0.02	0.61	$22.08	XXX	A+
70373-TC	Contrast x-ray of larynx	0.00	1.69	0.09	1.78	$64.43	XXX	A+
70380	X-ray exam of salivary gland	0.17	0.69	0.04	0.90	$32.58	XXX	A+
70380-26	X-ray exam of salivary gland	0.17	0.06	0.01	0.24	$8.69	XXX	A+
70380-TC	X-ray exam of salivary gland	0.00	0.63	0.03	0.66	$23.89	XXX	A+
70390	X-ray exam of salivary duct	0.38	1.82	0.11	2.31	$83.62	XXX	A+
70390-26	X-ray exam of salivary duct	0.38	0.13	0.02	0.53	$19.19	XXX	A+
70390-TC	X-ray exam of salivary duct	0.00	1.69	0.09	1.78	$64.43	XXX	A+
70450	Ct head/brain w/o dye	0.85	4.78	0.25	5.88	$212.85	XXX	A+
70450-26	Ct head/brain w/o dye	0.85	0.30	0.04	1.19	$43.08	XXX	A+
70450-TC	Ct head/brain w/o dye	0.00	4.48	0.21	4.69	$169.77	XXX	A+
70460	Ct head/brain w/dye	1.13	5.77	0.30	7.20	$260.63	XXX	A+
70460-26	Ct head/brain w/dye	1.13	0.40	0.05	1.58	$57.19	XXX	A+
70460-TC	Ct head/brain w/dye	0.00	5.37	0.25	5.62	$203.44	XXX	A+
70470	Ct head/brain w/o&w dye	1.27	7.16	0.37	8.80	$318.55	XXX	A+
70470-26	Ct head/brain w/o&w dye	1.27	0.45	0.06	1.78	$64.43	XXX	A+
70470-TC	Ct head/brain w/o&w dye	0.00	6.71	0.31	7.02	$254.12	XXX	A+
70480	Ct orbit/ear/fossa w/o dye	1.28	4.93	0.27	6.48	$234.57	XXX	A+
70480-26	Ct orbit/ear/fossa w/o dye	1.28	0.45	0.06	1.79	$64.80	XXX	A+
70480-TC	Ct orbit/ear/fossa w/o dye	0.00	4.48	0.21	4.69	$169.77	XXX	A+

* **M** = multiple surgery adjustment applies
  Me = multiple endoscopy rules may apply
  B = bilateral surgery adjustment applies
  A = assistant-at-surgery restriction

A+ = assistant-at-surgery restriction unless medical necessity established with documentation
C = cosurgeons payable
C+ = cosurgeons payable if medical necessity established with documentation

T = team surgeons permitted
T+ = team surgeons payable if medical necessity established with documentation
S = indicates services that are not covered by Medicare.

CPT five-digit codes, two-digit numeric modifiers, and descriptions only are © 2001 American Medical Association

Relative value units

CPT Code and Modifier	Description	Work RVU	Non Facility Practice Expense RVU	Facility Practice Expense RVU	PLI RVU	Total Non Facility RVUs	Medicare Payment Non Facility	Total Facility RVUs	Medicare Payment Facility	Global Period	Payment Policy Indicators*
70481	Ct orbit/ear/fossa w/dye	1.38	5.85	5.85	0.31	7.54	$272.94	7.54	$272.94	XXX	A+
70481-26	Ct orbit/ear/fossa w/dye	1.38	0.48	0.48	0.06	1.92	$69.50	1.92	$69.50	XXX	A+
70481-TC	Ct orbit/ear/fossa w/dye	0.00	5.37	5.37	0.25	5.62	$203.44	5.62	$203.44	XXX	A+
70482	Ct orbit/ear/fossa w/o&w dye	1.45	7.22	7.22	0.37	9.04	$327.24	9.04	$327.24	XXX	A+
70482-26	Ct orbit/ear/fossa w/o&w dye	1.45	0.51	0.51	0.06	2.02	$73.12	2.02	$73.12	XXX	A+
70482-TC	Ct orbit/ear/fossa w/o&w dye	0.00	6.71	6.71	0.31	7.02	$254.12	7.02	$254.12	XXX	A+
70486	Ct maxillofacial w/o dye	1.14	4.88	4.88	0.26	6.28	$227.33	6.28	$227.33	XXX	A+
70486-26	Ct maxillofacial w/o dye	1.14	0.40	0.40	0.05	1.59	$57.56	1.59	$57.56	XXX	A+
70486-TC	Ct maxillofacial w/o dye	0.00	4.48	4.48	0.21	4.69	$169.77	4.69	$169.77	XXX	A+
70487	Ct maxillofacial w/dye	1.30	5.83	5.83	0.31	7.44	$269.32	7.44	$269.32	XXX	A+
70487-26	Ct maxillofacial w/dye	1.30	0.46	0.46	0.06	1.82	$65.88	1.82	$65.88	XXX	A+
70487-TC	Ct maxillofacial w/dye	0.00	5.37	5.37	0.25	5.62	$203.44	5.62	$203.44	XXX	A+
70488	Ct maxillofacial w/o&w dye	1.42	7.21	7.21	0.37	9.00	$325.79	9.00	$325.79	XXX	A+
70488-26	Ct maxillofacial w/o&w dye	1.42	0.50	0.50	0.06	1.98	$71.67	1.98	$71.67	XXX	A+
70488-TC	Ct maxillofacial w/o&w dye	0.00	6.71	6.71	0.31	7.02	$254.12	7.02	$254.12	XXX	A+
70490	Ct soft tissue neck w/o dye	1.28	4.93	4.93	0.27	6.48	$234.57	6.48	$234.57	XXX	A+
70490-26	Ct soft tissue neck w/o dye	1.28	0.45	0.45	0.06	1.79	$64.80	1.79	$64.80	XXX	A+
70490-TC	Ct soft tissue neck w/o dye	0.00	4.48	4.48	0.21	4.69	$169.77	4.69	$169.77	XXX	A+
70491	Ct soft tissue neck w/dye	1.38	5.85	5.85	0.31	7.54	$272.94	7.54	$272.94	XXX	A+
70491-26	Ct soft tissue neck w/dye	1.38	0.48	0.48	0.06	1.92	$69.50	1.92	$69.50	XXX	A+
70491-TC	Ct soft tissue neck w/dye	0.00	5.37	5.37	0.25	5.62	$203.44	5.62	$203.44	XXX	A+
70492	Ct sft tsue nck w/o & w/dye	1.45	7.22	7.22	0.37	9.04	$327.24	9.04	$327.24	XXX	A+
70492-26	Ct sft tsue nck w/o & w/dye	1.45	0.51	0.51	0.06	2.02	$73.12	2.02	$73.12	XXX	A+
70492-TC	Ct sft tsue nck w/o & w/dye	0.00	6.71	6.71	0.31	7.02	$254.12	7.02	$254.12	XXX	A+
70496	Ct angiography, head	1.75	7.41	7.41	0.56	9.72	$351.86	9.72	$351.86	XXX	A+
70496-26	Ct angiography, head	1.75	0.70	0.70	0.08	2.53	$91.58	2.53	$91.58	XXX	A+
70496-TC	Ct angiography, head	0.00	6.71	6.71	0.48	7.19	$260.27	7.19	$260.27	XXX	A+

Code	Description								
70498	Ct angiography, neck	1.75	7.41	7.41	0.56	9.72	$351.86	XXX	A+
70498-26	Ct angiography, neck	1.75	0.70	0.70	0.08	2.53	$91.58	XXX	A+
70498-TC	Ct angiography, neck	0.00	6.71	6.71	0.48	7.19	$260.27	XXX	A+
70540	Mri orbit/face/neck w/o dye	1.35	11.11	11.11	0.36	12.82	$464.07	XXX	A+
70540-26	Mri orbit/face/neck w/o dye	1.35	0.47	0.47	0.04	1.86	$67.33	XXX	A+
70540-TC	Mri orbit/face/neck w/o dye	0.00	10.64	10.64	0.32	10.96	$396.74	XXX	A+
70542	Mri orbit/face/neck w/dye	1.62	13.33	13.33	0.44	15.39	$557.11	XXX	A+
70542-26	Mri orbit/face/neck w/dye	1.62	0.57	0.57	0.05	2.24	$81.09	XXX	A+
70542-TC	Mri orbit/face/neck w/dye	0.00	12.76	12.76	0.39	13.15	$476.02	XXX	A+
70543	Mri orbt/fac/nck w/o&w dye	2.15	24.39	24.39	0.77	27.31	$988.60	XXX	A+
70543-26	Mri orbt/fac/nck w/o&w dye	2.15	0.75	0.75	0.07	2.97	$107.51	XXX	A+
70543-TC	Mri orbt/fac/nck w/o&w dye	0.00	23.64	23.64	0.70	24.34	$881.09	XXX	A+
70544	Mr angiography head w/o dye	1.20	11.06	11.06	0.54	12.80	$463.35	XXX	A+
70544-26	Mr angiography head w/o dye	1.20	0.42	0.42	0.05	1.67	$60.45	XXX	A+
70544-TC	Mr angiography head w/o dye	0.00	10.64	10.64	0.49	11.13	$402.90	XXX	A+
70545	Mr angiography head w/dye	1.20	11.06	11.06	0.54	12.80	$463.35	XXX	A+
70545-26	Mr angiography head w/dye	1.20	0.42	0.42	0.05	1.67	$60.45	XXX	A+
70545-TC	Mr angiography head w/dye	0.00	10.64	10.64	0.49	11.13	$402.90	XXX	A+
70546	Mr angiograph head w/o&w dye	1.80	21.92	21.92	0.57	24.29	$879.28	XXX	A+
70546-26	Mr angiograph head w/o&w dye	1.80	0.63	0.63	0.08	2.51	$90.86	XXX	A+
70546-TC	Mr angiograph head w/o&w dye	0.00	21.29	21.29	0.49	21.78	$788.42	XXX	A+
70547	Mr angiography neck w/o dye	1.20	11.06	11.06	0.54	12.80	$463.35	XXX	A+
70547-26	Mr angiography neck w/o dye	1.20	0.42	0.42	0.05	1.67	$60.45	XXX	A+
70547-TC	Mr angiography neck w/o dye	0.00	10.64	10.64	0.49	11.13	$402.90	XXX	A+
70548	Mr angiography neck w/dye	1.20	11.06	11.06	0.54	12.80	$463.35	XXX	A+
70548-26	Mr angiography neck w/dye	1.20	0.42	0.42	0.05	1.67	$60.45	XXX	A+
70548-TC	Mr angiography neck w/dye	0.00	10.64	10.64	0.49	11.13	$402.90	XXX	A+
70549	Mr angiograph neck w/o&w dye	1.80	21.92	21.92	0.57	24.29	$879.28	XXX	A+

* **M** = multiple surgery adjustment applies
Me = multiple endoscopy rules may apply
B = bilateral surgery adjustment applies
A = assistant-at-surgery restriction

A+ = assistant-at-surgery restriction unless medical necessity established with documentation
C = cosurgeons payable
C+ = cosurgeons payable if medical necessity established with documentation

T = team surgeons permitted
T+ = team surgeons payable if medical necessity established with documentation
§ = indicates services that are not covered by Medicare.

CPT five-digit codes, two-digit numeric modifiers, and descriptions only are © 2001 American Medical Association

Medicare RBRVS: The Physicians' Guide

Relative value units

CPT Code and Modifier	Description	Work RVU	Non Facility Practice Expense RVU	Facility Practice Expense RVU	PLI RVU	Total Non Facility RVUs	Medicare Payment Non Facility	Total Facility RVUs	Medicare Payment Facility	Global Period	Payment Policy Indicators*
70549-26	Mr angiograph neck w/o&w dye	1.80	0.63	0.63	0.08	2.51	$90.86	2.51	$90.86	XXX	A+
70549-TC	Mr angiograph neck w/o&w dye	0.00	21.29	21.29	0.49	21.78	$788.42	21.78	$788.42	XXX	A+
70551	Mri brain w/o dye	1.48	11.16	11.16	0.56	13.20	$477.83	13.20	$477.83	XXX	A+
70551-26	Mri brain w/o dye	1.48	0.52	0.52	0.07	2.07	$74.93	2.07	$74.93	XXX	A+
70551-TC	Mri brain w/o dye	0.00	10.64	10.64	0.49	11.13	$402.90	11.13	$402.90	XXX	A+
70552	Mri brain w/dye	1.78	13.40	13.40	0.66	15.84	$573.40	15.84	$573.40	XXX	A+
70552-26	Mri brain w/dye	1.78	0.64	0.64	0.08	2.50	$90.50	2.50	$90.50	XXX	A+
70552-TC	Mri brain w/dye	0.00	12.76	12.76	0.58	13.34	$482.90	13.34	$482.90	XXX	A+
70553	Mri brain w/o&w dye	2.36	24.47	24.47	1.19	28.02	$1,014.30	28.02	$1,014.30	XXX	A+
70553-26	Mri brain w/o&w dye	2.36	0.83	0.83	0.10	3.29	$119.10	3.29	$119.10	XXX	A+
70553-TC	Mri brain w/o&w dye	0.00	23.64	23.64	1.09	24.73	$895.21	24.73	$895.21	XXX	A+
71010	Chest x-ray	0.18	0.51	0.51	0.03	0.72	$26.06	0.72	$26.06	XXX	A+
71010-26	Chest x-ray	0.18	0.06	0.06	0.01	0.25	$9.05	0.25	$9.05	XXX	A+
71010-TC	Chest x-ray	0.00	0.45	0.45	0.02	0.47	$17.01	0.47	$17.01	XXX	A+
71015	Chest x-ray	0.21	0.57	0.57	0.03	0.81	$29.32	0.81	$29.32	XXX	A+
71015-26	Chest x-ray	0.21	0.07	0.07	0.01	0.29	$10.50	0.29	$10.50	XXX	A+
71015-TC	Chest x-ray	0.00	0.50	0.50	0.02	0.52	$18.82	0.52	$18.82	XXX	A+
71020	Chest x-ray	0.22	0.67	0.67	0.04	0.93	$33.67	0.93	$33.67	XXX	A+
71020-26	Chest x-ray	0.22	0.08	0.08	0.01	0.31	$11.22	0.31	$11.22	XXX	A+
71020-TC	Chest x-ray	0.00	0.59	0.59	0.03	0.62	$22.44	0.62	$22.44	XXX	A+
71021	Chest x-ray	0.27	0.79	0.79	0.05	1.11	$40.18	1.11	$40.18	XXX	A+
71021-26	Chest x-ray	0.27	0.09	0.09	0.01	0.37	$13.39	0.37	$13.39	XXX	A+
71021-TC	Chest x-ray	0.00	0.70	0.70	0.04	0.74	$26.79	0.74	$26.79	XXX	A+
71022	Chest x-ray	0.31	0.81	0.81	0.06	1.18	$42.72	1.18	$42.72	XXX	A+
71022-26	Chest x-ray	0.31	0.11	0.11	0.02	0.44	$15.93	0.44	$15.93	XXX	A+
71022-TC	Chest x-ray	0.00	0.70	0.70	0.04	0.74	$26.79	0.74	$26.79	XXX	A+
71023	Chest x-ray and fluoroscopy	0.38	0.88	0.88	0.06	1.32	$47.78	1.32	$47.78	XXX	A+

Code	Description								
71023-26	Chest x-ray and fluoroscopy	0.38	0.14	0.14	0.02	0.54	$19.55	$19.55	0.54	XXX	A+
71023-TC	Chest x-ray and fluoroscopy	0.00	0.74	0.74	0.04	0.78	$28.24	$28.24	0.78	XXX	A+
71030	Chest x-ray	0.31	0.85	0.85	0.05	1.21	$43.80	$43.80	1.21	XXX	A+
71030-26	Chest x-ray	0.31	0.11	0.11	0.01	0.43	$15.57	$15.57	0.43	XXX	A+
71030-TC	Chest x-ray	0.00	0.74	0.74	0.04	0.78	$28.24	$28.24	0.78	XXX	A+
71034	Chest x-ray and fluoroscopy	0.46	1.54	1.54	0.09	2.09	$75.66	$75.66	2.09	XXX	A+
71034-26	Chest x-ray and fluoroscopy	0.46	0.17	0.17	0.02	0.65	$23.53	$23.53	0.65	XXX	A+
71034-TC	Chest x-ray and fluoroscopy	0.00	1.37	1.37	0.07	1.44	$52.13	$52.13	1.44	XXX	A+
71035	Chest x-ray	0.18	0.56	0.56	0.03	0.77	$27.87	$27.87	0.77	XXX	A+
71035-26	Chest x-ray	0.18	0.06	0.06	0.01	0.25	$9.05	$9.05	0.25	XXX	A+
71035-TC	Chest x-ray	0.00	0.50	0.50	0.02	0.52	$18.82	$18.82	0.52	XXX	A+
71040	Contrast x-ray of bronchi	0.58	1.59	1.59	0.10	2.27	$82.17	$82.17	2.27	XXX	A+
71040-26	Contrast x-ray of bronchi	0.58	0.20	0.20	0.03	0.81	$29.32	$29.32	0.81	XXX	A+
71040-TC	Contrast x-ray of bronchi	0.00	1.39	1.39	0.07	1.46	$52.85	$52.85	1.46	XXX	A+
71060	Contrast x-ray of bronchi	0.74	2.35	2.35	0.14	3.23	$116.92	$116.92	3.23	XXX	A+
71060-26	Contrast x-ray of bronchi	0.74	0.26	0.26	0.03	1.03	$37.29	$37.29	1.03	XXX	A+
71060-TC	Contrast x-ray of bronchi	0.00	2.09	2.09	0.11	2.20	$79.64	$79.64	2.20	XXX	A+
71090	X-ray & pacemaker insertion	0.54	1.82	1.82	0.11	2.47	$89.41	$89.41	2.47	XXX	A+
71090-26	X-ray & pacemaker insertion	0.54	0.22	0.22	0.02	0.78	$28.24	$28.24	0.78	XXX	A+
71090-TC	X-ray & pacemaker insertion	0.00	1.60	1.60	0.09	1.69	$61.18	$61.18	1.69	XXX	A+
71100	X-ray exam of ribs	0.22	0.62	0.62	0.04	0.88	$31.86	$31.86	0.88	XXX	A+
71100-26	X-ray exam of ribs	0.22	0.08	0.08	0.01	0.31	$11.22	$11.22	0.31	XXX	A+
71100-TC	X-ray exam of ribs	0.00	0.54	0.54	0.03	0.57	$20.63	$20.63	0.57	XXX	A+
71101	X-ray exam of ribs/chest	0.27	0.72	0.72	0.04	1.03	$37.29	$37.29	1.03	XXX	A+
71101-26	X-ray exam of ribs/chest	0.27	0.09	0.09	0.01	0.37	$13.39	$13.39	0.37	XXX	A+
71101-TC	X-ray exam of ribs/chest	0.00	0.63	0.63	0.03	0.66	$23.89	$23.89	0.66	XXX	A+
71110	X-ray exam of ribs	0.27	0.83	0.83	0.05	1.15	$41.63	$41.63	1.15	XXX	A+
71110-26	X-ray exam of ribs	0.27	0.09	0.09	0.01	0.37	$13.39	$13.39	0.37	XXX	A+

*M = multiple surgery adjustment applies
Me = multiple endoscopy rules may apply
B = bilateral surgery adjustment applies
A = assistant-at-surgery restriction

A+ = assistant-at-surgery restriction unless medical necessity established with documentation
C = cosurgeons payable
C+ = cosurgeons payable if medical necessity established with documentation

T = team surgeons permitted
T+ = team surgeons payable if medical necessity established with documentation
§ = indicates services that are not covered by Medicare.

CPT five-digit codes, two-digit numeric modifiers, and descriptions only are © 2001 American Medical Association

Medicare RBRVS: The Physicians' Guide

Relative value units

CPT Code and Modifier	Description	Work RVU	Non Facility Practice Expense RVU	Facility Practice Expense RVU	PLI RVU	Total Non Facility RVUs	Medicare Payment Non Facility	Total Facility RVUs	Medicare Payment Facility	Global Period	Payment Policy Indicators*
71110-TC	X-ray exam of ribs	0.00	0.74	0.74	0.04	0.78	$28.24	0.78	$28.24	XXX	A+
71111	X-ray exam of ribs/ chest	0.32	0.95	0.95	0.06	1.33	$48.14	1.33	$48.14	XXX	A+
71111-26	X-ray exam of ribs/ chest	0.32	0.11	0.11	0.01	0.44	$15.93	0.44	$15.93	XXX	A+
71111-TC	X-ray exam of ribs/ chest	0.00	0.84	0.84	0.05	0.89	$32.22	0.89	$32.22	XXX	A+
71120	X-ray exam of breastbone	0.20	0.69	0.69	0.04	0.93	$33.67	0.93	$33.67	XXX	A+
71120-26	X-ray exam of breastbone	0.20	0.07	0.07	0.01	0.28	$10.14	0.28	$10.14	XXX	A+
71120-TC	X-ray exam of breastbone	0.00	0.62	0.62	0.03	0.65	$23.53	0.65	$23.53	XXX	A+
71130	X-ray exam of breastbone	0.22	0.75	0.75	0.04	1.01	$36.56	1.01	$36.56	XXX	A+
71130-26	X-ray exam of breastbone	0.22	0.08	0.08	0.01	0.31	$11.22	0.31	$11.22	XXX	A+
71130-TC	X-ray exam of breastbone	0.00	0.67	0.67	0.03	0.70	$25.34	0.70	$25.34	XXX	A+
71250	Ct thorax w/o dye	1.16	6.02	6.02	0.31	7.49	$271.13	7.49	$271.13	XXX	A+
71250-26	Ct thorax w/o dye	1.16	0.41	0.41	0.05	1.62	$58.64	1.62	$58.64	XXX	A+
71250-TC	Ct thorax w/o dye	0.00	5.61	5.61	0.26	5.87	$212.49	5.87	$212.49	XXX	A+
71260	Ct thorax w/dye	1.24	7.14	7.14	0.36	8.74	$316.38	8.74	$316.38	XXX	A+
71260-26	Ct thorax w/dye	1.24	0.43	0.43	0.05	1.72	$62.26	1.72	$62.26	XXX	A+
71260-TC	Ct thorax w/dye	0.00	6.71	6.71	0.31	7.02	$254.12	7.02	$254.12	XXX	A+
71270	Ct thorax w/o&w dye	1.38	8.88	8.88	0.44	10.70	$387.33	10.70	$387.33	XXX	A+
71270-26	Ct thorax w/o&w dye	1.38	0.48	0.48	0.06	1.92	$69.50	1.92	$69.50	XXX	A+
71270-TC	Ct thorax w/o&w dye	0.00	8.40	8.40	0.38	8.78	$317.83	8.78	$317.83	XXX	A+
71275	Ct angiography, chest	1.92	9.17	9.17	0.38	11.47	$415.20	11.47	$415.20	XXX	A+
71275-26	Ct angiography, chest	1.92	0.77	0.77	0.06	2.75	$99.55	2.75	$99.55	XXX	A+
71275-TC	Ct angiography, chest	0.00	8.40	8.40	0.32	8.72	$315.66	8.72	$315.66	XXX	A+
71550	Mri chest w/o dye	1.46	11.15	11.15	0.41	13.02	$471.31	13.02	$471.31	XXX	A+
71550-26	Mri chest w/o dye	1.46	0.51	0.51	0.04	2.01	$72.76	2.01	$72.76	XXX	A+
71550-TC	Mri chest w/o dye	0.00	10.64	10.64	0.37	11.01	$398.55	11.01	$398.55	XXX	A+
71551	Mri chest w/dye	1.73	13.36	13.36	0.49	15.58	$563.98	15.58	$563.98	XXX	A+
71551-26	Mri chest w/dye	1.73	0.60	0.60	0.06	2.39	$86.52	2.39	$86.52	XXX	A+

Code	Description								
71551-TC	Mri chest w/dye	0.00	12.76	12.76	13.19	$477.47	13.19	$477.47	XXX	A+
71552	Mri chest w/o&w dye	2.26	24.43	24.43	27.33	$989.32	27.33	$989.32	XXX	A+
71552-26	Mri chest w/o&w dye	2.26	0.79	0.79	3.13	$113.30	3.13	$113.30	XXX	A+
71552-TC	Mri chest w/o&w dye	0.00	23.64	23.64	24.20	$876.02	24.20	$876.02	XXX	A+
71555	Mri angio chest w or w/o dye	1.81	11.28	11.28	13.66	$494.48	13.66	$494.48	XXX	A+
71555-26	Mri angio chest w or w/o dye	1.81	0.64	0.64	2.53	$91.58	2.53	$91.58	XXX	A+
71555-TC	Mri angio chest w or w/o dye	0.00	10.64	10.64	11.13	$402.90	11.13	$402.90	XXX	A+
72010	X-ray exam of spine	0.45	1.13	1.13	1.66	$60.09	1.66	$60.09	XXX	A+
72010-26	X-ray exam of spine	0.45	0.16	0.16	0.64	$23.17	0.64	$23.17	XXX	A+
72010-TC	X-ray exam of spine	0.00	0.97	0.97	1.02	$36.92	1.02	$36.92	XXX	A+
72020	X-ray exam of spine	0.15	0.44	0.44	0.62	$22.44	0.62	$22.44	XXX	A+
72020-26	X-ray exam of spine	0.15	0.05	0.05	0.21	$7.60	0.21	$7.60	XXX	A+
72020-TC	X-ray exam of spine	0.00	0.39	0.39	0.41	$14.84	0.41	$14.84	XXX	A+
72040	X-ray exam of neck spine	0.22	0.65	0.65	0.91	$32.94	0.91	$32.94	XXX	A+
72040-26	X-ray exam of neck spine	0.22	0.08	0.08	0.31	$11.22	0.31	$11.22	XXX	A+
72040-TC	X-ray exam of neck spine	0.00	0.57	0.57	0.60	$21.72	0.60	$21.72	XXX	A+
72050	X-ray exam of neck spine	0.31	0.95	0.95	1.33	$48.14	1.33	$48.14	XXX	A+
72050-26	X-ray exam of neck spine	0.31	0.11	0.11	0.44	$15.93	0.44	$15.93	XXX	A+
72050-TC	X-ray exam of neck spine	0.00	0.84	0.84	0.89	$32.22	0.89	$32.22	XXX	A+
72052	X-ray exam of neck spine	0.36	1.20	1.20	1.63	$59.00	1.63	$59.00	XXX	A+
72052-26	X-ray exam of neck spine	0.36	0.13	0.13	0.51	$18.46	0.51	$18.46	XXX	A+
72052-TC	X-ray exam of neck spine	0.00	1.07	1.07	1.12	$40.54	1.12	$40.54	XXX	A+
72069	X-ray exam of trunk spine	0.22	0.56	0.56	0.82	$29.68	0.82	$29.68	XXX	A+
72069-26	X-ray exam of trunk spine	0.22	0.09	0.09	0.33	$11.95	0.33	$11.95	XXX	A+
72069-TC	X-ray exam of trunk spine	0.00	0.47	0.47	0.49	$17.74	0.49	$17.74	XXX	A+
72070	X-ray exam of thoracic spine	0.22	0.70	0.70	0.96	$34.75	0.96	$34.75	XXX	A+
72070-26	X-ray exam of thoracic spine	0.22	0.08	0.08	0.31	$11.22	0.31	$11.22	XXX	A+
72070-TC	X-ray exam of thoracic spine	0.00	0.62	0.62	0.65	$23.53	0.65	$23.53	XXX	A+

*M = multiple surgery adjustment applies
Me = multiple endoscopy rules may apply
B = bilateral surgery adjustment applies
A = assistant-at-surgery restriction

A+ = assistant-at-surgery restriction unless medical necessity established with documentation
C = cosurgeons payable
C+ = cosurgeons payable if medical necessity established with documentation

T = team surgeons permitted
T+ = team surgeons payable if medical necessity established with documentation
$ = indicates services that are not covered by Medicare.

CPT five-digit codes, two-digit numeric modifiers, and descriptions only are © 2001 American Medical Association

Medicare RBRVS: The Physicians' Guide

Relative value units

CPT Code and Modifier	Description	Work RVU	Non Facility Practice Expense RVU	Facility Practice Expense RVU	PLI RVU	Total Non Facility RVUs	Medicare Payment Non Facility	Total Facility RVUs	Medicare Payment Facility	Global Period	Payment Policy Indicators*
72072	X-ray exam of thoracic spine	0.22	0.78	0.78	0.05	1.05	$38.01	1.05	$38.01	XXX	A+
72072-26	X-ray exam of thoracic spine	0.22	0.08	0.08	0.01	0.31	$11.22	0.31	$11.22	XXX	A+
72072-TC	X-ray exam of thoracic spine	0.00	0.70	0.70	0.04	0.74	$26.79	0.74	$26.79	XXX	A+
72074	X-ray exam of thoracic spine	0.22	0.94	0.94	0.06	1.22	$44.16	1.22	$44.16	XXX	A+
72074-26	X-ray exam of thoracic spine	0.22	0.08	0.08	0.01	0.31	$11.22	0.31	$11.22	XXX	A+
72074-TC	X-ray exam of thoracic spine	0.00	0.86	0.86	0.05	0.91	$32.94	0.91	$32.94	XXX	A+
72080	X-ray exam of trunk spine	0.22	0.71	0.71	0.05	0.98	$35.48	0.98	$35.48	XXX	A+
72080-26	X-ray exam of trunk spine	0.22	0.08	0.08	0.02	0.32	$11.58	0.32	$11.58	XXX	A+
72080-TC	X-ray exam of trunk spine	0.00	0.63	0.63	0.03	0.66	$23.89	0.66	$23.89	XXX	A+
72090	X-ray exam of trunk spine	0.28	0.73	0.73	0.05	1.06	$38.37	1.06	$38.37	XXX	A+
72090-26	X-ray exam of trunk spine	0.28	0.10	0.10	0.02	0.40	$14.48	0.40	$14.48	XXX	A+
72090-TC	X-ray exam of trunk spine	0.00	0.63	0.63	0.03	0.66	$23.89	0.66	$23.89	XXX	A+
72100	X-ray exam of lower spine	0.22	0.71	0.71	0.05	0.98	$35.48	0.98	$35.48	XXX	A+
72100-26	X-ray exam of lower spine	0.22	0.08	0.08	0.02	0.32	$11.58	0.32	$11.58	XXX	A+
72100-TC	X-ray exam of lower spine	0.00	0.63	0.63	0.03	0.66	$23.89	0.66	$23.89	XXX	A+
72110	X-ray exam of lower spine	0.31	0.97	0.97	0.07	1.35	$48.87	1.35	$48.87	XXX	A+
72110-26	X-ray exam of lower spine	0.31	0.11	0.11	0.02	0.44	$15.93	0.44	$15.93	XXX	A+
72110-TC	X-ray exam of lower spine	0.00	0.86	0.86	0.05	0.91	$32.94	0.91	$32.94	XXX	A+
72114	X-ray exam of lower spine	0.36	1.26	1.26	0.08	1.70	$61.54	1.70	$61.54	XXX	A+
72114-26	X-ray exam of lower spine	0.36	0.13	0.13	0.03	0.52	$18.82	0.52	$18.82	XXX	A+
72114-TC	X-ray exam of lower spine	0.00	1.13	1.13	0.05	1.18	$42.72	1.18	$42.72	XXX	A+
72120	X-ray exam of lower spine	0.22	0.92	0.92	0.07	1.21	$43.80	1.21	$43.80	XXX	A+
72120-26	X-ray exam of lower spine	0.22	0.08	0.08	0.02	0.32	$11.58	0.32	$11.58	XXX	A+
72120-TC	X-ray exam of lower spine	0.00	0.84	0.84	0.05	0.89	$32.22	0.89	$32.22	XXX	A+
72125	Ct neck spine w/o dye	1.16	6.02	6.02	0.31	7.49	$271.13	7.49	$271.13	XXX	A+
72125-26	Ct neck spine w/o dye	1.16	0.41	0.41	0.05	1.62	$58.64	1.62	$58.64	XXX	A+
72125-TC	Ct neck spine w/o dye	0.00	5.61	5.61	0.26	5.87	$212.49	5.87	$212.49	XXX	A+

Code	Description								
72126	Ct neck spine w/dye	1.22	7.14	7.14	0.36	8.72	$315.66	XXX	A+
72126-26	Ct neck spine w/dye	1.22	0.43	0.43	0.05	1.70	$61.54	XXX	A+
72126-TC	Ct neck spine w/dye	0.00	6.71	6.71	0.31	7.02	$254.12	XXX	A+
72127	Ct neck spine w/o&w dye	1.27	8.85	8.85	0.44	10.56	$382.26	XXX	A+
72127-26	Ct neck spine w/o&w dye	1.27	0.45	0.45	0.06	1.78	$64.43	XXX	A+
72127-TC	Ct neck spine w/o&w dye	0.00	8.40	8.40	0.38	8.78	$317.83	XXX	A+
72128	Ct chest spine w/o dye	1.16	6.02	6.02	0.31	7.49	$271.13	XXX	A+
72128-26	Ct chest spine w/o dye	1.16	0.41	0.41	0.05	1.62	$58.64	XXX	A+
72128-TC	Ct chest spine w/o dye	0.00	5.61	5.61	0.26	5.87	$212.49	XXX	A+
72129	Ct chest spine w/dye	1.22	7.14	7.14	0.36	8.72	$315.66	XXX	A+
72129-26	Ct chest spine w/dye	1.22	0.43	0.43	0.05	1.70	$61.54	XXX	A+
72129-TC	Ct chest spine w/dye	0.00	6.71	6.71	0.31	7.02	$254.12	XXX	A+
72130	Ct chest spine w/o&w dye	1.27	8.85	8.85	0.44	10.56	$382.26	XXX	A+
72130-26	Ct chest spine w/o&w dye	1.27	0.45	0.45	0.06	1.78	$64.43	XXX	A+
72130-TC	Ct chest spine w/o&w dye	0.00	8.40	8.40	0.38	8.78	$317.83	XXX	A+
72131	Ct lumbar spine w/o dye	1.16	6.02	6.02	0.31	7.49	$271.13	XXX	A+
72131-26	Ct lumbar spine w/o dye	1.16	0.41	0.41	0.05	1.62	$58.64	XXX	A+
72131-TC	Ct lumbar spine w/o dye	0.00	5.61	5.61	0.26	5.87	$212.49	XXX	A+
72132	Ct lumbar spine w/dye	1.22	7.14	7.14	0.37	8.73	$316.02	XXX	A+
72132-26	Ct lumbar spine w/dye	1.22	0.43	0.43	0.06	1.71	$61.90	XXX	A+
72132-TC	Ct lumbar spine w/dye	0.00	6.71	6.71	0.31	7.02	$254.12	XXX	A+
72133	Ct lumbar spine w/o&w dye	1.27	8.85	8.85	0.44	10.56	$382.26	XXX	A+
72133-26	Ct lumbar spine w/o&w dye	1.27	0.45	0.45	0.06	1.78	$64.43	XXX	A+
72133-TC	Ct lumbar spine w/o&w dye	0.00	8.40	8.40	0.38	8.78	$317.83	XXX	A+
72141	Mri neck spine w/o dye	1.60	11.20	11.20	0.56	13.36	$483.62	XXX	A+
72141-26	Mri neck spine w/o dye	1.60	0.56	0.56	0.07	2.23	$80.72	XXX	A+
72141-TC	Mri neck spine w/o dye	0.00	10.64	10.64	0.49	11.13	$402.90	XXX	A+
72142	Mri neck spine w/dye	1.92	13.45	13.45	0.67	16.04	$580.64	XXX	A+

* **M** = multiple surgery adjustment applies
Me = multiple endoscopy rules may apply
B = bilateral surgery adjustment applies
A = assistant-at-surgery restriction

A+ = assistant-at-surgery restriction unless medical necessity established with documentation
C = cosurgeons payable
C+ = cosurgeons payable if medical necessity established with documentation

T = team surgeons permitted
T+ = team surgeons payable if medical necessity established with documentation
§ = indicates services that are not covered by Medicare.

325 CPT five-digit codes, two-digit numeric modifiers, and descriptions only are © 2001 American Medical Association

Medicare RBRVS: The Physicians' Guide

Relative value units

CPT Code and Modifier	Description	Work RVU	Non Facility Practice Expense RVU	Facility Practice Expense RVU	PLI RVU	Total Non Facility RVUs	Medicare Payment Non Facility	Total Facility RVUs	Medicare Payment Facility	Global Period	Payment Policy Indicators*
72142-26	Mri neck spine w/dye	1.92	0.69	0.69	0.09	2.70	$97.74	2.70	$97.74	XXX	A+
72142-TC	Mri neck spine w/dye	0.00	12.76	12.76	0.58	13.34	$482.90	13.34	$482.90	XXX	A+
72146	Mri chest spine w/o dye	1.60	12.38	12.38	0.60	14.58	$527.78	14.58	$527.78	XXX	A+
72146-26	Mri chest spine w/o dye	1.60	0.56	0.56	0.07	2.23	$80.72	2.23	$80.72	XXX	A+
72146-TC	Mri chest spine w/o dye	0.00	11.82	11.82	0.53	12.35	$447.06	12.35	$447.06	XXX	A+
72147	Mri chest spine w/dye	1.92	13.44	13.44	0.67	16.03	$580.27	16.03	$580.27	XXX	A+
72147-26	Mri chest spine w/dye	1.92	0.68	0.68	0.09	2.69	$97.38	2.69	$97.38	XXX	A+
72147-TC	Mri chest spine w/dye	0.00	12.76	12.76	0.58	13.34	$482.90	13.34	$482.90	XXX	A+
72148	Mri lumbar spine w/o dye	1.48	12.34	12.34	0.60	14.42	$521.99	14.42	$521.99	XXX	A+
72148-26	Mri lumbar spine w/o dye	1.48	0.52	0.52	0.07	2.07	$74.93	2.07	$74.93	XXX	A+
72148-TC	Mri lumbar spine w/o dye	0.00	11.82	11.82	0.53	12.35	$447.06	12.35	$447.06	XXX	A+
72149	Mri lumbar spine w/dye	1.78	13.40	13.40	0.67	15.85	$573.76	15.85	$573.76	XXX	A+
72149-26	Mri lumbar spine w/dye	1.78	0.64	0.64	0.09	2.51	$90.86	2.51	$90.86	XXX	A+
72149-TC	Mri lumbar spine w/dye	0.00	12.76	12.76	0.58	13.34	$482.90	13.34	$482.90	XXX	A+
72156	Mri neck spine w/o&w dye	2.57	24.55	24.55	1.20	28.32	$1,025.16	28.32	$1,025.16	XXX	A+
72156-26	Mri neck spine w/o&w dye	2.57	0.91	0.91	0.11	3.59	$129.96	3.59	$129.96	XXX	A+
72156-TC	Mri neck spine w/o&w dye	0.00	23.64	23.64	1.09	24.73	$895.21	24.73	$895.21	XXX	A+
72157	Mri chest spine w/o&w dye	2.57	24.54	24.54	1.20	28.31	$1,024.80	28.31	$1,024.80	XXX	A+
72157-26	Mri chest spine w/o&w dye	2.57	0.90	0.90	0.11	3.58	$129.59	3.58	$129.59	XXX	A+
72157-TC	Mri chest spine w/o&w dye	0.00	23.64	23.64	1.09	24.73	$895.21	24.73	$895.21	XXX	A+
72158	Mri lumbar spine w/o&w dye	2.36	24.47	24.47	1.20	28.03	$1,014.66	28.03	$1,014.66	XXX	A+
72158-26	Mri lumbar spine w/o&w dye	2.36	0.83	0.83	0.11	3.30	$119.46	3.30	$119.46	XXX	A+
72158-TC	Mri lumbar spine w/o&w dye	0.00	23.64	23.64	1.09	24.73	$895.21	24.73	$895.21	XXX	A+
72159 §	Mr angio spine w/o&w dye	1.80	12.54	12.54	0.61	14.95	$541.18	14.95	$541.18	XXX	
72159-26 §	Mr angio spine w/o&w dye	1.80	0.72	0.72	0.08	2.60	$94.12	2.60	$94.12	XXX	
72159-TC §	Mr angio spine w/o&w dye	0.00	11.82	11.82	0.53	12.35	$447.06	12.35	$447.06	XXX	
72170	X-ray exam of pelvis	0.17	0.56	0.56	0.03	0.76	$27.51	0.76	$27.51	XXX	A+

Code	Description								
72170-26	X-ray exam of pelvis	0.17	0.06	0.06	0.01	0.24	$8.69	XXX	A+
72170-TC	X-ray exam of pelvis	0.00	0.50	0.50	0.02	0.52	$18.82	XXX	A+
72190	X-ray exam of pelvis	0.21	0.70	0.70	0.04	0.95	$34.39	XXX	A+
72190-26	X-ray exam of pelvis	0.21	0.07	0.07	0.01	0.29	$10.50	XXX	A+
72190-TC	X-ray exam of pelvis	0.00	0.63	0.63	0.03	0.66	$23.89	XXX	A+
72191	Ct angiograph pelv w/o&w dye	1.81	8.78	8.78	0.38	10.97	$397.11	XXX	A+
72191-26	Ct angiograph pelv w/o&w dye	1.81	0.72	0.72	0.06	2.59	$93.76	XXX	A+
72191-TC	Ct angiograph pelv w/o&w dye	0.00	8.06	8.06	0.32	8.38	$303.35	XXX	A+
72192	Ct pelvis w/o dye	1.09	5.99	5.99	0.31	7.39	$267.51	XXX	A+
72192-26	Ct pelvis w/o dye	1.09	0.38	0.38	0.05	1.52	$55.02	XXX	A+
72192-TC	Ct pelvis w/o dye	0.00	5.61	5.61	0.26	5.87	$212.49	XXX	A+
72193	Ct pelvis w/dye	1.16	6.91	6.91	0.35	8.42	$304.80	XXX	A+
72193-26	Ct pelvis w/dye	1.16	0.41	0.41	0.05	1.62	$58.64	XXX	A+
72193-TC	Ct pelvis w/dye	0.00	6.50	6.50	0.30	6.80	$246.15	XXX	A+
72194	Ct pelvis w/o&w dye	1.22	8.49	8.49	0.41	10.12	$366.34	XXX	A+
72194-26	Ct pelvis w/o&w dye	1.22	0.43	0.43	0.05	1.70	$61.54	XXX	A+
72194-TC	Ct pelvis w/o&w dye	0.00	8.06	8.06	0.36	8.42	$304.80	XXX	A+
72195	Mri pelvis w/o dye	1.46	11.15	11.15	0.42	13.03	$471.68	XXX	A+
72195-26	Mri pelvis w/o dye	1.46	0.51	0.51	0.05	2.02	$73.12	XXX	A+
72195-TC	Mri pelvis w/o dye	0.00	10.64	10.64	0.37	11.01	$398.55	XXX	A+
72196	Mri pelvis w/dye	1.73	13.36	13.36	0.48	15.57	$563.62	XXX	A+
72196-26	Mri pelvis w/dye	1.73	0.60	0.60	0.05	2.38	$86.15	XXX	A+
72196-TC	Mri pelvis w/dye	0.00	12.76	12.76	0.43	13.19	$477.47	XXX	A+
72197	Mri pelvis w/o & w dye	2.26	24.43	24.43	0.84	27.53	$996.56	XXX	A+
72197-26	Mri pelvis w/o & w dye	2.26	0.79	0.79	0.08	3.13	$113.30	XXX	A+
72197-TC	Mri pelvis w/o & w dye	0.00	23.64	23.64	0.76	24.40	$883.26	XXX	A+
72198 §	Mr angio pelvis w/o&w dye	1.80	11.36	11.36	0.57	13.73	$497.02	XXX	
72198-26 §	Mr angio pelvis w/o&w dye	1.80	0.72	0.72	0.08	2.60	$94.12	XXX	

* **M** = multiple surgery adjustment applies
Me = multiple endoscopy rules may apply
B = bilateral surgery adjustment applies
A = assistant-at-surgery restriction

A+ = assistant-at-surgery restriction unless medical necessity established with documentation
C = cosurgeons payable
C+ = cosurgeons payable if medical necessity established with documentation

T = team surgeons permitted
T+ = team surgeons payable if medical necessity established with documentation
§ = indicates services that are not covered by Medicare.

327 CPT five-digit codes, two-digit numeric modifiers, and descriptions only are © 2001 American Medical Association

Medicare RBRVS: The Physicians' Guide

Relative value units

CPT Code and Modifier	Description	Work RVU	Non Facility Practice Expense RVU	Facility Practice Expense RVU	PLI RVU	Total Non Facility RVUs	Medicare Payment Non Facility	Total Facility RVUs	Medicare Payment Facility	Global Period	Payment Policy Indicators*
72198-TC §	Mr angio pelvis w/o&w dye	0.00	10.64	10.64	0.49	11.13	$402.90	11.13	$402.90	XXX	
72200	X-ray exam sacroiliac joints	0.17	0.56	0.56	0.03	0.76	$27.51	0.76	$27.51	XXX	A+
72200-26	X-ray exam sacroiliac joints	0.17	0.06	0.06	0.01	0.24	$8.69	0.24	$8.69	XXX	A+
72200-TC	X-ray exam sacroiliac joints	0.00	0.50	0.50	0.02	0.52	$18.82	0.52	$18.82	XXX	A+
72202	X-ray exam sacroiliac joints	0.19	0.66	0.66	0.04	0.89	$32.22	0.89	$32.22	XXX	A+
72202-26	X-ray exam sacroiliac joints	0.19	0.07	0.07	0.01	0.27	$9.77	0.27	$9.77	XXX	A+
72202-TC	X-ray exam sacroiliac joints	0.00	0.59	0.59	0.03	0.62	$22.44	0.62	$22.44	XXX	A+
72220	X-ray exam of tailbone	0.17	0.60	0.60	0.04	0.81	$29.32	0.81	$29.32	XXX	A+
72220-26	X-ray exam of tailbone	0.17	0.06	0.06	0.01	0.24	$8.69	0.24	$8.69	XXX	A+
72220-TC	X-ray exam of tailbone	0.00	0.54	0.54	0.03	0.57	$20.63	0.57	$20.63	XXX	A+
72240	Contrast x-ray of neck spine	0.91	4.82	4.82	0.25	5.98	$216.47	5.98	$216.47	XXX	A+
72240-26	Contrast x-ray of neck spine	0.91	0.31	0.31	0.04	1.26	$45.61	1.26	$45.61	XXX	A+
72240-TC	Contrast x-ray of neck spine	0.00	4.51	4.51	0.21	4.72	$170.86	4.72	$170.86	XXX	A+
72255	Contrast x-ray, thorax spine	0.91	4.41	4.41	0.22	5.54	$200.54	5.54	$200.54	XXX	A+
72255-26	Contrast x-ray, thorax spine	0.91	0.30	0.30	0.04	1.25	$45.25	1.25	$45.25	XXX	A+
72255-TC	Contrast x-ray, thorax spine	0.00	4.11	4.11	0.18	4.29	$155.29	4.29	$155.29	XXX	A+
72265	Contrast x-ray, lower spine	0.83	4.15	4.15	0.22	5.20	$188.24	5.20	$188.24	XXX	A+
72265-26	Contrast x-ray, lower spine	0.83	0.28	0.28	0.04	1.15	$41.63	1.15	$41.63	XXX	A+
72265-TC	Contrast x-ray, lower spine	0.00	3.87	3.87	0.18	4.05	$146.61	4.05	$146.61	XXX	A+
72270	Contrast x-ray of spine	1.33	6.25	6.25	0.34	7.92	$286.70	7.92	$286.70	XXX	A+
72270-26	Contrast x-ray of spine	1.33	0.46	0.46	0.07	1.86	$67.33	1.86	$67.33	XXX	A+
72270-TC	Contrast x-ray of spine	0.00	5.79	5.79	0.27	6.06	$219.37	6.06	$219.37	XXX	A+
72275	Epidurography	0.76	2.20	2.20	0.21	3.17	$114.75	3.17	$114.75	XXX	
72275-26	Epidurography	0.76	0.21	0.21	0.03	1.00	$36.20	1.00	$36.20	XXX	
72275-TC	Epidurography	0.00	1.99	1.99	0.18	2.17	$78.55	2.17	$78.55	XXX	
72285	X-ray c/t spine disk	1.16	8.35	8.35	0.42	9.93	$359.46	9.93	$359.46	XXX	A+
72285-26	X-ray c/t spine disk	1.16	0.39	0.39	0.06	1.61	$58.28	1.61	$58.28	XXX	A+

Code	Description							
72285-TC	X-ray c/t spine disk	0.00	7.96	0.36	8.32	$301.18	XXX	A+
72295	X-ray of lower spine disk	0.83	7.76	0.37	8.96	$324.34	XXX	A+
72295-26	X-ray of lower spine disk	0.83	0.29	0.04	1.16	$41.99	XXX	A+
72295-TC	X-ray of lower spine disk	0.00	7.47	0.33	7.80	$282.35	XXX	A+
73000	X-ray exam of collar bone	0.16	0.56	0.03	0.75	$27.15	XXX	A+
73000-26	X-ray exam of collar bone	0.16	0.06	0.01	0.23	$8.33	XXX	A+
73000-TC	X-ray exam of collar bone	0.00	0.50	0.02	0.52	$18.82	XXX	A+
73010	X-ray exam of shoulder blade	0.17	0.56	0.03	0.76	$27.51	XXX	A+
73010-26	X-ray exam of shoulder blade	0.17	0.06	0.01	0.24	$8.69	XXX	A+
73010-TC	X-ray exam of shoulder blade	0.00	0.50	0.02	0.52	$18.82	XXX	A+
73020	X-ray exam of shoulder	0.15	0.50	0.03	0.68	$24.62	XXX	A+
73020-26	X-ray exam of shoulder	0.15	0.05	0.01	0.21	$7.60	XXX	A+
73020-TC	X-ray exam of shoulder	0.00	0.45	0.02	0.47	$17.01	XXX	A+
73030	X-ray exam of shoulder	0.18	0.60	0.04	0.82	$29.68	XXX	A+
73030-26	X-ray exam of shoulder	0.18	0.06	0.01	0.25	$9.05	XXX	A+
73030-TC	X-ray exam of shoulder	0.00	0.54	0.03	0.57	$20.63	XXX	A+
73040	Contrast x-ray of shoulder	0.54	2.18	0.13	2.85	$103.17	XXX	A+
73040-26	Contrast x-ray of shoulder	0.54	0.19	0.03	0.76	$27.51	XXX	A+
73040-TC	Contrast x-ray of shoulder	0.00	1.99	0.10	2.09	$75.66	XXX	A+
73050	X-ray exam of shoulders	0.20	0.70	0.05	0.95	$34.39	XXX	A+
73050-26	X-ray exam of shoulders	0.20	0.07	0.02	0.29	$10.50	XXX	A+
73050-TC	X-ray exam of shoulders	0.00	0.63	0.03	0.66	$23.89	XXX	A+
73060	X-ray exam of humerus	0.17	0.60	0.04	0.81	$29.32	XXX	A+
73060-26	X-ray exam of humerus	0.17	0.06	0.01	0.24	$8.69	XXX	A+
73060-TC	X-ray exam of humerus	0.00	0.54	0.03	0.57	$20.63	XXX	A+
73070	X-ray exam of elbow	0.15	0.55	0.03	0.73	$26.43	XXX	A+
73070-26	X-ray exam of elbow	0.15	0.05	0.01	0.21	$7.60	XXX	A+
73070-TC	X-ray exam of elbow	0.00	0.50	0.02	0.52	$18.82	XXX	A+

* **M** = multiple surgery adjustment applies
Me = multiple endoscopy rules may apply
B = bilateral surgery adjustment applies
A = assistant-at-surgery restriction

A+ = assistant-at-surgery restriction unless medical necessity established with documentation
C = cosurgeons payable
C+ = cosurgeons payable if medical necessity established with documentation

T = team surgeons permitted
T+ = team surgeons payable if medical necessity established with documentation
§ = indicates services that are not covered by Medicare.

CPT five-digit codes, two-digit numeric modifiers, and descriptions only are © 2001 American Medical Association

Medicare RBRVS: The Physicians' Guide

Relative value units

CPT Code and Modifier	Description	Work RVU	Non Facility Practice Expense RVU	Facility Practice Expense RVU	PLI RVU	Total Non Facility RVUs	Medicare Payment Non Facility	Total Facility RVUs	Medicare Payment Facility	Global Period	Payment Policy Indicators*
73080	X-ray exam of elbow	0.17	0.60	0.60	0.04	0.81	$29.32	0.81	$29.32	XXX	A+
73080-26	X-ray exam of elbow	0.17	0.06	0.06	0.01	0.24	$8.69	0.24	$8.69	XXX	A+
73080-TC	X-ray exam of elbow	0.00	0.54	0.54	0.03	0.57	$20.63	0.57	$20.63	XXX	A+
73085	Contrast x-ray of elbow	0.54	2.19	2.19	0.13	2.86	$103.53	2.86	$103.53	XXX	A+
73085-26	Contrast x-ray of elbow	0.54	0.20	0.20	0.03	0.77	$27.87	0.77	$27.87	XXX	A+
73085-TC	Contrast x-ray of elbow	0.00	1.99	1.99	0.10	2.09	$75.66	2.09	$75.66	XXX	A+
73090	X-ray exam of forearm	0.16	0.56	0.56	0.03	0.75	$27.15	0.75	$27.15	XXX	A+
73090-26	X-ray exam of forearm	0.16	0.06	0.06	0.01	0.23	$8.33	0.23	$8.33	XXX	A+
73090-TC	X-ray exam of forearm	0.00	0.50	0.50	0.02	0.52	$18.82	0.52	$18.82	XXX	A+
73092	X-ray exam of arm, infant	0.16	0.53	0.53	0.03	0.72	$26.06	0.72	$26.06	XXX	A+
73092-26	X-ray exam of arm, infant	0.16	0.06	0.06	0.01	0.23	$8.33	0.23	$8.33	XXX	A+
73092-TC	X-ray exam of arm, infant	0.00	0.47	0.47	0.02	0.49	$17.74	0.49	$17.74	XXX	A+
73100	X-ray exam of wrist	0.16	0.53	0.53	0.04	0.73	$26.43	0.73	$26.43	XXX	A+
73100-26	X-ray exam of wrist	0.16	0.06	0.06	0.02	0.24	$8.69	0.24	$8.69	XXX	A+
73100-TC	X-ray exam of wrist	0.00	0.47	0.47	0.02	0.49	$17.74	0.49	$17.74	XXX	A+
73110	X-ray exam of wrist	0.17	0.57	0.57	0.03	0.77	$27.87	0.77	$27.87	XXX	A+
73110-26	X-ray exam of wrist	0.17	0.06	0.06	0.01	0.24	$8.69	0.24	$8.69	XXX	A+
73110-TC	X-ray exam of wrist	0.00	0.51	0.51	0.02	0.53	$19.19	0.53	$19.19	XXX	A+
73115	Contrast x-ray of wrist	0.54	1.70	1.70	0.11	2.35	$85.07	2.35	$85.07	XXX	A+
73115-26	Contrast x-ray of wrist	0.54	0.20	0.20	0.03	0.77	$27.87	0.77	$27.87	XXX	A+
73115-TC	Contrast x-ray of wrist	0.00	1.50	1.50	0.08	1.58	$57.19	1.58	$57.19	XXX	A+
73120	X-ray exam of hand	0.16	0.53	0.53	0.03	0.72	$26.06	0.72	$26.06	XXX	A+
73120-26	X-ray exam of hand	0.16	0.06	0.06	0.01	0.23	$8.33	0.23	$8.33	XXX	A+
73120-TC	X-ray exam of hand	0.00	0.47	0.47	0.02	0.49	$17.74	0.49	$17.74	XXX	A+
73130	X-ray exam of hand	0.17	0.57	0.57	0.03	0.77	$27.87	0.77	$27.87	XXX	A+
73130-26	X-ray exam of hand	0.17	0.06	0.06	0.01	0.24	$8.69	0.24	$8.69	XXX	A+
73130-TC	X-ray exam of hand	0.00	0.51	0.51	0.02	0.53	$19.19	0.53	$19.19	XXX	A+

Code	Description							
73140	X-ray exam of finger(s)	0.13	0.44	0.44	0.03	0.60	$21.72	$21.72	XXX	A+
73140-26	X-ray exam of finger(s)	0.13	0.05	0.05	0.01	0.19	$6.88	$6.88	XXX	A+
73140-TC	X-ray exam of finger(s)	0.00	0.39	0.39	0.02	0.41	$14.84	$14.84	XXX	A+
73200	Ct upper extremity w/o dye	1.09	5.09	5.09	0.26	6.44	$233.12	$233.12	XXX	A+
73200-26	Ct upper extremity w/o dye	1.09	0.38	0.38	0.05	1.52	$55.02	$55.02	XXX	A+
73200-TC	Ct upper extremity w/o dye	0.00	4.71	4.71	0.21	4.92	$178.10	$178.10	XXX	A+
73201	Ct upper extremity w/dye	1.16	6.02	6.02	0.31	7.49	$271.13	$271.13	XXX	A+
73201-26	Ct upper extremity w/dye	1.16	0.41	0.41	0.05	1.62	$58.64	$58.64	XXX	A+
73201-TC	Ct upper extremity w/dye	0.00	5.61	5.61	0.26	5.87	$212.49	$212.49	XXX	A+
73202	Ct uppr extremity w/o&w dye	1.22	7.48	7.48	0.38	9.08	$328.69	$328.69	XXX	A+
73202-26	Ct uppr extremity w/o&w dye	1.22	0.43	0.43	0.06	1.71	$61.90	$61.90	XXX	A+
73202-TC	Ct uppr extremity w/o&w dye	0.00	7.05	7.05	0.32	7.37	$266.79	$266.79	XXX	A+
73206	Ct angio upr extrm w/o&w dye	1.81	7.77	7.77	0.38	9.96	$360.54	$360.54	XXX	A+
73206-26	Ct angio upr extrm w/o&w dye	1.81	0.72	0.72	0.06	2.59	$93.76	$93.76	XXX	A+
73206-TC	Ct angio upr extrm w/o&w dye	0.00	7.05	7.05	0.32	7.37	$266.79	$266.79	XXX	A+
73218	Mri upper extremity w/o dye	1.35	11.11	11.11	0.36	12.82	$464.07	$464.07	XXX	A+
73218-26	Mri upper extremity w/o dye	1.35	0.47	0.47	0.04	1.86	$67.33	$67.33	XXX	A+
73218-TC	Mri upper extremity w/o dye	0.00	10.64	10.64	0.32	10.96	$396.74	$396.74	XXX	A+
73219	Mri upper extremity w/dye	1.62	13.33	13.33	0.44	15.39	$557.11	$557.11	XXX	A+
73219-26	Mri upper extremity w/dye	1.62	0.57	0.57	0.05	2.24	$81.09	$81.09	XXX	A+
73219-TC	Mri upper extremity w/dye	0.00	12.76	12.76	0.39	13.15	$476.02	$476.02	XXX	A+
73220	Mri uppr extremity w/o&w dye	2.15	24.39	24.39	0.78	27.32	$988.96	$988.96	XXX	A+
73220-26	Mri uppr extremity w/o&w dye	2.15	0.75	0.75	0.08	2.98	$107.87	$107.87	XXX	A+
73220-TC	Mri uppr extremity w/o&w dye	0.00	23.64	23.64	0.70	24.34	$881.09	$881.09	XXX	A+
73221	Mri joint upr extrem w/o dye	1.35	11.11	11.11	0.36	12.82	$464.07	$464.07	XXX	A+
73221-26	Mri joint upr extrem w/o dye	1.35	0.47	0.47	0.04	1.86	$67.33	$67.33	XXX	A+
73221-TC	Mri joint upr extrem w/o dye	0.00	10.64	10.64	0.32	10.96	$396.74	$396.74	XXX	A+
73222	Mri joint upr extrem w/ dye	1.62	13.33	13.33	0.44	15.39	$557.11	$557.11	XXX	A+

* **M** = multiple surgery adjustment applies
   Me = multiple endoscopy rules may apply
   B = bilateral surgery adjustment applies
   A = assistant-at-surgery restriction

A+ = assistant-at-surgery restriction unless medical necessity established with documentation
C = cosurgeons payable
C+ = cosurgeons payable if medical necessity established with documentation

T = team surgeons permitted
T+ = team surgeons payable if medical necessity established with documentation
$ = indicates services that are not covered by Medicare.

CPT five-digit codes, two-digit numeric modifiers, and descriptions only are © 2001 American Medical Association

Medicare RBRVS: The Physicians' Guide

Relative value units

CPT Code and Modifier	Description	Work RVU	Non Facility Practice Expense RVU	Facility Practice Expense RVU	PLI RVU	Total Non Facility RVUs	Medicare Payment Non Facility	Total Facility RVUs	Medicare Payment Facility	Global Period	Payment Policy Indicators*
73222-26	Mri joint upr extrem w/ dye	1.62	0.57	0.57	0.05	2.24	$81.09	2.24	$81.09	XXX	A+
73222-TC	Mri joint upr extrem w/ dye	0.00	12.76	12.76	0.39	13.15	$476.02	13.15	$476.02	XXX	A+
73223	Mri joint upr extr w/o&w dye	2.15	24.39	24.39	0.77	27.31	$988.60	27.31	$988.60	XXX	A+
73223-26	Mri joint upr extr w/o&w dye	2.15	0.75	0.75	0.07	2.97	$107.51	2.97	$107.51	XXX	A+
73223-TC	Mri joint upr extr w/o&w dye	0.00	23.64	23.64	0.70	24.34	$881.09	24.34	$881.09	XXX	A+
73225 §	Mr angio upr extr w/o&w dye	1.73	11.33	11.33	0.57	13.63	$493.40	13.63	$493.40	XXX	
73225-26 §	Mr angio upr extr w/o&w dye	1.73	0.69	0.69	0.08	2.50	$90.50	2.50	$90.50	XXX	A+
73225-TC §	Mr angio upr extr w/o&w dye	0.00	10.64	10.64	0.49	11.13	$402.90	11.13	$402.90	XXX	A+
73500	X-ray exam of hip	0.17	0.51	0.51	0.03	0.71	$25.70	0.71	$25.70	XXX	A+
73500-26	X-ray exam of hip	0.17	0.06	0.06	0.01	0.24	$8.69	0.24	$8.69	XXX	A+
73500-TC	X-ray exam of hip	0.00	0.45	0.45	0.02	0.47	$17.01	0.47	$17.01	XXX	A+
73510	X-ray exam of hip	0.21	0.61	0.61	0.05	0.87	$31.49	0.87	$31.49	XXX	A+
73510-26	X-ray exam of hip	0.21	0.07	0.07	0.02	0.30	$10.86	0.30	$10.86	XXX	A+
73510-TC	X-ray exam of hip	0.00	0.54	0.54	0.03	0.57	$20.63	0.57	$20.63	XXX	A+
73520	X-ray exam of hips	0.26	0.72	0.72	0.05	1.03	$37.29	1.03	$37.29	XXX	A+
73520-26	X-ray exam of hips	0.26	0.09	0.09	0.02	0.37	$13.39	0.37	$13.39	XXX	A+
73520-TC	X-ray exam of hips	0.00	0.63	0.63	0.03	0.66	$23.89	0.66	$23.89	XXX	A+
73525	Contrast x-ray of hip	0.54	2.19	2.19	0.13	2.86	$103.53	2.86	$103.53	XXX	A+
73525-26	Contrast x-ray of hip	0.54	0.20	0.20	0.03	0.77	$27.87	0.77	$27.87	XXX	A+
73525-TC	Contrast x-ray of hip	0.00	1.99	1.99	0.10	2.09	$75.66	2.09	$75.66	XXX	A+
73530	X-ray exam of hip	0.29	0.60	0.60	0.03	0.92	$33.30	0.92	$33.30	XXX	A+
73530-26	X-ray exam of hip	0.29	0.10	0.10	0.01	0.40	$14.48	0.40	$14.48	XXX	A+
73530-TC	X-ray exam of hip	0.00	0.50	0.50	0.02	0.52	$18.82	0.52	$18.82	XXX	A+
73540	X-ray exam of pelvis & hips	0.20	0.61	0.61	0.05	0.86	$31.13	0.86	$31.13	XXX	A+
73540-26	X-ray exam of pelvis & hips	0.20	0.07	0.07	0.02	0.29	$10.50	0.29	$10.50	XXX	A+
73540-TC	X-ray exam of pelvis & hips	0.00	0.54	0.54	0.03	0.57	$20.63	0.57	$20.63	XXX	A+
73542	X-ray exam, sacroiliac joint	0.59	2.16	2.16	0.13	2.88	$104.25	2.88	$104.25	XXX	

Code	Description							
73542-26	X-ray exam, sacroiliac joint	0.59	0.17	0.03	0.79	$28.60	0.79	$28.60	XXX
73542-TC	X-ray exam, sacroiliac joint	0.00	1.99	0.10	2.09	$75.66	2.09	$75.66	XXX
73550	X-ray exam of thigh	0.17	0.60	0.04	0.81	$29.32	0.81	$29.32	XXX	A+
73550-26	X-ray exam of thigh	0.17	0.06	0.01	0.24	$8.69	0.24	$8.69	XXX	A+
73550-TC	X-ray exam of thigh	0.00	0.54	0.03	0.57	$20.63	0.57	$20.63	XXX	A+
73560	X-ray exam of knee, 1 or 2	0.17	0.56	0.04	0.77	$27.87	0.77	$27.87	XXX	A+
73560-26	X-ray exam of knee, 1 or 2	0.17	0.06	0.02	0.25	$9.05	0.25	$9.05	XXX	A+
73560-TC	X-ray exam of knee, 1 or 2	0.00	0.50	0.02	0.52	$18.82	0.52	$18.82	XXX	A+
73562	X-ray exam of knee, 3	0.18	0.60	0.05	0.83	$30.05	0.83	$30.05	XXX	A+
73562-26	X-ray exam of knee, 3	0.18	0.06	0.02	0.26	$9.41	0.26	$9.41	XXX	A+
73562-TC	X-ray exam of knee, 3	0.00	0.54	0.03	0.57	$20.63	0.57	$20.63	XXX	A+
73564	X-ray exam, knee, 4 or more	0.22	0.67	0.05	0.94	$34.03	0.94	$34.03	XXX	A+
73564-26	X-ray exam, knee, 4 or more	0.22	0.08	0.02	0.32	$11.58	0.32	$11.58	XXX	A+
73564-TC	X-ray exam, knee, 4 or more	0.00	0.59	0.03	0.62	$22.44	0.62	$22.44	XXX	A+
73565	X-ray exam of knees	0.17	0.54	0.04	0.75	$27.15	0.75	$27.15	XXX	A+
73565-26	X-ray exam of knees	0.17	0.07	0.02	0.26	$9.41	0.26	$9.41	XXX	A+
73565-TC	X-ray exam of knees	0.00	0.47	0.02	0.49	$17.74	0.49	$17.74	XXX	A+
73580	Contrast x-ray of knee joint	0.54	2.68	0.15	3.37	$121.99	3.37	$121.99	XXX	A+
73580-26	Contrast x-ray of knee joint	0.54	0.19	0.03	0.76	$27.51	0.76	$27.51	XXX	A+
73580-TC	Contrast x-ray of knee joint	0.00	2.49	0.12	2.61	$94.48	2.61	$94.48	XXX	A+
73590	X-ray exam of lower leg	0.17	0.56	0.03	0.76	$27.51	0.76	$27.51	XXX	A+
73590-26	X-ray exam of lower leg	0.17	0.06	0.01	0.24	$8.69	0.24	$8.69	XXX	A+
73590-TC	X-ray exam of lower leg	0.00	0.50	0.02	0.52	$18.82	0.52	$18.82	XXX	A+
73592	X-ray exam of leg, infant	0.16	0.53	0.03	0.72	$26.06	0.72	$26.06	XXX	A+
73592-26	X-ray exam of leg, infant	0.16	0.06	0.01	0.23	$8.33	0.23	$8.33	XXX	A+
73592-TC	X-ray exam of leg, infant	0.00	0.47	0.02	0.49	$17.74	0.49	$17.74	XXX	A+
73600	X-ray exam of ankle	0.16	0.53	0.03	0.72	$26.06	0.72	$26.06	XXX	A+
73600-26	X-ray exam of ankle	0.16	0.06	0.01	0.23	$8.33	0.23	$8.33	XXX	A+

*M = multiple surgery adjustment applies
Me = multiple endoscopy rules may apply
B = bilateral surgery adjustment applies
A = assistant-at-surgery restriction

A+ = assistant-at-surgery restriction unless medical necessity established with documentation
C = cosurgeons payable
C+ = cosurgeons payable if medical necessity established with documentation

T = team surgeons permitted
T+ = team surgeons payable if medical necessity established with documentation
$ = indicates services that are not covered by Medicare.

333 CPT five-digit codes, two-digit numeric modifiers, and descriptions only are © 2001 American Medical Association

Medicare RBRVS: The Physicians' Guide

Relative value units

CPT Code and Modifier	Description	Work RVU	Non Facility Practice Expense RVU	Facility Practice Expense RVU	PLI RVU	Total Non Facility RVUs	Medicare Payment Non Facility	Total Facility RVUs	Medicare Payment Facility	Global Period	Payment Policy Indicators*
73600-TC	X-ray exam of ankle	0.00	0.47	0.47	0.02	0.49	$17.74	0.49	$17.74	XXX	A+
73610	X-ray exam of ankle	0.17	0.57	0.57	0.03	0.77	$27.87	0.77	$27.87	XXX	A+
73610-26	X-ray exam of ankle	0.17	0.06	0.06	0.01	0.24	$8.69	0.24	$8.69	XXX	A+
73610-TC	X-ray exam of ankle	0.00	0.51	0.51	0.02	0.53	$19.19	0.53	$19.19	XXX	A+
73615	Contrast x-ray of ankle	0.54	2.18	2.18	0.13	2.85	$103.17	2.85	$103.17	XXX	A+
73615-26	Contrast x-ray of ankle	0.54	0.19	0.19	0.03	0.76	$27.51	0.76	$27.51	XXX	A+
73615-TC	Contrast x-ray of ankle	0.00	1.99	1.99	0.10	2.09	$75.66	2.09	$75.66	XXX	A+
73620	X-ray exam of foot	0.16	0.53	0.53	0.03	0.72	$26.06	0.72	$26.06	XXX	A+
73620-26	X-ray exam of foot	0.16	0.06	0.06	0.01	0.23	$8.33	0.23	$8.33	XXX	A+
73620-TC	X-ray exam of foot	0.00	0.47	0.47	0.02	0.49	$17.74	0.49	$17.74	XXX	A+
73630	X-ray exam of foot	0.17	0.57	0.57	0.03	0.77	$27.87	0.77	$27.87	XXX	A+
73630-26	X-ray exam of foot	0.17	0.06	0.06	0.01	0.24	$8.69	0.24	$8.69	XXX	A+
73630-TC	X-ray exam of foot	0.00	0.51	0.51	0.02	0.53	$19.19	0.53	$19.19	XXX	A+
73650	X-ray exam of heel	0.16	0.51	0.51	0.03	0.70	$25.34	0.70	$25.34	XXX	A+
73650-26	X-ray exam of heel	0.16	0.06	0.06	0.01	0.23	$8.33	0.23	$8.33	XXX	A+
73650-TC	X-ray exam of heel	0.00	0.45	0.45	0.02	0.47	$17.01	0.47	$17.01	XXX	A+
73660	X-ray exam of toe(s)	0.13	0.44	0.44	0.03	0.60	$21.72	0.60	$21.72	XXX	A+
73660-26	X-ray exam of toe(s)	0.13	0.05	0.05	0.01	0.19	$6.88	0.19	$6.88	XXX	A+
73660-TC	X-ray exam of toe(s)	0.00	0.39	0.39	0.02	0.41	$14.84	0.41	$14.84	XXX	A+
73700	Ct lower extremity w/o dye	1.09	5.09	5.09	0.26	6.44	$233.12	6.44	$233.12	XXX	A+
73700-26	Ct lower extremity w/o dye	1.09	0.38	0.38	0.05	1.52	$55.02	1.52	$55.02	XXX	A+
73700-TC	Ct lower extremity w/o dye	0.00	4.71	4.71	0.21	4.92	$178.10	4.92	$178.10	XXX	A+
73701	Ct lower extremity w/dye	1.16	6.02	6.02	0.31	7.49	$271.13	7.49	$271.13	XXX	A+
73701-26	Ct lower extremity w/dye	1.16	0.41	0.41	0.05	1.62	$58.64	1.62	$58.64	XXX	A+
73701-TC	Ct lower extremity w/dye	0.00	5.61	5.61	0.26	5.87	$212.49	5.87	$212.49	XXX	A+
73702	Ct lwr extremity w/o&w dye	1.22	7.48	7.48	0.37	9.07	$328.33	9.07	$328.33	XXX	A+
73702-26	Ct lwr extremity w/o&w dye	1.22	0.43	0.43	0.05	1.70	$61.54	1.70	$61.54	XXX	A+

73702-TC	Ct lwr extremity w/o&w dye	0.00	7.05	7.05	0.32	7.37	$266.79	XXX	A+
73706	Ct angio lwr extr w/o&w dye	1.90	7.81	7.81	0.38	10.09	$365.25	XXX	A+
73706-26	Ct angio lwr extr w/o&w dye	1.90	0.76	0.76	0.06	2.72	$98.46	XXX	A+
73706-TC	Ct angio lwr extr w/o&w dye	0.00	7.05	7.05	0.32	7.37	$266.79	XXX	A+
73718	Mri lower extremity w/o dye	1.35	11.11	11.11	0.36	12.82	$464.07	XXX	A+
73718-26	Mri lower extremity w/o dye	1.35	0.47	0.47	0.04	1.86	$67.33	XXX	A+
73718-TC	Mri lower extremity w/o dye	0.00	10.64	10.64	0.32	10.96	$396.74	XXX	A+
73719	Mri lower extremity w/dye	1.62	13.32	13.32	0.44	15.38	$556.74	XXX	A+
73719-26	Mri lower extremity w/dye	1.62	0.56	0.56	0.05	2.23	$80.72	XXX	A+
73719-TC	Mri lower extremity w/dye	0.00	12.76	12.76	0.39	13.15	$476.02	XXX	A+
73720	Mri lwr extremity w/o&w dye	2.15	24.39	24.39	0.78	27.32	$988.96	XXX	A+
73720-26	Mri lwr extremity w/o&w dye	2.15	0.75	0.75	0.08	2.98	$107.87	XXX	A+
73720-TC	Mri lwr extremity w/o&w dye	0.00	23.64	23.64	0.70	24.34	$881.09	XXX	A+
73721	Mri joint of lwr extre w/o d	1.35	11.11	11.11	0.36	12.82	$464.07	XXX	A+
73721-26	Mri joint of lwr extre w/o d	1.35	0.47	0.47	0.04	1.86	$67.33	XXX	A+
73721-TC	Mri joint of lwr extre w/o d	0.00	10.64	10.64	0.32	10.96	$396.74	XXX	A+
73722	Mri joint of lwr extr w/dye	1.62	13.33	13.33	0.45	15.40	$557.47	XXX	A+
73722-26	Mri joint of lwr extr w/dye	1.62	0.57	0.57	0.06	2.25	$81.45	XXX	A+
73722-TC	Mri joint of lwr extr w/dye	0.00	12.76	12.76	0.39	13.15	$476.02	XXX	A+
73723	Mri joint lwr extr w/o&w dye	2.15	24.39	24.39	0.77	27.31	$988.60	XXX	A+
73723-26	Mri joint lwr extr w/o&w dye	2.15	0.75	0.75	0.07	2.97	$107.51	XXX	A+
73723-TC	Mri joint lwr extr w/o&w dye	0.00	23.64	23.64	0.70	24.34	$881.09	XXX	A+
73725	Mr ang lwr ext w or w/o dye	1.82	11.28	11.28	0.57	13.67	$494.84	XXX	A+
73725-26	Mr ang lwr ext w or w/o dye	1.82	0.64	0.64	0.08	2.54	$91.95	XXX	A+
73725-TC	Mr ang lwr ext w or w/o dye	0.00	10.64	10.64	0.49	11.13	$402.90	XXX	A+
74000	X-ray exam of abdomen	0.18	0.56	0.56	0.03	0.77	$27.87	XXX	A+
74000-26	X-ray exam of abdomen	0.18	0.06	0.06	0.01	0.25	$9.05	XXX	A+
74000-TC	X-ray exam of abdomen	0.00	0.50	0.50	0.02	0.52	$18.82	XXX	A+

* **M** = multiple surgery adjustment applies
Me = multiple endoscopy rules may apply
B = bilateral surgery adjustment applies
A = assistant-at-surgery restriction

A+ = assistant-at-surgery restriction unless medical necessity established with documentation
C = cosurgeons payable
C+ = cosurgeons payable if medical necessity established with documentation

T = team surgeons permitted
T+ = team surgeons payable if medical necessity established with documentation
$ = indicates services that are not covered by Medicare.

335   CPT five-digit codes, two-digit numeric modifiers, and descriptions only are © 2001 American Medical Association

Medicare RBRVS: The Physicians' Guide

Relative value units

CPT Code and Modifier	Description	Work RVU	Non Facility Practice Expense RVU	Facility Practice Expense RVU	PLI RVU	Total Non Facility RVUs	Medicare Payment Non Facility	Total Facility RVUs	Medicare Payment Facility	Global Period	Payment Policy Indicators*
74010	X-ray exam of abdomen	0.23	0.62	0.62	0.04	0.89	$32.22	0.89	$32.22	XXX	A+
74010-26	X-ray exam of abdomen	0.23	0.08	0.08	0.01	0.32	$11.58	0.32	$11.58	XXX	A+
74010-TC	X-ray exam of abdomen	0.00	0.54	0.54	0.03	0.57	$20.63	0.57	$20.63	XXX	A+
74020	X-ray exam of abdomen	0.27	0.68	0.68	0.04	0.99	$35.84	0.99	$35.84	XXX	A+
74020-26	X-ray exam of abdomen	0.27	0.09	0.09	0.01	0.37	$13.39	0.37	$13.39	XXX	A+
74020-TC	X-ray exam of abdomen	0.00	0.59	0.59	0.03	0.62	$22.44	0.62	$22.44	XXX	A+
74022	X-ray exam series, abdomen	0.32	0.81	0.81	0.05	1.18	$42.72	1.18	$42.72	XXX	A+
74022-26	X-ray exam series, abdomen	0.32	0.11	0.11	0.01	0.44	$15.93	0.44	$15.93	XXX	A+
74022-TC	X-ray exam series, abdomen	0.00	0.70	0.70	0.04	0.74	$26.79	0.74	$26.79	XXX	A+
74150	Ct abdomen w/o dye	1.19	5.79	5.79	0.30	7.28	$263.53	7.28	$263.53	XXX	A+
74150-26	Ct abdomen w/o dye	1.19	0.42	0.42	0.05	1.66	$60.09	1.66	$60.09	XXX	A+
74150-TC	Ct abdomen w/o dye	0.00	5.37	5.37	0.25	5.62	$203.44	5.62	$203.44	XXX	A+
74160	Ct abdomen w/dye	1.27	6.94	6.94	0.36	8.57	$310.23	8.57	$310.23	XXX	A+
74160-26	Ct abdomen w/dye	1.27	0.44	0.44	0.06	1.77	$64.07	1.77	$64.07	XXX	A+
74160-TC	Ct abdomen w/dye	0.00	6.50	6.50	0.30	6.80	$246.15	6.80	$246.15	XXX	A+
74170	Ct abdomen w/o&w dye	1.40	8.55	8.55	0.42	10.37	$375.39	10.37	$375.39	XXX	A+
74170-26	Ct abdomen w/o&w dye	1.40	0.49	0.49	0.06	1.95	$70.59	1.95	$70.59	XXX	A+
74170-TC	Ct abdomen w/o&w dye	0.00	8.06	8.06	0.36	8.42	$304.80	8.42	$304.80	XXX	A+
74175	Ct angio abdom w/o&w dye	1.90	8.82	8.82	0.38	11.10	$401.81	11.10	$401.81	XXX	A+
74175-26	Ct angio abdom w/o&w dye	1.90	0.76	0.76	0.06	2.72	$98.46	2.72	$98.46	XXX	A+
74175-TC	Ct angio abdom w/o&w dye	0.00	8.06	8.06	0.32	8.38	$303.35	8.38	$303.35	XXX	A+
74181	Mri abdomen w/o dye	1.46	11.15	11.15	0.41	13.02	$471.31	13.02	$471.31	XXX	A+
74181-26	Mri abdomen w/o dye	1.46	0.51	0.51	0.04	2.01	$72.76	2.01	$72.76	XXX	A+
74181-TC	Mri abdomen w/o dye	0.00	10.64	10.64	0.37	11.01	$398.55	11.01	$398.55	XXX	A+
74182	Mri abdomen w/dye	1.73	13.36	13.36	0.49	15.58	$563.98	15.58	$563.98	XXX	A+
74182-26	Mri abdomen w/dye	1.73	0.60	0.60	0.06	2.39	$86.52	2.39	$86.52	XXX	A+
74182-TC	Mri abdomen w/dye	0.00	12.76	12.76	0.43	13.19	$477.47	13.19	$477.47	XXX	A+

Code	Description								
74183	Mri abdomen w/o&w dye	2.26	24.43	24.43	0.84	27.53	$996.56	XXX	A+
74183-26	Mri abdomen w/o&w dye	2.26	0.79	0.79	0.08	3.13	$113.30	XXX	A+
74183-TC	Mri abdomen w/o&w dye	0.00	23.64	23.64	0.76	24.40	$883.26	XXX	A+
74185	Mri angio, abdom w or w/o dy	1.80	11.27	11.27	0.57	13.64	$493.76	XXX	A+
74185-26	Mri angio, abdom w or w/o dy	1.80	0.63	0.63	0.08	2.51	$90.86	XXX	A+
74185-TC	Mri angio, abdom w or w/o dy	0.00	10.64	10.64	0.49	11.13	$402.90	XXX	A+
74190	X-ray exam of peritoneum	0.48	1.41	1.41	0.08	1.97	$71.31	XXX	A+
74190-26	X-ray exam of peritoneum	0.48	0.17	0.17	0.02	0.67	$24.25	XXX	A+
74190-TC	X-ray exam of peritoneum	0.00	1.24	1.24	0.06	1.30	$47.06	XXX	A+
74210	Contrst x-ray exam of throat	0.36	1.26	1.26	0.07	1.69	$61.18	XXX	A+
74210-26	Contrst x-ray exam of throat	0.36	0.13	0.13	0.02	0.51	$18.46	XXX	A+
74210-TC	Contrst x-ray exam of throat	0.00	1.13	1.13	0.05	1.18	$42.72	XXX	A+
74220	Contrast x-ray, esophagus	0.46	1.29	1.29	0.07	1.82	$65.88	XXX	A+
74220-26	Contrast x-ray, esophagus	0.46	0.16	0.16	0.02	0.64	$23.17	XXX	A+
74220-TC	Contrast x-ray, esophagus	0.00	1.13	1.13	0.05	1.18	$42.72	XXX	A+
74230	Cine/video x-ray, throat/eso	0.53	1.43	1.43	0.08	2.04	$73.85	XXX	A+
74230-26	Cine/video x-ray, throat/eso	0.53	0.19	0.19	0.02	0.74	$26.79	XXX	A+
74230-TC	Cine/video x-ray, throat/eso	0.00	1.24	1.24	0.06	1.30	$47.06	XXX	A+
74235	Remove esophagus obstruction	1.19	2.90	2.90	0.17	4.26	$154.21	XXX	A+
74235-26	Remove esophagus obstruction	1.19	0.41	0.41	0.05	1.65	$59.73	XXX	A+
74235-TC	Remove esophagus obstruction	0.00	2.49	2.49	0.12	2.61	$94.48	XXX	A+
74240	X-ray exam, upper gi tract	0.69	1.63	1.63	0.10	2.42	$87.60	XXX	A+
74240-26	X-ray exam, upper gi tract	0.69	0.24	0.24	0.03	0.96	$34.75	XXX	A+
74240-TC	X-ray exam, upper gi tract	0.00	1.39	1.39	0.07	1.46	$52.85	XXX	A+
74241	X-ray exam, upper gi tract	0.69	1.65	1.65	0.10	2.44	$88.33	XXX	A+
74241-26	X-ray exam, upper gi tract	0.69	0.24	0.24	0.03	0.96	$34.75	XXX	A+
74241-TC	X-ray exam, upper gi tract	0.00	1.41	1.41	0.07	1.48	$53.57	XXX	A+
74245	X-ray exam, upper gi tract	0.91	2.58	2.58	0.15	3.64	$131.77	XXX	A+

* **M** = multiple surgery adjustment applies
Me = multiple endoscopy rules may apply
B = bilateral surgery adjustment applies
A = assistant-at-surgery restriction

A+ = assistant-at-surgery restriction unless medical necessity established with documentation
C = cosurgeons payable
C+ = cosurgeons payable if medical necessity established with documentation

T = team surgeons permitted
T+ = team surgeons payable if medical necessity established with documentation
$ = indicates services that are not covered by Medicare.

337 CPT five-digit codes, two-digit numeric modifiers, and descriptions only are © 2001 American Medical Association

Medicare RBRVS: The Physicians' Guide

Relative value units

CPT Code and Modifier	Description	Work RVU	Non Facility Practice Expense RVU	Facility Practice Expense RVU	PLI RVU	Total Non Facility RVUs	Medicare Payment Non Facility	Total Facility RVUs	Medicare Payment Facility	Global Period	Payment Policy Indicators*
74245-26	X-ray exam, upper gi tract	0.91	0.32	0.32	0.04	1.27	$45.97	1.27	$45.97	XXX	A+
74245-TC	X-ray exam, upper gi tract	0.00	2.26	2.26	0.11	2.37	$85.79	2.37	$85.79	XXX	A+
74246	Contrst x-ray uppr gi tract	0.69	1.80	1.80	0.11	2.60	$94.12	2.60	$94.12	XXX	A+
74246-26	Contrst x-ray uppr gi tract	0.69	0.24	0.24	0.03	0.96	$34.75	0.96	$34.75	XXX	A+
74246-TC	Contrst x-ray uppr gi tract	0.00	1.56	1.56	0.08	1.64	$59.37	1.64	$59.37	XXX	A+
74247	Contrst x-ray uppr gi tract	0.69	1.84	1.84	0.12	2.65	$95.93	2.65	$95.93	XXX	A+
74247-26	Contrst x-ray uppr gi tract	0.69	0.24	0.24	0.03	0.96	$34.75	0.96	$34.75	XXX	A+
74247-TC	Contrst x-ray uppr gi tract	0.00	1.60	1.60	0.09	1.69	$61.18	1.69	$61.18	XXX	A+
74249	Contrst x-ray uppr gi tract	0.91	2.76	2.76	0.16	3.83	$138.64	3.83	$138.64	XXX	A+
74249-26	Contrst x-ray uppr gi tract	0.91	0.32	0.32	0.04	1.27	$45.97	1.27	$45.97	XXX	A+
74249-TC	Contrst x-ray uppr gi tract	0.00	2.44	2.44	0.12	2.56	$92.67	2.56	$92.67	XXX	A+
74250	X-ray exam of small bowel	0.47	1.40	1.40	0.08	1.95	$70.59	1.95	$70.59	XXX	A+
74250-26	X-ray exam of small bowel	0.47	0.16	0.16	0.02	0.65	$23.53	0.65	$23.53	XXX	A+
74250-TC	X-ray exam of small bowel	0.00	1.24	1.24	0.06	1.30	$47.06	1.30	$47.06	XXX	A+
74251	X-ray exam of small bowel	0.69	1.48	1.48	0.09	2.26	$81.81	2.26	$81.81	XXX	A+
74251-26	X-ray exam of small bowel	0.69	0.24	0.24	0.03	0.96	$34.75	0.96	$34.75	XXX	A+
74251-TC	X-ray exam of small bowel	0.00	1.24	1.24	0.06	1.30	$47.06	1.30	$47.06	XXX	A+
74260	X-ray exam of small bowel	0.50	1.58	1.58	0.09	2.17	$78.55	2.17	$78.55	XXX	A+
74260-26	X-ray exam of small bowel	0.50	0.17	0.17	0.02	0.69	$24.98	0.69	$24.98	XXX	A+
74260-TC	X-ray exam of small bowel	0.00	1.41	1.41	0.07	1.48	$53.57	1.48	$53.57	XXX	A+
74270	Contrast x-ray exam of colon	0.69	1.86	1.86	0.12	2.67	$96.65	2.67	$96.65	XXX	A+
74270-26	Contrast x-ray exam of colon	0.69	0.24	0.24	0.03	0.96	$34.75	0.96	$34.75	XXX	A+
74270-TC	Contrast x-ray exam of colon	0.00	1.62	1.62	0.09	1.71	$61.90	1.71	$61.90	XXX	A+
74280	Contrast x-ray exam of colon	0.99	2.47	2.47	0.15	3.61	$130.68	3.61	$130.68	XXX	A+
74280-26	Contrast x-ray exam of colon	0.99	0.35	0.35	0.04	1.38	$49.95	1.38	$49.95	XXX	A+
74280-TC	Contrast x-ray exam of colon	0.00	2.12	2.12	0.11	2.23	$80.72	2.23	$80.72	XXX	A+
74283	Contrast x-ray exam of colon	2.02	3.14	3.14	0.21	5.37	$194.39	5.37	$194.39	XXX	A+

Code	Description								
74283-26	Contrast x-ray exam of colon	2.02	0.71	0.09	2.82	2.82	$102.08	XXX	A+
74283-TC	Contrast x-ray exam of colon	0.00	2.43	0.12	2.55	2.55	$92.31	XXX	A+
74290	Contrast x-ray, gallbladder	0.32	0.81	0.05	1.18	1.18	$42.72	XXX	A+
74290-26	Contrast x-ray, gallbladder	0.32	0.11	0.01	0.44	0.44	$15.93	XXX	A+
74290-TC	Contrast x-ray, gallbladder	0.00	0.70	0.04	0.74	0.74	$26.79	XXX	A+
74291	Contrast x-rays, gallbladder	0.20	0.46	0.03	0.69	0.69	$24.98	XXX	A+
74291-26	Contrast x-rays, gallbladder	0.20	0.07	0.01	0.28	0.28	$10.14	XXX	A+
74291-TC	Contrast x-rays, gallbladder	0.00	0.39	0.02	0.41	0.41	$14.84	XXX	A+
74300	X-ray bile ducts/pancreas	0.00	0.00	0.00	0.00	0.00	$0.00	XXX	A+
74300-26	X-ray bile ducts/pancreas	0.36	0.13	0.02	0.51	0.51	$18.46	XXX	A+
74300-TC	X-ray bile ducts/pancreas	0.00	0.00	0.00	0.00	0.00	$0.00	XXX	A+
74301	X-rays at surgery add-on	0.00	0.00	0.00	0.00	0.00	$0.00	ZZZ	A+
74301-26	X-rays at surgery add-on	0.21	0.07	0.01	0.29	0.29	$10.50	ZZZ	A+
74301-TC	X-rays at surgery add-on	0.00	0.00	0.00	0.00	0.00	$0.00	ZZZ	A+
74305	X-ray bile ducts/pancreas	0.42	0.89	0.06	1.37	1.37	$49.59	XXX	A+
74305-26	X-ray bile ducts/pancreas	0.42	0.15	0.02	0.59	0.59	$21.36	XXX	A+
74305-TC	X-ray bile ducts/pancreas	0.00	0.74	0.04	0.78	0.78	$28.24	XXX	A+
74320	Contrast x-ray of bile ducts	0.54	3.18	0.16	3.88	3.88	$140.45	XXX	A+
74320-26	Contrast x-ray of bile ducts	0.54	0.19	0.02	0.75	0.75	$27.15	XXX	A+
74320-TC	Contrast x-ray of bile ducts	0.00	2.99	0.14	3.13	3.13	$113.30	XXX	A+
74327	X-ray bile stone removal	0.70	1.91	0.12	2.73	2.73	$98.82	XXX	A+
74327-26	X-ray bile stone removal	0.70	0.24	0.03	0.97	0.97	$35.11	XXX	A+
74327-TC	X-ray bile stone removal	0.00	1.67	0.09	1.76	1.76	$63.71	XXX	A+
74328	Xray bile duct endoscopy	0.70	3.24	0.17	4.11	4.11	$148.78	XXX	A+
74328-26	Xray bile duct endoscopy	0.70	0.25	0.03	0.98	0.98	$35.48	XXX	A+
74328-TC	Xray bile duct endoscopy	0.00	2.99	0.14	3.13	3.13	$113.30	XXX	A+
74329	X-ray for pancreas endoscopy	0.70	3.24	0.17	4.11	4.11	$148.78	XXX	A+
74329-26	X-ray for pancreas endoscopy	0.70	0.25	0.03	0.98	0.98	$35.48	XXX	A+

* **M** = multiple surgery adjustment applies
Me = multiple endoscopy rules may apply
B = bilateral surgery adjustment applies
A = assistant-at-surgery restriction

A+ = assistant-at-surgery restriction unless medical necessity established with documentation
C = cosurgeons payable
C+ = cosurgeons payable if medical necessity established with documentation

T = team surgeons permitted
T+ = team surgeons payable if medical necessity established with documentation
§ = indicates services that are not covered by Medicare.

339 CPT five-digit codes, two-digit numeric modifiers, and descriptions only are © 2001 American Medical Association

Medicare RBRVS: The Physicians' Guide

Relative value units

CPT Code and Modifier	Description	Work RVU	Non Facility Practice Expense RVU	Facility Practice Expense RVU	PLI RVU	Total Non Facility RVUs	Medicare Payment Non Facility	Total Facility RVUs	Medicare Payment Facility	Global Period	Payment Policy Indicators*
74329-TC	X-ray for pancreas endoscopy	0.00	2.99	2.99	0.14	3.13	$113.30	3.13	$113.30	XXX	A+
74330	X-ray bile/panc endoscopy	0.90	3.31	3.31	0.18	4.39	$158.91	4.39	$158.91	XXX	A+
74330-26	X-ray bile/panc endoscopy	0.90	0.32	0.32	0.04	1.26	$45.61	1.26	$45.61	XXX	A+
74330-TC	X-ray bile/panc endoscopy	0.00	2.99	2.99	0.14	3.13	$113.30	3.13	$113.30	XXX	A+
74340	X-ray guide for GI tube	0.54	2.68	2.68	0.14	3.36	$121.63	3.36	$121.63	XXX	A+
74340-26	X-ray guide for GI tube	0.54	0.19	0.19	0.02	0.75	$27.15	0.75	$27.15	XXX	A+
74340-TC	X-ray guide for GI tube	0.00	2.49	2.49	0.12	2.61	$94.48	2.61	$94.48	XXX	A+
74350	X-ray guide, stomach tube	0.76	3.26	3.26	0.17	4.19	$151.67	4.19	$151.67	XXX	A+
74350-26	X-ray guide, stomach tube	0.76	0.27	0.27	0.03	1.06	$38.37	1.06	$38.37	XXX	A+
74350-TC	X-ray guide, stomach tube	0.00	2.99	2.99	0.14	3.13	$113.30	3.13	$113.30	XXX	A+
74355	X-ray guide, intestinal tube	0.76	2.75	2.75	0.15	3.66	$132.49	3.66	$132.49	XXX	A+
74355-26	X-ray guide, intestinal tube	0.76	0.26	0.26	0.03	1.05	$38.01	1.05	$38.01	XXX	A+
74355-TC	X-ray guide, intestinal tube	0.00	2.49	2.49	0.12	2.61	$94.48	2.61	$94.48	XXX	A+
74360	X-ray guide, GI dilation	0.54	3.18	3.18	0.16	3.88	$140.45	3.88	$140.45	XXX	A+
74360-26	X-ray guide, GI dilation	0.54	0.19	0.19	0.02	0.75	$27.15	0.75	$27.15	XXX	A+
74360-TC	X-ray guide, GI dilation	0.00	2.99	2.99	0.14	3.13	$113.30	3.13	$113.30	XXX	A+
74363	X-ray, bile duct dilation	0.88	6.10	6.10	0.31	7.29	$263.89	7.29	$263.89	XXX	A+
74363-26	X-ray, bile duct dilation	0.88	0.31	0.31	0.04	1.23	$44.53	1.23	$44.53	XXX	A+
74363-TC	X-ray, bile duct dilation	0.00	5.79	5.79	0.27	6.06	$219.37	6.06	$219.37	XXX	A+
74400	Contrst x-ray, urinary tract	0.49	1.77	1.77	0.11	2.37	$85.79	2.37	$85.79	XXX	A+
74400-26	Contrst x-ray, urinary tract	0.49	0.17	0.17	0.02	0.68	$24.62	0.68	$24.62	XXX	A+
74400-TC	Contrst x-ray, urinary tract	0.00	1.60	1.60	0.09	1.69	$61.18	1.69	$61.18	XXX	A+
74410	Contrst x-ray, urinary tract	0.49	2.02	2.02	0.11	2.62	$94.84	2.62	$94.84	XXX	A+
74410-26	Contrst x-ray, urinary tract	0.49	0.17	0.17	0.02	0.68	$24.62	0.68	$24.62	XXX	A+
74410-TC	Contrst x-ray, urinary tract	0.00	1.85	1.85	0.09	1.94	$70.23	1.94	$70.23	XXX	A+
74415	Contrst x-ray, urinary tract	0.49	2.18	2.18	0.12	2.79	$101.00	2.79	$101.00	XXX	A+
74415-26	Contrst x-ray, urinary tract	0.49	0.17	0.17	0.02	0.68	$24.62	0.68	$24.62	XXX	A+

Code	Description							
74415-TC	Contrst x-ray, urinary tract	0.00	2.01	2.01	0.10	2.11	2.11	$76.38	XXX	A+
74420	Contrst x-ray, urinary tract	0.36	2.62	2.62	0.14	3.12	3.12	$112.94	XXX	A+
74420-26	Contrst x-ray, urinary tract	0.36	0.13	0.13	0.02	0.51	0.51	$18.46	XXX	A+
74420-TC	Contrst x-ray, urinary tract	0.00	2.49	2.49	0.12	2.61	2.61	$94.48	XXX	A+
74425	Contrst x-ray, urinary tract	0.36	1.37	1.37	0.08	1.81	1.81	$65.52	XXX	A+
74425-26	Contrst x-ray, urinary tract	0.36	0.13	0.13	0.02	0.51	0.51	$18.46	XXX	A+
74425-TC	Contrst x-ray, urinary tract	0.00	1.24	1.24	0.06	1.30	1.30	$47.06	XXX	A+
74430	Contrast x-ray, bladder	0.32	1.11	1.11	0.07	1.50	1.50	$54.30	XXX	A+
74430-26	Contrast x-ray, bladder	0.32	0.11	0.11	0.02	0.45	0.45	$16.29	XXX	A+
74430-TC	Contrast x-ray, bladder	0.00	1.00	1.00	0.05	1.05	1.05	$38.01	XXX	A+
74440	X-ray, male genital tract	0.38	1.20	1.20	0.07	1.65	1.65	$59.73	XXX	A+
74440-26	X-ray, male genital tract	0.38	0.13	0.13	0.02	0.53	0.53	$19.19	XXX	A+
74440-TC	X-ray, male genital tract	0.00	1.07	1.07	0.05	1.12	1.12	$40.54	XXX	A+
74445	X-ray exam of penis	1.14	1.46	1.46	0.10	2.70	2.70	$97.74	XXX	A+
74445-26	X-ray exam of penis	1.14	0.39	0.39	0.05	1.58	1.58	$57.19	XXX	A+
74445-TC	X-ray exam of penis	0.00	1.07	1.07	0.05	1.12	1.12	$40.54	XXX	A+
74450	X-ray, urethra/bladder	0.33	1.51	1.51	0.09	1.93	1.93	$69.86	XXX	A+
74450-26	X-ray, urethra/bladder	0.33	0.12	0.12	0.02	0.47	0.47	$17.01	XXX	A+
74450-TC	X-ray, urethra/bladder	0.00	1.39	1.39	0.07	1.46	1.46	$52.85	XXX	A+
74455	X-ray, urethra/bladder	0.33	1.61	1.61	0.10	2.04	2.04	$73.85	XXX	A+
74455-26	X-ray, urethra/bladder	0.33	0.11	0.11	0.02	0.46	0.46	$16.65	XXX	A+
74455-TC	X-ray, urethra/bladder	0.00	1.50	1.50	0.08	1.58	1.58	$57.19	XXX	A+
74470	X-ray exam of kidney lesion	0.54	1.37	1.37	0.08	1.99	1.99	$72.04	XXX	A+
74470-26	X-ray exam of kidney lesion	0.54	0.19	0.19	0.02	0.75	0.75	$27.15	XXX	A+
74470-TC	X-ray exam of kidney lesion	0.00	1.18	1.18	0.06	1.24	1.24	$44.89	XXX	A+
74475	X-ray control, cath insert	0.54	4.06	4.06	0.20	4.80	4.80	$173.76	XXX	A+
74475-26	X-ray control, cath insert	0.54	0.19	0.19	0.02	0.75	0.75	$27.15	XXX	A+
74475-TC	X-ray control, cath insert	0.00	3.87	3.87	0.18	4.05	4.05	$146.61	XXX	A+

* **M** = multiple surgery adjustment applies
Me = multiple endoscopy rules may apply
B = bilateral surgery adjustment applies
A = assistant-at-surgery restriction

A+ = assistant-at-surgery restriction unless medical necessity established with documentation
C = cosurgeons payable
C+ = cosurgeons payable if medical necessity established with documentation

T = team surgeons permitted
T+ = team surgeons payable if medical necessity established with documentation
$ = indicates services that are not covered by Medicare.

CPT five-digit codes, two-digit numeric modifiers, and descriptions only are © 2001 American Medical Association

Medicare RBRVS: The Physicians' Guide

Relative value units

CPT Code and Modifier	Description	Work RVU	Non Facility Practice Expense RVU	Facility Practice Expense RVU	PLI RVU	Total Non Facility RVUs	Medicare Payment Non Facility	Total Facility RVUs	Medicare Payment Facility	Global Period	Payment Policy Indicators*
74480	X-ray control, cath insert	0.54	4.06	4.06	0.20	4.80	$173.76	4.80	$173.76	XXX	A+
74480-26	X-ray control, cath insert	0.54	0.19	0.19	0.02	0.75	$27.15	0.75	$27.15	XXX	A+
74480-TC	X-ray control, cath insert	0.00	3.87	3.87	0.18	4.05	$146.61	4.05	$146.61	XXX	A+
74485	X-ray guide, GU dilation	0.54	3.18	3.18	0.17	3.89	$140.81	3.89	$140.81	XXX	A+
74485-26	X-ray guide, GU dilation	0.54	0.19	0.19	0.03	0.76	$27.51	0.76	$27.51	XXX	A+
74485-TC	X-ray guide, GU dilation	0.00	2.99	2.99	0.14	3.13	$113.30	3.13	$113.30	XXX	A+
74710	X-ray measurement of pelvis	0.34	1.12	1.12	0.07	1.53	$55.38	1.53	$55.38	XXX	A+
74710-26	X-ray measurement of pelvis	0.34	0.12	0.12	0.02	0.48	$17.38	0.48	$17.38	XXX	A+
74710-TC	X-ray measurement of pelvis	0.00	1.00	1.00	0.05	1.05	$38.01	1.05	$38.01	XXX	A+
74740	X-ray, female genital tract	0.38	1.37	1.37	0.08	1.83	$66.24	1.83	$66.24	XXX	A+
74740-26	X-ray, female genital tract	0.38	0.13	0.13	0.02	0.53	$19.19	0.53	$19.19	XXX	A+
74740-TC	X-ray, female genital tract	0.00	1.24	1.24	0.06	1.30	$47.06	1.30	$47.06	XXX	A+
74742	X-ray, fallopian tube	0.61	3.23	3.23	0.16	4.00	$144.80	4.00	$144.80	XXX	A+
74742-26	X-ray, fallopian tube	0.61	0.24	0.24	0.02	0.87	$31.49	0.87	$31.49	XXX	A+
74742-TC	X-ray, fallopian tube	0.00	2.99	2.99	0.14	3.13	$113.30	3.13	$113.30	XXX	A+
74775	X-ray exam of perineum	0.62	1.62	1.62	0.10	2.34	$84.71	2.34	$84.71	XXX	A+
74775-26	X-ray exam of perineum	0.62	0.23	0.23	0.03	0.88	$31.86	0.88	$31.86	XXX	A+
74775-TC	X-ray exam of perineum	0.00	1.39	1.39	0.07	1.46	$52.85	1.46	$52.85	XXX	A+
75552	Heart mri for morph w/o dye	1.60	11.20	11.20	0.56	13.36	$483.62	13.36	$483.62	XXX	A+
75552-26	Heart mri for morph w/o dye	1.60	0.56	0.56	0.07	2.23	$80.72	2.23	$80.72	XXX	A+
75552-TC	Heart mri for morph w/o dye	0.00	10.64	10.64	0.49	11.13	$402.90	11.13	$402.90	XXX	A+
75553	Heart mri for morph w/dye	2.00	11.35	11.35	0.58	13.93	$504.25	13.93	$504.25	XXX	A+
75553-26	Heart mri for morph w/dye	2.00	0.71	0.71	0.09	2.80	$101.36	2.80	$101.36	XXX	A+
75553-TC	Heart mri for morph w/dye	0.00	10.64	10.64	0.49	11.13	$402.90	11.13	$402.90	XXX	A+
75554	Cardiac MRI/function	1.83	11.33	11.33	0.56	13.72	$496.65	13.72	$496.65	XXX	A+
75554-26	Cardiac MRI/function	1.83	0.69	0.69	0.07	2.59	$93.76	2.59	$93.76	XXX	A+
75554-TC	Cardiac MRI/function	0.00	10.64	10.64	0.49	11.13	$402.90	11.13	$402.90	XXX	A+

Code	Description							
75555	Cardiac MRI/limited study	1.74	11.32	0.56	13.62	$493.03	XXX	A+
75555-26	Cardiac MRI/limited study	1.74	0.68	0.07	2.49	$90.14	XXX	A+
75555-TC	Cardiac MRI/limited study	0.00	10.64	0.49	11.13	$402.90	XXX	A+
75600	Contrast x-ray exam of aorta	0.49	12.16	0.56	13.21	$478.19	XXX	A+
75600-26	Contrast x-ray exam of aorta	0.49	0.20	0.02	0.71	$25.70	XXX	A+
75600-TC	Contrast x-ray exam of aorta	0.00	11.96	0.54	12.50	$452.49	XXX	A+
75605	Contrast x-ray exam of aorta	1.14	12.39	0.59	14.12	$511.13	XXX	A+
75605-26	Contrast x-ray exam of aorta	1.14	0.43	0.05	1.62	$58.64	XXX	A+
75605-TC	Contrast x-ray exam of aorta	0.00	11.96	0.54	12.50	$452.49	XXX	A+
75625	Contrast x-ray exam of aorta	1.14	12.37	0.59	14.10	$510.41	XXX	A+
75625-26	Contrast x-ray exam of aorta	1.14	0.41	0.05	1.60	$57.92	XXX	A+
75625-TC	Contrast x-ray exam of aorta	0.00	11.96	0.54	12.50	$452.49	XXX	A+
75630	X-ray aorta, leg arteries	1.79	13.14	0.65	15.58	$563.98	XXX	A+
75630-26	X-ray aorta, leg arteries	1.79	0.67	0.08	2.54	$91.95	XXX	A+
75630-TC	X-ray aorta, leg arteries	0.00	12.47	0.57	13.04	$472.04	XXX	A+
75635	Ct angio abdominal arteries	2.40	9.02	0.41	11.83	$428.24	XXX	A+
75635-26	Ct angio abdominal arteries	2.40	0.96	0.09	3.45	$124.89	XXX	A+
75635-TC	Ct angio abdominal arteries	0.00	8.06	0.32	8.38	$303.35	XXX	A+
75650	Artery x-rays, head & neck	1.49	12.49	0.61	14.59	$528.15	XXX	A+
75650-26	Artery x-rays, head & neck	1.49	0.53	0.07	2.09	$75.66	XXX	A+
75650-TC	Artery x-rays, head & neck	0.00	11.96	0.54	12.50	$452.49	XXX	A+
75658	Artery x-rays, arm	1.31	12.44	0.60	14.35	$519.46	XXX	A+
75658-26	Artery x-rays, arm	1.31	0.48	0.06	1.85	$66.97	XXX	A+
75658-TC	Artery x-rays, arm	0.00	11.96	0.54	12.50	$452.49	XXX	A+
75660	Artery x-rays, head & neck	1.31	12.44	0.60	14.35	$519.46	XXX	A+
75660-26	Artery x-rays, head & neck	1.31	0.48	0.06	1.85	$66.97	XXX	A+
75660-TC	Artery x-rays, head & neck	0.00	11.96	0.54	12.50	$452.49	XXX	A+
75662	Artery x-rays, head & neck	1.66	12.60	0.62	14.88	$538.64	XXX	A+

* M = multiple surgery adjustment applies
   Me = multiple endoscopy rules may apply
   B = bilateral surgery adjustment applies
   A = assistant-at-surgery restriction

A+ = assistant-at-surgery restriction unless medical necessity established with documentation
C = cosurgeons payable
C+ = cosurgeons payable if medical necessity established with documentation

T = team surgeons permitted
T+ = team surgeons payable if medical necessity established with documentation
$ = indicates services that are not covered by Medicare.

343 CPT five-digit codes, two-digit numeric modifiers, and descriptions only are © 2001 American Medical Association

Medicare RBRVS: The Physicians' Guide

Relative value units

CPT Code and Modifier	Description	Work RVU	Non Facility Practice Expense RVU	Facility Practice Expense RVU	PLI RVU	Total Non Facility RVUs	Medicare Payment Non Facility	Total Facility RVUs	Medicare Payment Facility	Global Period	Payment Policy Indicators*
75662-26	Artery x-rays, head & neck	1.66	0.64	0.64	0.08	2.38	$86.15	2.38	$86.15	XXX	A+
75662-TC	Artery x-rays, head & neck	0.00	11.96	11.96	0.54	12.50	$452.49	12.50	$452.49	XXX	A+
75665	Artery x-rays, head & neck	1.31	12.43	12.43	0.61	14.35	$519.46	14.35	$519.46	XXX	A+
75665-26	Artery x-rays, head & neck	1.31	0.47	0.47	0.07	1.85	$66.97	1.85	$66.97	XXX	A+
75665-TC	Artery x-rays, head & neck	0.00	11.96	11.96	0.54	12.50	$452.49	12.50	$452.49	XXX	A+
75671	Artery x-rays, head & neck	1.66	12.55	12.55	0.62	14.83	$536.83	14.83	$536.83	XXX	A+
75671-26	Artery x-rays, head & neck	1.66	0.59	0.59	0.08	2.33	$84.34	2.33	$84.34	XXX	A+
75671-TC	Artery x-rays, head & neck	0.00	11.96	11.96	0.54	12.50	$452.49	12.50	$452.49	XXX	A+
75676	Artery x-rays, neck	1.31	12.43	12.43	0.61	14.35	$519.46	14.35	$519.46	XXX	A+
75676-26	Artery x-rays, neck	1.31	0.47	0.47	0.07	1.85	$66.97	1.85	$66.97	XXX	A+
75676-TC	Artery x-rays, neck	0.00	11.96	11.96	0.54	12.50	$452.49	12.50	$452.49	XXX	A+
75680	Artery x-rays, neck	1.66	12.55	12.55	0.62	14.83	$536.83	14.83	$536.83	XXX	A+
75680-26	Artery x-rays, neck	1.66	0.59	0.59	0.08	2.33	$84.34	2.33	$84.34	XXX	A+
75680-TC	Artery x-rays, neck	0.00	11.96	11.96	0.54	12.50	$452.49	12.50	$452.49	XXX	A+
75685	Artery x-rays, spine	1.31	12.43	12.43	0.60	14.34	$519.10	14.34	$519.10	XXX	A+
75685-26	Artery x-rays, spine	1.31	0.47	0.47	0.06	1.84	$66.61	1.84	$66.61	XXX	A+
75685-TC	Artery x-rays, spine	0.00	11.96	11.96	0.54	12.50	$452.49	12.50	$452.49	XXX	A+
75705	Artery x-rays, spine	2.18	12.75	12.75	0.65	15.58	$563.98	15.58	$563.98	XXX	A+
75705-26	Artery x-rays, spine	2.18	0.79	0.79	0.11	3.08	$111.49	3.08	$111.49	XXX	A+
75705-TC	Artery x-rays, spine	0.00	11.96	11.96	0.54	12.50	$452.49	12.50	$452.49	XXX	A+
75710	Artery x-rays, arm/leg	1.14	12.38	12.38	0.60	14.12	$511.13	14.12	$511.13	XXX	A+
75710-26	Artery x-rays, arm/leg	1.14	0.42	0.42	0.06	1.62	$58.64	1.62	$58.64	XXX	A+
75710-TC	Artery x-rays, arm/leg	0.00	11.96	11.96	0.54	12.50	$452.49	12.50	$452.49	XXX	A+
75716	Artery x-rays, arms/legs	1.31	12.43	12.43	0.60	14.34	$519.10	14.34	$519.10	XXX	A+
75716-26	Artery x-rays, arms/legs	1.31	0.47	0.47	0.06	1.84	$66.61	1.84	$66.61	XXX	A+
75716-TC	Artery x-rays, arms/legs	0.00	11.96	11.96	0.54	12.50	$452.49	12.50	$452.49	XXX	A+
75722	Artery x-rays, kidney	1.14	12.39	12.39	0.59	14.12	$511.13	14.12	$511.13	XXX	A+

Code	Description								
75722-26	Artery x-rays, kidney	1.14	0.43	0.43	0.05	1.62	$58.64	XXX	A+
75722-TC	Artery x-rays, kidney	0.00	11.96	11.96	0.54	12.50	$452.49	XXX	A+
75724	Artery x-rays, kidneys	1.49	12.56	12.56	0.59	14.64	$529.96	XXX	A+
75724-26	Artery x-rays, kidneys	1.49	0.60	0.60	0.05	2.14	$77.47	XXX	A+
75724-TC	Artery x-rays, kidneys	0.00	11.96	11.96	0.54	12.50	$452.49	XXX	A+
75726	Artery x-rays, abdomen	1.14	12.36	12.36	0.59	14.09	$510.05	XXX	A+
75726-26	Artery x-rays, abdomen	1.14	0.40	0.40	0.05	1.59	$57.56	XXX	A+
75726-TC	Artery x-rays, abdomen	0.00	11.96	11.96	0.54	12.50	$452.49	XXX	A+
75731	Artery x-rays, adrenal gland	1.14	12.36	12.36	0.59	14.09	$510.05	XXX	A+
75731-26	Artery x-rays, adrenal gland	1.14	0.40	0.40	0.05	1.59	$57.56	XXX	A+
75731-TC	Artery x-rays, adrenal gland	0.00	11.96	11.96	0.54	12.50	$452.49	XXX	A+
75733	Artery x-rays, adrenals	1.31	12.43	12.43	0.60	14.34	$519.10	XXX	A+
75733-26	Artery x-rays, adrenals	1.31	0.47	0.47	0.06	1.84	$66.61	XXX	A+
75733-TC	Artery x-rays, adrenals	0.00	11.96	11.96	0.54	12.50	$452.49	XXX	A+
75736	Artery x-rays, pelvis	1.14	12.37	12.37	0.59	14.10	$510.41	XXX	A+
75736-26	Artery x-rays, pelvis	1.14	0.41	0.41	0.05	1.60	$57.92	XXX	A+
75736-TC	Artery x-rays, pelvis	0.00	11.96	11.96	0.54	12.50	$452.49	XXX	A+
75741	Artery x-rays, lung	1.31	12.42	12.42	0.60	14.33	$518.73	XXX	A+
75741-26	Artery x-rays, lung	1.31	0.46	0.46	0.06	1.83	$66.24	XXX	A+
75741-TC	Artery x-rays, lung	0.00	11.96	11.96	0.54	12.50	$452.49	XXX	A+
75743	Artery x-rays, lungs	1.66	12.54	12.54	0.61	14.81	$536.11	XXX	A+
75743-26	Artery x-rays, lungs	1.66	0.58	0.58	0.07	2.31	$83.62	XXX	A+
75743-TC	Artery x-rays, lungs	0.00	11.96	11.96	0.54	12.50	$452.49	XXX	A+
75746	Artery x-rays, lung	1.14	12.36	12.36	0.59	14.09	$510.05	XXX	A+
75746-26	Artery x-rays, lung	1.14	0.40	0.40	0.05	1.59	$57.56	XXX	A+
75746-TC	Artery x-rays, lung	0.00	11.96	11.96	0.54	12.50	$452.49	XXX	A+
75756	Artery x-rays, chest	1.14	12.44	12.44	0.58	14.16	$512.58	XXX	A+
75756-26	Artery x-rays, chest	1.14	0.48	0.48	0.04	1.66	$60.09	XXX	A+

* **M** = multiple surgery adjustment applies
Me = multiple endoscopy rules may apply
B = bilateral surgery adjustment applies
A = assistant-at-surgery restriction

A+ = assistant-at-surgery restriction unless medical necessity established with documentation
C = cosurgeons payable
C+ = cosurgeons payable if medical necessity established with documentation

T = team surgeons permitted
T+ = team surgeons payable if medical necessity established with documentation
S = indicates services that are not covered by Medicare.

345 CPT five-digit codes, two-digit numeric modifiers, and descriptions only are © 2001 American Medical Association

Medicare RBRVS: The Physicians' Guide

Relative value units

CPT Code and Modifier	Description	Work RVU	Non Facility Practice Expense RVU	Facility Practice Expense RVU	PLI RVU	Total Non Facility RVUs	Medicare Payment Non Facility	Total Facility RVUs	Medicare Payment Facility	Global Period	Payment Policy Indicators*
75756-TC	Artery x-rays, chest	0.00	11.96	11.96	0.54	12.50	$452.49	12.50	$452.49	XXX	A+
75774	Artery x-ray, each vessel	0.36	12.09	12.09	0.56	13.01	$470.95	13.01	$470.95	ZZZ	A+
75774-26	Artery x-ray, each vessel	0.36	0.13	0.13	0.02	0.51	$18.46	0.51	$18.46	ZZZ	A+
75774-TC	Artery x-ray, each vessel	0.00	11.96	11.96	0.54	12.50	$452.49	12.50	$452.49	ZZZ	A+
75790	Visualize A-V shunt	1.84	1.93	1.93	0.16	3.93	$142.26	3.93	$142.26	XXX	A+
75790-26	Visualize A-V shunt	1.84	0.64	0.64	0.09	2.57	$93.03	2.57	$93.03	XXX	A+
75790-TC	Visualize A-V shunt	0.00	1.29	1.29	0.07	1.36	$49.23	1.36	$49.23	XXX	A+
75801	Lymph vessel x-ray, arm/leg	0.81	5.42	5.42	0.29	6.52	$236.02	6.52	$236.02	XXX	A+
75801-26	Lymph vessel x-ray, arm/leg	0.81	0.28	0.28	0.05	1.14	$41.27	1.14	$41.27	XXX	A+
75801-TC	Lymph vessel x-ray, arm/leg	0.00	5.14	5.14	0.24	5.38	$194.75	5.38	$194.75	XXX	A+
75803	Lymph vessel x-ray, arms/legs	1.17	5.55	5.55	0.29	7.01	$253.76	7.01	$253.76	XXX	A+
75803-26	Lymph vessel x-ray, arms/legs	1.17	0.41	0.41	0.05	1.63	$59.00	1.63	$59.00	XXX	A+
75803-TC	Lymph vessel x-ray, arms/legs	0.00	5.14	5.14	0.24	5.38	$194.75	5.38	$194.75	XXX	A+
75805	Lymph vessel x-ray, trunk	0.81	6.08	6.08	0.31	7.20	$260.63	7.20	$260.63	XXX	A+
75805-26	Lymph vessel x-ray, trunk	0.81	0.29	0.29	0.04	1.14	$41.27	1.14	$41.27	XXX	A+
75805-TC	Lymph vessel x-ray, trunk	0.00	5.79	5.79	0.27	6.06	$219.37	6.06	$219.37	XXX	A+
75807	Lymph vessel x-ray, trunk	1.17	6.20	6.20	0.32	7.69	$278.37	7.69	$278.37	XXX	A+
75807-26	Lymph vessel x-ray, trunk	1.17	0.41	0.41	0.05	1.63	$59.00	1.63	$59.00	XXX	A+
75807-TC	Lymph vessel x-ray, trunk	0.00	5.79	5.79	0.27	6.06	$219.37	6.06	$219.37	XXX	A+
75809	Nonvascular shunt, x-ray	0.47	0.91	0.91	0.06	1.44	$52.13	1.44	$52.13	XXX	A+
75809-26	Nonvascular shunt, x-ray	0.47	0.17	0.17	0.02	0.66	$23.89	0.66	$23.89	XXX	A+
75809-TC	Nonvascular shunt, x-ray	0.00	0.74	0.74	0.04	0.78	$28.24	0.78	$28.24	XXX	A+
75810	Vein x-ray, spleen/liver	1.14	12.36	12.36	0.60	14.10	$510.41	14.10	$510.41	XXX	A+
75810-26	Vein x-ray, spleen/liver	1.14	0.40	0.40	0.06	1.60	$57.92	1.60	$57.92	XXX	A+
75810-TC	Vein x-ray, spleen/liver	0.00	11.96	11.96	0.54	12.50	$452.49	12.50	$452.49	XXX	A+
75820	Vein x-ray, arm/leg	0.70	1.15	1.15	0.08	1.93	$69.86	1.93	$69.86	XXX	A+
75820-26	Vein x-ray, arm/leg	0.70	0.25	0.25	0.03	0.98	$35.48	0.98	$35.48	XXX	A+

Code	Description								
75820-TC	Vein x-ray, arm/leg	0.00	0.90	0.90	0.05	0.95	$34.39	XXX	A+
75822	Vein x-ray, arms/legs	1.06	0.77	1.77	0.12	2.95	$106.79	XXX	A+
75822-26	Vein x-ray, arms/legs	1.06	0.37	0.37	0.05	1.48	$53.57	XXX	A+
75822-TC	Vein x-ray, arms/legs	0.00	1.40	1.40	0.07	1.47	$53.21	XXX	A+
75825	Vein x-ray, trunk	1.14	12.36	12.36	0.60	14.10	$510.41	XXX	A+
75825-26	Vein x-ray, trunk	1.14	0.40	0.40	0.06	1.60	$57.92	XXX	A+
75825-TC	Vein x-ray, trunk	0.00	11.96	11.96	0.54	12.50	$452.49	XXX	A+
75827	Vein x-ray, chest	1.14	12.36	12.36	0.59	14.09	$510.05	XXX	A+
75827-26	Vein x-ray, chest	1.14	0.40	0.40	0.05	1.59	$57.56	XXX	A+
75827-TC	Vein x-ray, chest	0.00	11.96	11.96	0.54	12.50	$452.49	XXX	A+
75831	Vein x-ray, kidney	1.14	12.36	12.36	0.59	14.09	$510.05	XXX	A+
75831-26	Vein x-ray, kidney	1.14	0.40	0.40	0.05	1.59	$57.56	XXX	A+
75831-TC	Vein x-ray, kidney	0.00	11.96	11.96	0.54	12.50	$452.49	XXX	A+
75833	Vein x-ray, kidneys	1.49	12.49	12.48	0.61	14.59	$528.15	XXX	A+
75833-26	Vein x-ray, kidneys	1.49	0.53	0.52	0.07	2.09	$75.66	XXX	A+
75833-TC	Vein x-ray, kidneys	0.00	11.96	11.96	0.54	12.50	$452.49	XXX	A+
75840	Vein x-ray, adrenal gland	1.14	12.38	12.38	0.61	14.13	$511.49	XXX	A+
75840-26	Vein x-ray, adrenal gland	1.14	0.42	0.42	0.07	1.63	$59.00	XXX	A+
75840-TC	Vein x-ray, adrenal gland	0.00	11.96	11.96	0.54	12.50	$452.49	XXX	A+
75842	Vein x-ray, adrenal glands	1.49	12.48	12.48	0.61	14.58	$527.78	XXX	A+
75842-26	Vein x-ray, adrenal glands	1.49	0.52	0.52	0.07	2.08	$75.29	XXX	A+
75842-TC	Vein x-ray, adrenal glands	0.00	11.96	11.96	0.54	12.50	$452.49	XXX	A+
75860	Vein x-ray, neck	1.14	12.39	12.39	0.60	14.13	$511.49	XXX	A+
75860-26	Vein x-ray, neck	1.14	0.43	0.43	0.06	1.63	$59.00	XXX	A+
75860-TC	Vein x-ray, neck	0.00	11.96	11.96	0.54	12.50	$452.49	XXX	A+
75870	Vein x-ray, skull	1.14	12.38	12.38	0.60	14.12	$511.13	XXX	A+
75870-26	Vein x-ray, skull	1.14	0.42	0.42	0.06	1.62	$58.64	XXX	A+
75870-TC	Vein x-ray, skull	0.00	11.96	11.96	0.54	12.50	$452.49	XXX	A+

* **M** = multiple surgery adjustment applies
Me = multiple endoscopy rules may apply
B = bilateral surgery adjustment applies
A = assistant-at-surgery restriction

A+ = assistant-at-surgery restriction unless medical necessity established with documentation
C = cosurgeons payable
C+ = cosurgeons payable if medical necessity established with documentation

T = team surgeons permitted
T+ = team surgeons payable if medical necessity established with documentation
$ = indicates services that are not covered by Medicare.

CPT five-digit codes, two-digit numeric modifiers, and descriptions only are © 2001 American Medical Association

Medicare RBRVS: The Physicians' Guide

Relative value units

CPT Code and Modifier	Description	Work RVU	Non Facility Practice Expense RVU	Facility Practice Expense RVU	PLI RVU	Total Non Facility RVUs	Medicare Payment Non Facility	Total Facility RVUs	Medicare Payment Facility	Global Period	Payment Policy Indicators*
75872	Vein x-ray, skull	1.14	12.36	12.36	0.59	14.09	$510.05	14.09	$510.05	XXX	A+
75872-26	Vein x-ray, skull	1.14	0.40	0.40	0.05	1.59	$57.56	1.59	$57.56	XXX	A+
75872-TC	Vein x-ray, skull	0.00	11.96	11.96	0.54	12.50	$452.49	12.50	$452.49	XXX	A+
75880	Vein x-ray, eye socket	0.70	1.17	1.17	0.08	1.95	$70.59	1.95	$70.59	XXX	A+
75880-26	Vein x-ray, eye socket	0.70	0.27	0.27	0.03	1.00	$36.20	1.00	$36.20	XXX	A+
75880-TC	Vein x-ray, eye socket	0.00	0.90	0.90	0.05	0.95	$34.39	0.95	$34.39	XXX	A+
75885	Vein x-ray, liver	1.44	12.46	12.46	0.60	14.50	$524.89	14.50	$524.89	XXX	A+
75885-26	Vein x-ray, liver	1.44	0.50	0.50	0.06	2.00	$72.40	2.00	$72.40	XXX	A+
75885-TC	Vein x-ray, liver	0.00	11.96	11.96	0.54	12.50	$452.49	12.50	$452.49	XXX	A+
75887	Vein x-ray, liver	1.44	12.46	12.46	0.60	14.50	$524.89	14.50	$524.89	XXX	A+
75887-26	Vein x-ray, liver	1.44	0.50	0.50	0.06	2.00	$72.40	2.00	$72.40	XXX	A+
75887-TC	Vein x-ray, liver	0.00	11.96	11.96	0.54	12.50	$452.49	12.50	$452.49	XXX	A+
75889	Vein x-ray, liver	1.14	12.36	12.36	0.59	14.09	$510.05	14.09	$510.05	XXX	A+
75889-26	Vein x-ray, liver	1.14	0.40	0.40	0.05	1.59	$57.56	1.59	$57.56	XXX	A+
75889-TC	Vein x-ray, liver	0.00	11.96	11.96	0.54	12.50	$452.49	12.50	$452.49	XXX	A+
75891	Vein x-ray, liver	1.14	12.36	12.36	0.59	14.09	$510.05	14.09	$510.05	XXX	A+
75891-26	Vein x-ray, liver	1.14	0.40	0.40	0.05	1.59	$57.56	1.59	$57.56	XXX	A+
75891-TC	Vein x-ray, liver	0.00	11.96	11.96	0.54	12.50	$452.49	12.50	$452.49	XXX	A+
75893	Venous sampling by catheter	0.54	12.15	12.15	0.56	13.25	$479.64	13.25	$479.64	XXX	A+
75893-26	Venous sampling by catheter	0.54	0.19	0.19	0.02	0.75	$27.15	0.75	$27.15	XXX	A+
75893-TC	Venous sampling by catheter	0.00	11.96	11.96	0.54	12.50	$452.49	12.50	$452.49	XXX	A+
75894	X-rays, transcath therapy	1.31	23.38	23.38	1.12	25.81	$934.30	25.81	$934.30	XXX	A+
75894-26	X-rays, transcath therapy	1.31	0.46	0.46	0.07	1.84	$66.61	1.84	$66.61	XXX	A+
75894-TC	X-rays, transcath therapy	0.00	22.92	22.92	1.05	23.97	$867.69	23.97	$867.69	XXX	A+
75896	X-rays, transcath therapy	1.31	20.42	20.42	0.97	22.70	$821.72	22.70	$821.72	XXX	A+
75896-26	X-rays, transcath therapy	1.31	0.48	0.48	0.06	1.85	$66.97	1.85	$66.97	XXX	A+

Code	Description								
75896-TC	X-rays, transcath therapy	0.00	19.94	19.94	0.91	20.85	$754.75	$754.75	XXX	A+
75898	Follow-up angiography	1.65	1.60	1.60	0.12	3.37	$121.99	$121.99	XXX	A+
75898-26	Follow-up angiography	1.65	0.60	0.60	0.07	2.32	$83.98	$83.98	XXX	A+
75898-TC	Follow-up angiography	0.00	1.00	1.00	0.05	1.05	$38.01	$38.01	XXX	A+
75900	Arterial catheter exchange	0.49	20.09	20.09	0.94	21.52	$779.01	$779.01	XXX	A+
75900-26	Arterial catheter exchange	0.49	0.17	0.17	0.02	0.68	$24.62	$24.62	XXX	A+
75900-TC	Arterial catheter exchange	0.00	19.92	19.92	0.92	20.84	$754.39	$754.39	XXX	A+
75940	X-ray placement, vein filter	0.54	12.15	12.15	0.57	13.26	$480.00	$480.00	XXX	A+
75940-26	X-ray placement, vein filter	0.54	0.19	0.19	0.03	0.76	$27.51	$27.51	XXX	A+
75940-TC	X-ray placement, vein filter	0.00	11.96	11.96	0.54	12.50	$452.49	$452.49	XXX	A+
75945	Intravascular us	0.40	4.48	4.48	0.23	5.11	$184.98	$184.98	XXX	A+
75945-26	Intravascular us	0.40	0.15	0.15	0.03	0.58	$21.00	$21.00	XXX	A+
75945-TC	Intravascular us	0.00	4.33	4.33	0.20	4.53	$163.98	$163.98	XXX	A+
75946	Intravascular us add-on	0.40	2.32	2.32	0.14	2.86	$103.53	$103.53	ZZZ	A+
75946-26	Intravascular us add-on	0.40	0.14	0.14	0.03	0.57	$20.63	$20.63	ZZZ	A+
75946-TC	Intravascular us add-on	0.00	2.18	2.18	0.11	2.29	$82.90	$82.90	ZZZ	A+
75952 §	Endovasc repair abdom aorta	0.00	0.00	0.00	0.00	0.00	$0.00	$0.00	XXX	A+
75952-26	Endovasc repair abdom aorta	4.50	1.80	1.80	0.68	6.98	$252.67	$252.67	XXX	A+
75952-TC	Endovasc repair abdom aorta	0.00	0.00	0.00	0.00	0.00	$0.00	$0.00	XXX	A+
75953 §	Abdom aneurysm endovas rpr	0.00	0.00	0.00	0.00	0.00	$0.00	$0.00	XXX	A+
75953-26	Abdom aneurysm endovas rpr	1.36	0.54	0.54	0.68	2.58	$93.39	$93.39	XXX	A+
75953-TC	Abdom aneurysm endovas rpr	0.00	0.00	0.00	0.00	0.00	$0.00	$0.00	XXX	A+
75960	Transcatheter intro, stent	0.82	14.45	14.45	0.68	15.95	$577.38	$577.38	XXX	A+
75960-26	Transcatheter intro, stent	0.82	0.30	0.30	0.04	1.16	$41.99	$41.99	XXX	A+
75960-TC	Transcatheter intro, stent	0.00	14.15	14.15	0.64	14.79	$535.39	$535.39	XXX	A+
75961	Retrieval, broken catheter	4.25	11.46	11.46	0.64	16.35	$591.86	$591.86	XXX	A+
75961-26	Retrieval, broken catheter	4.25	1.49	1.49	0.18	5.92	$214.30	$214.30	XXX	A+
75961-TC	Retrieval, broken catheter	0.00	9.97	9.97	0.46	10.43	$377.56	$377.56	XXX	A+

* **M** = multiple surgery adjustment applies
Me = multiple endoscopy rules may apply
B = bilateral surgery adjustment applies
A = assistant-at-surgery restriction

A+ = assistant-at-surgery restriction unless medical necessity established with documentation
C = cosurgeons payable
C+ = cosurgeons payable if medical necessity established with documentation

T = team surgeons permitted
T+ = team surgeons payable if medical necessity established with documentation
§ = indicates services that are not covered by Medicare.

CPT five-digit codes, two-digit numeric modifiers, and descriptions only are © 2001 American Medical Association

Medicare RBRVS: The Physicians' Guide

Relative value units

CPT Code and Modifier	Description	Work RVU	Non Facility Practice Expense RVU	Facility Practice Expense RVU	PLI RVU	Total Non Facility RVUs	Medicare Payment Non Facility	Total Facility RVUs	Medicare Payment Facility	Global Period	Payment Policy Indicators*
75962	Repair arterial blockage	0.54	15.15	15.15	0.72	16.41	$594.03	16.41	$594.03	XXX	A+
75962-26	Repair arterial blockage	0.54	0.20	0.20	0.03	0.77	$27.87	0.77	$27.87	XXX	A+
75962-TC	Repair arterial blockage	0.00	14.95	14.95	0.69	15.64	$566.16	15.64	$566.16	XXX	A+
75964	Repair artery blockage, each	0.36	8.10	8.10	0.38	8.84	$320.00	8.84	$320.00	ZZZ	A+
75964-26	Repair artery blockage, each	0.36	0.13	0.13	0.02	0.51	$18.46	0.51	$18.46	ZZZ	A+
75964-TC	Repair artery blockage, each	0.00	7.97	7.97	0.36	8.33	$301.54	8.33	$301.54	ZZZ	A+
75966	Repair arterial blockage	1.31	15.45	15.45	0.75	17.51	$633.85	17.51	$633.85	XXX	A+
75966-26	Repair arterial blockage	1.31	0.50	0.50	0.06	1.87	$67.69	1.87	$67.69	XXX	A+
75966-TC	Repair arterial blockage	0.00	14.95	14.95	0.69	15.64	$566.16	15.64	$566.16	XXX	A+
75968	Repair artery blockage, each	0.36	8.11	8.11	0.37	8.84	$320.00	8.84	$320.00	ZZZ	A+
75968-26	Repair artery blockage, each	0.36	0.14	0.14	0.01	0.51	$18.46	0.51	$18.46	ZZZ	A+
75968-TC	Repair artery blockage, each	0.00	7.97	7.97	0.36	8.33	$301.54	8.33	$301.54	ZZZ	A+
75970	Vascular biopsy	0.83	11.26	11.26	0.54	12.63	$457.20	12.63	$457.20	XXX	A+
75970-26	Vascular biopsy	0.83	0.30	0.30	0.04	1.17	$42.35	1.17	$42.35	XXX	A+
75970-TC	Vascular biopsy	0.00	10.96	10.96	0.50	11.46	$414.84	11.46	$414.84	XXX	A+
75978	Repair venous blockage	0.54	15.14	15.14	0.71	16.39	$593.30	16.39	$593.30	XXX	A+
75978-26	Repair venous blockage	0.54	0.19	0.19	0.02	0.75	$27.15	0.75	$27.15	XXX	A+
75978-TC	Repair venous blockage	0.00	14.95	14.95	0.69	15.64	$566.16	15.64	$566.16	XXX	A+
75980	Contrast xray exam bile duct	1.44	5.64	5.64	0.30	7.38	$267.15	7.38	$267.15	XXX	A+
75980-26	Contrast xray exam bile duct	1.44	0.50	0.50	0.06	2.00	$72.40	2.00	$72.40	XXX	A+
75980-TC	Contrast xray exam bile duct	0.00	5.14	5.14	0.24	5.38	$194.75	5.38	$194.75	XXX	A+
75982	Contrast xray exam bile duct	1.44	6.29	6.29	0.33	8.06	$291.77	8.06	$291.77	XXX	A+
75982-26	Contrast xray exam bile duct	1.44	0.50	0.50	0.06	2.00	$72.40	2.00	$72.40	XXX	A+
75982-TC	Contrast xray exam bile duct	0.00	5.79	5.79	0.27	6.06	$219.37	6.06	$219.37	XXX	A+
75984	Xray control catheter change	0.72	2.10	2.10	0.12	2.94	$106.43	2.94	$106.43	XXX	A+
75984-26	Xray control catheter change	0.72	0.25	0.25	0.03	1.00	$36.20	1.00	$36.20	XXX	A+
75984-TC	Xray control catheter change	0.00	1.85	1.85	0.09	1.94	$70.23	1.94	$70.23	XXX	A+

Code	Description								
75989	Abscess drainage under x-ray	1.19	3.41	0.19	4.79	$173.39	4.79	$173.39	XXX	A+
75989-26	Abscess drainage under x-ray	1.19	0.42	0.05	1.66	$60.09	1.66	$60.09	XXX	A+
75989-TC	Abscess drainage under x-ray	0.00	2.99	0.14	3.13	$113.30	3.13	$113.30	XXX	A+
75992	Atherectomy, x-ray exam	0.54	15.15	0.71	16.40	$593.67	16.40	$593.67	XXX	A+
75992-26	Atherectomy, x-ray exam	0.54	0.20	0.02	0.76	$27.51	0.76	$27.51	XXX	A+
75992-TC	Atherectomy, x-ray exam	0.00	14.95	0.69	15.64	$566.16	15.64	$566.16	XXX	A+
75993	Atherectomy, x-ray exam	0.36	8.11	0.37	8.84	$320.00	8.84	$320.00	ZZZ	A+
75993-26	Atherectomy, x-ray exam	0.36	0.14	0.01	0.51	$18.46	0.51	$18.46	ZZZ	A+
75993-TC	Atherectomy, x-ray exam	0.00	7.97	0.36	8.33	$301.54	8.33	$301.54	ZZZ	A+
75994	Atherectomy, x-ray exam	1.31	15.45	0.75	17.51	$633.85	17.51	$633.85	XXX	A+
75994-26	Atherectomy, x-ray exam	1.31	0.50	0.06	1.87	$67.69	1.87	$67.69	XXX	A+
75994-TC	Atherectomy, x-ray exam	0.00	14.95	0.69	15.64	$566.16	15.64	$566.16	XXX	A+
75995	Atherectomy, x-ray exam	1.31	15.42	0.75	17.48	$632.76	17.48	$632.76	XXX	A+
75995-26	Atherectomy, x-ray exam	1.31	0.47	0.06	1.84	$66.61	1.84	$66.61	XXX	A+
75995-TC	Atherectomy, x-ray exam	0.00	14.95	0.69	15.64	$566.16	15.64	$566.16	XXX	A+
75996	Atherectomy, x-ray exam	0.36	8.09	0.37	8.82	$319.28	8.82	$319.28	ZZZ	A+
75996-26	Atherectomy, x-ray exam	0.36	0.12	0.01	0.49	$17.74	0.49	$17.74	ZZZ	A+
75996-TC	Atherectomy, x-ray exam	0.00	7.97	0.36	8.33	$301.54	8.33	$301.54	ZZZ	A+
76000	Fluoroscope examination	0.17	1.31	0.07	1.55	$56.11	1.55	$56.11	XXX	A+
76000-26	Fluoroscope examination	0.17	0.07	0.01	0.25	$9.05	0.25	$9.05	XXX	A+
76000-TC	Fluoroscope examination	0.00	1.24	0.06	1.30	$47.06	1.30	$47.06	XXX	A+
76001	Fluoroscope exam, extensive	0.67	2.73	0.15	3.55	$128.51	3.55	$128.51	XXX	A+
76001-26	Fluoroscope exam, extensive	0.67	0.24	0.03	0.94	$34.03	0.94	$34.03	XXX	A+
76001-TC	Fluoroscope exam, extensive	0.00	2.49	0.12	2.61	$94.48	2.61	$94.48	XXX	A+
76003	Needle localization by x-ray	0.54	1.43	0.09	2.06	$74.57	2.06	$74.57	XXX	A+
76003-26	Needle localization by x-ray	0.54	0.19	0.03	0.76	$27.51	0.76	$27.51	XXX	A+
76003-TC	Needle localization by x-ray	0.00	1.24	0.06	1.30	$47.06	1.30	$47.06	XXX	A+
76005	Fluoroguide for spine inject	0.60	1.41	0.09	2.10	$76.02	2.10	$76.02	XXX	A+

* **M** = multiple surgery adjustment applies
Me = multiple endoscopy rules may apply
B = bilateral surgery adjustment applies
A = assistant-at-surgery restriction

A+ = assistant-at-surgery restriction unless medical necessity established with documentation
C = cosurgeons payable
C+ = cosurgeons payable if medical necessity established with documentation

T = team surgeons permitted
T+ = team surgeons payable if medical necessity established with documentation
$ = indicates services that are not covered by Medicare.

351 CPT five-digit codes, two-digit numeric modifiers, and descriptions only are © 2001 American Medical Association

Medicare RBRVS: The Physicians' Guide

Relative value units

CPT Code and Modifier	Description	Work RVU	Non Facility Practice Expense RVU	Facility Practice Expense RVU	PLI RVU	Total Non Facility RVUs	Medicare Payment Non Facility	Total Facility RVUs	Medicare Payment Facility	Global Period	Payment Policy Indicators*
76005-26	Fluoroguide for spine inject	0.60	0.17	0.17	0.03	0.80	$28.96	0.80	$28.96	XXX	
76005-TC	Fluoroguide for spine inject	0.00	1.24	1.24	0.06	1.30	$47.06	1.30	$47.06	XXX	
76006	X-ray stress view	0.41	0.20	0.20	0.04	0.65	$23.53	0.65	$23.53	XXX	A+
76010	X-ray, nose to rectum	0.18	0.56	0.56	0.03	0.77	$27.87	0.77	$27.87	XXX	A+
76010-26	X-ray, nose to rectum	0.18	0.06	0.06	0.01	0.25	$9.05	0.25	$9.05	XXX	A+
76010-TC	X-ray, nose to rectum	0.00	0.50	0.50	0.02	0.52	$18.82	0.52	$18.82	XXX	A+
76012 §	Percut vertebroplasty fluor	0.00	0.00	0.00	0.00	0.00	$0.00	0.00	$0.00	XXX	A+
76012-26	Percut vertebroplasty fluor	1.31	0.52	0.52	0.23	2.06	$74.57	2.06	$74.57	XXX	A+
76012-TC	Percut vertebroplasty fluor	0.00	0.00	0.00	0.00	0.00	$0.00	0.00	$0.00	XXX	A+
76013 §	Percut vertebroplasty, ct	0.00	0.00	0.00	0.00	0.00	$0.00	0.00	$0.00	XXX	A+
76013-26	Percut vertebroplasty, ct	1.38	0.55	0.55	0.48	2.41	$87.24	2.41	$87.24	XXX	A+
76013-TC	Percut vertebroplasty, ct	0.00	0.00	0.00	0.00	0.00	$0.00	0.00	$0.00	XXX	A+
76020	X-rays for bone age	0.19	0.57	0.57	0.03	0.79	$28.60	0.79	$28.60	XXX	A+
76020-26	X-rays for bone age	0.19	0.07	0.07	0.01	0.27	$9.77	0.27	$9.77	XXX	A+
76020-TC	X-rays for bone age	0.00	0.50	0.50	0.02	0.52	$18.82	0.52	$18.82	XXX	A+
76040	X-rays, bone evaluation	0.27	0.84	0.84	0.07	1.18	$42.72	1.18	$42.72	XXX	A+
76040-26	X-rays, bone evaluation	0.27	0.10	0.10	0.03	0.40	$14.48	0.40	$14.48	XXX	A+
76040-TC	X-rays, bone evaluation	0.00	0.74	0.74	0.04	0.78	$28.24	0.78	$28.24	XXX	A+
76061	X-rays, bone survey	0.45	1.11	1.11	0.07	1.63	$59.00	1.63	$59.00	XXX	A+
76061-26	X-rays, bone survey	0.45	0.16	0.16	0.02	0.63	$22.81	0.63	$22.81	XXX	A+
76061-TC	X-rays, bone survey	0.00	0.95	0.95	0.05	1.00	$36.20	1.00	$36.20	XXX	A+
76062	X-rays, bone survey	0.54	1.56	1.56	0.09	2.19	$79.28	2.19	$79.28	XXX	A+
76062-26	X-rays, bone survey	0.54	0.19	0.19	0.02	0.75	$27.15	0.75	$27.15	XXX	A+
76062-TC	X-rays, bone survey	0.00	1.37	1.37	0.07	1.44	$52.13	1.44	$52.13	XXX	A+
76065	X-rays, bone evaluation	0.70	0.95	0.95	0.05	1.70	$61.54	1.70	$61.54	XXX	A+
76065-26	X-rays, bone evaluation	0.70	0.25	0.25	0.01	0.96	$34.75	0.96	$34.75	XXX	A+
76065-TC	X-rays, bone evaluation	0.00	0.70	0.70	0.04	0.74	$26.79	0.74	$26.79	XXX	A+

Code	Description							
76066	Joint survey, single view	0.31	1.17	0.07	1.55	$56.11	XXX	A+
76066-26	Joint survey, single view	0.31	0.11	0.02	0.44	$15.93	XXX	A+
76066-TC	Joint survey, single view	0.00	1.06	0.05	1.11	$40.18	XXX	A+
76070 §	CT scan, bone density study	0.25	2.90	0.14	3.29	$119.10	XXX	
76070-26 §	CT scan, bone density study	0.25	0.10	0.01	0.36	$13.03	XXX	
76070-TC §	CT scan, bone density study	0.00	2.80	0.13	2.93	$106.06	XXX	
76075	Us exam, abdom, limited	0.30	3.05	0.15	3.50	$126.70	XXX	A+
76075-26	Us exam, abdom, limited	0.30	0.11	0.01	0.42	$15.20	XXX	A+
76075-TC	Us exam, abdom, limited	0.00	2.94	0.14	3.08	$111.49	XXX	A+
76076	Dual energy x-ray study	0.22	0.80	0.05	1.07	$38.73	XXX	A+
76076-26	Dual energy x-ray study	0.22	0.08	0.01	0.31	$11.22	XXX	A+
76076-TC	Dual energy x-ray study	0.00	0.72	0.04	0.76	$27.51	XXX	A+
76078	Radiographic absorptiometry	0.20	0.80	0.05	1.05	$38.01	XXX	A+
76078-26	Radiographic absorptiometry	0.20	0.08	0.01	0.29	$10.50	XXX	A+
76078-TC	Radiographic absorptiometry	0.00	0.72	0.04	0.76	$27.51	XXX	A+
76080	X-ray exam of fistula	0.54	1.19	0.07	1.80	$65.16	XXX	A+
76080-26	X-ray exam of fistula	0.54	0.19	0.02	0.75	$27.15	XXX	A+
76080-TC	X-ray exam of fistula	0.00	1.00	0.05	1.05	$38.01	XXX	A+
76085	Computer mammogram add-on	0.06	NA	0.02	0.49	$17.74	NA	ZZZ	A+
76085-26	Computer mammogram add-on	0.06	0.02	0.01	0.09	$3.26	$3.26	ZZZ	A+
76085-TC	Computer mammogram add-on	0.00	NA	0.01	0.40	$14.48	NA	XXX	A+
76086	X-ray of mammary duct	0.36	2.62	0.14	3.12	$112.94	XXX	A+
76086-26	X-ray of mammary duct	0.36	0.13	0.02	0.51	$18.46	XXX	A+
76086-TC	X-ray of mammary duct	0.00	2.49	0.12	2.61	$94.48	XXX	A+
76088	X-ray of mammary ducts	0.45	3.64	0.18	4.27	$154.57	XXX	A+
76088-26	X-ray of mammary ducts	0.45	0.16	0.02	0.63	$22.81	XXX	A+
76088-TC	X-ray of mammary ducts	0.00	3.48	0.16	3.64	$131.77	XXX	A+
76090	Mammogram, one breast	0.70	1.25	0.08	2.03	$73.48	XXX	A+

* **M** = multiple surgery adjustment applies
Me = multiple endoscopy rules may apply
B = bilateral surgery adjustment applies
A = assistant-at-surgery restriction

A+ = assistant-at-surgery restriction unless medical necessity established with documentation
C = cosurgeons payable
C+ = cosurgeons payable if medical necessity established with documentation

T = team surgeons permitted
T+ = team surgeons payable if medical necessity established with documentation
§ = indicates services that are not covered by Medicare.

353   CPT five-digit codes, two-digit numeric modifiers, and descriptions only are © 2001 American Medical Association

Medicare RBRVS: The Physicians' Guide

Relative value units

CPT Code and Modifier	Description	Work RVU	Non Facility Practice Expense RVU	Facility Practice Expense RVU	PLI RVU	Total Non Facility RVUs	Medicare Payment Non Facility	Total Facility RVUs	Medicare Payment Facility	Global Period	Payment Policy Indicators*
76090-26	Mammogram, one breast	0.70	0.25	0.25	0.03	0.98	$35.48	0.98	$35.48	XXX	A+
76090-TC	Mammogram, one breast	0.00	1.00	1.00	0.05	1.05	$38.01	1.05	$38.01	XXX	A+
76091	Mammogram, both breasts	0.87	1.54	1.54	0.09	2.50	$90.50	2.50	$90.50	XXX	A+
76091-26	Mammogram, both breasts	0.87	0.30	0.30	0.03	1.20	$43.44	1.20	$43.44	XXX	A+
76091-TC	Mammogram, both breasts	0.00	1.24	1.24	0.06	1.30	$47.06	1.30	$47.06	XXX	A+
76092	Mammogram, screening	0.70	1.47	NA	0.09	2.26	$81.81	NA	NA	XXX	A+
76092-26	Mammogram, screening	0.70	0.25	0.25	0.03	0.98	$35.48	0.98	$35.48	XXX	A+
76092-TC	Mammogram, screening	0.00	1.22	NA	0.06	1.28	$46.33	NA	NA	XXX	A+
76093	Magnetic image, breast	1.63	17.31	17.31	0.83	19.77	$715.66	19.77	$715.66	XXX	A+
76093-26	Magnetic image, breast	1.63	0.57	0.57	0.07	2.27	$82.17	2.27	$82.17	XXX	A+
76093-TC	Magnetic image, breast	0.00	16.74	16.74	0.76	17.50	$633.49	17.50	$633.49	XXX	A+
76094	Magnetic image, both breasts	1.63	23.28	23.28	1.10	26.01	$941.54	26.01	$941.54	XXX	A+
76094-26	Magnetic image, both breasts	1.63	0.57	0.57	0.07	2.27	$82.17	2.27	$82.17	XXX	A+
76094-TC	Magnetic image, both breasts	0.00	22.71	22.71	1.03	23.74	$859.37	23.74	$859.37	XXX	A+
76095	Stereotactic breast biopsy	1.59	7.36	7.36	0.40	9.35	$338.46	9.35	$338.46	XXX	A+
76095-26	Stereotactic breast biopsy	1.59	0.56	0.56	0.09	2.24	$81.09	2.24	$81.09	XXX	A+
76095-TC	Stereotactic breast biopsy	0.00	6.80	6.80	0.31	7.11	$257.38	7.11	$257.38	XXX	A+
76096	X-ray of needle wire, breast	0.56	1.44	1.44	0.09	2.09	$75.66	2.09	$75.66	XXX	A+
76096-26	X-ray of needle wire, breast	0.56	0.20	0.20	0.03	0.79	$28.60	0.79	$28.60	XXX	A+
76096-TC	X-ray of needle wire, breast	0.00	1.24	1.24	0.06	1.30	$47.06	1.30	$47.06	XXX	A+
76098	X-ray exam, breast specimen	0.16	0.45	0.45	0.03	0.64	$23.17	0.64	$23.17	XXX	A+
76098-26	X-ray exam, breast specimen	0.16	0.06	0.06	0.01	0.23	$8.33	0.23	$8.33	XXX	A+
76098-TC	X-ray exam, breast specimen	0.00	0.39	0.39	0.02	0.41	$14.84	0.41	$14.84	XXX	A+
76100	X-ray exam of body section	0.58	1.38	1.38	0.09	2.05	$74.21	2.05	$74.21	XXX	A+
76100-26	X-ray exam of body section	0.58	0.20	0.20	0.03	0.81	$29.32	0.81	$29.32	XXX	A+
76100-TC	X-ray exam of body section	0.00	1.18	1.18	0.06	1.24	$44.89	1.24	$44.89	XXX	A+
76101	Complex body section x-ray	0.58	1.55	1.55	0.10	2.23	$80.72	2.23	$80.72	XXX	A+

Code	Description								
76101-26	Complex body section x-ray	0.58	0.20	0.20	0.03	0.81	0.81	$29.32	XXX	A+
76101-TC	Complex body section x-ray	0.00	1.35	1.35	0.07	1.42	1.42	$51.40	XXX	A+
76102	Complex body section x-rays	0.58	1.84	1.84	0.12	2.54	2.54	$91.95	XXX	A+
76102-26	Complex body section x-rays	0.58	0.20	0.20	0.03	0.81	0.81	$29.32	XXX	A+
76102-TC	Complex body section x-rays	0.00	1.64	1.64	0.09	1.73	1.73	$62.62	XXX	A+
76120	Cine/video x-rays	0.38	1.14	1.14	0.07	1.59	1.59	$57.56	XXX	A+
76120-26	Cine/video x-rays	0.38	0.14	0.14	0.02	0.54	0.54	$19.55	XXX	A+
76120-TC	Cine/video x-rays	0.00	1.00	1.00	0.05	1.05	1.05	$38.01	XXX	A+
76125	Cine/video x-rays add-on	0.27	0.84	0.84	0.05	1.16	1.16	$41.99	ZZZ	A+
76125-26	Cine/video x-rays add-on	0.27	0.10	0.10	0.01	0.38	0.38	$13.76	ZZZ	A+
76125-TC	Cine/video x-rays add-on	0.00	0.74	0.74	0.04	0.78	0.78	$28.24	ZZZ	A+
76150	X-ray exam, dry process	0.00	0.39	0.39	0.02	0.41	0.41	$14.84	XXX	A+
76350	Special x-ray contrast study	0.00	0.00	0.00	0.00	0.00	0.00	$0.00	XXX	A+
76355	CAT scan for localization	1.21	8.28	8.28	0.41	9.90	9.90	$358.37	XXX	A+
76355-26	CAT scan for localization	1.21	0.44	0.44	0.06	1.71	1.71	$61.90	XXX	A+
76355-TC	CAT scan for localization	0.00	7.84	7.84	0.35	8.19	8.19	$296.47	XXX	A+
76360	CAT scan for needle biopsy	1.16	8.24	8.24	0.40	9.80	9.80	$354.75	XXX	A+
76360-26	CAT scan for needle biopsy	1.16	0.40	0.40	0.05	1.61	1.61	$58.28	XXX	A+
76360-TC	CAT scan for needle biopsy	0.00	7.84	7.84	0.35	8.19	8.19	$296.47	XXX	A+
76362	Cat scan for tissue ablation	4.00	9.24	9.24	1.38	14.62	14.62	$529.23	XXX	A+
76362-26	Cat scan for tissue ablation	4.00	1.40	1.40	0.17	5.57	5.57	$201.63	XXX	A+
76362-TC	Cat scan for tissue ablation	0.00	7.84	7.84	1.21	9.05	9.05	$327.60	XXX	A+
76370	CAT scan for therapy guide	0.85	3.10	3.10	0.17	4.12	4.12	$149.14	XXX	A+
76370-26	CAT scan for therapy guide	0.85	0.30	0.30	0.04	1.19	1.19	$43.08	XXX	A+
76370-TC	CAT scan for therapy guide	0.00	2.80	2.80	0.13	2.93	2.93	$106.06	XXX	A+
76375	3d/holograph reconstr add-on	0.16	3.42	3.42	0.16	3.74	3.74	$135.39	XXX	A+
76375-26	3d/holograph reconstr add-on	0.16	0.06	0.06	0.01	0.23	0.23	$8.33	XXX	A+
76375-TC	3d/holograph reconstr add-on	0.00	3.36	3.36	0.15	3.51	3.51	$127.06	XXX	A+

*M = multiple surgery adjustment applies
Me = multiple endoscopy rules may apply
B = bilateral surgery adjustment applies
A = assistant-at-surgery restriction

A+ = assistant-at-surgery restriction unless medical necessity established with documentation
C = cosurgeons payable
C+ = cosurgeons payable if medical necessity established with documentation

T = team surgeons permitted
T+ = team surgeons payable if medical necessity established with documentation
§ = indicates services that are not covered by Medicare.

CPT five-digit codes, two-digit numeric modifiers, and descriptions only are © 2001 American Medical Association

Medicare RBRVS: The Physicians' Guide

Relative value units

CPT Code and Modifier	Description	Work RVU	Non Facility Practice Expense RVU	Facility Practice Expense RVU	PLI RVU	Total Non Facility RVUs	Medicare Payment Non Facility	Total Facility RVUs	Medicare Payment Facility	Global Period	Payment Policy Indicators*
76380	CAT scan follow-up study	0.98	3.66	3.66	0.19	4.83	$174.84	4.83	$174.84	XXX	A+
76380-26	CAT scan follow-up study	0.98	0.34	0.34	0.04	1.36	$49.23	1.36	$49.23	XXX	A+
76380-TC	CAT scan follow-up study	0.00	3.32	3.32	0.15	3.47	$125.61	3.47	$125.61	XXX	A+
76390	Mr spectroscopy	1.40	11.14	11.14	0.55	13.09	$473.85	13.09	$473.85	XXX	A+
76390-26	Mr spectroscopy	1.40	0.50	0.50	0.06	1.96	$70.95	1.96	$70.95	XXX	A+
76390-TC	Mr spectroscopy	0.00	10.64	10.64	0.49	11.13	$402.90	11.13	$402.90	XXX	A+
76393	Mr guidance for needle place	1.50	11.16	11.16	0.53	13.19	$477.47	13.19	$477.47	XXX	A+
76393-26	Mr guidance for needle place	1.50	0.52	0.52	0.07	2.09	$75.66	2.09	$75.66	XXX	A+
76393-TC	Mr guidance for needle place	0.00	10.64	10.64	0.46	11.10	$401.81	11.10	$401.81	XXX	A+
76394	Mri for tissue ablation	4.25	12.13	12.13	1.43	17.81	$644.71	17.81	$644.71	XXX	A+
76394-26	Mri for tissue ablation	4.25	1.49	1.49	0.14	5.88	$212.85	5.88	$212.85	XXX	A+
76394-TC	Mri for tissue ablation	0.00	10.64	10.64	1.29	11.93	$431.86	11.93	$431.86	XXX	A+
76400	Magnetic image, bone marrow	1.60	11.20	11.20	0.56	13.36	$483.62	13.36	$483.62	XXX	A+
76400-26	Magnetic image, bone marrow	1.60	0.56	0.56	0.07	2.23	$80.72	2.23	$80.72	XXX	A+
76400-TC	Magnetic image, bone marrow	0.00	10.64	10.64	0.49	11.13	$402.90	11.13	$402.90	XXX	A+
76490	Us for tissue ablation	2.00	2.13	2.13	0.36	4.49	$162.53	4.49	$162.53	XXX	A+
76490-26	Us for tissue ablation	2.00	0.69	0.69	0.12	2.81	$101.72	2.81	$101.72	XXX	A+
76490-TC	Us for tissue ablation	0.00	1.44	1.44	0.24	1.68	$60.81	1.68	$60.81	XXX	A+
76499	Radiographic procedure	0.00	0.00	0.00	0.00	0.00	$0.00	0.00	$0.00	XXX	A+
76499-26	Radiographic procedure	0.00	0.00	0.00	0.00	0.00	$0.00	0.00	$0.00	XXX	A+
76499-TC	Radiographic procedure	0.00	0.00	0.00	0.00	0.00	$0.00	0.00	$0.00	XXX	A+

Radiology: Diagnostic ultrasound

CPT Code and Modifier	Description	Work RVU	Non Facility Practice Expense RVU	Facility Practice Expense RVU	PLI RVU	Total Non Facility RVUs	Medicare Payment Non Facility	Total Facility RVUs	Medicare Payment Facility	Global Period	Payment Policy Indicators*
76506	Echo exam of head	0.63	1.61	1.61	0.10	2.34	$84.71	2.34	$84.71	XXX	A+
76506-26	Echo exam of head	0.63	0.26	0.26	0.03	0.92	$33.30	0.92	$33.30	XXX	A+
76506-TC	Echo exam of head	0.00	1.35	1.35	0.07	1.42	$51.40	1.42	$51.40	XXX	A+
76511	Echo exam of eye	0.94	2.37	2.37	0.08	3.39	$122.72	3.39	$122.72	XXX	A+
76511-26	Echo exam of eye	0.94	0.45	0.45	0.02	1.41	$51.04	1.41	$51.04	XXX	A+

Code	Description								
76511-TC	Echo exam of eye	0.00	1.92	1.92	0.06	1.98	$71.67	XXX	A+
76512	Echo exam of eye	0.66	2.49	2.49	0.09	3.24	$117.29	XXX	A+
76512-26	Echo exam of eye	0.66	0.31	0.31	0.01	0.98	$35.48	XXX	A+
76512-TC	Echo exam of eye	0.00	2.18	2.18	0.08	2.26	$81.81	XXX	A+
76513	Echo exam of eye, water bath	0.66	2.90	2.90	0.09	3.65	$132.13	XXX	A+
76513-26	Echo exam of eye, water bath	0.66	0.32	0.32	0.01	0.99	$35.84	XXX	A+
76513-TC	Echo exam of eye, water bath	0.00	2.58	2.58	0.08	2.66	$96.29	XXX	A+
76516	Echo exam of eye	0.54	2.04	2.04	0.07	2.65	$95.93	XXX	A+
76516-26	Echo exam of eye	0.54	0.26	0.26	0.01	0.81	$29.32	XXX	A+
76516-TC	Echo exam of eye	0.00	1.78	1.78	0.06	1.84	$66.61	XXX	A+
76519	Echo exam of eye	0.54	1.91	1.91	0.07	2.52	$91.22	XXX	A+
76519-26	Echo exam of eye	0.54	0.26	0.26	0.01	0.81	$29.32	XXX	A+
76519-TC	Echo exam of eye	0.00	1.65	1.65	0.06	1.71	$61.90	XXX	A+
76529	Echo exam of eye	0.57	2.70	2.70	0.08	3.35	$121.27	XXX	A+
76529-26	Echo exam of eye	0.57	0.27	0.27	0.01	0.85	$30.77	XXX	A+
76529-TC	Echo exam of eye	0.00	2.43	2.43	0.07	2.50	$90.50	XXX	A+
76536	Us exam of head and neck	0.56	1.55	1.55	0.09	2.20	$79.64	XXX	A+
76536-26	Us exam of head and neck	0.56	0.20	0.20	0.02	0.78	$28.24	XXX	A+
76536-TC	Us exam of head and neck	0.00	1.35	1.35	0.07	1.42	$51.40	XXX	A+
76604	Us exam, chest, b-scan	0.55	1.43	1.43	0.08	2.06	$74.57	XXX	A+
76604-26	Us exam, chest, b-scan	0.55	0.19	0.19	0.02	0.76	$27.51	XXX	A+
76604-TC	Us exam, chest, b-scan	0.00	1.24	1.24	0.06	1.30	$47.06	XXX	A+
76645	Us exam, breast(s)	0.54	1.19	1.19	0.08	1.81	$65.52	XXX	A+
76645-26	Us exam, breast(s)	0.54	0.19	0.19	0.03	0.76	$27.51	XXX	A+
76645-TC	Us exam, breast(s)	0.00	1.00	1.00	0.05	1.05	$38.01	XXX	A+
76700	Us exam, abdom, complete	0.81	2.15	2.15	0.13	3.09	$111.86	XXX	A+
76700-26	Us exam, abdom, complete	0.81	0.28	0.28	0.04	1.13	$40.91	XXX	A+
76700-TC	Us exam, abdom, complete	0.00	1.87	1.87	0.09	1.96	$70.95	XXX	A+

* **M** = multiple surgery adjustment applies
Me = multiple endoscopy rules may apply
B = bilateral surgery adjustment applies
A = assistant-at-surgery restriction

A+ = assistant-at-surgery restriction unless medical necessity established with documentation
C = cosurgeons payable
C+ = cosurgeons payable if medical necessity established with documentation

T = team surgeons permitted
T+ = team surgeons payable if medical necessity established with documentation
S = indicates services that are not covered by Medicare.

CPT five-digit codes, two-digit numeric modifiers, and descriptions only are © 2001 American Medical Association

Medicare RBRVS: The Physicians' Guide

Relative value units

CPT Code and Modifier	Description	Work RVU	Non Facility Practice Expense RVU	Facility Practice Expense RVU	PLI RVU	Total Non Facility RVUs	Medicare Payment Non Facility	Total Facility RVUs	Medicare Payment Facility	Global Period	Payment Policy Indicators*
76705	Us exam, abdom, limited	0.59	1.56	1.56	0.10	2.25	$81.45	2.25	$81.45	XXX	A+
76705-26	Us exam, abdom, limited	0.59	0.21	0.21	0.03	0.83	$30.05	0.83	$30.05	XXX	A+
76705-TC	Us exam, abdom, limited	0.00	1.35	1.35	0.07	1.42	$51.40	1.42	$51.40	XXX	A+
76770	Us exam abdo back wall, comp	0.74	2.13	2.13	0.12	2.99	$108.24	2.99	$108.24	XXX	A+
76770-26	Us exam abdo back wall, comp	0.74	0.26	0.26	0.03	1.03	$37.29	1.03	$37.29	XXX	A+
76770-TC	Us exam abdo back wall, comp	0.00	1.87	1.87	0.09	1.96	$70.95	1.96	$70.95	XXX	A+
76775	Us exam abdo back wall, lim	0.58	1.55	1.55	0.10	2.23	$80.72	2.23	$80.72	XXX	A+
76775-26	Us exam abdo back wall, lim	0.58	0.20	0.20	0.03	0.81	$29.32	0.81	$29.32	XXX	A+
76775-TC	Us exam abdo back wall, lim	0.00	1.35	1.35	0.07	1.42	$51.40	1.42	$51.40	XXX	A+
76778	Us exam kidney transplant	0.74	2.13	2.13	0.12	2.99	$108.24	2.99	$108.24	XXX	A+
76778-26	Us exam kidney transplant	0.74	0.26	0.26	0.03	1.03	$37.29	1.03	$37.29	XXX	A+
76778-TC	Us exam kidney transplant	0.00	1.87	1.87	0.09	1.96	$70.95	1.96	$70.95	XXX	A+
76800	Us exam, spinal canal	1.13	1.73	1.73	0.11	2.97	$107.51	2.97	$107.51	XXX	A+
76800-26	Us exam, spinal canal	1.13	0.38	0.38	0.04	1.55	$56.11	1.55	$56.11	XXX	A+
76800-TC	Us exam, spinal canal	0.00	1.35	1.35	0.07	1.42	$51.40	1.42	$51.40	XXX	A+
76805	Us exam, pg uterus, compl	0.99	2.35	2.35	0.14	3.48	$125.97	3.48	$125.97	XXX	A+
76805-26	Us exam, pg uterus, compl	0.99	0.36	0.36	0.04	1.39	$50.32	1.39	$50.32	XXX	A+
76805-TC	Us exam, pg uterus, compl	0.00	1.99	1.99	0.10	2.09	$75.66	2.09	$75.66	XXX	A+
76810	Us exam, pg uterus, mult	1.97	4.74	4.74	0.25	6.96	$251.95	6.96	$251.95	XXX	A+
76810-26	Us exam, pg uterus, mult	1.97	0.75	0.75	0.07	2.79	$101.00	2.79	$101.00	XXX	A+
76810-TC	Us exam, pg uterus, mult	0.00	3.99	3.99	0.18	4.17	$150.95	4.17	$150.95	XXX	A+
76815	Us exam, pg uterus limit	0.65	1.60	1.60	0.09	2.34	$84.71	2.34	$84.71	XXX	A+
76815-26	Us exam, pg uterus limit	0.65	0.25	0.25	0.02	0.92	$33.30	0.92	$33.30	XXX	A+
76815-TC	Us exam, pg uterus limit	0.00	1.35	1.35	0.07	1.42	$51.40	1.42	$51.40	XXX	A+
76816	Us exam pg uterus repeat	0.57	1.28	1.28	0.07	1.92	$69.50	1.92	$69.50	XXX	A+
76816-26	Us exam pg uterus repeat	0.57	0.22	0.22	0.02	0.81	$29.32	0.81	$29.32	XXX	A+
76816-TC	Us exam pg uterus repeat	0.00	1.06	1.06	0.05	1.11	$40.18	1.11	$40.18	XXX	A+

Code	Description								
76818	Fetal biophy profile w/nst	1.05	1.94	0.12	3.11	$112.58	3.11	$112.58	XXX	A+
76818-26	Fetal biophy profile w/nst	1.05	0.41	0.04	1.50	$54.30	1.50	$54.30	XXX	A+
76818-TC	Fetal biophy profile w/nst	0.00	1.53	0.08	1.61	$58.28	1.61	$58.28	XXX	A+
76819	Fetal biophys profil w/o nst	0.77	1.83	0.10	2.70	$97.74	2.70	$97.74	XXX	A+
76819-26	Fetal biophys profil w/o nst	0.77	0.30	0.02	1.09	$39.46	1.09	$39.46	XXX	A+
76819-TC	Fetal biophys profil w/o nst	0.00	1.53	0.08	1.61	$58.28	1.61	$58.28	XXX	A+
76825	Echo exam of fetal heart	1.67	2.50	0.15	4.32	$156.38	4.32	$156.38	XXX	A+
76825-26	Echo exam of fetal heart	1.67	0.63	0.06	2.36	$85.43	2.36	$85.43	XXX	A+
76825-TC	Echo exam of fetal heart	0.00	1.87	0.09	1.96	$70.95	1.96	$70.95	XXX	A+
76826	Echo exam of fetal heart	0.83	0.97	0.07	1.87	$67.69	1.87	$67.69	XXX	A+
76826-26	Echo exam of fetal heart	0.83	0.30	0.03	1.16	$41.99	1.16	$41.99	XXX	A+
76826-TC	Echo exam of fetal heart	0.00	0.67	0.04	0.71	$25.70	0.71	$25.70	XXX	A+
76827	Echo exam of fetal heart	0.58	1.85	0.12	2.55	$92.31	2.55	$92.31	XXX	A+
76827-26	Echo exam of fetal heart	0.58	0.22	0.02	0.82	$29.68	0.82	$29.68	XXX	A+
76827-TC	Echo exam of fetal heart	0.00	1.63	0.10	1.73	$62.62	1.73	$62.62	XXX	A+
76828	Echo exam of fetal heart	0.56	1.29	0.09	1.94	$70.23	1.94	$70.23	XXX	A+
76828-26	Echo exam of fetal heart	0.56	0.23	0.02	0.81	$29.32	0.81	$29.32	XXX	A+
76828-TC	Echo exam of fetal heart	0.00	1.06	0.07	1.13	$40.91	1.13	$40.91	XXX	A+
76830	Us exam, transvaginal	0.69	1.68	0.11	2.48	$89.77	2.48	$89.77	XXX	A+
76830-26	Us exam, transvaginal	0.69	0.24	0.03	0.96	$34.75	0.96	$34.75	XXX	A+
76830-TC	Us exam, transvaginal	0.00	1.44	0.08	1.52	$55.02	1.52	$55.02	XXX	A+
76831	Echo exam, uterus	0.72	1.71	0.10	2.53	$91.58	2.53	$91.58	XXX	A+
76831-26	Echo exam, uterus	0.72	0.27	0.02	1.01	$36.56	1.01	$36.56	XXX	A+
76831-TC	Echo exam, uterus	0.00	1.44	0.08	1.52	$55.02	1.52	$55.02	XXX	A+
76856	Us exam, pelvic, complete	0.69	1.68	0.11	2.48	$89.77	2.48	$89.77	XXX	A+
76856-26	Us exam, pelvic, complete	0.69	0.24	0.03	0.96	$34.75	0.96	$34.75	XXX	A+
76856-TC	Us exam, pelvic, complete	0.00	1.44	0.08	1.52	$55.02	1.52	$55.02	XXX	A+
76857	Us exam, pelvic, limited	0.38	1.13	0.07	1.58	$57.19	1.58	$57.19	XXX	A+

* **M** = multiple surgery adjustment applies
Me = multiple endoscopy rules may apply
B = bilateral surgery adjustment applies
A = assistant-at-surgery restriction

A+ = assistant-at-surgery restriction unless medical necessity established with documentation
C = cosurgeons payable
C+ = cosurgeons payable if medical necessity established with documentation

T = team surgeons permitted
T+ = team surgeons payable if medical necessity established with documentation
$ = indicates services that are not covered by Medicare.

CPT five-digit codes, two-digit numeric modifiers, and descriptions only are © 2001 American Medical Association

Medicare RBRVS: The Physicians' Guide

Relative value units

CPT Code and Modifier	Description	Work RVU	Non Facility Practice Expense RVU	Facility Practice Expense RVU	PLI RVU	Total Non Facility RVUs	Medicare Payment Non Facility	Total Facility RVUs	Medicare Payment Facility	Global Period	Payment Policy Indicators*
76857-26	Us exam, pelvic, limited	0.38	0.13	0.13	0.02	0.53	$19.19	0.53	$19.19	XXX	A+
76857-TC	Us exam, pelvic, limited	0.00	1.00	1.00	0.05	1.05	$38.01	1.05	$38.01	XXX	A+
76870	Us exam, scrotum	0.64	1.66	1.66	0.11	2.41	$87.24	2.41	$87.24	XXX	A+
76870-26	Us exam, scrotum	0.64	0.22	0.22	0.03	0.89	$32.22	0.89	$32.22	XXX	A+
76870-TC	Us exam, scrotum	0.00	1.44	1.44	0.08	1.52	$55.02	1.52	$55.02	XXX	A+
76872	Echo exam, transrectal	0.69	1.68	1.68	0.12	2.49	$90.14	2.49	$90.14	XXX	A+
76872-26	Echo exam, transrectal	0.69	0.24	0.24	0.04	0.97	$35.11	0.97	$35.11	XXX	A+
76872-TC	Echo exam, transrectal	0.00	1.44	1.44	0.08	1.52	$55.02	1.52	$55.02	XXX	A+
76873	Echograp trans r, pros study	1.55	2.53	2.53	0.21	4.29	$155.29	4.29	$155.29	XXX	
76873-26	Echograp trans r, pros study	1.55	0.54	0.54	0.08	2.17	$78.55	2.17	$78.55	XXX	
76873-TC	Echograp trans r, pros study	0.00	1.99	1.99	0.13	2.12	$76.74	2.12	$76.74	XXX	
76880	Us exam, extremity	0.59	1.56	1.56	0.10	2.25	$81.45	2.25	$81.45	XXX	A+
76880-26	Us exam, extremity	0.59	0.21	0.21	0.03	0.83	$30.05	0.83	$30.05	XXX	A+
76880-TC	Us exam, extremity	0.00	1.35	1.35	0.07	1.42	$51.40	1.42	$51.40	XXX	A+
76885	Us exam infant hips, dynamic	0.74	1.70	1.70	0.11	2.55	$92.31	2.55	$92.31	XXX	A+
76885-26	Us exam infant hips, dynamic	0.74	0.26	0.26	0.03	1.03	$37.29	1.03	$37.29	XXX	A+
76885-TC	Us exam infant hips, dynamic	0.00	1.44	1.44	0.08	1.52	$55.02	1.52	$55.02	XXX	A+
76886	Us exam infant hips, static	0.62	1.57	1.57	0.10	2.29	$82.90	2.29	$82.90	XXX	A+
76886-26	Us exam infant hips, static	0.62	0.22	0.22	0.03	0.87	$31.49	0.87	$31.49	XXX	A+
76886-TC	Us exam infant hips, static	0.00	1.35	1.35	0.07	1.42	$51.40	1.42	$51.40	XXX	A+
76930	Echo guide, cardiocentesis	0.67	1.71	1.71	0.10	2.48	$89.77	2.48	$89.77	XXX	A+
76930-26	Echo guide, cardiocentesis	0.67	0.27	0.27	0.02	0.96	$34.75	0.96	$34.75	XXX	A+
76930-TC	Echo guide, cardiocentesis	0.00	1.44	1.44	0.08	1.52	$55.02	1.52	$55.02	XXX	A+
76932	Echo guide for heart biopsy	0.67	1.71	1.71	0.10	2.48	$89.77	2.48	$89.77	XXX	A+
76932-26	Echo guide for heart biopsy	0.67	0.27	0.27	0.02	0.96	$34.75	0.96	$34.75	XXX	A+
76932-TC	Echo guide for heart biopsy	0.00	1.44	1.44	0.08	1.52	$55.02	1.52	$55.02	XXX	A+
76936	Echo guide for artery repair	1.99	6.68	6.68	0.39	9.06	$327.96	9.06	$327.96	XXX	A+

Code	Description							
76936-26	Echo guide for artery repair	1.99	0.70	0.70	0.11	2.80	$101.36	XXX	A+
76936-TC	Echo guide for artery repair	0.00	5.98	5.98	0.28	6.26	$226.61	XXX	A+
76941	Echo guide for transfusion	1.34	1.98	1.98	0.13	3.45	$124.89	XXX	A+
76941-26	Echo guide for transfusion	1.34	0.53	0.53	0.06	1.93	$69.86	XXX	A+
76941-TC	Echo guide for transfusion	0.00	1.45	1.45	0.07	1.52	$55.02	XXX	A+
76942	Echo guide for biopsy	0.67	1.67	1.67	0.12	2.46	$89.05	XXX	A+
76942-26	Echo guide for biopsy	0.67	0.23	0.23	0.04	0.94	$34.03	XXX	A+
76942-TC	Echo guide for biopsy	0.00	1.44	1.44	0.08	1.52	$55.02	XXX	A+
76945	Echo guide, villus sampling	0.67	1.69	1.69	0.10	2.46	$89.05	XXX	A+
76945-26	Echo guide, villus sampling	0.67	0.24	0.24	0.03	0.94	$34.03	XXX	A+
76945-TC	Echo guide, villus sampling	0.00	1.45	1.45	0.07	1.52	$55.02	XXX	A+
76946	Echo guide for amniocentesis	0.38	1.59	1.59	0.09	2.06	$74.57	XXX	A+
76946-26	Echo guide for amniocentesis	0.38	0.15	0.15	0.01	0.54	$19.55	XXX	A+
76946-TC	Echo guide for amniocentesis	0.00	1.44	1.44	0.08	1.52	$55.02	XXX	A+
76948	Echo guide, ova aspiration	0.38	1.57	1.57	0.10	2.05	$74.21	XXX	A+
76948-26	Echo guide, ova aspiration	0.38	0.13	0.13	0.02	0.53	$19.19	XXX	A+
76948-TC	Echo guide, ova aspiration	0.00	1.44	1.44	0.08	1.52	$55.02	XXX	A+
76950	Echo guidance radiotherapy	0.58	1.45	1.45	0.09	2.12	$76.74	XXX	A+
76950-26	Echo guidance radiotherapy	0.58	0.21	0.21	0.03	0.82	$29.68	XXX	A+
76950-TC	Echo guidance radiotherapy	0.00	1.24	1.24	0.06	1.30	$47.06	XXX	A+
76965	Echo guidance radiotherapy	1.34	5.75	5.75	0.31	7.40	$267.87	XXX	A+
76965-26	Echo guidance radiotherapy	1.34	0.46	0.46	0.07	1.87	$67.69	XXX	A+
76965-TC	Echo guidance radiotherapy	0.00	5.29	5.29	0.24	5.53	$200.18	XXX	A+
76970	Ultrasound exam follow-up	0.40	1.14	1.14	0.07	1.61	$58.28	XXX	A+
76970-26	Ultrasound exam follow-up	0.40	0.14	0.14	0.02	0.56	$20.27	XXX	A+
76970-TC	Ultrasound exam follow-up	0.00	1.00	1.00	0.05	1.05	$38.01	XXX	A+
76975	GI endoscopic ultrasound	0.81	1.73	1.73	0.11	2.65	$95.93	XXX	A+
76975-26	GI endoscopic ultrasound	0.81	0.29	0.29	0.03	1.13	$40.91	XXX	A+

* **M** = multiple surgery adjustment applies
Me = multiple endoscopy rules may apply
B = bilateral surgery adjustment applies
A = assistant-at-surgery restriction

A+ = assistant-at-surgery restriction unless medical necessity established with documentation
C = cosurgeons payable
C+ = cosurgeons payable if medical necessity established with documentation

T = team surgeons permitted
T+ = team surgeons payable if medical necessity established with documentation
§ = indicates services that are not covered by Medicare.

CPT five-digit codes, two-digit numeric modifiers, and descriptions only are © 2001 American Medical Association

Medicare RBRVS: The Physicians' Guide

Relative value units

CPT Code and Modifier	Description	Work RVU	Non Facility Practice Expense RVU	Facility Practice Expense RVU	PLI RVU	Total Non Facility RVUs	Medicare Payment Non Facility	Total Facility RVUs	Medicare Payment Facility	Global Period	Payment Policy Indicators*
76975-TC	GI endoscopic ultrasound	0.00	1.44	1.44	0.08	1.52	$55.02	1.52	$55.02	XXX	A+
76977	Us bone density measure	0.05	0.80	0.80	0.05	0.90	$32.58	0.90	$32.58	XXX	A+
76977-26	Us bone density measure	0.05	0.02	0.02	0.01	0.08	$2.90	0.08	$2.90	XXX	A+
76977-TC	Us bone density measure	0.00	0.78	0.78	0.04	0.82	$29.68	0.82	$29.68	XXX	A+
76986	Ultrasound guide intraoper	1.20	2.91	2.91	0.19	4.30	$155.66	4.30	$155.66	XXX	A+
76986-26	Ultrasound guide intraoper	1.20	0.42	0.42	0.07	1.69	$61.18	1.69	$61.18	XXX	A+
76986-TC	Ultrasound guide intraoper	0.00	2.49	2.49	0.12	2.61	$94.48	2.61	$94.48	XXX	A+
76999	Echo examination procedure	0.00	0.00	0.00	0.00	0.00	$0.00	0.00	$0.00	XXX	A+
76999-26	Echo examination procedure	0.00	0.00	0.00	0.00	0.00	$0.00	0.00	$0.00	XXX	A+
76999-TC	Echo examination procedure	0.00	0.00	0.00	0.00	0.00	$0.00	0.00	$0.00	XXX	A+

Radiology: Radiation oncology

CPT Code and Modifier	Description	Work RVU	Non Facility Practice Expense RVU	Facility Practice Expense RVU	PLI RVU	Total Non Facility RVUs	Medicare Payment Non Facility	Total Facility RVUs	Medicare Payment Facility	Global Period	Payment Policy Indicators*
77261	Radiation therapy planning	1.39	0.56	0.56	0.06	2.01	$72.76	2.01	$72.76	XXX	A+
77262	Radiation therapy planning	2.11	0.82	0.82	0.09	3.02	$109.32	3.02	$109.32	XXX	A+
77263	Radiation therapy planning	3.14	1.23	1.23	0.13	4.50	$162.90	4.50	$162.90	XXX	A+
77280	Set radiation therapy field	0.70	3.55	3.55	0.18	4.43	$160.36	4.43	$160.36	XXX	A+
77280-26	Set radiation therapy field	0.70	0.25	0.25	0.03	0.98	$35.48	0.98	$35.48	XXX	A+
77280-TC	Set radiation therapy field	0.00	3.30	3.30	0.15	3.45	$124.89	3.45	$124.89	XXX	A+
77285	Set radiation therapy field	1.05	5.67	5.67	0.29	7.01	$253.76	7.01	$253.76	XXX	A+
77285-26	Set radiation therapy field	1.05	0.38	0.38	0.04	1.47	$53.21	1.47	$53.21	XXX	A+
77285-TC	Set radiation therapy field	0.00	5.29	5.29	0.25	5.54	$200.54	5.54	$200.54	XXX	A+
77290	Set radiation therapy field	1.56	6.74	6.74	0.35	8.65	$313.12	8.65	$313.12	XXX	A+
77290-26	Set radiation therapy field	1.56	0.56	0.56	0.06	2.18	$78.91	2.18	$78.91	XXX	A+
77290-TC	Set radiation therapy field	0.00	6.18	6.18	0.29	6.47	$234.21	6.47	$234.21	XXX	A+
77295	Set radiation therapy field	4.57	28.18	28.18	1.41	34.16	$1,236.56	34.16	$1,236.56	XXX	A+
77295-26	Set radiation therapy field	4.57	1.65	1.65	0.18	6.40	$231.67	6.40	$231.67	XXX	A+
77295-TC	Set radiation therapy field	0.00	26.53	26.53	1.23	27.76	$1,004.89	27.76	$1,004.89	XXX	A+
77299	Radiation therapy planning	0.00	0.00	0.00	0.00	0.00	$0.00	0.00	$0.00	XXX	A+

Code	Description								
77299-26	Radiation therapy planning	0.00	0.00	0.00	0.00	0.00	$0.00	XXX	A+
77299-TC	Radiation therapy planning	0.00	0.00	0.00	0.00	0.00	$0.00	XXX	A+
77300	Radiation therapy dose plan	0.62	1.50	1.50	0.09	2.21	$80.00	XXX	A+
77300-26	Radiation therapy dose plan	0.62	0.22	0.22	0.03	0.87	$31.49	XXX	A+
77300-TC	Radiation therapy dose plan	0.00	1.28	1.28	0.06	1.34	$48.51	XXX	A+
77301	Radiotherapy dos plan, imrt	8.00	29.72	29.72	1.41	39.13	$1,416.47	XXX	A+
77301-26	Radiotherapy dos plan, imrt	8.00	3.19	3.19	0.18	11.37	$411.58	XXX	A+
77301-TC	Radiotherapy dos plan, imrt	0.00	26.53	26.53	1.23	27.76	$1,004.89	XXX	A+
77305	Radiation therapy dose plan	0.70	2.01	2.01	0.12	2.83	$102.44	XXX	A+
77305-26	Radiation therapy dose plan	0.70	0.25	0.25	0.03	0.98	$35.48	XXX	A+
77305-TC	Radiation therapy dose plan	0.00	1.76	1.76	0.09	1.85	$66.97	XXX	A+
77310	Radiation therapy dose plan	1.05	2.59	2.59	0.15	3.79	$137.19	XXX	A+
77310-26	Radiation therapy dose plan	1.05	0.38	0.38	0.04	1.47	$53.21	XXX	A+
77310-TC	Radiation therapy dose plan	0.00	2.21	2.21	0.11	2.32	$83.98	XXX	A+
77315	Radiation therapy dose plan	1.56	3.09	3.09	0.18	4.83	$174.84	XXX	A+
77315-26	Radiation therapy dose plan	1.56	0.56	0.56	0.06	2.18	$78.91	XXX	A+
77315-TC	Radiation therapy dose plan	0.00	2.53	2.53	0.12	2.65	$95.93	XXX	A+
77321	Radiation therapy port plan	0.95	4.18	4.18	0.21	5.34	$193.30	XXX	A+
77321-26	Radiation therapy port plan	0.95	0.34	0.34	0.04	1.33	$48.14	XXX	A+
77321-TC	Radiation therapy port plan	0.00	3.84	3.84	0.17	4.01	$145.16	XXX	A+
77326	Radiation therapy dose plan	0.93	2.58	2.58	0.15	3.66	$132.49	XXX	A+
77326-26	Radiation therapy dose plan	0.93	0.34	0.34	0.04	1.31	$47.42	XXX	A+
77326-TC	Radiation therapy dose plan	0.00	2.24	2.24	0.11	2.35	$85.07	XXX	A+
77327	Radiation therapy dose plan	1.39	3.80	3.80	0.21	5.40	$195.48	XXX	A+
77327-26	Radiation therapy dose plan	1.39	0.50	0.50	0.06	1.95	$70.59	XXX	A+
77327-TC	Radiation therapy dose plan	0.00	3.30	3.30	0.15	3.45	$124.89	XXX	A+
77328	Radiation therapy dose plan	2.09	5.46	5.46	0.30	7.85	$284.16	XXX	A+
77328-26	Radiation therapy dose plan	2.09	0.75	0.75	0.09	2.93	$106.06	XXX	A+

* **M** = multiple surgery adjustment applies
Me = multiple endoscopy rules may apply
B = bilateral surgery adjustment applies
A = assistant-at-surgery restriction

A+ = assistant-at-surgery restriction unless medical necessity established with documentation
C = cosurgeons payable
C+ = cosurgeons payable if medical necessity established with documentation

T = team surgeons permitted
T+ = team surgeons payable if medical necessity established with documentation
§ = indicates services that are not covered by Medicare.

Medicare RBRVS: The Physicians' Guide

Relative value units

CPT Code and Modifier	Description	Work RVU	Non Facility Practice Expense RVU	Facility Practice Expense RVU	PLI RVU	Total Non Facility RVUs	Medicare Payment Non Facility	Total Facility RVUs	Medicare Payment Facility	Global Period	Payment Policy Indicators*
77328-TC	Radiation therapy dose plan	0.00	4.71	4.71	0.21	4.92	$178.10	4.92	$178.10	XXX	A+
77331	Special radiation dosimetry	0.87	0.79	0.79	0.06	1.72	$62.26	1.72	$62.26	XXX	A+
77331-26	Special radiation dosimetry	0.87	0.31	0.31	0.04	1.22	$44.16	1.22	$44.16	XXX	A+
77331-TC	Special radiation dosimetry	0.00	0.48	0.48	0.02	0.50	$18.10	0.50	$18.10	XXX	A+
77332	Radiation treatment aid(s)	0.54	1.47	1.47	0.08	2.09	$75.66	2.09	$75.66	XXX	A+
77332-26	Radiation treatment aid(s)	0.54	0.19	0.19	0.02	0.75	$27.15	0.75	$27.15	XXX	A+
77332-TC	Radiation treatment aid(s)	0.00	1.28	1.28	0.06	1.34	$48.51	1.34	$48.51	XXX	A+
77333	Radiation treatment aid(s)	0.84	2.10	2.10	0.13	3.07	$111.13	3.07	$111.13	XXX	A+
77333-26	Radiation treatment aid(s)	0.84	0.30	0.30	0.04	1.18	$42.72	1.18	$42.72	XXX	A+
77333-TC	Radiation treatment aid(s)	0.00	1.80	1.80	0.09	1.89	$68.42	1.89	$68.42	XXX	A+
77334	Radiation treatment aid(s)	1.24	3.54	3.54	0.19	4.97	$179.91	4.97	$179.91	XXX	A+
77334-26	Radiation treatment aid(s)	1.24	0.45	0.45	0.05	1.74	$62.99	1.74	$62.99	XXX	A+
77334-TC	Radiation treatment aid(s)	0.00	3.09	3.09	0.14	3.23	$116.92	3.23	$116.92	XXX	A+
77336	Radiation physics consult	0.00	2.83	2.83	0.13	2.96	$107.15	2.96	$107.15	XXX	A+
77370	Radiation physics consult	0.00	3.31	3.31	0.15	3.46	$125.25	3.46	$125.25	XXX	A+
77399	External radiation dosimetry	0.00	0.00	0.00	0.00	0.00	$0.00	0.00	$0.00	XXX	A+
77399-26	External radiation dosimetry	0.00	0.00	0.00	0.00	0.00	$0.00	0.00	$0.00	XXX	A+
77399-TC	External radiation dosimetry	0.00	0.00	0.00	0.00	0.00	$0.00	0.00	$0.00	XXX	A+
77401	Radiation treatment delivery	0.00	1.68	1.68	0.09	1.77	$64.07	1.77	$64.07	XXX	A+
77402	Radiation treatment delivery	0.00	1.68	1.68	0.09	1.77	$64.07	1.77	$64.07	XXX	A+
77403	Radiation treatment delivery	0.00	1.68	1.68	0.09	1.77	$64.07	1.77	$64.07	XXX	A+
77404	Radiation treatment delivery	0.00	1.68	1.68	0.09	1.77	$64.07	1.77	$64.07	XXX	A+
77406	Radiation treatment delivery	0.00	1.68	1.68	0.09	1.77	$64.07	1.77	$64.07	XXX	A+
77407	Radiation treatment delivery	0.00	1.98	1.98	0.10	2.08	$75.29	2.08	$75.29	XXX	A+
77408	Radiation treatment delivery	0.00	1.98	1.98	0.10	2.08	$75.29	2.08	$75.29	XXX	A+
77409	Radiation treatment delivery	0.00	1.98	1.98	0.10	2.08	$75.29	2.08	$75.29	XXX	A+
77411	Radiation treatment delivery	0.00	1.98	1.98	0.10	2.08	$75.29	2.08	$75.29	XXX	A+

Code	Description								
77412	Radiation treatment delivery	0.00	2.21	2.21	0.11	2.32	2.32	$83.98	XXX	A+
77413	Radiation treatment delivery	0.00	2.21	2.21	0.11	2.32	2.32	$83.98	XXX	A+
77414	Radiation treatment delivery	0.00	2.21	2.21	0.11	2.32	2.32	$83.98	XXX	A+
77416	Radiation treatment delivery	0.00	2.21	2.21	0.11	2.32	2.32	$83.98	XXX	A+
77417	Radiology port film(s)	0.00	0.56	0.56	0.03	0.59	0.59	$21.36	XXX	A+
77418	Radiation tx delivery, imrt	0.00	16.07	16.07	0.11	16.18	16.18	$585.70	XXX	A+
77427	Radiation tx management, x5	3.31	1.19	1.19	0.14	4.64	4.64	$167.96	XXX	
77431	Radiation therapy management	1.81	0.73	0.73	0.07	2.61	2.61	$94.48	XXX	A+
77432	Stereotactic radiation trmt	7.93	3.25	3.25	0.33	11.51	11.51	$416.65	XXX	A+
77470	Special radiation treatment	2.09	11.34	11.34	0.58	14.01	14.01	$507.15	XXX	A+
77470-26	Special radiation treatment	2.09	0.75	0.75	0.09	2.93	2.93	$106.06	XXX	A+
77470-TC	Special radiation treatment	0.00	10.59	10.59	0.49	11.08	11.08	$401.09	XXX	A+
77499	Radiation therapy management	0.00	0.00	0.00	0.00	0.00	0.00	$0.00	XXX	A+
77499-26	Radiation therapy management	0.00	0.00	0.00	0.00	0.00	0.00	$0.00	XXX	A+
77499-TC	Radiation therapy management	0.00	0.00	0.00	0.00	0.00	0.00	$0.00	XXX	A+
77520	Proton trmt, simple w/o comp	0.00	0.00	0.00	0.00	0.00	0.00	$0.00	XXX	
77522	Proton trmt, simple w/comp	0.00	0.00	0.00	0.00	0.00	0.00	$0.00	XXX	
77523	Proton trmt, intermediate	0.00	0.00	0.00	0.00	0.00	0.00	$0.00	XXX	
77525	Proton treatment, complex	0.00	0.00	0.00	0.00	0.00	0.00	$0.00	XXX	
77600	Hyperthermia treatment	1.56	3.44	3.44	0.21	5.21	5.21	$188.60	XXX	A+
77600-26	Hyperthermia treatment	1.56	0.55	0.55	0.08	2.19	2.19	$79.28	XXX	A+
77600-TC	Hyperthermia treatment	0.00	2.89	2.89	0.13	3.02	3.02	$109.32	XXX	A+
77605	Hyperthermia treatment	2.09	4.62	4.62	0.31	7.02	7.02	$254.12	XXX	A+
77605-26	Hyperthermia treatment	2.09	0.76	0.76	0.13	2.98	2.98	$107.87	XXX	A+
77605-TC	Hyperthermia treatment	0.00	3.86	3.86	0.18	4.04	4.04	$146.24	XXX	A+
77610	Hyperthermia treatment	1.56	3.44	3.44	0.20	5.20	5.20	$188.24	XXX	A+
77610-26	Hyperthermia treatment	1.56	0.55	0.55	0.07	2.18	2.18	$78.91	XXX	A+
77610-TC	Hyperthermia treatment	0.00	2.89	2.89	0.13	3.02	3.02	$109.32	XXX	A+

* **M** = multiple surgery adjustment applies
Me = multiple endoscopy rules may apply
B = bilateral surgery adjustment applies
A = assistant-at-surgery restriction

A+ = assistant-at-surgery restriction unless medical necessity established with documentation
C = cosurgeons payable
C+ = cosurgeons payable if medical necessity established with documentation

T = team surgeons permitted
T+ = team surgeons payable if medical necessity established with documentation
§ = indicates services that are not covered by Medicare.

CPT five-digit codes, two-digit numeric modifiers, and descriptions only are © 2001 American Medical Association

Medicare RBRVS: The Physicians' Guide

Relative value units

CPT Code and Modifier	Description	Work RVU	Non Facility Practice Expense RVU	Facility Practice Expense RVU	PLI RVU	Total Non Facility RVUs	Medicare Payment Non Facility	Total Facility RVUs	Medicare Payment Facility	Global Period	Payment Policy Indicators*
77615	Hyperthermia treatment	2.09	4.60	4.60	0.27	6.96	$251.95	6.96	$251.95	XXX	A+
77615-26	Hyperthermia treatment	2.09	0.74	0.74	0.09	2.92	$105.70	2.92	$105.70	XXX	A+
77615-TC	Hyperthermia treatment	0.00	3.86	3.86	0.18	4.04	$146.24	4.04	$146.24	XXX	A+
77620	Hyperthermia treatment	1.56	3.47	3.47	0.19	5.22	$188.96	5.22	$188.96	XXX	A+
77620-26	Hyperthermia treatment	1.56	0.58	0.58	0.06	2.20	$79.64	2.20	$79.64	XXX	A+
77620-TC	Hyperthermia treatment	0.00	2.89	2.89	0.13	3.02	$109.32	3.02	$109.32	XXX	A+
77750	Infuse radioactive materials	4.91	3.04	3.04	0.23	8.18	$296.11	8.18	$296.11	090	A+
77750-26	Infuse radioactive materials	4.91	1.77	1.77	0.17	6.85	$247.96	6.85	$247.96	090	A+
77750-TC	Infuse radioactive materials	0.00	1.27	1.27	0.06	1.33	$48.14	1.33	$48.14	090	A+
77761	Apply intrcav radiat simple	3.81	3.51	3.51	0.28	7.60	$275.11	7.60	$275.11	090	A+
77761-26	Apply intrcav radiat simple	3.81	1.13	1.13	0.16	5.10	$184.62	5.10	$184.62	090	A+
77761-TC	Apply intrcav radiat simple	0.00	2.38	2.38	0.12	2.50	$90.50	2.50	$90.50	090	A+
77762	Apply intrcav radiat interm	5.72	5.42	5.42	0.38	11.52	$417.01	11.52	$417.01	090	A+
77762-26	Apply intrcav radiat interm	5.72	1.99	1.99	0.22	7.93	$287.06	7.93	$287.06	090	A+
77762-TC	Apply intrcav radiat interm	0.00	3.43	3.43	0.16	3.59	$129.96	3.59	$129.96	090	A+
77763	Apply intrcav radiat compl	8.57	7.38	7.38	0.53	16.48	$596.56	16.48	$596.56	090	A+
77763-26	Apply intrcav radiat compl	8.57	3.12	3.12	0.34	12.03	$435.48	12.03	$435.48	090	A+
77763-TC	Apply intrcav radiat compl	0.00	4.26	4.26	0.19	4.45	$161.09	4.45	$161.09	090	A+
77776	Apply interstit radiat simpl	4.66	3.72	3.72	0.35	8.73	$316.02	8.73	$316.02	090	A+
77776-26	Apply interstit radiat simpl	4.66	1.65	1.65	0.24	6.55	$237.10	6.55	$237.10	090	A+ C
77776-TC	Apply interstit radiat simpl	0.00	2.07	2.07	0.11	2.18	$78.91	2.18	$78.91	090	A+
77777	Apply interstit radiat inter	7.48	6.37	6.37	0.50	14.35	$519.46	14.35	$519.46	090	A+
77777-26	Apply interstit radiat inter	7.48	2.35	2.35	0.32	10.15	$367.42	10.15	$367.42	090	A+ C
77777-TC	Apply interstit radiat inter	0.00	4.02	4.02	0.18	4.20	$152.04	4.20	$152.04	090	A+
77778	Apply iterstit radiat compl	11.19	8.90	8.90	0.69	20.78	$752.22	20.78	$752.22	090	A+
77778-26	Apply iterstit radiat compl	11.19	4.02	4.02	0.47	15.68	$567.60	15.68	$567.60	090	A+ C
77778-TC	Apply iterstit radiat compl	0.00	4.88	4.88	0.22	5.10	$184.62	5.10	$184.62	090	A+

Code	Description							
77781	High intensity brachytherapy	1.66	19.88	0.95	22.49	$814.12	22.49	$814.12	090	A+
77781-26	High intensity brachytherapy	1.66	0.60	0.07	2.33	$84.34	2.33	$84.34	090	A+
77781-TC	High intensity brachytherapy	0.00	19.28	0.88	20.16	$729.78	20.16	$729.78	090	A+
77782	High intensity brachytherapy	2.49	20.18	0.98	23.65	$856.11	23.65	$856.11	090	A+
77782-26	High intensity brachytherapy	2.49	0.90	0.10	3.49	$126.34	3.49	$126.34	090	A+
77782-TC	High intensity brachytherapy	0.00	19.28	0.88	20.16	$729.78	20.16	$729.78	090	A+
77783	High intensity brachytherapy	3.73	20.62	1.03	25.38	$918.74	25.38	$918.74	090	A+
77783-26	High intensity brachytherapy	3.73	1.34	0.15	5.22	$188.96	5.22	$188.96	090	A+
77783-TC	High intensity brachytherapy	0.00	19.28	0.88	20.16	$729.78	20.16	$729.78	090	A+
77784	High intensity brachytherapy	5.61	21.30	1.10	28.01	$1,013.94	28.01	$1,013.94	090	A+
77784-26	High intensity brachytherapy	5.61	2.02	0.22	7.85	$284.16	7.85	$284.16	090	A+
77784-TC	High intensity brachytherapy	0.00	19.28	0.88	20.16	$729.78	20.16	$729.78	090	A+
77789	Apply surface radiation	1.12	0.84	0.05	2.01	$72.76	2.01	$72.76	090	A+
77789-26	Apply surface radiation	1.12	0.41	0.03	1.56	$56.47	1.56	$56.47	090	A+
77789-TC	Apply surface radiation	0.00	0.43	0.02	0.45	$16.29	0.45	$16.29	090	A+
77790	Radiation handling	1.05	0.86	0.06	1.97	$71.31	1.97	$71.31	XXX	A+
77790-26	Radiation handling	1.05	0.38	0.04	1.47	$53.21	1.47	$53.21	XXX	A+
77790-TC	Radiation handling	0.00	0.48	0.02	0.50	$18.10	0.50	$18.10	XXX	A+
77799	Radium/radioisotope therapy	0.00	0.00	0.00	0.00	$0.00	0.00	$0.00	XXX	A+
77799-26	Radium/radioisotope therapy	0.00	0.00	0.00	0.00	$0.00	0.00	$0.00	XXX	A+
77799-TC	Radium/radioisotope therapy	0.00	0.00	0.00	0.00	$0.00	0.00	$0.00	XXX	A+
78000	Thyroid, single uptake	0.19	0.99	0.06	1.24	$44.89	1.24	$44.89	XXX	A+
78000-26	Thyroid, single uptake	0.19	0.07	0.01	0.27	$9.77	0.27	$9.77	XXX	A+
78000-TC	Thyroid, single uptake	0.00	0.92	0.05	0.97	$35.11	0.97	$35.11	XXX	A+
78001	Thyroid, multiple uptakes	0.26	1.33	0.07	1.66	$60.09	1.66	$60.09	XXX	A+
78001-26	Thyroid, multiple uptakes	0.26	0.09	0.01	0.36	$13.03	0.36	$13.03	XXX	A+
78001-TC	Thyroid, multiple uptakes	0.00	1.24	0.06	1.30	$47.06	1.30	$47.06	XXX	A+
78003	Thyroid suppress/stimul	0.33	1.04	0.06	1.43	$51.76	1.43	$51.76	XXX	A+

* **M** = multiple surgery adjustment applies
Me = multiple endoscopy rules may apply
B = bilateral surgery adjustment applies
A = assistant-at-surgery restriction

A+ = assistant-at-surgery restriction unless medical necessity established with documentation
C = cosurgeons payable
C+ = cosurgeons payable if medical necessity established with documentation

T = team surgeons permitted
T+ = team surgeons payable if medical necessity established with documentation
$ = indicates services that are not covered by Medicare.

367 CPT five-digit codes, two-digit numeric modifiers, and descriptions only are © 2001 American Medical Association

Medicare RBRVS: The Physicians' Guide

Relative value units

CPT Code and Modifier	Description	Work RVU	Non Facility Practice Expense RVU	Facility Practice Expense RVU	PLI RVU	Total Non Facility RVUs	Medicare Payment Non Facility	Total Facility RVUs	Medicare Payment Facility	Global Period	Payment Policy Indicators*
78003-26	Thyroid suppress/stimul	0.33	0.12	0.12	0.01	0.46	$16.65	0.46	$16.65	XXX	A+
78003-TC	Thyroid suppress/stimul	0.00	0.92	0.92	0.05	0.97	$35.11	0.97	$35.11	XXX	A+
78006	Thyroid imaging with uptake	0.49	2.44	2.44	0.13	3.06	$110.77	3.06	$110.77	XXX	A+
78006-26	Thyroid imaging with uptake	0.49	0.18	0.18	0.02	0.69	$24.98	0.69	$24.98	XXX	A+
78006-TC	Thyroid imaging with uptake	0.00	2.26	2.26	0.11	2.37	$85.79	2.37	$85.79	XXX	A+
78007	Thyroid image, mult uptakes	0.50	2.62	2.62	0.14	3.26	$118.01	3.26	$118.01	XXX	A+
78007-26	Thyroid image, mult uptakes	0.50	0.18	0.18	0.02	0.70	$25.34	0.70	$25.34	XXX	A+
78007-TC	Thyroid image, mult uptakes	0.00	2.44	2.44	0.12	2.56	$92.67	2.56	$92.67	XXX	A+
78010	Thyroid imaging	0.39	1.87	1.87	0.11	2.37	$85.79	2.37	$85.79	XXX	A+
78010-26	Thyroid imaging	0.39	0.14	0.14	0.02	0.55	$19.91	0.55	$19.91	XXX	A+
78010-TC	Thyroid imaging	0.00	1.73	1.73	0.09	1.82	$65.88	1.82	$65.88	XXX	A+
78011	Thyroid imaging with flow	0.45	2.45	2.45	0.13	3.03	$109.68	3.03	$109.68	XXX	A+
78011-26	Thyroid imaging with flow	0.45	0.16	0.16	0.02	0.63	$22.81	0.63	$22.81	XXX	A+
78011-TC	Thyroid imaging with flow	0.00	2.29	2.29	0.11	2.40	$86.88	2.40	$86.88	XXX	A+
78015	Thyroid met imaging	0.67	2.68	2.68	0.15	3.50	$126.70	3.50	$126.70	XXX	A+
78015-26	Thyroid met imaging	0.67	0.24	0.24	0.03	0.94	$34.03	0.94	$34.03	XXX	A+
78015-TC	Thyroid met imaging	0.00	2.44	2.44	0.12	2.56	$92.67	2.56	$92.67	XXX	A+
78016	Thyroid met imaging/studies	0.82	3.62	3.62	0.18	4.62	$167.24	4.62	$167.24	XXX	A+
78016-26	Thyroid met imaging/studies	0.82	0.31	0.31	0.03	1.16	$41.99	1.16	$41.99	XXX	A+
78016-TC	Thyroid met imaging/studies	0.00	3.31	3.31	0.15	3.46	$125.25	3.46	$125.25	XXX	A+
78018	Thyroid met imaging, body	0.86	5.47	5.47	0.27	6.60	$238.91	6.60	$238.91	XXX	A+
78018-26	Thyroid met imaging, body	0.86	0.32	0.32	0.03	1.21	$43.80	1.21	$43.80	XXX	A+
78018-TC	Thyroid met imaging, body	0.00	5.15	5.15	0.24	5.39	$195.11	5.39	$195.11	XXX	A+
78020	Thyroid met uptake	0.60	1.47	1.47	0.14	2.21	$80.00	2.21	$80.00	ZZZ	A+
78020-26	Thyroid met uptake	0.60	0.23	0.23	0.02	0.85	$30.77	0.85	$30.77	ZZZ	A+
78020-TC	Thyroid met uptake	0.00	1.24	1.24	0.12	1.36	$49.23	1.36	$49.23	ZZZ	A+
78070	Parathyroid nuclear imaging	0.82	2.03	2.03	0.12	2.97	$107.51	2.97	$107.51	XXX	A+

Code	Description								
78070-26	Parathyroid nuclear imaging	0.82	0.30	0.30	0.03	1.15	$41.63	XXX	A+
78070-TC	Parathyroid nuclear imaging	0.00	1.73	1.73	0.09	1.82	$65.88	XXX	A+
78075	Adrenal nuclear imaging	0.74	5.44	5.44	0.27	6.45	$233.48	XXX	A+
78075-26	Adrenal nuclear imaging	0.74	0.29	0.29	0.03	1.06	$38.37	XXX	A+
78075-TC	Adrenal nuclear imaging	0.00	5.15	5.15	0.24	5.39	$195.11	XXX	A+
78099	Endocrine nuclear procedure	0.00	0.00	0.00	0.00	0.00	$0.00	XXX	A+
78099-26	Endocrine nuclear procedure	0.00	0.00	0.00	0.00	0.00	$0.00	XXX	A+
78099-TC	Endocrine nuclear procedure	0.00	0.00	0.00	0.00	0.00	$0.00	XXX	A+
78102	Bone marrow imaging, ltd	0.55	2.15	2.15	0.12	2.82	$102.08	XXX	A+
78102-26	Bone marrow imaging, ltd	0.55	0.21	0.21	0.02	0.78	$28.24	XXX	A+
78102-TC	Bone marrow imaging, ltd	0.00	1.94	1.94	0.10	2.04	$73.85	XXX	A+
78103	Bone marrow imaging, mult	0.75	3.28	3.28	0.17	4.20	$152.04	XXX	A+
78103-26	Bone marrow imaging, mult	0.75	0.27	0.27	0.03	1.05	$38.01	XXX	A+
78103-TC	Bone marrow imaging, mult	0.00	3.01	3.01	0.14	3.15	$114.03	XXX	A+
78104	Bone marrow imaging, body	0.80	4.16	4.16	0.21	5.17	$187.15	XXX	A+
78104-26	Bone marrow imaging, body	0.80	0.29	0.29	0.03	1.12	$40.54	XXX	A+
78104-TC	Bone marrow imaging, body	0.00	3.87	3.87	0.18	4.05	$146.61	XXX	A+
78110	Plasma volume, single	0.19	0.97	0.97	0.06	1.22	$44.16	XXX	A+
78110-26	Plasma volume, single	0.19	0.07	0.07	0.01	0.27	$9.77	XXX	A+
78110-TC	Plasma volume, single	0.00	0.90	0.90	0.05	0.95	$34.39	XXX	A+
78111	Plasma volume, multiple	0.22	2.52	2.52	0.13	2.87	$103.89	XXX	A+
78111-26	Plasma volume, multiple	0.22	0.08	0.08	0.01	0.31	$11.22	XXX	A+
78111-TC	Plasma volume, multiple	0.00	2.44	2.44	0.12	2.56	$92.67	XXX	A+
78120	Red cell mass, single	0.23	1.73	1.73	0.10	2.06	$74.57	XXX	A+
78120-26	Red cell mass, single	0.23	0.09	0.09	0.01	0.33	$11.95	XXX	A+
78120-TC	Red cell mass, single	0.00	1.64	1.64	0.09	1.73	$62.62	XXX	A+
78121	Red cell mass, multiple	0.32	2.88	2.88	0.13	3.33	$120.54	XXX	A+
78121-26	Red cell mass, multiple	0.32	0.12	0.12	0.01	0.45	$16.29	XXX	A+

* **M** = multiple surgery adjustment applies
   Me = multiple endoscopy rules may apply
   B = bilateral surgery adjustment applies
   A = assistant-at-surgery restriction

A+ = assistant-at-surgery restriction unless medical necessity established with documentation
C = cosurgeons payable
C+ = cosurgeons payable if medical necessity established with documentation

T = team surgeons permitted
T+ = team surgeons payable if medical necessity established with documentation
§ = indicates services that are not covered by Medicare.

369 CPT five-digit codes, two-digit numeric modifiers, and descriptions only are © 2001 American Medical Association

Medicare RBRVS: The Physicians' Guide

Relative value units

CPT Code and Modifier	Description	Work RVU	Non Facility Practice Expense RVU	Facility Practice Expense RVU	PLI RVU	Total Non Facility RVUs	Medicare Payment Non Facility	Total Facility RVUs	Medicare Payment Facility	Global Period	Payment Policy Indicators*
78121-TC	Red cell mass, multiple	0.00	2.76	2.76	0.12	2.88	$104.25	2.88	$104.25	XXX	A+
78122	Blood volume	0.45	4.54	4.54	0.22	5.21	$188.60	5.21	$188.60	XXX	A+
78122-26	Blood volume	0.45	0.17	0.17	0.02	0.64	$23.17	0.64	$23.17	XXX	A+
78122-TC	Blood volume	0.00	4.37	4.37	0.20	4.57	$165.43	4.57	$165.43	XXX	A+
78130	Red cell survival study	0.61	2.93	2.93	0.15	3.69	$133.58	3.69	$133.58	XXX	A+
78130-26	Red cell survival study	0.61	0.22	0.22	0.03	0.86	$31.13	0.86	$31.13	XXX	A+
78130-TC	Red cell survival study	0.00	2.71	2.71	0.12	2.83	$102.44	2.83	$102.44	XXX	A+
78135	Red cell survival kinetics	0.64	4.86	4.86	0.24	5.74	$207.78	5.74	$207.78	XXX	A+
78135-26	Red cell survival kinetics	0.64	0.23	0.23	0.03	0.90	$32.58	0.90	$32.58	XXX	A+
78135-TC	Red cell survival kinetics	0.00	4.63	4.63	0.21	4.84	$175.20	4.84	$175.20	XXX	A+
78140	Red cell sequestration	0.61	3.95	3.95	0.20	4.76	$172.31	4.76	$172.31	XXX	A+
78140-26	Red cell sequestration	0.61	0.21	0.21	0.03	0.85	$30.77	0.85	$30.77	XXX	A+
78140-TC	Red cell sequestration	0.00	3.74	3.74	0.17	3.91	$141.54	3.91	$141.54	XXX	A+
78160	Plasma iron turnover	0.33	3.60	3.60	0.19	4.12	$149.14	4.12	$149.14	XXX	A+
78160-26	Plasma iron turnover	0.33	0.12	0.12	0.03	0.48	$17.38	0.48	$17.38	XXX	A+
78160-TC	Plasma iron turnover	0.00	3.48	3.48	0.16	3.64	$131.77	3.64	$131.77	XXX	A+
78162	Iron absorption exam	0.45	3.22	3.22	0.15	3.82	$138.28	3.82	$138.28	XXX	A+
78162-26	Iron absorption exam	0.45	0.18	0.18	0.01	0.64	$23.17	0.64	$23.17	XXX	A+
78162-TC	Iron absorption exam	0.00	3.04	3.04	0.14	3.18	$115.11	3.18	$115.11	XXX	A+
78170	Red cell iron utilization	0.41	5.19	5.19	0.27	5.87	$212.49	5.87	$212.49	XXX	A+
78170-26	Red cell iron utilization	0.41	0.15	0.15	0.04	0.60	$21.72	0.60	$21.72	XXX	A+
78170-TC	Red cell iron utilization	0.00	5.04	5.04	0.23	5.27	$190.77	5.27	$190.77	XXX	A+
78172	Total body iron estimation	0.00	0.00	0.00	0.00	0.00	$0.00	0.00	$0.00	XXX	A+
78172-26	Total body iron estimation	0.53	0.20	0.20	0.02	0.75	$27.15	0.75	$27.15	XXX	A+
78172-TC	Total body iron estimation	0.00	0.00	0.00	0.00	0.00	$0.00	0.00	$0.00	XXX	A+
78185	Spleen imaging	0.40	2.39	2.39	0.13	2.92	$105.70	2.92	$105.70	XXX	A+
78185-26	Spleen imaging	0.40	0.15	0.15	0.02	0.57	$20.63	0.57	$20.63	XXX	A+

Code	Description								
78185-TC	Spleen imaging	0.00	2.24	2.24	0.11	2.35	$85.07	XXX	A+
78190	Platelet survival, kinetics	1.09	5.83	5.83	0.31	7.23	$261.72	XXX	A+
78190-26	Platelet survival, kinetics	1.09	0.40	0.40	0.06	1.55	$56.11	XXX	A+
78190-TC	Platelet survival, kinetics	0.00	5.43	5.43	0.25	5.68	$205.61	XXX	A+
78191	Platelet survival	0.61	7.19	7.19	0.34	8.14	$294.66	XXX	A+
78191-26	Platelet survival	0.61	0.22	0.22	0.03	0.86	$31.13	XXX	A+
78191-TC	Platelet survival	0.00	6.97	6.97	0.31	7.28	$263.53	XXX	A+
78195	Lymph system imaging	1.20	4.31	4.31	0.23	5.74	$207.78	XXX	A+
78195-26	Lymph system imaging	1.20	0.44	0.44	0.05	1.69	$61.18	XXX	A+
78195-TC	Lymph system imaging	0.00	3.87	3.87	0.18	4.05	$146.61	XXX	A+
78199	Blood/lymph nuclear exam	0.00	0.00	0.00	0.00	0.00	$0.00	XXX	A+
78199-26	Blood/lymph nuclear exam	0.00	0.00	0.00	0.00	0.00	$0.00	XXX	A+
78199-TC	Blood/lymph nuclear exam	0.00	0.00	0.00	0.00	0.00	$0.00	XXX	A+
78201	Liver imaging	0.44	2.40	2.40	0.13	2.97	$107.51	XXX	A+
78201-26	Liver imaging	0.44	0.16	0.16	0.02	0.62	$22.44	XXX	A+
78201-TC	Liver imaging	0.00	2.24	2.24	0.11	2.35	$85.07	XXX	A+
78202	Liver imaging with flow	0.51	2.93	2.93	0.14	3.58	$129.59	XXX	A+
78202-26	Liver imaging with flow	0.51	0.19	0.19	0.02	0.72	$26.06	XXX	A+
78202-TC	Liver imaging with flow	0.00	2.74	2.74	0.12	2.86	$103.53	XXX	A+
78205	Liver imaging (3D)	0.71	5.87	5.87	0.29	6.87	$248.69	XXX	A+
78205-26	Liver imaging (3D)	0.71	0.26	0.26	0.03	1.00	$36.20	XXX	A+
78205-TC	Liver imaging (3D)	0.00	5.61	5.61	0.26	5.87	$212.49	XXX	A+
78206	Liver image (3d) w/flow	0.96	5.96	5.96	0.13	7.05	$255.20	XXX	A+
78206-26	Liver image (3d) w/flow	0.96	0.35	0.35	0.04	1.35	$48.87	XXX	A+
78206-TC	Liver image (3d) w/flow	0.00	5.61	5.61	0.09	5.70	$206.34	XXX	A+
78215	Liver and spleen imaging	0.49	2.97	2.97	0.14	3.60	$130.32	XXX	A+
78215-26	Liver and spleen imaging	0.49	0.18	0.18	0.02	0.69	$24.98	XXX	A+
78215-TC	Liver and spleen imaging	0.00	2.79	2.79	0.12	2.91	$105.34	XXX	A+

* **M** = multiple surgery adjustment applies
   Me = multiple endoscopy rules may apply
   B = bilateral surgery adjustment applies
   A = assistant-at-surgery restriction

A+ = assistant-at-surgery restriction unless medical necessity established with documentation
C = cosurgeons payable
C+ = cosurgeons payable if medical necessity established with documentation

T = team surgeons permitted
T+ = team surgeons payable if medical necessity established with documentation
§ = indicates services that are not covered by Medicare.

CPT five-digit codes, two-digit numeric modifiers, and descriptions only are © 2001 American Medical Association

Medicare RBRVS: The Physicians' Guide

Relative value units

CPT Code and Modifier	Description	Work RVU	Non Facility Practice Expense RVU	Facility Practice Expense RVU	PLI RVU	Total Non Facility RVUs	Medicare Payment Non Facility	Total Facility RVUs	Medicare Payment Facility	Global Period	Payment Policy Indicators*
78216	Liver & spleen image/flow	0.57	3.52	3.52	0.17	4.26	$154.21	4.26	$154.21	XXX	A+
78216-26	Liver & spleen image/flow	0.57	0.21	0.21	0.02	0.80	$28.96	0.80	$28.96	XXX	A+
78216-TC	Liver & spleen image/flow	0.00	3.31	3.31	0.15	3.46	$125.25	3.46	$125.25	XXX	A+
78220	Liver function study	0.49	3.72	3.72	0.18	4.39	$158.91	4.39	$158.91	XXX	A+
78220-26	Liver function study	0.49	0.18	0.18	0.02	0.69	$24.98	0.69	$24.98	XXX	A+
78220-TC	Liver function study	0.00	3.54	3.54	0.16	3.70	$133.94	3.70	$133.94	XXX	A+
78223	Hepatobiliary imaging	0.84	3.78	3.78	0.20	4.82	$174.48	4.82	$174.48	XXX	A+
78223-26	Hepatobiliary imaging	0.84	0.30	0.30	0.04	1.18	$42.72	1.18	$42.72	XXX	A+
78223-TC	Hepatobiliary imaging	0.00	3.48	3.48	0.16	3.64	$131.77	3.64	$131.77	XXX	A+
78230	Salivary gland imaging	0.45	2.23	2.23	0.13	2.81	$101.72	2.81	$101.72	XXX	A+
78230-26	Salivary gland imaging	0.45	0.16	0.16	0.02	0.63	$22.81	0.63	$22.81	XXX	A+
78230-TC	Salivary gland imaging	0.00	2.07	2.07	0.11	2.18	$78.91	2.18	$78.91	XXX	A+
78231	Serial salivary imaging	0.52	3.21	3.21	0.16	3.89	$140.81	3.89	$140.81	XXX	A+
78231-26	Serial salivary imaging	0.52	0.20	0.20	0.02	0.74	$26.79	0.74	$26.79	XXX	A+
78231-TC	Serial salivary imaging	0.00	3.01	3.01	0.14	3.15	$114.03	3.15	$114.03	XXX	A+
78232	Salivary gland function exam	0.47	3.54	3.54	0.16	4.17	$150.95	4.17	$150.95	XXX	A+
78232-26	Salivary gland function exam	0.47	0.18	0.18	0.01	0.66	$23.89	0.66	$23.89	XXX	A+
78232-TC	Salivary gland function exam	0.00	3.36	3.36	0.15	3.51	$127.06	3.51	$127.06	XXX	A+
78258	Esophageal motility study	0.74	3.01	3.01	0.15	3.90	$141.18	3.90	$141.18	XXX	A+
78258-26	Esophageal motility study	0.74	0.27	0.27	0.03	1.04	$37.65	1.04	$37.65	XXX	A+
78258-TC	Esophageal motility study	0.00	2.74	2.74	0.12	2.86	$103.53	2.86	$103.53	XXX	A+
78261	Gastric mucosa imaging	0.69	4.15	4.15	0.21	5.05	$182.81	5.05	$182.81	XXX	A+
78261-26	Gastric mucosa imaging	0.69	0.26	0.26	0.03	0.98	$35.48	0.98	$35.48	XXX	A+
78261-TC	Gastric mucosa imaging	0.00	3.89	3.89	0.18	4.07	$147.33	4.07	$147.33	XXX	A+
78262	Gastroesophageal reflux exam	0.68	4.29	4.29	0.21	5.18	$187.51	5.18	$187.51	XXX	A+
78262-26	Gastroesophageal reflux exam	0.68	0.25	0.25	0.03	0.96	$34.75	0.96	$34.75	XXX	A+
78262-TC	Gastroesophageal reflux exam	0.00	4.04	4.04	0.18	4.22	$152.76	4.22	$152.76	XXX	A+

Code	Description							
78264	Gastric emptying study	0.78	4.20	4.20	0.21	5.19	$187.87	5.19	$187.87	XXX	A+
78264-26	Gastric emptying study	0.78	0.28	0.28	0.03	1.09	$39.46	1.09	$39.46	XXX	A+
78264-TC	Gastric emptying study	0.00	3.92	3.92	0.18	4.10	$148.42	4.10	$148.42	XXX	A+
78270	Vit B-12 absorption exam	0.20	1.54	1.54	0.09	1.83	$66.24	1.83	$66.24	XXX	A+
78270-26	Vit B-12 absorption exam	0.20	0.07	0.07	0.01	0.28	$10.14	0.28	$10.14	XXX	A+
78270-TC	Vit B-12 absorption exam	0.00	1.47	1.47	0.08	1.55	$56.11	1.55	$56.11	XXX	A+
78271	Vit B-12 absorp exam, IF	0.20	1.63	1.63	0.09	1.92	$69.50	1.92	$69.50	XXX	A+
78271-26	Vit B-12 absorp exam, IF	0.20	0.07	0.07	0.01	0.28	$10.14	0.28	$10.14	XXX	A+
78271-TC	Vit B-12 absorp exam, IF	0.00	1.56	1.56	0.08	1.64	$59.37	1.64	$59.37	XXX	A+
78272	Vit B-12 absorp, combined	0.27	2.30	2.30	0.12	2.69	$97.38	2.69	$97.38	XXX	A+
78272-26	Vit B-12 absorp, combined	0.27	0.10	0.10	0.01	0.38	$13.76	0.38	$13.76	XXX	A+
78272-TC	Vit B-12 absorp, combined	0.00	2.20	2.20	0.11	2.31	$83.62	2.31	$83.62	XXX	A+
78278	Acute GI blood loss imaging	0.99	4.98	4.98	0.25	6.22	$225.16	6.22	$225.16	XXX	A+
78278-26	Acute GI blood loss imaging	0.99	0.35	0.35	0.04	1.38	$49.95	1.38	$49.95	XXX	A+
78278-TC	Acute GI blood loss imaging	0.00	4.63	4.63	0.21	4.84	$175.20	4.84	$175.20	XXX	A+
78282	GI protein loss exam	0.00	0.00	0.00	0.00	0.00	$0.00	0.00	$0.00	XXX	A+
78282-26	GI protein loss exam	0.38	0.13	0.13	0.02	0.53	$19.19	0.53	$19.19	XXX	A+
78282-TC	GI protein loss exam	0.00	0.00	0.00	0.00	0.00	$0.00	0.00	$0.00	XXX	A+
78290	Meckel's divert exam	0.68	3.13	3.13	0.16	3.97	$143.71	3.97	$143.71	XXX	A+
78290-26	Meckel's divert exam	0.68	0.24	0.24	0.03	0.95	$34.39	0.95	$34.39	XXX	A+
78290-TC	Meckel's divert exam	0.00	2.89	2.89	0.13	3.02	$109.32	3.02	$109.32	XXX	A+
78291	Leveen/shunt patency exam	0.88	3.23	3.23	0.17	4.28	$154.93	4.28	$154.93	XXX	A+
78291-26	Leveen/shunt patency exam	0.88	0.32	0.32	0.04	1.24	$44.89	1.24	$44.89	XXX	A+
78291-TC	Leveen/shunt patency exam	0.00	2.91	2.91	0.13	3.04	$110.05	3.04	$110.05	XXX	A+
78299	GI nuclear procedure	0.00	0.00	0.00	0.00	0.00	$0.00	0.00	$0.00	XXX	A+
78299-26	GI nuclear procedure	0.00	0.00	0.00	0.00	0.00	$0.00	0.00	$0.00	XXX	A+
78299-TC	GI nuclear procedure	0.00	0.00	0.00	0.00	0.00	$0.00	0.00	$0.00	XXX	A+
78300	Bone imaging, limited area	0.62	2.58	2.58	0.15	3.35	$121.27	3.35	$121.27	XXX	A+

* **M** = multiple surgery adjustment applies
Me = multiple endoscopy rules may apply
B = bilateral surgery adjustment applies
A = assistant-at-surgery restriction

A+ = assistant-at-surgery restriction unless medical necessity established with documentation
C = cosurgeons payable
C+ = cosurgeons payable if medical necessity established with documentation

T = team surgeons permitted
T+ = team surgeons payable if medical necessity established with documentation
§ = indicates services that are not covered by Medicare.

CPT five-digit codes, two-digit numeric modifiers, and descriptions only are © 2001 American Medical Association

Medicare RBRVS: The Physicians' Guide

Relative value units

CPT Code and Modifier	Description	Work RVU	Non Facility Practice Expense RVU	Facility Practice Expense RVU	PLI RVU	Total Non Facility RVUs	Medicare Payment Non Facility	Total Facility RVUs	Medicare Payment Facility	Global Period	Payment Policy Indicators*
78300-26	Bone imaging, limited area	0.62	0.22	0.22	0.03	0.87	$31.49	0.87	$31.49	XXX	A+
78300-TC	Bone imaging, limited area	0.00	2.36	2.36	0.12	2.48	$89.77	2.48	$89.77	XXX	A+
78305	Bone imaging, multiple areas	0.83	3.78	3.78	0.19	4.80	$173.76	4.80	$173.76	XXX	A+
78305-26	Bone imaging, multiple areas	0.83	0.30	0.30	0.03	1.16	$41.99	1.16	$41.99	XXX	A+
78305-TC	Bone imaging, multiple areas	0.00	3.48	3.48	0.16	3.64	$131.77	3.64	$131.77	XXX	A+
78306	Bone imaging, whole body	0.86	4.37	4.37	0.22	5.45	$197.29	5.45	$197.29	XXX	M A+
78306-26	Bone imaging, whole body	0.86	0.31	0.31	0.04	1.21	$43.80	1.21	$43.80	XXX	M A+
78306-TC	Bone imaging, whole body	0.00	4.06	4.06	0.18	4.24	$153.48	4.24	$153.48	XXX	M A+
78315	Bone imaging, 3 phase	1.02	4.91	4.91	0.25	6.18	$223.71	6.18	$223.71	XXX	A+
78315-26	Bone imaging, 3 phase	1.02	0.37	0.37	0.04	1.43	$51.76	1.43	$51.76	XXX	A+
78315-TC	Bone imaging, 3 phase	0.00	4.54	4.54	0.21	4.75	$171.95	4.75	$171.95	XXX	A+
78320	Bone imaging (3D)	1.04	6.00	6.00	0.30	7.34	$265.70	7.34	$265.70	XXX	M A+
78320-26	Bone imaging (3D)	1.04	0.39	0.39	0.04	1.47	$53.21	1.47	$53.21	XXX	M A+
78320-TC	Bone imaging (3D)	0.00	5.61	5.61	0.26	5.87	$212.49	5.87	$212.49	XXX	M A+
78350	Bone mineral, single photon	0.22	0.80	0.80	0.05	1.07	$38.73	1.07	$38.73	XXX	A+
78350-26	Bone mineral, single photon	0.22	0.08	0.08	0.01	0.31	$11.22	0.31	$11.22	XXX	A+
78350-TC	Bone mineral, single photon	0.00	0.72	0.72	0.04	0.76	$27.51	0.76	$27.51	XXX	A+
78351 §	Bone mineral, dual photon	0.30	1.64	0.12	0.01	1.95	$70.59	0.43	$15.57	XXX	
78399	Musculoskeletal nuclear exam	0.00	0.00	0.00	0.00	0.00	$0.00	0.00	$0.00	XXX	A+
78399-26	Musculoskeletal nuclear exam	0.00	0.00	0.00	0.00	0.00	$0.00	0.00	$0.00	XXX	A+
78399-TC	Musculoskeletal nuclear exam	0.00	0.00	0.00	0.00	0.00	$0.00	0.00	$0.00	XXX	A+
78414	Non-imaging heart function	0.00	0.00	0.00	0.00	0.00	$0.00	0.00	$0.00	XXX	A+
78414-26	Non-imaging heart function	0.45	0.16	0.16	0.02	0.63	$22.81	0.63	$22.81	XXX	A+
78414-TC	Non-imaging heart function	0.00	0.00	0.00	0.00	0.00	$0.00	0.00	$0.00	XXX	A+
78428	Cardiac shunt imaging	0.78	2.46	2.46	0.14	3.38	$122.35	3.38	$122.35	XXX	A+
78428-26	Cardiac shunt imaging	0.78	0.32	0.32	0.03	1.13	$40.91	1.13	$40.91	XXX	A+
78428-TC	Cardiac shunt imaging	0.00	2.14	2.14	0.11	2.25	$81.45	2.25	$81.45	XXX	A+

Code	Description							
78445	Vascular flow imaging	0.49	1.94	1.94	0.11	2.54	$91.95	$91.95	XXX	A+
78445-26	Vascular flow imaging	0.49	0.18	0.18	0.02	0.69	$24.98	$24.98	XXX	A+
78445-TC	Vascular flow imaging	0.00	1.76	1.76	0.09	1.85	$66.97	$66.97	XXX	A+
78455	Venous thrombosis study	0.73	4.04	4.04	0.20	4.97	$179.91	$179.91	XXX	A+
78455-26	Venous thrombosis study	0.73	0.26	0.26	0.03	1.02	$36.92	$36.92	XXX	A+
78455-TC	Venous thrombosis study	0.00	3.78	3.78	0.17	3.95	$142.99	$142.99	XXX	A+
78456	Acute venous thrombus image	1.00	4.15	4.15	0.28	5.43	$196.56	$196.56	XXX	
78456-26	Acute venous thrombus image	1.00	0.37	0.37	0.04	1.41	$51.04	$51.04	XXX	
78456-TC	Acute venous thrombus image	0.00	3.78	3.78	0.24	4.02	$145.52	$145.52	XXX	A+
78457	Venous thrombosis imaging	0.77	2.81	2.81	0.15	3.73	$135.02	$135.02	XXX	A+
78457-26	Venous thrombosis imaging	0.77	0.28	0.28	0.03	1.08	$39.10	$39.10	XXX	A+
78457-TC	Venous thrombosis imaging	0.00	2.53	2.53	0.12	2.65	$95.93	$95.93	XXX	A+
78458	Ven thrombosis images, bilat	0.90	4.17	4.17	0.20	5.27	$190.77	$190.77	XXX	A+
78458-26	Ven thrombosis images, bilat	0.90	0.35	0.35	0.03	1.28	$46.33	$46.33	XXX	A+
78458-TC	Ven thrombosis images, bilat	0.00	3.82	3.82	0.17	3.99	$144.43	$144.43	XXX	A+
78459-26 §	Heart muscle imaging (PET)	1.88	0.75	0.75	0.08	2.71	$98.10	$98.10	XXX	A+
78460	Heart muscle blood, single	0.86	2.55	2.55	0.14	3.55	$128.51	$128.51	XXX	A+
78460-26	Heart muscle blood, single	0.86	0.31	0.31	0.03	1.20	$43.44	$43.44	XXX	A+
78460-TC	Heart muscle blood, single	0.00	2.24	2.24	0.11	2.35	$85.07	$85.07	XXX	A+
78461	Heart muscle blood, multiple	1.23	4.94	4.94	0.26	6.43	$232.76	$232.76	XXX	A+
78461-26	Heart muscle blood, multiple	1.23	0.46	0.46	0.05	1.74	$62.99	$62.99	XXX	A+
78461-TC	Heart muscle blood, multiple	0.00	4.48	4.48	0.21	4.69	$169.77	$169.77	XXX	A+
78464	Heart image (3d), single	1.09	7.12	7.12	0.35	8.56	$309.87	$309.87	XXX	A+
78464-26	Heart image (3d), single	1.09	0.41	0.41	0.04	1.54	$55.75	$55.75	XXX	A+
78464-TC	Heart image (3d), single	0.00	6.71	6.71	0.31	7.02	$254.12	$254.12	XXX	A+
78465	Heart image (3d), multiple	1.46	11.76	11.76	0.56	13.78	$498.82	$498.82	XXX	A+
78465-26	Heart image (3d), multiple	1.46	0.56	0.56	0.05	2.07	$74.93	$74.93	XXX	A+
78465-TC	Heart image (3d), multiple	0.00	11.20	11.20	0.51	11.71	$423.89	$423.89	XXX	A+

* **M** = multiple surgery adjustment applies
Me = multiple endoscopy rules may apply
B = bilateral surgery adjustment applies
A = assistant-at-surgery restriction

A+ = assistant-at-surgery restriction unless medical necessity established with documentation
C = cosurgeons payable
C+ = cosurgeons payable if medical necessity established with documentation

T = team surgeons permitted
T+ = team surgeons payable if medical necessity established with documentation
$ = indicates services that are not covered by Medicare.

CPT five-digit codes, two-digit numeric modifiers, and descriptions only are © 2001 American Medical Association

Medicare RBRVS: The Physicians' Guide

Relative value units

CPT Code and Modifier	Description	Work RVU	Non Facility Practice Expense RVU	Facility Practice Expense RVU	PLI RVU	Total Non Facility RVUs	Medicare Payment Non Facility	Total Facility RVUs	Medicare Payment Facility	Global Period	Payment Policy Indicators*
78466	Heart infarct image	0.69	2.75	2.75	0.15	3.59	$129.96	3.59	$129.96	XXX	A+
78466-26	Heart infarct image	0.69	0.26	0.26	0.03	0.98	$35.48	0.98	$35.48	XXX	A+
78466-TC	Heart infarct image	0.00	2.49	2.49	0.12	2.61	$94.48	2.61	$94.48	XXX	A+
78468	Heart infarct image (ef)	0.80	3.78	3.78	0.19	4.77	$172.67	4.77	$172.67	XXX	A+
78468-26	Heart infarct image (ef)	0.80	0.30	0.30	0.03	1.13	$40.91	1.13	$40.91	XXX	A+
78468-TC	Heart infarct image (ef)	0.00	3.48	3.48	0.16	3.64	$131.77	3.64	$131.77	XXX	A+
78469	Heart infarct image (3D)	0.92	5.31	5.31	0.26	6.49	$234.93	6.49	$234.93	XXX	A+
78469-26	Heart infarct image (3D)	0.92	0.35	0.35	0.03	1.30	$47.06	1.30	$47.06	XXX	A+
78469-TC	Heart infarct image (3D)	0.00	4.96	4.96	0.23	5.19	$187.87	5.19	$187.87	XXX	A+
78472	Gated heart, planar, single	0.98	5.60	5.60	0.29	6.87	$248.69	6.87	$248.69	XXX	A+
78472-26	Gated heart, planar, single	0.98	0.37	0.37	0.04	1.39	$50.32	1.39	$50.32	XXX	A+
78472-TC	Gated heart, planar, single	0.00	5.23	5.23	0.25	5.48	$198.37	5.48	$198.37	XXX	A+
78473	Gated heart, multiple	1.47	8.40	8.40	0.40	10.27	$371.77	10.27	$371.77	XXX	A+
78473-26	Gated heart, multiple	1.47	0.56	0.56	0.05	2.08	$75.29	2.08	$75.29	XXX	A+
78473-TC	Gated heart, multiple	0.00	7.84	7.84	0.35	8.19	$296.47	8.19	$296.47	XXX	A+
78478	Heart wall motion add-on	0.62	1.72	1.72	0.10	2.44	$88.33	2.44	$88.33	ZZZ	A+
78478-26	Heart wall motion add-on	0.62	0.24	0.24	0.02	0.88	$31.86	0.88	$31.86	ZZZ	A+
78478-TC	Heart wall motion add-on	0.00	1.48	1.48	0.08	1.56	$56.47	1.56	$56.47	ZZZ	A+
78480	Heart function add-on	0.62	1.72	1.72	0.10	2.44	$88.33	2.44	$88.33	ZZZ	A+
78480-26	Heart function add-on	0.62	0.24	0.24	0.02	0.88	$31.86	0.88	$31.86	ZZZ	A+
78480-TC	Heart function add-on	0.00	1.48	1.48	0.08	1.56	$56.47	1.56	$56.47	ZZZ	A+
78481	Heart first pass, single	0.98	5.35	5.35	0.26	6.59	$238.55	6.59	$238.55	XXX	A+
78481-26	Heart first pass, single	0.98	0.39	0.39	0.03	1.40	$50.68	1.40	$50.68	XXX	A+
78481-TC	Heart first pass, single	0.00	4.96	4.96	0.23	5.19	$187.87	5.19	$187.87	XXX	A+
78483	Heart first pass, multiple	1.47	8.05	8.05	0.39	9.91	$358.73	9.91	$358.73	XXX	A+
78483-26	Heart first pass, multiple	1.47	0.58	0.58	0.05	2.10	$76.02	2.10	$76.02	XXX	A+
78483-TC	Heart first pass, multiple	0.00	7.47	7.47	0.34	7.81	$282.72	7.81	$282.72	XXX	A+

Code	Description							
78491-26 §	Heart image (pet), single	1.50	0.60	0.05	2.15	$77.83	$77.83	XXX
78492-26 §	Heart image (pet), multiple	1.87	0.75	0.06	2.68	$97.01	$97.01	XXX
78494	Heart image, spect	1.19	7.15	0.29	8.63	$312.40	$312.40	XXX	A+
78494-26	Heart image, spect	1.19	0.44	0.04	1.67	$60.45	$60.45	XXX	A+
78494-TC	Heart image, spect	0.00	6.71	0.25	6.96	$251.95	$251.95	XXX	A+
78496	Heart first pass add-on	0.50	6.91	0.27	7.68	$278.01	$278.01	ZZZ	A+
78496-26	Heart first pass add-on	0.50	0.20	0.02	0.72	$26.06	$26.06	ZZZ	A+
78496-TC	Heart first pass add-on	0.00	6.71	0.25	6.96	$251.95	$251.95	ZZZ	A+
78499	Cardiovascular nuclear exam	0.00	0.00	0.00	0.00	$0.00	$0.00	XXX	A+
78499-26	Cardiovascular nuclear exam	0.00	0.00	0.00	0.00	$0.00	$0.00	XXX	A+
78499-TC	Cardiovascular nuclear exam	0.00	0.00	0.00	0.00	$0.00	$0.00	XXX	A+
78580	Lung perfusion imaging	0.74	3.53	0.18	4.45	$161.09	$161.09	XXX	A+
78580-26	Lung perfusion imaging	0.74	0.27	0.03	1.04	$37.65	$37.65	XXX	A+
78580-TC	Lung perfusion imaging	0.00	3.26	0.15	3.41	$123.44	$123.44	XXX	A+
78584	Lung V/Q image single breath	0.99	3.39	0.18	4.56	$165.07	$165.07	XXX	A+
78584-26	Lung V/Q image single breath	0.99	0.35	0.04	1.38	$49.95	$49.95	XXX	A+
78584-TC	Lung V/Q image single breath	0.00	3.04	0.14	3.18	$115.11	$115.11	XXX	A+
78585	Lung V/Q imaging	1.09	5.74	0.30	7.13	$258.10	$258.10	XXX	A+
78585-26	Lung V/Q imaging	1.09	0.39	0.05	1.53	$55.38	$55.38	XXX	A+
78585-TC	Lung V/Q imaging	0.00	5.35	0.25	5.60	$202.72	$202.72	XXX	A+
78586	Aerosol lung image, single	0.40	2.60	0.14	3.14	$113.67	$113.67	XXX	A+
78586-26	Aerosol lung image, single	0.40	0.14	0.02	0.56	$20.27	$20.27	XXX	A+
78586-TC	Aerosol lung image, single	0.00	2.46	0.12	2.58	$93.39	$93.39	XXX	A+
78587	Aerosol lung image, multiple	0.49	2.84	0.14	3.47	$125.61	$125.61	XXX	A+
78587-26	Aerosol lung image, multiple	0.49	0.18	0.02	0.69	$24.98	$24.98	XXX	A+
78587-TC	Aerosol lung image, multiple	0.00	2.66	0.12	2.78	$100.63	$100.63	XXX	A+
78588	Perfusion lung image	1.09	3.43	0.20	4.72	$170.86	$170.86	XXX	A+
78588-26	Perfusion lung image	1.09	0.39	0.05	1.53	$55.38	$55.38	XXX	A+

* **M** = multiple surgery adjustment applies
Me = multiple endoscopy rules may apply
B = bilateral surgery adjustment applies
A = assistant-at-surgery restriction

A+ = assistant-at-surgery restriction unless medical necessity established with documentation
C = cosurgeons payable
C+ = cosurgeons payable if medical necessity established with documentation

T = team surgeons permitted
T+ = team surgeons payable if medical necessity established with documentation
$ = indicates services that are not covered by Medicare.

377 CPT five-digit codes, two-digit numeric modifiers, and descriptions only are © 2001 American Medical Association

Medicare RBRVS: The Physicians' Guide

Relative value units

CPT Code and Modifier	Description	Work RVU	Non Facility Practice Expense RVU	Facility Practice Expense RVU	PLI RVU	Total Non Facility RVUs	Medicare Payment Non Facility	Total Facility RVUs	Medicare Payment Facility	Global Period	Payment Policy Indicators*
78588-TC	Perfusion lung image	0.00	3.04	3.04	0.15	3.19	$115.48	3.19	$115.48	XXX	A+
78591	Vent image, 1 breath, 1 proj	0.40	2.86	2.86	0.14	3.40	$123.08	3.40	$123.08	XXX	A+
78591-26	Vent image, 1 breath, 1 proj	0.40	0.15	0.15	0.02	0.57	$20.63	0.57	$20.63	XXX	A+
78591-TC	Vent image, 1 breath, 1 proj	0.00	2.71	2.71	0.12	2.83	$102.44	2.83	$102.44	XXX	A+
78593	Vent image, 1 proj, gas	0.49	3.46	3.46	0.17	4.12	$149.14	4.12	$149.14	XXX	A+
78593-26	Vent image, 1 proj, gas	0.49	0.18	0.18	0.02	0.69	$24.98	0.69	$24.98	XXX	A+
78593-TC	Vent image, 1 proj, gas	0.00	3.28	3.28	0.15	3.43	$124.16	3.43	$124.16	XXX	A+
78594	Vent image, mult proj, gas	0.53	4.92	4.92	0.23	5.68	$205.61	5.68	$205.61	XXX	A+
78594-26	Vent image, mult proj, gas	0.53	0.19	0.19	0.02	0.74	$26.79	0.74	$26.79	XXX	A+
78594-TC	Vent image, mult proj, gas	0.00	4.73	4.73	0.21	4.94	$178.82	4.94	$178.82	XXX	A+
78596	Lung differential function	1.27	7.17	7.17	0.36	8.80	$318.55	8.80	$318.55	XXX	A+
78596-26	Lung differential function	1.27	0.46	0.46	0.05	1.78	$64.43	1.78	$64.43	XXX	A+
78596-TC	Lung differential function	0.00	6.71	6.71	0.31	7.02	$254.12	7.02	$254.12	XXX	A+
78599	Respiratory nuclear exam	0.00	0.00	0.00	0.00	0.00	$0.00	0.00	$0.00	XXX	A+
78599-26	Respiratory nuclear exam	0.00	0.00	0.00	0.00	0.00	$0.00	0.00	$0.00	XXX	A+
78599-TC	Respiratory nuclear exam	0.00	0.00	0.00	0.00	0.00	$0.00	0.00	$0.00	XXX	A+
78600	Brain imaging, ltd static	0.44	2.90	2.90	0.14	3.48	$125.97	3.48	$125.97	XXX	A+
78600-26	Brain imaging, ltd static	0.44	0.16	0.16	0.02	0.62	$22.44	0.62	$22.44	XXX	A+
78600-TC	Brain imaging, ltd static	0.00	2.74	2.74	0.12	2.86	$103.53	2.86	$103.53	XXX	A+
78601	Brain imaging, ltd w/ flow	0.51	3.41	3.41	0.17	4.09	$148.05	4.09	$148.05	XXX	A+
78601-26	Brain imaging, ltd w/ flow	0.51	0.18	0.18	0.02	0.71	$25.70	0.71	$25.70	XXX	A+
78601-TC	Brain imaging, ltd w/ flow	0.00	3.23	3.23	0.15	3.38	$122.35	3.38	$122.35	XXX	A+
78605	Brain imaging, complete	0.53	3.42	3.42	0.17	4.12	$149.14	4.12	$149.14	XXX	A+
78605-26	Brain imaging, complete	0.53	0.19	0.19	0.02	0.74	$26.79	0.74	$26.79	XXX	A+
78605-TC	Brain imaging, complete	0.00	3.23	3.23	0.15	3.38	$122.35	3.38	$122.35	XXX	A+
78606	Brain imaging, compl w/flow	0.64	3.90	3.90	0.20	4.74	$171.58	4.74	$171.58	XXX	A+
78606-26	Brain imaging, compl w/flow	0.64	0.23	0.23	0.03	0.90	$32.58	0.90	$32.58	XXX	A+

Code	Description							
78606-TC	Brain imaging, compl w/flow	0.00	3.67	3.67	0.17	3.84	$139.00	XXX	A+
78607	Brain imaging (3D)	1.23	6.70	6.70	0.34	8.27	$299.37	XXX	A+
78607-26	Brain imaging (3D)	1.23	0.47	0.47	0.05	1.75	$63.35	XXX	A+
78607-TC	Brain imaging (3D)	0.00	6.23	6.23	0.29	6.52	$236.02	XXX	A+
78610	Brain flow imaging only	0.30	1.61	1.61	0.09	2.00	$72.40	XXX	A+
78610-26	Brain flow imaging only	0.30	0.11	0.11	0.01	0.42	$15.20	XXX	A+
78610-TC	Brain flow imaging only	0.00	1.50	1.50	0.08	1.58	$57.19	XXX	A+
78615	Cerebral vascular flow image	0.42	3.81	3.81	0.19	4.42	$160.00	XXX	A+
78615-26	Cerebral vascular flow image	0.42	0.16	0.16	0.02	0.60	$21.72	XXX	A+
78615-TC	Cerebral vascular flow image	0.00	3.65	3.65	0.17	3.82	$138.28	XXX	A+
78630	Cerebrospinal fluid scan	0.68	5.02	5.02	0.25	5.95	$215.39	XXX	A+
78630-26	Cerebrospinal fluid scan	0.68	0.24	0.24	0.03	0.95	$34.39	XXX	A+
78630-TC	Cerebrospinal fluid scan	0.00	4.78	4.78	0.22	5.00	$181.00	XXX	A+
78635	CSF ventriculography	0.61	2.67	2.67	0.14	3.42	$123.80	XXX	A+
78635-26	CSF ventriculography	0.61	0.25	0.25	0.02	0.88	$31.86	XXX	A+
78635-TC	CSF ventriculography	0.00	2.42	2.42	0.12	2.54	$91.95	XXX	A+
78645	CSF shunt evaluation	0.57	3.47	3.47	0.17	4.21	$152.40	XXX	A+
78645-26	CSF shunt evaluation	0.57	0.21	0.21	0.02	0.80	$28.96	XXX	A+
78645-TC	CSF shunt evaluation	0.00	3.26	3.26	0.15	3.41	$123.44	XXX	A+
78647	Cerebrospinal fluid scan	0.90	5.94	5.94	0.29	7.13	$258.10	XXX	A+
78647-26	Cerebrospinal fluid scan	0.90	0.33	0.33	0.03	1.26	$45.61	XXX	A+
78647-TC	Cerebrospinal fluid scan	0.00	5.61	5.61	0.26	5.87	$212.49	XXX	A+
78650	CSF leakage imaging	0.61	4.63	4.63	0.22	5.46	$197.65	XXX	A+
78650-26	CSF leakage imaging	0.61	0.22	0.22	0.02	0.85	$30.77	XXX	A+
78650-TC	CSF leakage imaging	0.00	4.41	4.41	0.20	4.61	$166.88	XXX	A+
78660	Nuclear exam of tear flow	0.53	2.20	2.20	0.12	2.85	$103.17	XXX	A+
78660-26	Nuclear exam of tear flow	0.53	0.19	0.19	0.02	0.74	$26.79	XXX	A+
78660-TC	Nuclear exam of tear flow	0.00	2.01	2.01	0.10	2.11	$76.38	XXX	A+

* **M** = multiple surgery adjustment applies
Me = multiple endoscopy rules may apply
B = bilateral surgery adjustment applies
A = assistant-at-surgery restriction

A+ = assistant-at-surgery restriction unless medical necessity established with documentation
C = cosurgeons payable
C+ = cosurgeons payable if medical necessity established with documentation

T = team surgeons permitted
T+ = team surgeons payable if medical necessity established with documentation
$ = indicates services that are not covered by Medicare.

Medicare RBRVS: The Physicians' Guide

Relative value units

CPT Code and Modifier	Description	Work RVU	Non Facility Practice Expense RVU	Facility Practice Expense RVU	PLI RVU	Total Non Facility RVUs	Medicare Payment Non Facility	Total Facility RVUs	Medicare Payment Facility	Global Period	Payment Policy Indicators*
78699	Nervous system nuclear exam	0.00	0.00	0.00	0.00	0.00	$0.00	0.00	$0.00	XXX	A+
78699-26	Nervous system nuclear exam	0.00	0.00	0.00	0.00	0.00	$0.00	0.00	$0.00	XXX	A+
78699-TC	Nervous system nuclear exam	0.00	0.00	0.00	0.00	0.00	$0.00	0.00	$0.00	XXX	A+
78700	Kidney imaging, static	0.45	3.05	3.05	0.15	3.65	$132.13	3.65	$132.13	XXX	A+
78700-26	Kidney imaging, static	0.45	0.16	0.16	0.02	0.63	$22.81	0.63	$22.81	XXX	A+
78700-TC	Kidney imaging, static	0.00	2.89	2.89	0.13	3.02	$109.32	3.02	$109.32	XXX	A+
78701	Kidney imaging with flow	0.49	3.55	3.55	0.17	4.21	$152.40	4.21	$152.40	XXX	A+
78701-26	Kidney imaging with flow	0.49	0.17	0.17	0.02	0.68	$24.62	0.68	$24.62	XXX	A+
78701-TC	Kidney imaging with flow	0.00	3.38	3.38	0.15	3.53	$127.78	3.53	$127.78	XXX	A+
78704	Imaging renogram	0.74	4.03	4.03	0.20	4.97	$179.91	4.97	$179.91	XXX	A+
78704-26	Imaging renogram	0.74	0.27	0.27	0.03	1.04	$37.65	1.04	$37.65	XXX	A+
78704-TC	Imaging renogram	0.00	3.76	3.76	0.17	3.93	$142.26	3.93	$142.26	XXX	A+
78707	Kidney flow/function image	0.96	4.59	4.59	0.23	5.78	$209.23	5.78	$209.23	XXX	A+
78707-26	Kidney flow/function image	0.96	0.35	0.35	0.04	1.35	$48.87	1.35	$48.87	XXX	A+
78707-TC	Kidney flow/function image	0.00	4.24	4.24	0.19	4.43	$160.36	4.43	$160.36	XXX	A+
78708	Kidney flow/function image	1.21	4.68	4.68	0.24	6.13	$221.90	6.13	$221.90	XXX	A+
78708-26	Kidney flow/function image	1.21	0.44	0.44	0.05	1.70	$61.54	1.70	$61.54	XXX	A+
78708-TC	Kidney flow/function image	0.00	4.24	4.24	0.19	4.43	$160.36	4.43	$160.36	XXX	A+
78709	Kidney flow/function image	1.41	4.75	4.75	0.25	6.41	$232.04	6.41	$232.04	XXX	A+
78709-26	Kidney flow/function image	1.41	0.51	0.51	0.06	1.98	$71.67	1.98	$71.67	XXX	A+
78709-TC	Kidney flow/function image	0.00	4.24	4.24	0.19	4.43	$160.36	4.43	$160.36	XXX	A+
78710	Kidney imaging (3D)	0.66	5.84	5.84	0.29	6.79	$245.79	6.79	$245.79	XXX	A+
78710-26	Kidney imaging (3D)	0.66	0.23	0.23	0.03	0.92	$33.30	0.92	$33.30	XXX	A+
78710-TC	Kidney imaging (3D)	0.00	5.61	5.61	0.26	5.87	$212.49	5.87	$212.49	XXX	A+
78715	Renal vascular flow exam	0.30	1.61	1.61	0.09	2.00	$72.40	2.00	$72.40	XXX	A+
78715-26	Renal vascular flow exam	0.30	0.11	0.11	0.01	0.42	$15.20	0.42	$15.20	XXX	A+
78715-TC	Renal vascular flow exam	0.00	1.50	1.50	0.08	1.58	$57.19	1.58	$57.19	XXX	A+

Code	Description								
78725	Kidney function study	0.38	1.83	1.83	0.10	2.31	$83.62	XXX	A+
78725-26	Kidney function study	0.38	0.14	0.14	0.01	0.53	$19.19	XXX	A+
78725-TC	Kidney function study	0.00	1.69	1.69	0.09	1.78	$64.43	XXX	A+
78730	Urinary bladder retention	0.36	1.52	1.52	0.09	1.97	$71.31	XXX	A+
78730-26	Urinary bladder retention	0.36	0.13	0.13	0.02	0.51	$18.46	XXX	A+
78730-TC	Urinary bladder retention	0.00	1.39	1.39	0.07	1.46	$52.85	XXX	A+
78740	Ureteral reflux study	0.57	2.22	2.22	0.12	2.91	$105.34	XXX	A+
78740-26	Ureteral reflux study	0.57	0.21	0.21	0.02	0.80	$28.96	XXX	A+
78740-TC	Ureteral reflux study	0.00	2.01	2.01	0.10	2.11	$76.38	XXX	A+
78760	Testicular imaging	0.66	2.77	2.77	0.15	3.58	$129.59	XXX	A+
78760-26	Testicular imaging	0.66	0.23	0.23	0.03	0.92	$33.30	XXX	A+
78760-TC	Testicular imaging	0.00	2.54	2.54	0.12	2.66	$96.29	XXX	A+
78761	Testicular imaging/flow	0.71	3.30	3.30	0.17	4.18	$151.31	XXX	A+
78761-26	Testicular imaging/flow	0.71	0.26	0.26	0.03	1.00	$36.20	XXX	A+
78761-TC	Testicular imaging/flow	0.00	3.04	3.04	0.14	3.18	$115.11	XXX	A+
78799	Genitourinary nuclear exam	0.00	0.00	0.00	0.00	0.00	$0.00	XXX	A+
78799-26	Genitourinary nuclear exam	0.00	0.00	0.00	0.00	0.00	$0.00	XXX	A+
78799-TC	Genitourinary nuclear exam	0.00	0.00	0.00	0.00	0.00	$0.00	XXX	A+
78800	Tumor imaging, limited area	0.66	3.46	3.46	0.18	4.30	$155.66	XXX	A+
78800-26	Tumor imaging, limited area	0.66	0.23	0.23	0.03	0.92	$33.30	XXX	A+
78800-TC	Tumor imaging, limited area	0.00	3.23	3.23	0.15	3.38	$122.35	XXX	A+
78801	Tumor imaging, mult areas	0.79	4.30	4.30	0.21	5.30	$191.86	XXX	A+
78801-26	Tumor imaging, mult areas	0.79	0.29	0.29	0.03	1.11	$40.18	XXX	A+
78801-TC	Tumor imaging, mult areas	0.00	4.01	4.01	0.18	4.19	$151.67	XXX	A+
78802	Tumor imaging, whole body	0.86	5.57	5.57	0.28	6.71	$242.90	XXX	M A+
78802-26	Tumor imaging, whole body	0.86	0.32	0.32	0.03	1.21	$43.80	XXX	A+
78802-TC	Tumor imaging, whole body	0.00	5.25	5.25	0.25	5.50	$199.10	XXX	M A+
78803	Tumor imaging (3D)	1.09	6.64	6.64	0.33	8.06	$291.77	XXX	M A+

*M = multiple surgery adjustment applies
Me = multiple endoscopy rules may apply
B = bilateral surgery adjustment applies
A = assistant-at-surgery restriction

A+ = assistant-at-surgery restriction unless medical necessity established with documentation
C = cosurgeons payable
C+ = cosurgeons payable if medical necessity established with documentation

T = team surgeons permitted
T+ = team surgeons payable if medical necessity established with documentation
$ = indicates services that are not covered by Medicare.

381   CPT five-digit codes, two-digit numeric modifiers, and descriptions only are © 2001 American Medical Association

Medicare RBRVS: The Physicians' Guide

Relative value units

CPT Code and Modifier	Description	Work RVU	Non Facility Practice Expense RVU	Facility Practice Expense RVU	PLI RVU	Total Non Facility RVUs	Medicare Payment Non Facility	Total Facility RVUs	Medicare Payment Facility	Global Period	Payment Policy Indicators*
78803-26	Tumor imaging (3D)	1.09	0.41	0.41	0.04	1.54	$55.75	1.54	$55.75	XXX	M A+
78803-TC	Tumor imaging (3D)	0.00	6.23	6.23	0.29	6.52	$236.02	6.52	$236.02	XXX	M A+
78805	Abscess imaging, ltd area	0.73	3.50	3.50	0.18	4.41	$159.64	4.41	$159.64	XXX	A+
78805-26	Abscess imaging, ltd area	0.73	0.27	0.27	0.03	1.03	$37.29	1.03	$37.29	XXX	A+
78805-TC	Abscess imaging, ltd area	0.00	3.23	3.23	0.15	3.38	$122.35	3.38	$122.35	XXX	A+
78806	Abscess imaging, whole body	0.86	6.43	6.43	0.32	7.61	$275.48	7.61	$275.48	XXX	M A+
78806-26	Abscess imaging, whole body	0.86	0.32	0.32	0.03	1.21	$43.80	1.21	$43.80	XXX	M A+
78806-TC	Abscess imaging, whole body	0.00	6.11	6.11	0.29	6.40	$231.67	6.40	$231.67	XXX	M A+
78807	Nuclear localization/abscess	1.09	6.66	6.66	0.33	8.08	$292.49	8.08	$292.49	XXX	M A+
78807-26	Nuclear localization/abscess	1.09	0.43	0.43	0.04	1.56	$56.47	1.56	$56.47	XXX	M A+
78807-TC	Nuclear localization/abscess	0.00	6.23	6.23	0.29	6.52	$236.02	6.52	$236.02	XXX	M A+
78810-26 §	Tumor imaging (PET)	1.93	0.77	0.77	0.09	2.79	$101.00	2.79	$101.00	XXX	
78890 §	Nuclear medicine data proc	0.05	1.26	1.26	0.06	1.37	$49.59	1.37	$49.59	XXX	
78890-26 §	Nuclear medicine data proc	0.05	0.02	0.02	0.01	0.08	$2.90	0.08	$2.90	XXX	
78890-TC §	Nuclear medicine data proc	0.00	1.24	1.24	0.05	1.29	$46.70	1.29	$46.70	XXX	
78891 §	Nuclear med data proc	0.10	2.53	2.53	0.12	2.75	$99.55	2.75	$99.55	XXX	
78891-26 §	Nuclear med data proc	0.10	0.04	0.04	0.01	0.15	$5.43	0.15	$5.43	XXX	
78891-TC §	Nuclear med data proc	0.00	2.49	2.49	0.11	2.60	$94.12	2.60	$94.12	XXX	
78999	Nuclear diagnostic exam	0.00	0.00	0.00	0.00	0.00	$0.00	0.00	$0.00	XXX	A+
78999-26	Nuclear diagnostic exam	0.00	0.00	0.00	0.00	0.00	$0.00	0.00	$0.00	XXX	A+
78999-TC	Nuclear diagnostic exam	0.00	0.00	0.00	0.00	0.00	$0.00	0.00	$0.00	XXX	A+
79000	Init hyperthyroid therapy	1.80	3.14	3.14	0.19	5.13	$185.70	5.13	$185.70	XXX	A+
79000-26	Init hyperthyroid therapy	1.80	0.65	0.65	0.07	2.52	$91.22	2.52	$91.22	XXX	
79000-TC	Init hyperthyroid therapy	0.00	2.49	2.49	0.12	2.61	$94.48	2.61	$94.48	XXX	A+
79001	Repeat hyperthyroid therapy	1.05	1.63	1.63	0.10	2.78	$100.63	2.78	$100.63	XXX	A+
79001-26	Repeat hyperthyroid therapy	1.05	0.39	0.39	0.04	1.48	$53.57	1.48	$53.57	XXX	A+
79001-TC	Repeat hyperthyroid therapy	0.00	1.24	1.24	0.06	1.30	$47.06	1.30	$47.06	XXX	A+

79020	Thyroid ablation	1.81	3.13	3.13	0.19	5.13	$185.70	XXX	A+
79020-26	Thyroid ablation	1.81	0.64	0.64	0.07	2.52	$91.22	XXX	A+
79020-TC	Thyroid ablation	0.00	2.49	2.49	0.12	2.61	$94.48	XXX	A+
79030	Thyroid ablation, carcinoma	2.10	3.26	3.26	0.20	5.56	$201.27	XXX	A+
79030-26	Thyroid ablation, carcinoma	2.10	0.77	0.77	0.08	2.95	$106.79	XXX	A+
79030-TC	Thyroid ablation, carcinoma	0.00	2.49	2.49	0.12	2.61	$94.48	XXX	A+
79035	Thyroid metastatic therapy	2.52	3.43	3.43	0.21	6.16	$222.99	XXX	A+
79035-26	Thyroid metastatic therapy	2.52	0.94	0.94	0.09	3.55	$128.51	XXX	A+
79035-TC	Thyroid metastatic therapy	0.00	2.49	2.49	0.12	2.61	$94.48	XXX	A+
79100	Hematopoetic nuclear therapy	1.32	3.00	3.00	0.17	4.49	$162.53	XXX	A+
79100-26	Hematopoetic nuclear therapy	1.32	0.51	0.51	0.05	1.88	$68.05	XXX	A+
79100-TC	Hematopoetic nuclear therapy	0.00	2.49	2.49	0.12	2.61	$94.48	XXX	A+
79200	Intracavitary nuclear trmt	1.99	3.23	3.23	0.19	5.41	$195.84	XXX	A+
79200-26	Intracavitary nuclear trmt	1.99	0.74	0.74	0.07	2.80	$101.36	XXX	A+
79200-TC	Intracavitary nuclear trmt	0.00	2.49	2.49	0.12	2.61	$94.48	XXX	A+
79300	Interstitial nuclear therapy	0.00	0.00	0.00	0.00	0.00	$0.00	XXX	A+
79300-26	Interstitial nuclear therapy	1.60	0.68	0.68	0.07	2.35	$85.07	XXX	A+
79300-TC	Interstitial nuclear therapy	0.00	0.00	0.00	0.00	0.00	$0.00	XXX	A+
79400	Nonhemato nuclear therapy	1.96	3.22	3.22	0.20	5.38	$194.75	XXX	A+
79400-26	Nonhemato nuclear therapy	1.96	0.73	0.73	0.08	2.77	$100.27	XXX	A+
79400-TC	Nonhemato nuclear therapy	0.00	2.49	2.49	0.12	2.61	$94.48	XXX	A+
79420	Intravascular nuclear ther	0.00	0.00	0.00	0.00	0.00	$0.00	XXX	A+
79420-26	Intravascular nuclear ther	1.51	0.54	0.54	0.06	2.11	$76.38	XXX	A+
79420-TC	Intravascular nuclear ther	0.00	0.00	0.00	0.00	0.00	$0.00	XXX	A+
79440	Nuclear joint therapy	1.99	3.29	3.29	0.20	5.48	$198.37	XXX	A+
79440-26	Nuclear joint therapy	1.99	0.80	0.80	0.08	2.87	$103.89	XXX	A+
79440-TC	Nuclear joint therapy	0.00	2.49	2.49	0.12	2.61	$94.48	XXX	A+

* **M** = multiple surgery adjustment applies
Me = multiple endoscopy rules may apply
B = bilateral surgery adjustment applies
A = assistant-at-surgery restriction

A+ = assistant-at-surgery restriction unless medical necessity established with documentation
C = cosurgeons payable
C+ = cosurgeons payable if medical necessity established with documentation

T = team surgeons permitted
T+ = team surgeons payable if medical necessity established with documentation
$ = indicates services that are not covered by Medicare.

CPT five-digit codes, two-digit numeric modifiers, and descriptions only are © 2001 American Medical Association

Relative value units

CPT Code and Modifier	Description	Work RVU	Non Facility Practice Expense RVU	Facility Practice Expense RVU	PLI RVU	Total Non Facility RVUs	Medicare Payment Non Facility	Total Facility RVUs	Medicare Payment Facility	Global Period	Payment Policy Indicators*
79900	Provide ther radiopharm(s)	0.00	0.00	0.00	0.00	0.00	$0.00	0.00	$0.00	XXX	A+
79999	Nuclear medicine therapy	0.00	0.00	0.00	0.00	0.00	$0.00	0.00	$0.00	XXX	A+
79999-26	Nuclear medicine therapy	0.00	0.00	0.00	0.00	0.00	$0.00	0.00	$0.00	XXX	A+
79999-TC	Nuclear medicine therapy	0.00	0.00	0.00	0.00	0.00	$0.00	0.00	$0.00	XXX	A+
Pathology and laboratory: Consultations (Clinical Pathology)											
80500	Lab pathology consultation	0.37	0.21	0.17	0.01	0.59	$21.36	0.55	$19.91	XXX	A+
80502	Lab pathology consultation	1.33	0.63	0.61	0.05	2.01	$72.76	1.99	$72.04	XXX	A+
Pathology and laboratory: Chemistry											
83020-26	Hemoglobin electrophoresis	0.37	0.17	0.17	0.01	0.55	$19.91	0.55	$19.91	XXX	A+
83912-26	Genetic examination	0.37	0.17	0.17	0.01	0.55	$19.91	0.55	$19.91	XXX	A+
84165-26	Assay of serum proteins	0.37	0.17	0.17	0.01	0.55	$19.91	0.55	$19.91	XXX	A+
84181-26	Western blot test	0.37	0.15	0.15	0.01	0.53	$19.19	0.53	$19.19	XXX	A+
84182-26	Protein, western blot test	0.37	0.15	0.15	0.01	0.53	$19.19	0.53	$19.19	XXX	A+
Pathology and laboratory: Hematology and coagulation											
85060	Blood smear interpretation	0.45	0.19	0.19	0.02	0.66	$23.89	0.66	$23.89	XXX	A+
85097	Bone marrow interpretation	0.94	1.75	0.43	0.03	2.72	$98.46	1.40	$50.68	XXX	A+
85390-26	Fibrinolysins screen	0.37	0.12	0.12	0.01	0.50	$18.10	0.50	$18.10	XXX	A+
85576-26	Blood platelet aggregation	0.37	0.16	0.16	0.01	0.54	$19.55	0.54	$19.55	XXX	A+
Pathology and laboratory: Immunology											
86077	Physician blood bank service	0.94	0.48	0.43	0.03	1.45	$52.49	1.40	$50.68	XXX	A+
86078	Physician blood bank service	0.94	0.51	0.43	0.03	1.48	$53.57	1.40	$50.68	XXX	A+
86079	Physician blood bank service	0.94	0.50	0.44	0.03	1.47	$53.21	1.41	$51.04	XXX	A+
86255-26	Fluorescent antibody, screen	0.37	0.17	0.17	0.01	0.55	$19.91	0.55	$19.91	XXX	A+
86256-26	Fluorescent antibody, titer	0.37	0.17	0.17	0.01	0.55	$19.91	0.55	$19.91	XXX	A+
86320-26	Serum immunoelectrophoresis	0.37	0.17	0.17	0.01	0.55	$19.91	0.55	$19.91	XXX	A+
86325-26	Other immunoelectrophoresis	0.37	0.17	0.17	0.01	0.55	$19.91	0.55	$19.91	XXX	A+

Code	Description							
86327-26	Immunoelectrophoresis assay	0.42	0.20	0.01	0.63	$22.81	0.63	$22.81	XXX	A+
86334-26	Immunofixation procedure	0.37	0.17	0.01	0.55	$19.91	0.55	$19.91	XXX	A+
86485	Skin test, candida	0.00	0.00	0.00	0.00	$0.00	0.00	$0.00	XXX	A+
86490	Coccidioidomycosis skin test	0.00	0.28	0.02	0.30	$10.86	0.30	$10.86	XXX	A+
86510	Histoplasmosis skin test	0.00	0.30	0.02	0.32	$11.58	0.32	$11.58	XXX	A+
86580	TB intradermal test	0.00	0.24	0.02	0.26	$9.41	0.26	$9.41	XXX	A+
86585	TB tine test	0.00	0.19	0.01	0.20	$7.24	0.20	$7.24	XXX	A+
86586	Skin test, unlisted	0.00	0.00	0.00	0.00	$0.00	0.00	$0.00	XXX	A+

Pathology and laboratory: Microbiology

87164-26	Dark field examination	0.37	0.12	0.01	0.50	$18.10	0.49	$17.74	XXX	A+
87207-26	Smear, special stain	0.37	0.18	0.01	0.56	$20.27	0.55	$19.91	XXX	A+

Pathology and laboratory: Anatomic pathology

88104	Cytopathology, fluids	0.56	0.72	0.04	1.32	$47.78	1.32	$47.78	XXX	A+
88104-26	Cytopathology, fluids	0.56	0.26	0.02	0.84	$30.41	0.84	$30.41	XXX	A+
88104-TC	Cytopathology, fluids	0.00	0.46	0.02	0.48	$17.38	0.48	$17.38	XXX	A+
88106	Cytopathology, fluids	0.56	0.72	0.04	1.32	$47.78	1.32	$47.78	XXX	A+
88106-26	Cytopathology, fluids	0.56	0.26	0.02	0.84	$30.41	0.84	$30.41	XXX	A+
88106-TC	Cytopathology, fluids	0.00	0.46	0.02	0.48	$17.38	0.48	$17.38	XXX	A+
88107	Cytopathology, fluids	0.76	1.01	0.05	1.82	$65.88	1.82	$65.88	XXX	A+
88107-26	Cytopathology, fluids	0.76	0.35	0.03	1.14	$41.27	1.14	$41.27	XXX	A+
88107-TC	Cytopathology, fluids	0.00	0.66	0.02	0.68	$24.62	0.68	$24.62	XXX	A+
88108	Cytopath, concentrate tech	0.56	0.94	0.04	1.54	$55.75	1.54	$55.75	XXX	A+
88108-26	Cytopath, concentrate tech	0.56	0.26	0.02	0.84	$30.41	0.84	$30.41	XXX	A+
88108-TC	Cytopath, concentrate tech	0.00	0.68	0.02	0.70	$25.34	0.70	$25.34	XXX	A+
88125	Forensic cytopathology	0.26	0.30	0.02	0.58	$21.00	0.58	$21.00	XXX	A+
88125-26	Forensic cytopathology	0.26	0.12	0.01	0.39	$14.12	0.39	$14.12	XXX	A+
88125-TC	Forensic cytopathology	0.00	0.18	0.01	0.19	$6.88	0.19	$6.88	XXX	A+

*M = multiple surgery adjustment applies
Me = multiple endoscopy rules may apply
B = bilateral surgery adjustment applies
A = assistant-at-surgery restriction

A+ = assistant-at-surgery restriction unless medical necessity established with documentation
C = cosurgeons payable
C+ = cosurgeons payable if medical necessity established with documentation

T = team surgeons permitted
T+ = team surgeons payable if medical necessity established with documentation
$ = indicates services that are not covered by Medicare.

CPT five-digit codes, two-digit numeric modifiers, and descriptions only are © 2001 American Medical Association

Medicare RBRVS: The Physicians' Guide

Relative value units

CPT Code and Modifier	Description	Work RVU	Non Facility Practice Expense RVU	Facility Practice Expense RVU	PLI RVU	Total Non Facility RVUs	Medicare Payment Non Facility	Total Facility RVUs	Medicare Payment Facility	Global Period	Payment Policy Indicators*
88141	Cytopath, c/v, interpret	0.42	0.19	0.19	0.01	0.62	$22.44	0.62	$22.44	XXX	A+
88160	Cytopath smear, other source	0.50	1.01	1.01	0.04	1.55	$56.11	1.55	$56.11	XXX	A+
88160-26	Cytopath smear, other source	0.50	0.23	0.23	0.02	0.75	$27.15	0.75	$27.15	XXX	A+
88160-TC	Cytopath smear, other source	0.00	0.78	0.78	0.02	0.80	$28.96	0.80	$28.96	XXX	A+
88161	Cytopath smear, other source	0.50	1.22	1.22	0.04	1.76	$63.71	1.76	$63.71	XXX	A+
88161-26	Cytopath smear, other source	0.50	0.23	0.23	0.02	0.75	$27.15	0.75	$27.15	XXX	A+
88161-TC	Cytopath smear, other source	0.00	0.99	0.99	0.02	1.01	$36.56	1.01	$36.56	XXX	A+
88162	Cytopath smear, other source	0.76	0.73	0.73	0.05	1.54	$55.75	1.54	$55.75	XXX	A+
88162-26	Cytopath smear, other source	0.76	0.35	0.35	0.03	1.14	$41.27	1.14	$41.27	XXX	A+
88162-TC	Cytopath smear, other source	0.00	0.38	0.38	0.02	0.40	$14.48	0.40	$14.48	XXX	A+
88172	Cytopathology eval of fna	0.60	0.68	0.68	0.04	1.32	$47.78	1.32	$47.78	XXX	A+
88172-26	Cytopathology eval of fna	0.60	0.28	0.28	0.02	0.90	$32.58	0.90	$32.58	XXX	A+
88172-TC	Cytopathology eval of fna	0.00	0.40	0.40	0.02	0.42	$15.20	0.42	$15.20	XXX	A+
88173	Cytopath eval, fna, report	1.39	1.80	1.80	0.07	3.26	$118.01	3.26	$118.01	XXX	A+
88173-26	Cytopath eval, fna, report	1.39	0.64	0.64	0.05	2.08	$75.29	2.08	$75.29	XXX	A+
88173-TC	Cytopath eval, fna, report	0.00	1.16	1.16	0.02	1.18	$42.72	1.18	$42.72	XXX	A+
88180	Cell marker study	0.36	0.60	0.60	0.03	0.99	$35.84	0.99	$35.84	XXX	A+
88180-26	Cell marker study	0.36	0.17	0.17	0.01	0.54	$19.55	0.54	$19.55	XXX	A+
88180-TC	Cell marker study	0.00	0.43	0.43	0.02	0.45	$16.29	0.45	$16.29	XXX	A+
88182	Cell marker study	0.77	1.81	1.81	0.06	2.64	$95.57	2.64	$95.57	XXX	A+
88182-26	Cell marker study	0.77	0.36	0.36	0.03	1.16	$41.99	1.16	$41.99	XXX	A+
88182-TC	Cell marker study	0.00	1.45	1.45	0.03	1.48	$53.57	1.48	$53.57	XXX	A+
88199	Cytopathology procedure	0.00	0.00	0.00	0.00	0.00	$0.00	0.00	$0.00	XXX	A+
88199-26	Cytopathology procedure	0.00	0.00	0.00	0.00	0.00	$0.00	0.00	$0.00	XXX	A+
88199-TC	Cytopathology procedure	0.00	0.00	0.00	0.00	0.00	$0.00	0.00	$0.00	XXX	A+
88291	Cyto/molecular report	0.52	0.23	0.23	0.02	0.77	$27.87	0.77	$27.87	XXX	A+
88299	Cytogenetic study	0.00	0.00	0.00	0.00	0.00	$0.00	0.00	$0.00	XXX	A+

Pathology and laboratory: Surgical pathology

Code	Description							
88300	Surgical path, gross	0.08	0.34	0.02	0.44	$15.93	XXX	A+
88300-26	Surgical path, gross	0.08	0.04	0.01	0.13	$4.71	XXX	A+
88300-TC	Surgical path, gross	0.00	0.30	0.01	0.31	$11.22	XXX	A+
88302	Tissue exam by pathologist	0.13	0.73	0.03	0.89	$32.22	XXX	A+
88302-26	Tissue exam by pathologist	0.13	0.06	0.01	0.20	$7.24	XXX	A+
88302-TC	Tissue exam by pathologist	0.00	0.67	0.02	0.69	$24.98	XXX	A+
88304	Tissue exam by pathologist	0.22	0.95	0.03	1.20	$43.44	XXX	A+
88304-26	Tissue exam by pathologist	0.22	0.10	0.01	0.33	$11.95	XXX	A+
88304-TC	Tissue exam by pathologist	0.00	0.85	0.02	0.87	$31.49	XXX	A+
88305	Tissue exam by pathologist	0.75	1.78	0.05	2.58	$93.39	XXX	A+
88305-26	Tissue exam by pathologist	0.75	0.35	0.02	1.12	$40.54	XXX	A+
88305-TC	Tissue exam by pathologist	0.00	1.43	0.03	1.46	$52.85	XXX	A+
88307	Tissue exam by pathologist	1.59	2.71	0.11	4.41	$159.64	XXX	A+
88307-26	Tissue exam by pathologist	1.59	0.74	0.06	2.39	$86.52	XXX	A+
88307-TC	Tissue exam by pathologist	0.00	1.97	0.05	2.02	$73.12	XXX	A+
88309	Tissue exam by pathologist	2.28	3.40	0.13	5.81	$210.32	XXX	A+
88309-26	Tissue exam by pathologist	2.28	1.05	0.08	3.41	$123.44	XXX	A+
88309-TC	Tissue exam by pathologist	0.00	2.35	0.05	2.40	$86.88	XXX	A+
88311	Decalcify tissue	0.24	0.21	0.02	0.47	$17.01	XXX	A+
88311-26	Decalcify tissue	0.24	0.11	0.01	0.36	$13.03	XXX	A+
88311-TC	Decalcify tissue	0.00	0.10	0.01	0.11	$3.98	XXX	A+
88312	Special stains	0.54	1.69	0.03	2.26	$81.81	XXX	A+
88312-26	Special stains	0.54	0.25	0.02	0.81	$29.32	XXX	A+
88312-TC	Special stains	0.00	1.44	0.01	1.45	$52.49	XXX	A+
88313	Special stains	0.24	1.47	0.02	1.73	$62.62	XXX	A+
88313-26	Special stains	0.24	0.11	0.01	0.36	$13.03	XXX	A+
88313-TC	Special stains	0.00	1.36	0.01	1.37	$49.59	XXX	A+

* **M** = multiple surgery adjustment applies
Me = multiple endoscopy rules may apply
B = bilateral surgery adjustment applies
A = assistant-at-surgery restriction

A+ = assistant-at-surgery restriction unless medical necessity established with documentation
C = cosurgeons payable
C+ = cosurgeons payable if medical necessity established with documentation

T = team surgeons permitted
T+ = team surgeons payable if medical necessity established with documentation
§ = indicates services that are not covered by Medicare.

CPT five-digit codes, two-digit numeric modifiers, and descriptions only are © 2001 American Medical Association

Medicare RBRVS: The Physicians' Guide

Relative value units

CPT Code and Modifier	Description	Work RVU	Non Facility Practice Expense RVU	Facility Practice Expense RVU	PLI RVU	Total Non Facility RVUs	Medicare Payment Non Facility	Total Facility RVUs	Medicare Payment Facility	Global Period	Payment Policy Indicators*
88314	Histochemical stain	0.45	0.86	0.86	0.04	1.35	$48.87	1.35	$48.87	XXX	A+
88314-26	Histochemical stain	0.45	0.20	0.20	0.02	0.67	$24.25	0.67	$24.25	XXX	A+
88314-TC	Histochemical stain	0.00	0.66	0.66	0.02	0.68	$24.62	0.68	$24.62	XXX	A+
88318	Chemical histochemistry	0.42	0.59	0.59	0.02	1.03	$37.29	1.03	$37.29	XXX	A+
88318-26	Chemical histochemistry	0.42	0.20	0.20	0.01	0.63	$22.81	0.63	$22.81	XXX	A+
88318-TC	Chemical histochemistry	0.00	0.39	0.39	0.01	0.40	$14.48	0.40	$14.48	XXX	A+
88319	Enzyme histochemistry	0.53	2.45	2.45	0.04	3.02	$109.32	3.02	$109.32	XXX	A+
88319-26	Enzyme histochemistry	0.53	0.24	0.24	0.02	0.79	$28.60	0.79	$28.60	XXX	A+
88319-TC	Enzyme histochemistry	0.00	2.21	2.21	0.02	2.23	$80.72	2.23	$80.72	XXX	A+
88321	Microslide consultation	1.30	0.62	0.60	0.04	1.96	$70.95	1.94	$70.23	XXX	A+
88323	Microslide consultation	1.35	1.37	1.37	0.07	2.79	$101.00	2.79	$101.00	XXX	A+
88323-26	Microslide consultation	1.35	0.63	0.63	0.05	2.03	$73.48	2.03	$73.48	XXX	A+
88323-TC	Microslide consultation	0.00	0.74	0.74	0.02	0.76	$27.51	0.76	$27.51	XXX	A+
88325	Comprehensive review of data	2.22	0.98	0.98	0.08	3.28	$118.73	3.28	$118.73	XXX	A+
88329	Path consult introp	0.67	0.39	0.31	0.02	1.08	$39.10	1.00	$36.20	XXX	A+
88331	Path consult intraop, 1 bloc	1.19	0.87	0.87	0.07	2.13	$77.10	2.13	$77.10	XXX	A+
88331-26	Path consult intraop, 1 bloc	1.19	0.55	0.55	0.04	1.78	$64.43	1.78	$64.43	XXX	A+
88331-TC	Path consult intraop, 1 bloc	0.00	0.32	0.32	0.03	0.35	$12.67	0.35	$12.67	XXX	A+
88332	Path consult intraop, addl	0.59	0.47	0.47	0.04	1.10	$39.82	1.10	$39.82	XXX	A+
88332-26	Path consult intraop, addl	0.59	0.27	0.27	0.02	0.88	$31.86	0.88	$31.86	XXX	A+
88332-TC	Path consult intraop, addl	0.00	0.20	0.20	0.02	0.22	$7.96	0.22	$7.96	XXX	A+
88342	Immunocytochemistry	0.85	1.43	1.43	0.05	2.33	$84.34	2.33	$84.34	XXX	A+
88342-26	Immunocytochemistry	0.85	0.39	0.39	0.03	1.27	$45.97	1.27	$45.97	XXX	A+
88342-TC	Immunocytochemistry	0.00	1.04	1.04	0.02	1.06	$38.37	1.06	$38.37	XXX	A+
88346	Immunofluorescent study	0.86	1.20	1.20	0.05	2.11	$76.38	2.11	$76.38	XXX	A+
88346-26	Immunofluorescent study	0.86	0.39	0.39	0.03	1.28	$46.33	1.28	$46.33	XXX	A+
88346-TC	Immunofluorescent study	0.00	0.81	0.81	0.02	0.83	$30.05	0.83	$30.05	XXX	A+

Code	Description								
88347	Immunofluorescent study	0.86	1.90	0.05	2.81	$101.72	2.81	$101.72	XXX	A+
88347-26	Immunofluorescent study	0.86	0.38	0.03	1.27	$45.97	1.27	$45.97	XXX	A+
88347-TC	Immunofluorescent study	0.00	1.52	0.02	1.54	$55.75	1.54	$55.75	XXX	A+
88348	Electron microscopy	1.51	6.96	0.11	8.58	$310.59	8.58	$310.59	XXX	A+
88348-26	Electron microscopy	1.51	0.69	0.05	2.25	$81.45	2.25	$81.45	XXX	A+
88348-TC	Electron microscopy	0.00	6.27	0.06	6.33	$229.14	6.33	$229.14	XXX	A+
88349	Scanning electron microscopy	0.76	8.51	0.08	9.35	$338.46	9.35	$338.46	XXX	A+
88349-26	Scanning electron microscopy	0.76	0.35	0.03	1.14	$41.27	1.14	$41.27	XXX	A+
88349-TC	Scanning electron microscopy	0.00	8.16	0.05	8.21	$297.20	8.21	$297.20	XXX	A+
88355	Analysis, skeletal muscle	1.85	2.41	0.12	4.38	$158.55	4.38	$158.55	XXX	A+
88355-26	Analysis, skeletal muscle	1.85	0.86	0.07	2.78	$100.63	2.78	$100.63	XXX	A+
88355-TC	Analysis, skeletal muscle	0.00	1.55	0.05	1.60	$57.92	1.60	$57.92	XXX	A+
88356	Analysis, nerve	3.02	4.96	0.16	8.14	$294.66	8.14	$294.66	XXX	A+
88356-26	Analysis, nerve	3.02	1.37	0.10	4.49	$162.53	4.49	$162.53	XXX	A+
88356-TC	Analysis, nerve	0.00	3.59	0.06	3.65	$132.13	3.65	$132.13	XXX	A+
88358	Analysis, tumor	2.82	1.76	0.16	4.74	$171.58	4.74	$171.58	XXX	A+
88358-26	Analysis, tumor	2.82	1.30	0.10	4.22	$152.76	4.22	$152.76	XXX	A+
88358-TC	Analysis, tumor	0.00	0.46	0.06	0.52	$18.82	0.52	$18.82	XXX	A+
88362	Nerve teasing preparations	2.17	3.36	0.12	5.65	$204.53	5.65	$204.53	XXX	A+
88362-26	Nerve teasing preparations	2.17	0.99	0.07	3.23	$116.92	3.23	$116.92	XXX	A+
88362-TC	Nerve teasing preparations	0.00	2.37	0.05	2.42	$87.60	2.42	$87.60	XXX	A+
88365	Tissue hybridization	0.93	2.03	0.05	3.01	$108.96	3.01	$108.96	XXX	A+
88365-26	Tissue hybridization	0.93	0.43	0.03	1.39	$50.32	1.39	$50.32	XXX	A+
88365-TC	Tissue hybridization	0.00	1.60	0.02	1.62	$58.64	1.62	$58.64	XXX	A+
88371-26	Protein, western blot tissue	0.37	0.15	0.01	0.53	$19.19	0.52	$18.82	XXX	A+
88372-26	Protein analysis w/probe	0.37	0.17	0.01	0.55	$19.91	0.55	$19.91	XXX	A+
88380	Microdissection	0.00	0.00	0.00	0.00	$0.00	0.00	$0.00	XXX	A+
88380-26	Microdissection	0.00	0.00	0.00	0.00	$0.00	0.00	$0.00	XXX	A+

* **M** = multiple surgery adjustment applies
Me = multiple endoscopy rules may apply
B = bilateral surgery adjustment applies
A = assistant-at-surgery restriction

A+ = assistant-at-surgery restriction unless medical necessity established with documentation
C = cosurgeons payable
C+ = cosurgeons payable if medical necessity established with documentation

T = team surgeons permitted
T+ = team surgeons payable if medical necessity established with documentation
§ = indicates services that are not covered by Medicare.

CPT five-digit codes, two-digit numeric modifiers, and descriptions only are © 2001 American Medical Association

Medicare RBRVS: The Physicians' Guide

Relative value units

CPT Code and Modifier	Description	Work RVU	Non Facility Practice Expense RVU	Facility Practice Expense RVU	PLI RVU	Total Non Facility RVUs	Medicare Payment Non Facility	Total Facility RVUs	Medicare Payment Facility	Global Period	Payment Policy Indicators*
88380-TC	Microdissection	0.00	0.00	0.00	0.00	0.00	$0.00	0.00	$0.00	XXX	A+
88399	Surgical pathology procedure	0.00	0.00	0.00	0.00	0.00	$0.00	0.00	$0.00	XXX	A+
88399-26	Surgical pathology procedure	0.00	0.00	0.00	0.00	0.00	$0.00	0.00	$0.00	XXX	A+
88399-TC	Surgical pathology procedure	0.00	0.00	0.00	0.00	0.00	$0.00	0.00	$0.00	XXX	A+

Pathology and laboratory: Other procedures

CPT Code and Modifier	Description	Work RVU	Non Facility Practice Expense RVU	Facility Practice Expense RVU	PLI RVU	Total Non Facility RVUs	Medicare Payment Non Facility	Total Facility RVUs	Medicare Payment Facility	Global Period	Payment Policy Indicators*
89060-26	Exam synovial fluid crystals	0.37	0.18	0.17	0.01	0.56	$20.27	0.55	$19.91	XXX	A+
89100	Sample intestinal contents	0.60	2.29	0.23	0.02	2.91	$105.34	0.85	$30.77	XXX	A+
89105	Sample intestinal contents	0.50	2.25	0.18	0.02	2.77	$100.27	0.70	$25.34	XXX	A+
89130	Sample stomach contents	0.45	2.21	0.13	0.02	2.68	$97.01	0.60	$21.72	XXX	A+
89132	Sample stomach contents	0.19	1.15	0.05	0.01	1.35	$48.87	0.25	$9.05	XXX	A+
89135	Sample stomach contents	0.79	2.53	0.25	0.03	3.35	$121.27	1.07	$38.73	XXX	A+
89136	Sample stomach contents	0.21	2.05	0.08	0.01	2.27	$82.17	0.30	$10.86	XXX	A+
89140	Sample stomach contents	0.94	2.36	0.19	0.03	3.33	$120.54	1.16	$41.99	XXX	A+
89141	Sample stomach contents	0.85	3.14	0.40	0.03	4.02	$145.52	1.28	$46.33	XXX	A+
89350	Sputum specimen collection	0.00	0.39	0.39	0.02	0.41	$14.84	0.41	$14.84	XXX	A+
89360	Collect sweat for test	0.00	0.43	0.43	0.02	0.45	$16.29	0.45	$16.29	XXX	A+
89399	Pathology lab procedure	0.00	0.00	0.00	0.00	0.00	$0.00	0.00	$0.00	XXX	A+
89399-26	Pathology lab procedure	0.00	0.00	0.00	0.00	0.00	$0.00	0.00	$0.00	XXX	A+
89399-TC	Pathology lab procedure	0.00	0.00	0.00	0.00	0.00	$0.00	0.00	$0.00	XXX	A+

Medicine: Therapeutic or diagnostic infusions (excludes chemotherapy)

CPT Code and Modifier	Description	Work RVU	Non Facility Practice Expense RVU	Facility Practice Expense RVU	PLI RVU	Total Non Facility RVUs	Medicare Payment Non Facility	Total Facility RVUs	Medicare Payment Facility	Global Period	Payment Policy Indicators*
90471	Immunization admin	0.00	0.10	0.10	0.01	0.11	$3.98	0.11	$3.98	XXX	A+
90472	Immunization admin, each add	0.00	0.10	0.10	0.01	0.11	$3.98	0.11	$3.98	ZZZ	A+
90780	IV infusion therapy, 1 hour	0.00	1.06	1.06	0.06	1.12	$40.54	1.12	$40.54	XXX	A+
90781	IV infusion, additional hour	0.00	0.53	0.53	0.03	0.56	$20.27	0.56	$20.27	ZZZ	A+

Medicine: Therapeutic or diagnostic injections

CPT Code and Modifier	Description	Work RVU	Non Facility Practice Expense RVU	Facility Practice Expense RVU	PLI RVU	Total Non Facility RVUs	Medicare Payment Non Facility	Total Facility RVUs	Medicare Payment Facility	Global Period	Payment Policy Indicators*
90782	Injection, sc/im	0.00	0.10	0.10	0.01	0.11	$3.98	0.11	$3.98	XXX	A+
90783	Injection, ia	0.00	0.39	0.39	0.02	0.41	$14.84	0.41	$14.84	XXX	A+

Code	Description								
90784	Injection, iv	0.00	0.45	0.03	0.48	$17.38	0.48	$17.38	XXX	A+
90788	Injection of antibiotic	0.00	0.11	0.01	0.12	$4.34	0.12	$4.34	XXX	A+
90799	Ther/prophylactic/dx inject	0.00	0.00	0.00	0.00	$0.00	0.00	$0.00	XXX	A+

Medicine: Psychiatry

Code	Description								
90801	Psy dx interview	2.80	1.14	0.06	4.00	$144.80	3.79	$137.19	XXX	A+
90802	Intac psy dx interview	3.01	1.17	0.07	4.25	$153.85	4.07	$147.33	XXX	A+
90804	Psytx, office, 20-30 min	1.21	0.53	0.03	1.77	$64.07	1.64	$59.37	XXX	A+
90805	Psytx, off, 20-30 min w/e&m	1.37	0.59	0.03	1.99	$72.04	1.84	$66.61	XXX	A+
90806	Psytx, off, 45-50 min	1.86	0.75	0.04	2.65	$95.93	2.52	$91.22	XXX	A+
90807	Psytx, off, 45-50 min w/e&m	2.02	0.79	0.05	2.86	$103.53	2.73	$98.82	XXX	A+
90808	Psytx, office, 75-80 min	2.79	1.06	0.07	3.92	$141.90	3.79	$137.19	XXX	A+
90809	Psytx, off, 75-80, w/e&m	2.95	1.11	0.07	4.13	$149.50	3.99	$144.43	XXX	A+
90810	Intac psytx, off, 20-30 min	1.32	0.56	0.03	1.91	$69.14	1.79	$64.80	XXX	A+
90811	Intac psytx, 20-30, w/e&m	1.48	0.63	0.03	2.14	$77.47	1.99	$72.04	XXX	A+
90812	Intac psytx, off, 45-50 min	1.97	0.80	0.05	2.82	$102.08	2.71	$98.10	XXX	A+
90813	Intac psytx, 45-50 min w/e&m	2.13	0.87	0.05	3.05	$110.41	2.89	$104.62	XXX	A+
90814	Intac psytx, off, 75-80 min	2.90	1.15	0.07	4.12	$149.14	3.98	$144.07	XXX	A+
90815	Intac psytx, 75-80 w/e&m	3.06	1.15	0.07	4.28	$154.93	4.15	$150.23	XXX	A+
90816	Psytx, hosp, 20-30 min	1.25	0.57	0.03	1.85	$66.97	1.71	$61.90	XXX	A+
90817	Psytx, hosp, 20-30 min w/e&m	1.41	0.62	0.03	2.06	$74.57	1.89	$68.42	XXX	A+
90818	Psytx, hosp, 45-50 min	1.89	0.80	0.04	2.73	$98.82	2.58	$93.39	XXX	A+
90819	Psytx, hosp, 45-50 min w/e&m	2.05	0.83	0.05	2.93	$106.06	2.76	$99.91	XXX	A+
90821	Psytx, hosp, 75-80 min	2.83	1.11	0.06	4.00	$144.80	3.86	$139.73	XXX	A+
90822	Psytx, hosp, 75-80 min w/e&m	2.99	1.30	0.07	4.36	$157.83	4.03	$145.88	XXX	A+
90823	Intac psytx, hosp, 20-30 min	1.36	0.65	0.03	2.04	$73.85	1.84	$66.61	XXX	A+
90824	Intac psytx, hsp 20-30 w/e&m	1.52	0.70	0.03	2.25	$81.45	2.05	$74.21	XXX	A+
90826	Intac psytx, hosp, 45-50 min	2.01	0.89	0.04	2.94	$106.43	2.73	$98.82	XXX	A+
90827	Intac psytx, hsp 45-50 w/e&m	2.16	0.91	0.05	3.12	$112.94	2.91	$105.34	XXX	A+

* **M** = multiple surgery adjustment applies
Me = multiple endoscopy rules may apply
B = bilateral surgery adjustment applies
A = assistant-at-surgery restriction

A+ = assistant-at-surgery restriction unless medical necessity established with documentation
C = cosurgeons payable
C+ = cosurgeons payable if medical necessity established with documentation

T = team surgeons permitted
T+ = team surgeons payable if medical necessity established with documentation
§ = indicates services that are not covered by Medicare.

CPT five-digit codes, two-digit numeric modifiers, and descriptions only are © 2001 American Medical Association

Medicare RBRVS: The Physicians' Guide

Relative value units

CPT Code and Modifier	Description	Work RVU	Non Facility Practice Expense RVU	Facility Practice Expense RVU	PLI RVU	Total Non Facility RVUs	Medicare Payment Non Facility	Total Facility RVUs	Medicare Payment Facility	Global Period	Payment Policy Indicators*
90828	Intac psytx, hosp, 75-80 min	2.94	1.90	1.02	0.07	4.91	$177.74	4.03	$145.88	XXX	A+
90829	Intac psytx, hsp 75-80 w/e&m	3.10	1.23	1.02	0.07	4.40	$159.28	4.19	$151.67	XXX	A+
90845	Psychoanalysis	1.79	0.71	0.57	0.04	2.54	$91.95	2.40	$86.88	XXX	A+
90846	Family psytx w/o patient	1.83	0.73	0.62	0.04	2.60	$94.12	2.49	$90.14	XXX	A+
90847	Family psytx w/patient	2.21	0.86	0.75	0.05	3.12	$112.94	3.01	$108.96	XXX	A+
90849	Multiple family group psytx	0.59	0.31	0.20	0.01	0.91	$32.94	0.80	$28.96	XXX	A+
90853	Group psychotherapy	0.59	0.35	0.20	0.01	0.95	$34.39	0.80	$28.96	XXX	A+
90857	Intac group psytx	0.63	0.37	0.21	0.02	1.02	$36.92	0.86	$31.13	XXX	A+
90862	Medication management	0.95	0.44	0.31	0.02	1.41	$51.04	1.28	$46.33	XXX	A+
90865	Narcosynthesis	2.84	1.70	0.94	0.07	4.61	$166.88	3.85	$139.37	XXX	A+
90870	Electroconvulsive therapy	1.88	0.74	0.74	0.04	2.66	$96.29	2.66	$96.29	000	A+
90871	Electroconvulsive therapy	2.72	NA	1.04	0.06	NA	NA	3.82	$138.28	000	
90875 §	Psychophysiological therapy	1.20	0.90	0.48	0.03	2.13	$77.10	1.71	$61.90	XXX	
90876 §	Psychophysiological therapy	1.90	1.18	0.76	0.04	3.12	$112.94	2.70	$97.74	XXX	
90880	Hypnotherapy	2.19	0.91	0.71	0.05	3.15	$114.03	2.95	$106.79	XXX	A+
90885 §	Psy evaluation of records	0.97	0.39	0.39	0.02	1.38	$49.95	1.38	$49.95	XXX	
90887 §	Consultation with family	1.48	0.83	0.59	0.03	2.34	$84.71	2.10	$76.02	XXX	
90899	Psychiatric service/therapy	0.00	0.00	0.00	0.00	0.00	$0.00	0.00	$0.00	XXX	A+

Medicine: Biofeedback

CPT Code and Modifier	Description	Work RVU	Non Facility Practice Expense RVU	Facility Practice Expense RVU	PLI RVU	Total Non Facility RVUs	Medicare Payment Non Facility	Total Facility RVUs	Medicare Payment Facility	Global Period	Payment Policy Indicators*
90901	Biofeedback train, any meth	0.41	0.82	0.17	0.02	1.25	$45.25	0.60	$21.72	XXX	A+
90911	Biofeedback peri/uro/rectal	0.89	0.87	0.39	0.04	1.80	$65.16	1.32	$47.78	000	A+
90918	ESRD related services, month	11.18	5.53	5.53	0.30	17.01	$615.75	17.01	$615.75	000	A+
90919	ESRD related services, month	8.54	4.53	4.53	0.24	13.31	$481.81	13.31	$481.81	XXX	A+
90920	ESRD related services, month	7.27	4.02	4.02	0.19	11.48	$415.57	11.48	$415.57	XXX	A+
90921	ESRD related services, month	4.47	2.96	2.96	0.12	7.55	$273.30	7.55	$273.30	XXX	A+
90922	ESRD related services, day	0.37	0.17	0.17	0.01	0.55	$19.91	0.55	$19.91	XXX	A+
90923	ESRD related services, day	0.28	0.15	0.15	0.01	0.44	$15.93	0.44	$15.93	XXX	A+

Code	Description								
90924	ESRD related services, day	0.24	0.13	0.01	0.38	$13.76	0.38	XXX	A+
90925	ESRD related services, day	0.15	0.10	0.01	0.26	$9.41	0.26	XXX	A+
90935	Hemodialysis, one evaluation	1.22	0.86	0.03	NA	NA	2.11	000	A+
90937	Hemodialysis, repeated eval	2.11	1.20	0.06	NA	NA	3.37	000	A+
90945	Dialysis, one evaluation	1.28	0.89	0.04	NA	NA	2.21	000	A+
90947	Dialysis, repeated eval	2.16	1.24	0.06	NA	NA	3.46	000	A+
90997	Hemoperfusion	1.84	1.10	0.05	NA	NA	2.99	000	A+
90999	Dialysis procedure	0.00	0.00	0.00	0.00	$0.00	0.00	XXX	A+

Medicine: Gastroenterelogy

Code	Description								
91000	Esophageal intubation	0.73	0.32	0.04	1.09	$39.46	1.09	000	A+
91000-26	Esophageal intubation	0.73	0.25	0.03	1.01	$36.56	1.01	000	A+
91000-TC	Esophageal intubation	0.00	0.07	0.01	0.08	$2.90	0.08	000	A+
91010	Esophagus motility study	1.25	2.60	0.10	3.95	$142.99	3.95	000	A+
91010-26	Esophagus motility study	1.25	0.46	0.05	1.76	$63.71	1.76	000	A+
91010-TC	Esophagus motility study	0.00	2.14	0.05	2.19	$79.28	2.19	000	A+
91011	Esophagus motility study	1.50	2.71	0.10	4.31	$156.02	4.31	000	A+
91011-26	Esophagus motility study	1.50	0.55	0.05	2.10	$76.02	2.10	000	A+
91011-TC	Esophagus motility study	0.00	2.16	0.05	2.21	$80.00	2.21	000	A+
91012	Esophagus motility study	1.46	2.35	0.12	3.93	$142.26	3.93	000	A+
91012-26	Esophagus motility study	1.46	0.54	0.06	2.06	$74.57	2.06	000	A+
91012-TC	Esophagus motility study	0.00	1.81	0.06	1.87	$67.69	1.87	000	A+
91020	Gastric motility	1.44	2.96	0.11	4.51	$163.26	4.51	000	A+
91020-26	Gastric motility	1.44	0.51	0.06	2.01	$72.76	2.01	000	A+
91020-TC	Gastric motility	0.00	2.45	0.05	2.50	$90.50	2.50	000	A+
91030	Acid perfusion of esophagus	0.91	2.27	0.05	3.23	$116.92	3.23	000	A+
91030-26	Acid perfusion of esophagus	0.91	0.34	0.03	1.28	$46.33	1.28	000	A+
91030-TC	Acid perfusion of esophagus	0.00	1.93	0.02	1.95	$70.59	1.95	000	A+
91032	Esophagus, acid reflux test	1.21	2.26	0.10	3.57	$129.23	3.57	000	A+

* **M** = multiple surgery adjustment applies
Me = multiple endoscopy rules may apply
B = bilateral surgery adjustment applies
A = assistant-at-surgery restriction

A+ = assistant-at-surgery restriction unless medical necessity established with documentation
C = cosurgeons payable
C+ = cosurgeons payable if medical necessity established with documentation

T = team surgeons permitted
T+ = team surgeons payable if medical necessity established with documentation
§ = indicates services that are not covered by Medicare.

CPT five-digit codes, two-digit numeric modifiers, and descriptions only are © 2001 American Medical Association

Medicare RBRVS: The Physicians' Guide

Relative value units

CPT Code and Modifier	Description	Work RVU	Non Facility Practice Expense RVU	Facility Practice Expense RVU	PLI RVU	Total Non Facility RVUs	Medicare Payment Non Facility	Total Facility RVUs	Medicare Payment Facility	Global Period	Payment Policy Indicators*
91032-26	Esophagus, acid reflux test	1.21	0.44	0.44	0.05	1.70	$61.54	1.70	$61.54	000	A+
91032-TC	Esophagus, acid reflux test	0.00	1.82	1.82	0.05	1.87	$67.69	1.87	$67.69	000	A+
91033	Prolonged acid reflux test	1.30	2.64	2.64	0.14	4.08	$147.69	4.08	$147.69	000	A+
91033-26	Prolonged acid reflux test	1.30	0.48	0.48	0.05	1.83	$66.24	1.83	$66.24	000	A+
91033-TC	Prolonged acid reflux test	0.00	2.16	2.16	0.09	2.25	$81.45	2.25	$81.45	000	A+
91052	Gastric analysis test	0.79	2.19	2.19	0.05	3.03	$109.68	3.03	$109.68	000	A+
91052-26	Gastric analysis test	0.79	0.29	0.29	0.03	1.11	$40.18	1.11	$40.18	000	A+
91052-TC	Gastric analysis test	0.00	1.90	1.90	0.02	1.92	$69.50	1.92	$69.50	000	A+
91055	Gastric intubation for smear	0.94	2.22	2.22	0.06	3.22	$116.56	3.22	$116.56	000	A+
91055-26	Gastric intubation for smear	0.94	0.28	0.28	0.04	1.26	$45.61	1.26	$45.61	000	A+
91055-TC	Gastric intubation for smear	0.00	1.94	1.94	0.02	1.96	$70.95	1.96	$70.95	000	A+
91060	Gastric saline load test	0.45	0.28	0.28	0.04	0.77	$27.87	0.77	$27.87	000	A+
91060-26	Gastric saline load test	0.45	0.15	0.15	0.02	0.62	$22.44	0.62	$22.44	000	A+
91060-TC	Gastric saline load test	0.00	0.13	0.13	0.02	0.15	$5.43	0.15	$5.43	000	A+
91065	Breath hydrogen test	0.20	4.55	4.55	0.03	4.78	$173.03	4.78	$173.03	000	A+
91065-26	Breath hydrogen test	0.20	0.07	0.07	0.01	0.28	$10.14	0.28	$10.14	000	A+
91065-TC	Breath hydrogen test	0.00	4.48	4.48	0.02	4.50	$162.90	4.50	$162.90	000	A+
91100	Pass intestine bleeding tube	1.08	NA	0.48	0.06	NA	NA	1.62	$58.64	000	A+
91105	Gastric intubation treatment	0.37	NA	0.21	0.02	NA	NA	0.60	$21.72	000	A+
91122	Anal pressure record	1.77	2.77	2.77	0.17	4.71	$170.50	4.71	$170.50	000	A+
91122-26	Anal pressure record	1.77	0.63	0.63	0.10	2.50	$90.50	2.50	$90.50	000	A+
91122-TC	Anal pressure record	0.00	2.14	2.14	0.07	2.21	$80.00	2.21	$80.00	000	A+
91132	Electrogastrography	0.00	0.00	0.00	0.00	0.00	$0.00	0.00	$0.00	XXX	A+
91132-26	Electrogastrography	0.52	0.21	0.21	0.03	0.76	$27.51	0.76	$27.51	XXX	A+
91132-TC	Electrogastrography	0.00	0.00	0.00	0.00	0.00	$0.00	0.00	$0.00	XXX	A+
91133	Electrogastrography w/test	0.00	0.00	0.00	0.00	0.00	$0.00	0.00	$0.00	XXX	A+
91133-26	Electrogastrography w/test	0.66	0.26	0.26	0.03	0.95	$34.39	0.95	$34.39	XXX	A+

Code	Description										
91133-TC	Electrogastrography w/test	0.00	0.00	0.00	0.00	$0.00	0.00	$0.00	XXX		A+
91299	Gastroenterology procedure	0.00	0.00	0.00	0.00	$0.00	0.00	$0.00	XXX		A+
91299-26	Gastroenterology procedure	0.00	0.00	0.00	0.00	$0.00	0.00	$0.00	XXX		A+
91299-TC	Gastroenterology procedure	0.00	0.00	0.00	0.00	$0.00	0.00	$0.00	XXX		A+

Medicine: Ophthalmology

Code	Description										
92002	Eye exam, new patient	0.88	0.96	0.38	0.02	1.86	$67.33	1.28	$46.33	XXX	A+
92004	Eye exam, new patient	1.67	1.71	0.73	0.03	3.41	$123.44	2.43	$87.96	XXX	A+
92012	Eye exam established pat	0.67	1.01	0.31	0.01	1.69	$61.18	0.99	$35.84	XXX	A+
92014	Eye exam & treatment	1.10	1.40	0.50	0.02	2.52	$91.22	1.62	$58.64	XXX	A+
92015 §	Refraction	0.38	1.51	0.15	0.01	1.90	$68.78	0.54	$19.55	XXX	
92018	New eye exam & treatment	2.50	NA	1.14	0.03	NA	NA	3.67	$132.85	XXX	A+
92019	Eye exam & treatment	1.31	NA	0.61	0.03	NA	NA	1.95	$70.59	XXX	A+
92020	Special eye evaluation	0.37	0.95	0.17	0.01	1.33	$48.14	0.55	$19.91	XXX	A+
92060	Special eye evaluation	0.69	0.74	0.74	0.02	1.45	$52.49	1.45	$52.49	XXX	A+
92060-26	Special eye evaluation	0.69	0.31	0.31	0.01	1.01	$36.56	1.01	$36.56	XXX	A+
92060-TC	Special eye evaluation	0.00	0.43	0.43	0.01	0.44	$15.93	0.44	$15.93	XXX	A+
92065	Orthoptic/pleoptic training	0.37	1.19	1.19	0.02	1.58	$57.19	1.58	$57.19	XXX	A+
92065-26	Orthoptic/pleoptic training	0.37	0.15	0.15	0.01	0.53	$19.19	0.53	$19.19	XXX	A+
92065-TC	Orthoptic/pleoptic training	0.00	1.04	1.04	0.01	1.05	$38.01	1.05	$38.01	XXX	A+
92070	Fitting of contact lens	0.70	1.12	0.34	0.01	1.83	$66.24	1.05	$38.01	XXX	A+
92081	Visual field examination(s)	0.36	1.84	1.84	0.02	2.22	$80.36	2.22	$80.36	XXX	A+
92081-26	Visual field examination(s)	0.36	0.16	0.16	0.01	0.53	$19.19	0.53	$19.19	XXX	A+
92081-TC	Visual field examination(s)	0.00	1.68	1.68	0.01	1.69	$61.18	1.69	$61.18	XXX	A+
92082	Visual field examination(s)	0.44	0.85	0.85	0.02	1.31	$47.42	1.31	$47.42	XXX	A+
92082-26	Visual field examination(s)	0.44	0.20	0.20	0.01	0.65	$23.53	0.65	$23.53	XXX	A+
92082-TC	Visual field examination(s)	0.00	0.65	0.65	0.01	0.66	$23.89	0.66	$23.89	XXX	A+
92083	Visual field examination(s)	0.50	1.51	1.51	0.02	2.03	$73.48	2.03	$73.48	XXX	A+
92083-26	Visual field examination(s)	0.50	0.23	0.23	0.01	0.74	$26.79	0.74	$26.79	XXX	A+

* **M** = multiple surgery adjustment applies
Me = multiple endoscopy rules may apply
B = bilateral surgery adjustment applies
A = assistant-at-surgery restriction

A+ = assistant-at-surgery restriction unless medical necessity established with documentation
C = cosurgeons payable
C+ = cosurgeons payable if medical necessity established with documentation

T = team surgeons permitted
T+ = team surgeons payable if medical necessity established with documentation
§ = indicates services that are not covered by Medicare.

395 CPT five-digit codes, two-digit numeric modifiers, and descriptions only are © 2001 American Medical Association

Medicare RBRVS: The Physicians' Guide

Relative value units

CPT Code and Modifier	Description	Work RVU	Non Facility Practice Expense RVU	Facility Practice Expense RVU	PLI RVU	Total Non Facility RVUs	Medicare Payment Non Facility	Total Facility RVUs	Medicare Payment Facility	Global Period	Payment Policy Indicators*
92083-TC	Visual field examination(s)	0.00	1.28	1.28	0.01	1.29	$46.70	1.29	$46.70	XXX	A+
92100	Serial tonometry exam(s)	0.92	0.75	0.40	0.02	1.69	$61.18	1.34	$48.51	XXX	A+
92120	Tonography & eye evaluation	0.81	0.81	0.31	0.02	1.64	$59.37	1.14	$41.27	XXX	A+
92130	Water provocation tonography	0.81	0.92	0.32	0.02	1.75	$63.35	1.15	$41.63	XXX	A+
92135	Opthalmic dx imaging	0.35	1.48	1.48	0.02	1.85	$66.97	1.85	$66.97	XXX	A
92135-26	Opthalmic dx imaging	0.35	0.17	0.17	0.01	0.53	$19.19	0.53	$19.19	XXX	A
92135-TC	Opthalmic dx imaging	0.00	1.31	1.31	0.01	1.32	$47.78	1.32	$47.78	XXX	A
92136	Ophthalmic biometry	0.54	1.52	1.52	0.07	2.13	$77.10	2.13	$77.10	XXX	A+
92136-26	Ophthalmic biometry	0.54	0.22	0.22	0.01	0.77	$27.87	0.77	$27.87	XXX	A+
92136-TC	Ophthalmic biometry	0.00	1.30	1.30	0.06	1.36	$49.23	1.36	$49.23	XXX	A+
92140	Glaucoma provocative tests	0.50	1.01	0.22	0.01	1.52	$55.02	0.73	$26.43	XXX	A+
92225	Special eye exam, initial	0.38	0.23	0.17	0.01	0.62	$22.44	0.56	$20.27	XXX	A+
92226	Special eye exam, subsequent	0.33	0.22	0.15	0.01	0.56	$20.27	0.49	$17.74	XXX	A+
92230	Eye exam with photos	0.60	1.73	0.21	0.02	2.35	$85.07	0.83	$30.05	XXX	A+
92235	Eye exam with photos	0.81	2.62	2.62	0.07	3.50	$126.70	3.50	$126.70	XXX	A+
92235-26	Eye exam with photos	0.81	0.39	0.39	0.02	1.22	$44.16	1.22	$44.16	XXX	A+
92235-TC	Eye exam with photos	0.00	2.23	2.23	0.05	2.28	$82.53	2.28	$82.53	XXX	A+
92240	Icg angiography	1.10	5.24	5.24	0.07	6.41	$232.04	6.41	$232.04	XXX	A+
92240-26	Icg angiography	1.10	0.53	0.53	0.02	1.65	$59.73	1.65	$59.73	XXX	A+
92240-TC	Icg angiography	0.00	4.71	4.71	0.05	4.76	$172.31	4.76	$172.31	XXX	A+
92250	Eye exam with photos	0.44	1.37	1.37	0.02	1.83	$66.24	1.83	$66.24	XXX	A+
92250-26	Eye exam with photos	0.44	0.20	0.20	0.01	0.65	$23.53	0.65	$23.53	XXX	A+
92250-TC	Eye exam with photos	0.00	1.17	1.17	0.01	1.18	$42.72	1.18	$42.72	XXX	A+
92260	Ophthalmoscopy/dynamometry	0.20	0.24	0.10	0.01	0.45	$16.29	0.31	$11.22	XXX	A+
92265	Eye muscle evaluation	0.81	1.23	1.23	0.04	2.08	$75.29	2.08	$75.29	XXX	A+
92265-26	Eye muscle evaluation	0.81	0.38	0.38	0.02	1.21	$43.80	1.21	$43.80	XXX	A+
92265-TC	Eye muscle evaluation	0.00	0.85	0.85	0.02	0.87	$31.49	0.87	$31.49	XXX	A+

Code	Description								
92270	Electro-oculography	0.81	1.15	0.05	2.01	$72.76	2.01	XXX	A+
92270-26	Electro-oculography	0.81	0.37	0.03	1.21	$43.80	1.21	XXX	A+
92270-TC	Electro-oculography	0.00	0.78	0.02	0.80	$28.96	0.80	XXX	A+
92275	Electroretinography	1.01	1.25	0.04	2.30	$83.26	2.30	XXX	A+
92275-26	Electroretinography	1.01	0.46	0.02	1.49	$53.94	1.49	XXX	A+
92275-TC	Electroretinography	0.00	0.79	0.02	0.81	$29.32	0.81	XXX	A+
92283	Color vision examination	0.17	0.74	0.02	0.93	$33.67	0.93	XXX	A+
92283-26	Color vision examination	0.17	0.07	0.01	0.25	$9.05	0.25	XXX	A+
92283-TC	Color vision examination	0.00	0.67	0.01	0.68	$24.62	0.68	XXX	A+
92284	Dark adaptation eye exam	0.24	1.75	0.02	2.01	$72.76	2.01	XXX	A+
92284-26	Dark adaptation eye exam	0.24	0.09	0.01	0.34	$12.31	0.34	XXX	A+
92284-TC	Dark adaptation eye exam	0.00	1.66	0.01	1.67	$60.45	1.67	XXX	A+
92285	Eye photography	0.20	0.80	0.02	1.02	$36.92	1.02	XXX	A+
92285-26	Eye photography	0.20	0.09	0.01	0.30	$10.86	0.30	XXX	A+
92285-TC	Eye photography	0.00	0.71	0.01	0.72	$26.06	0.72	XXX	A+
92286	Internal eye photography	0.66	3.00	0.03	3.69	$133.58	3.69	XXX	A+
92286-26	Internal eye photography	0.66	0.32	0.01	0.99	$35.84	0.99	XXX	A+
92286-TC	Internal eye photography	0.00	2.68	0.02	2.70	$97.74	2.70	XXX	A+
92287	Internal eye photography	0.81	3.16	0.02	3.99	$144.43	1.14	XXX	A+
92310 §	Contact lens fitting	1.17	1.10	0.03	2.30	$83.26	1.67	XXX	
92311	Contact lens fitting	1.08	1.17	0.03	2.28	$82.53	1.42	XXX	A+
92312	Contact lens fitting	1.26	1.17	0.03	2.46	$89.05	1.74	XXX	A+
92313	Contact lens fitting	0.92	1.21	0.02	2.15	$77.83	1.27	XXX	A+
92314 §	Prescription of contact lens	0.69	0.91	0.01	1.61	$58.28	0.98	XXX	
92315	Prescription of contact lens	0.45	0.95	0.01	1.41	$51.04	0.63	XXX	A+
92316	Prescription of contact lens	0.68	1.03	0.01	1.72	$62.26	0.99	XXX	A+
92317	Prescription of contact lens	0.45	0.97	0.01	1.43	$51.76	0.64	XXX	A+
92325	Modification of contact lens	0.00	0.38	0.01	0.39	$14.12	0.39	XXX	A+

*M = multiple surgery adjustment applies
Me = multiple endoscopy rules may apply
B = bilateral surgery adjustment applies
A = assistant-at-surgery restriction

A+ = assistant-at-surgery restriction unless medical necessity established with documentation
C = cosurgeons payable
C+ = cosurgeons payable if medical necessity established with documentation

T = team surgeons permitted
T+ = team surgeons payable if medical necessity established with documentation
§ = indicates services that are not covered by Medicare.

397 CPT five-digit codes, two-digit numeric modifiers, and descriptions only are © 2001 American Medical Association

Medicare RBRVS: The Physicians' Guide

Relative value units

CPT Code and Modifier	Description	Work RVU	Non Facility Practice Expense RVU	Facility Practice Expense RVU	PLI RVU	Total Non Facility RVUs	Medicare Payment Non Facility	Total Facility RVUs	Medicare Payment Facility	Global Period	Payment Policy Indicators*
92326	Replacement of contact lens	0.00	1.55	1.55	0.05	1.60	$57.92	1.60	$57.92	XXX	A+
92330	Fitting of artificial eye	1.08	1.01	0.38	0.04	2.13	$77.10	1.50	$54.30	XXX	A+
92335	Fitting of artificial eye	0.45	0.99	0.17	0.01	1.45	$52.49	0.63	$22.81	XXX	A+
92340 §	Fitting of spectacles	0.37	0.68	0.15	0.01	1.06	$38.37	0.53	$19.19	XXX	
92341 §	Fitting of spectacles	0.47	0.72	0.19	0.01	1.20	$43.44	0.67	$24.25	XXX	
92342 §	Fitting of spectacles	0.53	0.74	0.21	0.01	1.28	$46.33	0.75	$27.15	XXX	
92352 §	Special spectacles fitting	0.37	0.68	0.15	0.01	1.06	$38.37	0.53	$19.19	XXX	
92353 §	Special spectacles fitting	0.50	0.73	0.20	0.02	1.25	$45.25	0.72	$26.06	XXX	
92354 §	Special spectacles fitting	0.00	8.41	8.41	0.08	8.49	$307.33	8.49	$307.33	XXX	
92355 §	Special spectacles fitting	0.00	4.11	4.11	0.01	4.12	$149.14	4.12	$149.14	XXX	
92358 §	Eye prosthesis service	0.00	0.92	0.92	0.04	0.96	$34.75	0.96	$34.75	XXX	
92370 §	Repair & adjust spectacles	0.32	0.54	0.13	0.02	0.88	$31.86	0.47	$17.01	XXX	
92371 §	Repair & adjust spectacles	0.00	0.59	0.59	0.02	0.61	$22.08	0.61	$22.08	XXX	
92392 §	Supply of low vision aids	0.00	3.84	3.84	0.02	3.86	$139.73	3.86	$139.73	XXX	
92393 §	Supply of artificial eye	0.00	11.92	11.92	0.47	12.39	$448.51	12.39	$448.51	XXX	
92395 §	Supply of spectacles	0.00	1.30	1.30	0.08	1.38	$49.95	1.38	$49.95	XXX	
92396 §	Supply of contact lenses	0.00	2.19	2.19	0.06	2.25	$81.45	2.25	$81.45	XXX	
92499	Eye service or procedure	0.00	0.00	0.00	0.00	0.00	$0.00	0.00	$0.00	XXX	A+
92499-26	Eye service or procedure	0.00	0.00	0.00	0.00	0.00	$0.00	0.00	$0.00	XXX	A+
92499-TC	Eye service or procedure	0.00	0.00	0.00	0.00	0.00	$0.00	0.00	$0.00	XXX	A+
Medicine: Special otorhinolaryngologic services											
92502	Ear and throat examination	1.51	NA	1.28	0.06	NA	NA	2.85	$103.17	000	A+
92504	Ear microscopy examination	0.18	1.10	0.09	0.01	1.29	$46.70	0.28	$10.14	XXX	A+
92506	Speech/hearing evaluation	0.86	1.72	0.43	0.04	2.62	$94.84	1.33	$48.14	XXX	A+
92507	Speech/hearing therapy	0.52	1.54	0.28	0.02	2.08	$75.29	0.82	$29.68	XXX	A+
92508	Speech/hearing therapy	0.26	1.77	0.15	0.01	2.04	$73.85	0.42	$15.20	XXX	A+
92510	Rehab for ear implant	1.50	2.11	0.83	0.06	3.67	$132.85	2.39	$86.52	XXX	A+

Code	Description								
92511	Nasopharyngoscopy	0.84	1.36	0.42	0.03	2.23	$80.72	1.29	$46.70	000	A+
92512	Nasal function studies	0.55	1.13	0.17	0.02	1.70	$61.54	0.74	$26.79	XXX	A+
92516	Facial nerve function test	0.43	0.94	0.24	0.02	1.39	$50.32	0.69	$24.98	XXX	A+
92520	Laryngeal function studies	0.76	0.52	0.43	0.03	1.31	$47.42	1.22	$44.16	XXX	A+
92525 §	Oral function evaluation	1.50	1.69	0.60	0.07	3.26	$118.01	2.17	$78.55	XXX	
92526	Oral function therapy	0.55	1.55	0.27	0.02	2.12	$76.74	0.84	$30.41	XXX	A+
92541	Spontaneous nystagmus test	0.40	1.45	1.45	0.04	1.89	$68.42	1.89	$68.42	XXX	A+
92541-26	Spontaneous nystagmus test	0.40	0.20	0.20	0.02	0.62	$22.44	0.62	$22.44	XXX	A+
92541-TC	Spontaneous nystagmus test	0.00	1.25	1.25	0.02	1.27	$45.97	1.27	$45.97	XXX	A+
92542	Positional nystagmus test	0.33	1.39	1.39	0.03	1.75	$63.35	1.75	$63.35	XXX	A+
92542-26	Positional nystagmus test	0.33	0.17	0.17	0.01	0.51	$18.46	0.51	$18.46	XXX	A+
92542-TC	Positional nystagmus test	0.00	1.22	1.22	0.02	1.24	$44.89	1.24	$44.89	XXX	A+
92543	Caloric vestibular test	0.10	0.39	0.39	0.02	0.51	$18.46	0.51	$18.46	XXX	A+
92543-26	Caloric vestibular test	0.10	0.05	0.05	0.01	0.16	$5.79	0.16	$5.79	XXX	A+
92543-TC	Caloric vestibular test	0.00	0.34	0.34	0.01	0.35	$12.67	0.35	$12.67	XXX	A+
92544	Optokinetic nystagmus test	0.26	1.35	1.35	0.03	1.64	$59.37	1.64	$59.37	XXX	A+
92544-26	Optokinetic nystagmus test	0.26	0.13	0.13	0.01	0.40	$14.48	0.40	$14.48	XXX	A+
92544-TC	Optokinetic nystagmus test	0.00	1.22	1.22	0.02	1.24	$44.89	1.24	$44.89	XXX	A+
92545	Oscillating tracking test	0.23	1.32	1.32	0.03	1.58	$57.19	1.58	$57.19	XXX	A+
92545-26	Oscillating tracking test	0.23	0.12	0.12	0.01	0.36	$13.03	0.36	$13.03	XXX	A+
92545-TC	Oscillating tracking test	0.00	1.20	1.20	0.02	1.22	$44.16	1.22	$44.16	XXX	A+
92546	Sinusoidal rotational test	0.29	2.22	2.22	0.03	2.54	$91.95	2.54	$91.95	XXX	A+
92546-26	Sinusoidal rotational test	0.29	0.14	0.14	0.01	0.44	$15.93	0.44	$15.93	XXX	A+
92546-TC	Sinusoidal rotational test	0.00	2.08	2.08	0.02	2.10	$76.02	2.10	$76.02	XXX	A+
92547	Supplemental electrical test	0.00	1.21	1.21	0.05	1.26	$45.61	1.26	$45.61	ZZZ	A+
92548	Posturography	0.50	2.09	2.09	0.13	2.72	$98.46	2.72	$98.46	XXX	A+
92548-26	Posturography	0.50	0.28	0.28	0.02	0.80	$28.96	0.80	$28.96	XXX	A+
92548-TC	Posturography	0.00	1.81	1.81	0.11	1.92	$69.50	1.92	$69.50	XXX	A+

* **M** = multiple surgery adjustment applies
Me = multiple endoscopy rules may apply
B = bilateral surgery adjustment applies
A = assistant-at-surgery restriction

A+ = assistant-at-surgery restriction unless medical necessity established with documentation
C = cosurgeons payable
C+ = cosurgeons payable if medical necessity established with documentation

T = team surgeons permitted
T+ = team surgeons payable if medical necessity established with documentation
§ = indicates services that are not covered by Medicare.

CPT five-digit codes, two-digit numeric modifiers, and descriptions only are © 2001 American Medical Association

Medicare RBRVS: The Physicians' Guide

Relative value units

CPT Code and Modifier	Description	Work RVU	Non Facility Practice Expense RVU	Facility Practice Expense RVU	PLI RVU	Total Non Facility RVUs	Medicare Payment Non Facility	Total Facility RVUs	Medicare Payment Facility	Global Period	Payment Policy Indicators*
92552	Pure tone audiometry, air	0.00	0.42	0.42	0.03	0.45	$16.29	0.45	$16.29	XXX	A+
92553	Audiometry, air & bone	0.00	0.62	0.62	0.05	0.67	$24.25	0.67	$24.25	XXX	A+
92555	Speech threshold audiometry	0.00	0.36	0.36	0.03	0.39	$14.12	0.39	$14.12	XXX	A+
92556	Speech audiometry, complete	0.00	0.54	0.54	0.05	0.59	$21.36	0.59	$21.36	XXX	A+
92557	Comprehensive hearing test	0.00	1.13	1.13	0.10	1.23	$44.53	1.23	$44.53	XXX	A+
92561	Bekesy audiometry, diagnosis	0.00	0.68	0.68	0.05	0.73	$26.43	0.73	$26.43	XXX	A+
92562	Loudness balance test	0.00	0.39	0.39	0.03	0.42	$15.20	0.42	$15.20	XXX	A+
92563	Tone decay hearing test	0.00	0.36	0.36	0.03	0.39	$14.12	0.39	$14.12	XXX	A+
92564	Sisi hearing test	0.00	0.45	0.45	0.04	0.49	$17.74	0.49	$17.74	XXX	A+
92565	Stenger test, pure tone	0.00	0.38	0.38	0.03	0.41	$14.84	0.41	$14.84	XXX	A+
92567	Tympanometry	0.00	0.50	0.50	0.05	0.55	$19.91	0.55	$19.91	XXX	A+
92568	Acoustic reflex testing	0.00	0.36	0.36	0.03	0.39	$14.12	0.39	$14.12	XXX	A+
92569	Acoustic reflex decay test	0.00	0.39	0.39	0.03	0.42	$15.20	0.42	$15.20	XXX	A+
92571	Filtered speech hearing test	0.00	0.37	0.37	0.03	0.40	$14.48	0.40	$14.48	XXX	A+
92572	Staggered spondaic word test	0.00	0.08	0.08	0.01	0.09	$3.26	0.09	$3.26	XXX	A+
92573	Lombard test	0.00	0.33	0.33	0.03	0.36	$13.03	0.36	$13.03	XXX	A+
92575	Sensorineural acuity test	0.00	0.28	0.28	0.02	0.30	$10.86	0.30	$10.86	XXX	A+
92576	Synthetic sentence test	0.00	0.42	0.42	0.04	0.46	$16.65	0.46	$16.65	XXX	A+
92577	Stenger test, speech	0.00	0.68	0.68	0.06	0.74	$26.79	0.74	$26.79	XXX	A+
92579	Visual audiometry (vra)	0.00	0.69	0.69	0.05	0.74	$26.79	0.74	$26.79	XXX	A+
92582	Conditioning play audiometry	0.00	0.69	0.69	0.05	0.74	$26.79	0.74	$26.79	XXX	A+
92583	Select picture audiometry	0.00	0.84	0.84	0.07	0.91	$32.94	0.91	$32.94	XXX	A+
92584	Electrocochleography	0.00	2.35	2.35	0.17	2.52	$91.22	2.52	$91.22	XXX	A+
92585	Auditor evoke potent, compre	0.50	1.98	1.98	0.14	2.62	$94.84	2.62	$94.84	XXX	A+
92585-26	Auditor evoke potent, compre	0.50	0.23	0.23	0.02	0.75	$27.15	0.75	$27.15	XXX	A+
92585-TC	Auditor evoke potent, compre	0.00	1.75	1.75	0.12	1.87	$67.69	1.87	$67.69	XXX	A+
92586	Auditor evoke potent, limit	0.00	1.75	1.75	0.12	1.87	$67.69	1.87	$67.69	XXX	A+

Code	Description								
92587	Evoked auditory test	0.13	1.31	1.31	0.10	1.54	$55.75	1.54	$55.75	XXX	A+
92587-26	Evoked auditory test	0.13	0.07	1.31	0.01	1.54	$7.60	0.21	$7.60	XXX	A+
92587-TC	Evoked auditory test	0.00	1.24	1.24	0.09	1.33	$48.14	1.33	$48.14	XXX	A+
92588	Evoked auditory test	0.36	1.58	1.58	0.12	2.06	$74.57	2.06	$74.57	XXX	A+
92588-26	Evoked auditory test	0.36	0.18	0.18	0.01	0.55	$19.91	0.55	$19.91	XXX	A+
92588-TC	Evoked auditory test	0.00	1.40	1.40	0.11	1.51	$54.66	1.51	$54.66	XXX	A+
92589	Auditory function test(s)	0.00	0.51	0.51	0.05	0.56	$20.27	0.56	$20.27	XXX	A+
92596	Ear protector evaluation	0.00	0.56	0.56	0.05	0.61	$22.08	0.61	$22.08	XXX	A+
92599	ENT procedure/service	0.00	0.00	0.00	0.00	0.00	$0.00	0.00	$0.00	XXX	A+
92599-26	ENT procedure/service	0.00	0.00	0.00	0.00	0.00	$0.00	0.00	$0.00	XXX	A+
92599-TC	ENT procedure/service	0.00	0.00	0.00	0.00	0.00	$0.00	0.00	$0.00	XXX	A+

Medicine: Cardiovascular

Code	Description								
92950	Heart/lung resuscitation cpr	3.80	1.59	1.18	0.21	5.60	$202.72	5.19	$187.87	000	A+
92953	Temporary external pacing	0.23	NA	0.23	0.01	NA	NA	0.47	$17.01	000	A+
92960	Cardioversion electric, ext	2.25	2.23	0.91	0.08	4.56	$165.07	3.24	$117.29	000	A+
92961	Cardioversion, electric, int	4.60	NA	1.85	0.17	NA	NA	6.62	$239.64	000	
92970	Cardioassist, internal	3.52	NA	1.27	0.17	NA	NA	4.96	$179.55	000	A+
92971	Cardioassist, external	1.77	NA	0.86	0.06	NA	NA	2.69	$97.38	000	A+
92973	Percut coronary thrombectomy	3.28	NA	1.37	0.17	NA	NA	4.82	$174.48	ZZZ	A+
92974	Cath place, cardio brachytx	3.00	NA	1.26	1.18	NA	NA	5.44	$196.92	ZZZ	A+
92975	Dissolve clot, heart vessel	7.25	NA	3.01	0.22	NA	NA	10.48	$379.37	000	M
92977	Dissolve clot, heart vessel	0.00	7.65	7.65	0.38	8.03	$290.68	8.03	$290.68	XXX	A+
92978	Intravasc us, heart add-on	1.80	5.09	5.09	0.26	7.15	$258.82	7.15	$258.82	ZZZ	A+
92978-26	Intravasc us, heart add-on	1.80	0.76	0.76	0.06	2.62	$94.84	2.62	$94.84	ZZZ	A+
92978-TC	Intravasc us, heart add-on	0.00	4.33	4.33	0.20	4.53	$163.98	4.53	$163.98	ZZZ	A+
92979	Intravasc us, heart add-on	1.44	2.76	2.76	0.15	4.35	$157.47	4.35	$157.47	ZZZ	A+
92979-26	Intravasc us, heart add-on	1.44	0.58	0.58	0.04	2.06	$74.57	2.06	$74.57	ZZZ	A+
92979-TC	Intravasc us, heart add-on	0.00	2.18	2.18	0.11	2.29	$82.90	2.29	$82.90	ZZZ	A+

* **M** = multiple surgery adjustment applies
Me = multiple endoscopy rules may apply
B = bilateral surgery adjustment applies
A = assistant-at-surgery restriction

A+ = assistant-at-surgery restriction unless medical necessity established with documentation
C = cosurgeons payable
C+ = cosurgeons payable if medical necessity established with documentation

T = team surgeons permitted
T+ = team surgeons payable if medical necessity established with documentation
$ = indicates services that are not covered by Medicare.

CPT five-digit codes, two-digit numeric modifiers, and descriptions only are © 2001 American Medical Association

Medicare RBRVS: The Physicians' Guide

Relative value units

CPT Code and Modifier	Description	Work RVU	Non Facility Practice Expense RVU	Facility Practice Expense RVU	PLI RVU	Total Non Facility RVUs	Medicare Payment Non Facility	Total Facility RVUs	Medicare Payment Facility	Global Period	Payment Policy Indicators*
92980	Insert intracoronary stent	14.84	NA	6.22	0.78	NA	NA	21.84	$790.59	000	A+
92981	Insert intracoronary stent	4.17	NA	1.75	0.21	NA	NA	6.13	$221.90	ZZZ	A+
92982	Coronary artery dilation	10.98	NA	4.59	0.57	NA	NA	16.14	$584.26	000	M A+
92984	Coronary artery dilation	2.97	NA	1.24	0.16	NA	NA	4.37	$158.19	ZZZ	A+
92986	Revision of aortic valve	21.80	NA	10.43	1.14	NA	NA	33.37	$1,207.97	090	M A+
92987	Revision of mitral valve	22.70	NA	10.85	1.18	NA	NA	34.73	$1,257.20	090	M A+
92990	Revision of pulmonary valve	17.34	NA	8.41	0.90	NA	NA	26.65	$964.71	090	M A+
92992	Revision of heart chamber	0.00	0.00	0.00	0.00	0.00	$0.00	0.00	$0.00	090	M
92993	Revision of heart chamber	0.00	0.00	0.00	0.00	0.00	$0.00	0.00	$0.00	090	M
92995	Coronary atherectomy	12.09	NA	5.06	0.63	NA	NA	17.78	$643.62	000	M A+
92996	Coronary atherectomy add-on	3.26	NA	1.37	0.17	NA	NA	4.80	$173.76	ZZZ	A+
92997	Pul art balloon repr, percut	12.00	NA	4.55	0.63	NA	NA	17.18	$621.90	000	M A+
92998	Pul art balloon repr, percut	6.00	NA	2.06	0.31	NA	NA	8.37	$302.99	ZZZ	A+
93000	Electrocardiogram, complete	0.17	0.50	0.50	0.03	0.70	$25.34	0.70	$25.34	XXX	A+
93005	Electrocardiogram, tracing	0.00	0.43	0.43	0.02	0.45	$16.29	0.45	$16.29	XXX	A+
93010	Electrocardiogram report	0.17	0.07	0.07	0.01	0.25	$9.05	0.25	$9.05	XXX	A+
93012	Transmission of ecg	0.00	2.24	2.24	0.15	2.39	$86.52	2.39	$86.52	XXX	A+
93014	Report on transmitted ecg	0.52	0.19	0.19	0.02	0.73	$26.43	0.73	$26.43	XXX	A+
93015	Cardiovascular stress test	0.75	1.90	1.90	0.11	2.76	$99.91	2.76	$99.91	XXX	A+
93016	Cardiovascular stress test	0.45	0.18	0.18	0.01	0.64	$23.17	0.64	$23.17	XXX	A+
93017	Cardiovascular stress test	0.00	1.60	1.60	0.09	1.69	$61.18	1.69	$61.18	XXX	A+
93018	Cardiovascular stress test	0.30	0.12	0.12	0.01	0.43	$15.57	0.43	$15.57	XXX	A+
93024	Cardiac drug stress test	1.17	1.55	1.55	0.11	2.83	$102.44	2.83	$102.44	XXX	A+
93024-26	Cardiac drug stress test	1.17	0.48	0.48	0.04	1.69	$61.18	1.69	$61.18	XXX	A+
93024-TC	Cardiac drug stress test	0.00	1.07	1.07	0.07	1.14	$41.27	1.14	$41.27	XXX	A+
93025	Microvolt t-wave assess	0.75	6.42	6.42	0.11	7.28	$263.53	7.28	$263.53	XXX	A+
93040	Rhythm ECG with report	0.16	0.19	0.19	0.02	0.37	$13.39	0.37	$13.39	XXX	A+

Code	Description								
93041	Rhythm ECG, tracing	0.00	0.14	0.14	0.15	$5.43	$5.43	XXX	A+
93042	Rhythm ECG, report	0.16	0.05	0.05	0.01	$7.96	$7.96	XXX	A+
93224	ECG monitor/report, 24 hrs	0.52	3.47	3.47	4.20	$152.04	$152.04	XXX	A+
93225	ECG monitor/record, 24 hrs	0.00	1.18	1.18	1.25	$45.25	$45.25	XXX	A+
93226	ECG monitor/report, 24 hrs	0.00	2.08	2.08	2.20	$79.64	$79.64	XXX	A+
93227	ECG monitor/review, 24 hrs	0.52	0.21	0.21	0.75	$27.15	$27.15	XXX	A+
93230	ECG monitor/report, 24 hrs	0.52	3.72	3.72	4.46	$161.45	$161.45	XXX	A+
93231	Ecg monitor/record, 24 hrs	0.00	1.44	1.44	1.53	$55.38	$55.38	XXX	A+
93232	ECG monitor/report, 24 hrs	0.00	2.07	2.07	2.18	$78.91	$78.91	XXX	A+
93233	ECG monitor/review, 24 hrs	0.52	0.21	0.21	0.75	$27.15	$27.15	XXX	A+
93235	ECG monitor/report, 24 hrs	0.45	2.66	2.66	3.24	$117.29	$117.29	XXX	A+
93236	ECG monitor/report, 24 hrs	0.00	2.49	2.49	2.61	$94.48	$94.48	XXX	A+
93237	ECG monitor/review, 24 hrs	0.45	0.17	0.17	0.63	$22.81	$22.81	XXX	A+
93268	ECG record/review	0.52	3.62	3.62	4.38	$158.55	$158.55	XXX	A+
93270	ECG recording	0.00	1.18	1.18	1.25	$45.25	$45.25	XXX	A+
93271	Ecg/monitoring and analysis	0.00	2.24	2.24	2.39	$86.52	$86.52	XXX	A+
93272	Ecg/review, interpret only	0.52	0.20	0.20	0.74	$26.79	$26.79	XXX	A+
93278	ECG/signal-averaged	0.25	1.19	1.19	1.54	$55.75	$55.75	XXX	A+
93278-26	ECG/signal-averaged	0.25	0.10	0.10	0.36	$13.03	$13.03	XXX	A+
93278-TC	ECG/signal-averaged	0.00	1.09	1.09	1.18	$42.72	$42.72	XXX	A+
93303	Echo transthoracic	1.30	4.16	4.16	5.69	$205.97	$205.97	XXX	A+
93303-26	Echo transthoracic	1.30	0.50	0.50	1.84	$66.61	$66.61	XXX	A+
93303-TC	Echo transthoracic	0.00	3.66	3.66	3.85	$139.37	$139.37	XXX	A+
93304	Echo transthoracic	0.75	2.15	2.15	3.03	$109.68	$109.68	XXX	A+
93304-26	Echo transthoracic	0.75	0.30	0.30	1.07	$38.73	$38.73	XXX	A+
93304-TC	Echo transthoracic	0.00	1.85	1.85	1.96	$70.95	$70.95	XXX	A+
93307	Echo exam of heart	0.92	4.04	4.04	5.18	$187.51	$187.51	XXX	A+
93307-26	Echo exam of heart	0.92	0.38	0.38	1.33	$48.14	$48.14	XXX	A+

* **M** = multiple surgery adjustment applies
Me = multiple endoscopy rules may apply
B = bilateral surgery adjustment applies
A = assistant-at-surgery restriction

A+ = assistant-at-surgery restriction unless medical necessity established with documentation
C = cosurgeons payable
C+ = cosurgeons payable if medical necessity established with documentation

T = team surgeons permitted
T+ = team surgeons payable if medical necessity established with documentation
$ = indicates services that are not covered by Medicare.

403   CPT five-digit codes, two-digit numeric modifiers, and descriptions only are © 2001 American Medical Association

Medicare RBRVS: The Physicians' Guide

Relative value units

CPT Code and Modifier	Description	Work RVU	Non Facility Practice Expense RVU	Facility Practice Expense RVU	PLI RVU	Total Non Facility RVUs	Medicare Payment Non Facility	Total Facility RVUs	Medicare Payment Facility	Global Period	Payment Policy Indicators*
93307-TC	Echo exam of heart	0.00	3.66	3.66	0.19	3.85	$139.37	3.85	$139.37	XXX	A+
93308	Echo exam of heart	0.53	2.07	2.07	0.13	2.73	$98.82	2.73	$98.82	XXX	A+
93308-26	Echo exam of heart	0.53	0.22	0.22	0.02	0.77	$27.87	0.77	$27.87	XXX	A+
93308-TC	Echo exam of heart	0.00	1.85	1.85	0.11	1.96	$70.95	1.96	$70.95	XXX	A+
93312	Echo transesophageal	2.20	4.45	4.45	0.32	6.97	$252.31	6.97	$252.31	XXX	A+
93312-26	Echo transesophageal	2.20	0.86	0.86	0.08	3.14	$113.67	3.14	$113.67	XXX	A+
93312-TC	Echo transesophageal	0.00	3.59	3.59	0.24	3.83	$138.64	3.83	$138.64	XXX	A+
93313	Echo transesophageal	0.95	5.29	0.22	0.05	6.29	$227.69	1.22	$44.16	XXX	A+
93314	Echo transesophageal	1.25	4.10	4.10	0.28	5.63	$203.80	5.63	$203.80	XXX	A+
93314-26	Echo transesophageal	1.25	0.51	0.51	0.04	1.80	$65.16	1.80	$65.16	XXX	A+
93314-TC	Echo transesophageal	0.00	3.59	3.59	0.24	3.83	$138.64	3.83	$138.64	XXX	A+
93315	Echo transesophageal	2.78	4.70	4.70	0.34	7.82	$283.08	7.82	$283.08	XXX	A+
93315-26	Echo transesophageal	2.78	1.11	1.11	0.10	3.99	$144.43	3.99	$144.43	XXX	A+
93315-TC	Echo transesophageal	0.00	3.59	3.59	0.24	3.83	$138.64	3.83	$138.64	XXX	A+
93316	Echo transesophageal	0.95	6.39	0.25	0.05	7.39	$267.51	1.25	$45.25	XXX	A+
93317	Echo transesophageal	1.83	4.31	4.31	0.30	6.44	$233.12	6.44	$233.12	XXX	A+
93317-26	Echo transesophageal	1.83	0.72	0.72	0.06	2.61	$94.48	2.61	$94.48	XXX	A+
93317-TC	Echo transesophageal	0.00	3.59	3.59	0.24	3.83	$138.64	3.83	$138.64	XXX	A+
93318	Echo transesophageal intraop	0.00	0.00	0.00	0.00	0.00	$0.00	0.00	$0.00	XXX	A+
93318-26	Echo transesophageal intraop	2.20	0.88	0.88	0.06	3.14	$113.67	3.14	$113.67	XXX	A+
93318-TC	Echo transesophageal intraop	0.00	0.00	0.00	0.00	0.00	$0.00	0.00	$0.00	XXX	A+
93320	Doppler echo exam, heart	0.38	1.79	1.79	0.11	2.28	$82.53	2.28	$82.53	ZZZ	A+
93320-26	Doppler echo exam, heart	0.38	0.16	0.16	0.01	0.55	$19.91	0.55	$19.91	ZZZ	A+
93320-TC	Doppler echo exam, heart	0.00	1.63	1.63	0.10	1.73	$62.62	1.73	$62.62	ZZZ	A+
93321	Doppler echo exam, heart	0.15	1.12	1.12	0.08	1.35	$48.87	1.35	$48.87	ZZZ	A+
93321-26	Doppler echo exam, heart	0.15	0.06	0.06	0.01	0.22	$7.96	0.22	$7.96	ZZZ	A
93321-TC	Doppler echo exam, heart	0.00	1.06	1.06	0.07	1.13	$40.91	1.13	$40.91	ZZZ	A+

Code	Description									
93325	Doppler color flow add-on	0.07	2.78	2.78	0.18	3.03	3.03	$109.68	ZZZ		A+
93325-26	Doppler color flow add-on	0.07	0.03	0.03	0.01	0.11	0.11	$3.98	ZZZ		A+
93325-TC	Doppler color flow add-on	0.00	2.75	2.75	0.17	2.92	2.92	$105.70	ZZZ		A+
93350	Echo transthoracic	1.48	2.28	2.28	0.13	3.89	3.89	$140.81	XXX		A+
93350-26	Echo transthoracic	1.48	0.61	0.61	0.02	2.11	2.11	$76.38	XXX		A+
93350-TC	Echo transthoracic	0.00	1.67	1.67	0.11	1.78	1.78	$64.43	XXX		A+
93501	Right heart catheterization	3.02	17.23	17.23	1.03	21.28	21.28	$770.32	000	M	A+
93501-26	Right heart catheterization	3.02	1.24	1.24	0.16	4.42	4.42	$160.00	000	M	A+
93501-TC	Right heart catheterization	0.00	15.99	15.99	0.87	16.86	16.86	$610.32	000		A+
93503	Insert/place heart catheter	2.91	NA	NA	0.16	NA	NA	$136.83	000		A+
93505	Biopsy of heart lining	4.38	3.67	3.67	0.36	8.41	8.41	$304.44	000	M	A+
93505-26	Biopsy of heart lining	4.38	1.80	1.80	0.23	6.41	6.41	$232.04	000	M	A+
93505-TC	Biopsy of heart lining	0.00	1.87	1.87	0.13	2.00	2.00	$72.40	000		A+
93508	Cath placement, angiography	4.10	13.64	13.64	0.75	18.49	18.49	$669.32	000	M	A+
93508-26	Cath placement, angiography	4.10	1.71	1.71	0.21	6.02	6.02	$217.92	000	M	A+
93508-TC	Cath placement, angiography	0.00	11.93	11.93	0.54	12.47	12.47	$451.40	000		A+
93510	Left heart catheterization	4.33	36.77	36.77	2.13	43.23	43.23	$1,564.89	000	M	A+
93510-26	Left heart catheterization	4.33	1.82	1.82	0.22	6.37	6.37	$230.59	000	M	A+
93510-TC	Left heart catheterization	0.00	34.95	34.95	1.91	36.86	36.86	$1,334.30	000		A+
93511	Left heart catheterization	5.03	36.12	36.12	2.11	43.26	43.26	$1,565.98	000	M	A+
93511-26	Left heart catheterization	5.03	2.10	2.10	0.26	7.39	7.39	$267.51	000	M	A+
93511-TC	Left heart catheterization	0.00	34.02	34.02	1.85	35.87	35.87	$1,298.47	000		A+
93514	Left heart catheterization	7.05	36.79	36.79	2.22	46.06	46.06	$1,667.34	000	M	A+
93514-26	Left heart catheterization	7.05	2.77	2.77	0.37	10.19	10.19	$368.87	000	M	A+
93514-TC	Left heart catheterization	0.00	34.02	34.02	1.85	35.87	35.87	$1,298.47	000		A+
93524	Left heart catheterization	6.95	47.32	47.32	2.79	57.06	57.06	$2,065.53	000	M	A+
93524-26	Left heart catheterization	6.95	2.86	2.86	0.36	10.17	10.17	$368.15	000	M	A+
93524-TC	Left heart catheterization	0.00	44.46	44.46	2.43	46.89	46.89	$1,697.38	000		A+

* **M** = multiple surgery adjustment applies
Me = multiple endoscopy rules may apply
B = bilateral surgery adjustment applies
A = assistant-at-surgery restriction

A+ = assistant-at-surgery restriction unless medical necessity established with documentation
C = cosurgeons payable
C+ = cosurgeons payable if medical necessity established with documentation

T = team surgeons permitted
T+ = team surgeons payable if medical necessity established with documentation
§ = indicates services that are not covered by Medicare.

CPT five-digit codes, two-digit numeric modifiers, and descriptions only are © 2001 American Medical Association

Medicare RBRVS: The Physicians' Guide

Relative value units

CPT Code and Modifier	Description	Work RVU	Non Facility Practice Expense RVU	Facility Practice Expense RVU	PLI RVU	Total Non Facility RVUs	Medicare Payment Non Facility	Total Facility RVUs	Medicare Payment Facility	Global Period	Payment Policy Indicators*
93526	Rt & Lt heart catheters	5.99	48.18	48.18	2.81	56.98	$2,062.63	56.98	$2,062.63	000	M A+
93526-26	Rt & Lt heart catheters	5.99	2.50	2.50	0.31	8.80	$318.55	8.80	$318.55	000	M A+
93526-TC	Rt & Lt heart catheters	0.00	45.68	45.68	2.50	48.18	$1,744.08	48.18	$1,744.08	000	A+
93527	Rt & Lt heart catheters	7.28	47.49	47.49	2.81	57.58	$2,084.35	57.58	$2,084.35	000	M A+
93527-26	Rt & Lt heart catheters	7.28	3.03	3.03	0.38	10.69	$386.97	10.69	$386.97	000	M A+
93527-TC	Rt & Lt heart catheters	0.00	44.46	44.46	2.43	46.89	$1,697.38	46.89	$1,697.38	000	A+
93528	Rt & Lt heart catheters	9.00	48.27	48.27	2.90	60.17	$2,178.11	60.17	$2,178.11	000	M A+
93528-26	Rt & Lt heart catheters	9.00	3.81	3.81	0.47	13.28	$480.73	13.28	$480.73	000	M A+
93528-TC	Rt & Lt heart catheters	0.00	44.46	44.46	2.43	46.89	$1,697.38	46.89	$1,697.38	000	A+
93529	Rt&lt heart catheterization	4.80	46.46	46.46	2.68	53.94	$1,952.58	53.94	$1,952.58	000	M A+
93529-26	Rt&lt heart catheterization	4.80	2.00	2.00	0.25	7.05	$255.20	7.05	$255.20	000	M A+
93529-TC	Rt&lt heart catheterization	0.00	44.46	44.46	2.43	46.89	$1,697.38	46.89	$1,697.38	000	A+
93530	Rt heart cath, congenital	4.23	17.59	17.59	1.11	22.93	$830.05	22.93	$830.05	000	M A+
93530-26	Rt heart cath, congenital	4.23	1.60	1.60	0.24	6.07	$219.73	6.07	$219.73	000	M A+
93530-TC	Rt heart cath, congenital	0.00	15.99	15.99	0.87	16.86	$610.32	16.86	$610.32	000	A+
93531	R & l heart cath, congenital	8.35	48.92	48.92	2.96	60.23	$2,180.28	60.23	$2,180.28	000	M A+
93531-26	R & l heart cath, congenital	8.35	3.24	3.24	0.46	12.05	$436.20	12.05	$436.20	000	M A+
93531-TC	R & l heart cath, congenital	0.00	45.68	45.68	2.50	48.18	$1,744.08	48.18	$1,744.08	000	A+
93532	R & l heart cath, congenital	10.00	48.58	48.58	2.95	61.53	$2,227.34	61.53	$2,227.34	000	M A+
93532-26	R & l heart cath, congenital	10.00	4.12	4.12	0.52	14.64	$529.96	14.64	$529.96	000	M A+
93532-TC	R & l heart cath, congenital	0.00	44.46	44.46	2.43	46.89	$1,697.38	46.89	$1,697.38	000	A+
93533	R & l heart cath, congenital	6.70	47.01	47.01	2.86	56.57	$2,047.79	56.57	$2,047.79	000	M A+
93533-26	R & l heart cath, congenital	6.70	2.55	2.55	0.43	9.68	$350.41	9.68	$350.41	000	M A+
93533-TC	R & l heart cath, congenital	0.00	44.46	44.46	2.43	46.89	$1,697.38	46.89	$1,697.38	000	A+
93539	Injection, cardiac cath	0.40	0.84	0.17	0.01	1.25	$45.25	0.58	$21.00	000	A+
93540	Injection, cardiac cath	0.43	0.86	0.18	0.01	1.30	$47.06	0.62	$22.44	000	A+
93541	Injection for lung angiogram	0.29	NA	0.12	0.01	NA	NA	0.42	$15.20	000	A+

Code	Description									
93542	Injection for heart x-rays	0.29	NA	0.12	0.01	NA	0.42	$15.20	000	A+
93543	Injection for heart x-rays	0.29	0.55	0.12	0.01	0.85	0.42	$15.20	000	A+
93544	Injection for aortography	0.25	0.53	0.10	0.01	0.79	0.36	$13.03	000	A+
93545	Inject for coronary x-rays	0.40	0.85	0.17	0.01	1.26	0.58	$21.00	000	A+
93555	Imaging, cardiac cath	0.81	6.27	6.27	0.31	7.39	7.39	$267.51	XXX	A+
93555-26	Imaging, cardiac cath	0.81	0.34	0.34	0.03	1.18	1.18	$42.72	XXX	A+
93555-TC	Imaging, cardiac cath	0.00	5.93	5.93	0.28	6.21	6.21	$224.80	XXX	A+
93556	Imaging, cardiac cath	0.83	9.71	9.71	0.45	10.99	10.99	$397.83	XXX	A+
93556-26	Imaging, cardiac cath	0.83	0.35	0.35	0.03	1.21	1.21	$43.80	XXX	A+
93556-TC	Imaging, cardiac cath	0.00	9.36	9.36	0.42	9.78	9.78	$354.03	XXX	A+
93561	Cardiac output measurement	0.50	0.67	0.67	0.07	1.24	1.24	$44.89	000	A+
93561-26	Cardiac output measurement	0.50	0.16	0.16	0.02	0.68	0.68	$24.62	000	A+
93561-TC	Cardiac output measurement	0.00	0.51	0.51	0.05	0.56	0.56	$20.27	000	A+
93562	Cardiac output measurement	0.16	0.34	0.34	0.04	0.54	0.54	$19.55	000	A+
93562-26	Cardiac output measurement	0.16	0.05	0.05	0.01	0.22	0.22	$7.96	000	A+
93562-TC	Cardiac output measurement	0.00	0.29	0.29	0.03	0.32	0.32	$11.58	000	A+
93571	Heart flow reserve measure	1.80	5.06	5.06	0.31	7.17	7.17	$259.55	ZZZ	A+
93571-26	Heart flow reserve measure	1.80	0.73	0.73	0.11	2.64	2.64	$95.57	ZZZ	A+
93571-TC	Heart flow reserve measure	0.00	4.33	4.33	0.20	4.53	4.53	$163.98	ZZZ	A+
93572	Heart flow reserve measure	1.44	2.70	2.70	0.28	4.42	4.42	$160.00	ZZZ	A+
93572-26	Heart flow reserve measure	1.44	0.52	0.52	0.17	2.13	2.13	$77.10	ZZZ	A+
93572-TC	Heart flow reserve measure	0.00	2.18	2.18	0.11	2.29	2.29	$82.90	ZZZ	A+
93600	Bundle of His recording	2.12	2.74	2.74	0.22	5.08	5.08	$183.89	000	A+
93600-26	Bundle of His recording	2.12	0.89	0.89	0.11	3.12	3.12	$112.94	000	A+
93600-TC	Bundle of His recording	0.00	1.85	1.85	0.11	1.96	1.96	$70.95	000	A+
93602	Intra-atrial recording	2.12	1.94	1.94	0.18	4.24	4.24	$153.48	000	A+
93602-26	Intra-atrial recording	2.12	0.88	0.88	0.12	3.12	3.12	$112.94	000	A+
93602-TC	Intra-atrial recording	0.00	1.06	1.06	0.06	1.12	1.12	$40.54	000	A+

* **M** = multiple surgery adjustment applies
Me = multiple endoscopy rules may apply
B = bilateral surgery adjustment applies
A = assistant-at-surgery restriction

A+ = assistant-at-surgery restriction unless medical necessity established with documentation
C = cosurgeons payable
C+ = cosurgeons payable if medical necessity established with documentation

T = team surgeons permitted
T+ = team surgeons payable if medical necessity established with documentation
$ = indicates services that are not covered by Medicare.

CPT five-digit codes, two-digit numeric modifiers, and descriptions only are © 2001 American Medical Association

Medicare RBRVS: The Physicians' Guide

Relative value units

CPT Code and Modifier	Description	Work RVU	Non Facility Practice Expense RVU	Facility Practice Expense RVU	PLI RVU	Total Non Facility RVUs	Medicare Payment Non Facility	Total Facility RVUs	Medicare Payment Facility	Global Period	Payment Policy Indicators*
93603	Right ventricular recording	2.12	2.46	2.46	0.20	4.78	$173.03	4.78	$173.03	000	A+
93603-26	Right ventricular recording	2.12	0.86	0.86	0.11	3.09	$111.86	3.09	$111.86	000	A+
93603-TC	Right ventricular recording	0.00	1.60	1.60	0.09	1.69	$61.18	1.69	$61.18	000	A+
93609	Map tachycardia, add-on	4.81	4.59	4.59	0.66	10.06	$364.16	10.06	$364.16	ZZZ	A+
93609-26	Map tachycardia, add-on	4.81	2.01	2.01	0.52	7.34	$265.70	7.34	$265.70	ZZZ	A+
93609-TC	Map tachycardia, add-on	0.00	2.58	2.58	0.14	2.72	$98.46	2.72	$98.46	ZZZ	A+
93610	Intra-atrial pacing	3.02	2.52	2.52	0.25	5.79	$209.59	5.79	$209.59	000	A+
93610-26	Intra-atrial pacing	3.02	1.23	1.23	0.17	4.42	$160.00	4.42	$160.00	000	A+
93610-TC	Intra-atrial pacing	0.00	1.29	1.29	0.08	1.37	$49.59	1.37	$49.59	000	A+
93612	Intraventricular pacing	3.02	2.76	2.76	0.26	6.04	$218.64	6.04	$218.64	000	A+
93612-26	Intraventricular pacing	3.02	1.23	1.23	0.17	4.42	$160.00	4.42	$160.00	000	A+
93612-TC	Intraventricular pacing	0.00	1.53	1.53	0.09	1.62	$58.64	1.62	$58.64	000	A+
93613	Electrophys map, 3d, add-on	0.00	0.00	0.00	0.00	0.00	$0.00	0.00	$0.00	XXX	A+
93613-26	Electrophys map, 3d, add-on	7.00	2.79	2.79	0.52	10.31	$373.21	10.31	$373.21	XXX	A+
93613-TC	Electrophys map, 3d, add-on	0.00	0.00	0.00	0.00	0.00	$0.00	0.00	$0.00	XXX	A+
93615	Esophageal recording	0.99	0.66	0.66	0.05	1.70	$61.54	1.70	$61.54	000	A+
93615-26	Esophageal recording	0.99	0.36	0.36	0.03	1.38	$49.95	1.38	$49.95	000	A+
93615-TC	Esophageal recording	0.00	0.30	0.30	0.02	0.32	$11.58	0.32	$11.58	000	A+
93616	Esophageal recording	1.49	0.80	0.80	0.08	2.37	$85.79	2.37	$85.79	000	A+
93616-26	Esophageal recording	1.49	0.50	0.50	0.06	2.05	$74.21	2.05	$74.21	000	A+
93616-TC	Esophageal recording	0.00	0.30	0.30	0.02	0.32	$11.58	0.32	$11.58	000	A+
93618	Heart rhythm pacing	4.26	5.54	5.54	0.42	10.22	$369.96	10.22	$369.96	000	A+
93618-26	Heart rhythm pacing	4.26	1.78	1.78	0.22	6.26	$226.61	6.26	$226.61	000	A+
93618-TC	Heart rhythm pacing	0.00	3.76	3.76	0.20	3.96	$143.35	3.96	$143.35	000	A+
93619	Electrophysiology evaluation	7.32	10.32	10.32	0.77	18.41	$666.43	18.41	$666.43	000	A+
93619-26	Electrophysiology evaluation	7.32	3.00	3.00	0.38	10.70	$387.33	10.70	$387.33	000	A+
93619-TC	Electrophysiology evaluation	0.00	7.32	7.32	0.39	7.71	$279.10	7.71	$279.10	000	A+

Code	Description								
93620	Electrophysiology evaluation	11.59	13.33	1.04	25.96	$939.73	25.96	$939.73	000	A+
93620-26	Electrophysiology evaluation	11.59	4.82	0.60	17.01	$615.75	17.01	$615.75	000	A+
93620-TC	Electrophysiology evaluation	0.00	8.51	0.44	8.95	$323.98	8.95	$323.98	000	A+
93621	Electrophysiology evaluation	0.00	0.00	0.00	0.00	$0.00	0.00	$0.00	ZZZ	A+
93621-26	Electrophysiology evaluation	2.10	0.88	0.15	3.13	$113.30	3.13	$113.30	ZZZ	A+
93621-TC	Electrophysiology evaluation	0.00	0.00	0.00	0.00	$0.00	0.00	$0.00	ZZZ	A+
93622	Electrophysiology evaluation	0.00	0.00	0.00	0.00	$0.00	0.00	$0.00	ZZZ	A+
93622-26	Electrophysiology evaluation	3.10	1.30	0.67	5.07	$183.53	5.07	$183.53	ZZZ	A+
93622-TC	Electrophysiology evaluation	0.00	0.00	0.00	0.00	$0.00	0.00	$0.00	ZZZ	A+
93623	Stimulation, pacing heart	0.00	0.00	0.00	0.00	$0.00	0.00	$0.00	ZZZ	A+
93623-26	Stimulation, pacing heart	2.85	1.19	0.15	4.19	$151.67	4.19	$151.67	ZZZ	A+
93623-TC	Stimulation, pacing heart	0.00	0.00	0.00	0.00	$0.00	0.00	$0.00	ZZZ	A+
93624	Electrophysiologic study	4.81	3.87	0.36	9.04	$327.24	9.04	$327.24	000	A+
93624-26	Electrophysiologic study	4.81	1.99	0.25	7.05	$255.20	7.05	$255.20	000	A+
93624-TC	Electrophysiologic study	0.00	1.88	0.11	1.99	$72.04	1.99	$72.04	000	A+
93631	Heart pacing, mapping	7.60	8.65	1.17	17.42	$630.59	17.42	$630.59	000	A+
93631-26	Heart pacing, mapping	7.60	2.81	0.66	11.07	$400.73	11.07	$400.73	000	A+
93631-TC	Heart pacing, mapping	0.00	5.84	0.51	6.35	$229.86	6.35	$229.86	000	A+
93640	Evaluation heart device	3.52	8.27	0.53	12.32	$445.97	12.32	$445.97	000	A+
93640-26	Evaluation heart device	3.52	1.46	0.18	5.16	$186.79	5.16	$186.79	000	A+
93640-TC	Evaluation heart device	0.00	6.81	0.35	7.16	$259.19	7.16	$259.19	000	A+
93641	Electrophysiology evaluation	5.93	9.28	0.66	15.87	$574.48	15.87	$574.48	000	A+
93641-26	Electrophysiology evaluation	5.93	2.47	0.31	8.71	$315.30	8.71	$315.30	000	A+
93641-TC	Electrophysiology evaluation	0.00	6.81	0.35	7.16	$259.19	7.16	$259.19	000	A+
93642	Electrophysiology evaluation	4.89	8.85	0.51	14.25	$515.84	14.25	$515.84	000	A+
93642-26	Electrophysiology evaluation	4.89	2.04	0.16	7.09	$256.65	7.09	$256.65	000	A+
93642-TC	Electrophysiology evaluation	0.00	6.81	0.35	7.16	$259.19	7.16	$259.19	000	A+
93650	Ablate heart dysrhythm focus	10.51	NA	0.55	NA	NA	15.38	$556.74	000	A+

* **M** = multiple surgery adjustment applies
Me = multiple endoscopy rules may apply
B = bilateral surgery adjustment applies
A = assistant-at-surgery restriction

A+ = assistant-at-surgery restriction unless medical necessity established with documentation
C = cosurgeons payable
C+ = cosurgeons payable if medical necessity established with documentation

T = team surgeons permitted
T+ = team surgeons payable if medical necessity established with documentation
§ = indicates services that are not covered by Medicare.

CPT five-digit codes, two-digit numeric modifiers, and descriptions only are © 2001 American Medical Association

Medicare RBRVS: The Physicians' Guide

Relative value units

CPT Code and Modifier	Description	Work RVU	Non Facility Practice Expense RVU	Facility Practice Expense RVU	PLI RVU	Total Non Facility RVUs	Medicare Payment Non Facility	Total Facility RVUs	Medicare Payment Facility	Global Period	Payment Policy Indicators*
93651	Ablate heart dysrhythm focus	16.25	NA	6.78	0.85	NA	NA	23.88	$864.44	000	A+
93652	Ablate heart dysrhythm focus	17.68	NA	7.36	0.92	NA	NA	25.96	$939.73	000	A+
93660	Tilt table evaluation	1.89	2.39	2.39	0.08	4.36	$157.83	4.36	$157.83	000	A+
93660-26	Tilt table evaluation	1.89	0.79	0.79	0.06	2.74	$99.19	2.74	$99.19	000	A+
93660-TC	Tilt table evaluation	0.00	1.60	1.60	0.02	1.62	$58.64	1.62	$58.64	000	A+
93662 §	Intracardiac ecg (ice)	0.00	0.00	0.00	0.00	0.00	$0.00	0.00	$0.00	ZZZ	A+
93662-26	Intracardiac ecg (ice)	2.80	1.12	1.12	0.41	4.33	$156.74	4.33	$156.74	ZZZ	A+
93662-TC §	Intracardiac ecg (ice)	0.00	0.00	0.00	0.00	0.00	$0.00	0.00	$0.00	XXX	A+
93701	Bioimpedance, thoracic	0.17	0.78	0.78	0.02	0.97	$35.11	0.97	$35.11	XXX	A+
93701-26	Bioimpedance, thoracic	0.17	0.07	0.07	0.01	0.25	$9.05	0.25	$9.05	XXX	A+
93701-TC	Bioimpedance, thoracic	0.00	0.71	0.71	0.01	0.72	$26.06	0.72	$26.06	XXX	A+
93720	Total body plethysmography	0.17	0.73	0.73	0.06	0.96	$34.75	0.96	$34.75	XXX	A+
93721	Plethysmography tracing	0.00	0.67	0.67	0.05	0.72	$26.06	0.72	$26.06	XXX	A+
93722	Plethysmography report	0.17	0.06	0.06	0.01	0.24	$8.69	0.24	$8.69	XXX	A+
93724	Analyze pacemaker system	4.89	5.80	5.80	0.38	11.07	$400.73	11.07	$400.73	000	A+
93724-26	Analyze pacemaker system	4.89	2.04	2.04	0.18	7.11	$257.38	7.11	$257.38	000	A+
93724-TC	Analyze pacemaker system	0.00	3.76	3.76	0.20	3.96	$143.35	3.96	$143.35	000	A+
93727	Analyze ilr system	0.52	0.21	0.21	0.05	0.78	$28.24	0.78	$28.24	XXX	
93731	Analyze pacemaker system	0.45	0.66	0.66	0.05	1.16	$41.99	1.16	$41.99	XXX	A+
93731-26	Analyze pacemaker system	0.45	0.19	0.19	0.02	0.66	$23.89	0.66	$23.89	XXX	A+
93731-TC	Analyze pacemaker system	0.00	0.47	0.47	0.03	0.50	$18.10	0.50	$18.10	XXX	A+
93732	Analyze pacemaker system	0.92	0.87	0.87	0.06	1.85	$66.97	1.85	$66.97	XXX	A+
93732-26	Analyze pacemaker system	0.92	0.38	0.38	0.03	1.33	$48.14	1.33	$48.14	XXX	A+
93732-TC	Analyze pacemaker system	0.00	0.49	0.49	0.03	0.52	$18.82	0.52	$18.82	XXX	A+
93733	Telephone analy, pacemaker	0.17	0.76	0.76	0.06	0.99	$35.84	0.99	$35.84	XXX	A+
93733-26	Telephone analy, pacemaker	0.17	0.07	0.07	0.01	0.25	$9.05	0.25	$9.05	XXX	A+
93733-TC	Telephone analy, pacemaker	0.00	0.69	0.69	0.05	0.74	$26.79	0.74	$26.79	XXX	A+

Code	Description								
93734	Analyze pacemaker system	0.38	0.49	0.49	0.03	0.90	$32.58	$32.58	0.90	XXX	A+
93734-26	Analyze pacemaker system	0.38	0.16	0.16	0.01	0.55	$19.91	$19.91	0.55	XXX	A+
93734-TC	Analyze pacemaker system	0.00	0.33	0.33	0.02	0.35	$12.67	$12.67	0.35	XXX	A+
93735	Analyze pacemaker system	0.74	0.72	0.72	0.06	1.52	$55.02	$55.02	1.52	XXX	A+
93735-26	Analyze pacemaker system	0.74	0.30	0.30	0.03	1.07	$38.73	$38.73	1.07	XXX	A+
93735-TC	Analyze pacemaker system	0.00	0.42	0.42	0.03	0.45	$16.29	$16.29	0.45	XXX	A+
93736	Telephone analy, pacemaker	0.15	0.66	0.66	0.06	0.87	$31.49	$31.49	0.87	XXX	A+
93736-26	Telephone analy, pacemaker	0.15	0.06	0.06	0.01	0.22	$7.96	$7.96	0.22	XXX	A+
93736-TC	Telephone analy, pacemaker	0.00	0.60	0.60	0.05	0.65	$23.53	$23.53	0.65	XXX	A+
93740 §	Temperature gradient studies	0.16	0.21	0.21	0.02	0.39	$14.12	$14.12	0.39	XXX	
93740-26 §	Temperature gradient studies	0.16	0.06	0.06	0.01	0.23	$8.33	$8.33	0.23	XXX	
93740-TC §	Temperature gradient studies	0.00	0.15	0.15	0.01	0.16	$5.79	$5.79	0.16	XXX	
93741	Analyze ht pace device sngl	0.80	0.96	0.96	0.05	1.81	$65.52	$65.52	1.81	XXX	
93741-26	Analyze ht pace device sngl	0.80	0.33	0.33	0.02	1.15	$41.63	$41.63	1.15	XXX	
93741-TC	Analyze ht pace device sngl	0.00	0.63	0.63	0.03	0.66	$23.89	$23.89	0.66	XXX	
93742	Analyze ht pace device sngl	0.91	1.01	1.01	0.05	1.97	$71.31	$71.31	1.97	XXX	
93742-26	Analyze ht pace device sngl	0.91	0.38	0.38	0.02	1.31	$47.42	$47.42	1.31	XXX	
93742-TC	Analyze ht pace device sngl	0.00	0.63	0.63	0.03	0.66	$23.89	$23.89	0.66	XXX	
93743	Analyze ht pace device dual	1.03	1.13	1.13	0.06	2.22	$80.36	$80.36	2.22	XXX	
93743-26	Analyze ht pace device dual	1.03	0.43	0.43	0.03	1.49	$53.94	$53.94	1.49	XXX	
93743-TC	Analyze ht pace device dual	0.00	0.70	0.70	0.03	0.73	$26.43	$26.43	0.73	XXX	
93744	Analyze ht pace device dual	1.18	1.12	1.12	0.06	2.36	$85.43	$85.43	2.36	XXX	
93744-26	Analyze ht pace device dual	1.18	0.49	0.49	0.03	1.70	$61.54	$61.54	1.70	XXX	
93744-TC	Analyze ht pace device dual	0.00	0.63	0.63	0.03	0.66	$23.89	$23.89	0.66	XXX	
93770 §	Measure venous pressure	0.16	0.09	0.09	0.02	0.27	$9.77	$9.77	0.27	XXX	
93770-26 §	Measure venous pressure	0.16	0.06	0.06	0.01	0.23	$8.33	$8.33	0.23	XXX	
93770-TC §	Measure venous pressure	0.00	0.03	0.03	0.01	0.04	$1.45	$1.45	0.04	XXX	
93797	Cardiac rehab	0.18	0.33	0.07	0.01	0.52	$18.82	$9.41	0.26	000	A+

* **M** = multiple surgery adjustment applies
Me = multiple endoscopy rules may apply
B = bilateral surgery adjustment applies
A = assistant-at-surgery restriction

A+ = assistant-at-surgery restriction unless medical necessity established with documentation
C = cosurgeons payable
C+ = cosurgeons payable if medical necessity established with documentation

T = team surgeons permitted
T+ = team surgeons payable if medical necessity established with documentation
§ = indicates services that are not covered by Medicare.

411 CPT five-digit codes, two-digit numeric modifiers, and descriptions only are © 2001 American Medical Association

Medicare RBRVS: The Physicians' Guide

Relative value units

CPT Code and Modifier	Description	Work RVU	Non Facility Practice Expense RVU	Facility Practice Expense RVU	PLI RVU	Total Non Facility RVUs	Medicare Payment Non Facility	Total Facility RVUs	Medicare Payment Facility	Global Period	Payment Policy Indicators*
93798	Cardiac rehab/monitor	0.28	0.44	0.11	0.01	0.73	$26.43	0.40	$14.48	000	A+
93799	Cardiovascular procedure	0.00	0.00	0.00	0.00	0.00	$0.00	0.00	$0.00	XXX	A+
93799-26	Cardiovascular procedure	0.00	0.00	0.00	0.00	0.00	$0.00	0.00	$0.00	XXX	A+
93799-TC	Cardiovascular procedure	0.00	0.00	0.00	0.00	0.00	$0.00	0.00	$0.00	XXX	A+

Medicine: Noninvasive vascular diagnostic studies

CPT Code and Modifier	Description	Work RVU	Non Facility Practice Expense RVU	Facility Practice Expense RVU	PLI RVU	Total Non Facility RVUs	Medicare Payment Non Facility	Total Facility RVUs	Medicare Payment Facility	Global Period	Payment Policy Indicators*
93875	Extracranial study	0.22	1.13	1.13	0.10	1.45	$52.49	1.45	$52.49	XXX	A+
93875-26	Extracranial study	0.22	0.08	0.08	0.01	0.31	$11.22	0.31	$11.22	XXX	A+
93875-TC	Extracranial study	0.00	1.05	1.05	0.09	1.14	$41.27	1.14	$41.27	XXX	A+
93880	Extracranial study	0.60	3.76	3.76	0.33	4.69	$169.77	4.69	$169.77	XXX	A+
93880-26	Extracranial study	0.60	0.22	0.22	0.04	0.86	$31.13	0.86	$31.13	XXX	A+
93880-TC	Extracranial study	0.00	3.54	3.54	0.29	3.83	$138.64	3.83	$138.64	XXX	A+
93882	Extracranial study	0.40	2.50	2.50	0.22	3.12	$112.94	3.12	$112.94	XXX	A+
93882-26	Extracranial study	0.40	0.15	0.15	0.04	0.59	$21.36	0.59	$21.36	XXX	A+
93882-TC	Extracranial study	0.00	2.35	2.35	0.18	2.53	$91.58	2.53	$91.58	XXX	A+
93886	Intracranial study	0.94	4.40	4.40	0.37	5.71	$206.70	5.71	$206.70	XXX	A+
93886-26	Intracranial study	0.94	0.40	0.40	0.05	1.39	$50.32	1.39	$50.32	XXX	A+
93886-TC	Intracranial study	0.00	4.00	4.00	0.32	4.32	$156.38	4.32	$156.38	XXX	A+
93888	Intracranial study	0.62	2.91	2.91	0.26	3.79	$137.19	3.79	$137.19	XXX	A+
93888-26	Intracranial study	0.62	0.24	0.24	0.04	0.90	$32.58	0.90	$32.58	XXX	A+
93888-TC	Intracranial study	0.00	2.67	2.67	0.22	2.89	$104.62	2.89	$104.62	XXX	A+
93922	Extremity study	0.25	1.18	1.18	0.13	1.56	$56.47	1.56	$56.47	XXX	A+
93922-26	Extremity study	0.25	0.09	0.09	0.02	0.36	$13.03	0.36	$13.03	XXX	A+
93922-TC	Extremity study	0.00	1.09	1.09	0.11	1.20	$43.44	1.20	$43.44	XXX	A+
93923	Extremity study	0.45	2.24	2.24	0.22	2.91	$105.34	2.91	$105.34	XXX	A+
93923-26	Extremity study	0.45	0.16	0.16	0.04	0.65	$23.53	0.65	$23.53	XXX	A+
93923-TC	Extremity study	0.00	2.08	2.08	0.18	2.26	$81.81	2.26	$81.81	XXX	A+

93924	Extremity study	0.50	2.43	2.43	0.26	3.19	3.19	$115.48	$115.48	XXX	A+
93924-26	Extremity study	0.50	0.18	0.18	0.05	0.73	0.73	$26.43	$26.43	XXX	A+
93924-TC	Extremity study	0.00	2.25	2.25	0.21	2.46	2.46	$89.05	$89.05	XXX	A+
93925	Lower extremity study	0.58	3.76	3.76	0.33	4.67	4.67	$169.05	$169.05	XXX	A+
93925-26	Lower extremity study	0.58	0.21	0.21	0.04	0.83	0.83	$30.05	$30.05	XXX	A+
93925-TC	Lower extremity study	0.00	3.55	3.55	0.29	3.84	3.84	$139.00	$139.00	XXX	A+
93926	Lower extremity study	0.39	2.51	2.51	0.22	3.12	3.12	$112.94	$112.94	XXX	A+
93926-26	Lower extremity study	0.39	0.14	0.14	0.03	0.56	0.56	$20.27	$20.27	XXX	A+
93926-TC	Lower extremity study	0.00	2.37	2.37	0.19	2.56	2.56	$92.67	$92.67	XXX	A+
93930	Upper extremity study	0.46	3.93	3.93	0.34	4.73	4.73	$171.22	$171.22	XXX	A+
93930-26	Upper extremity study	0.46	0.16	0.16	0.03	0.65	0.65	$23.53	$23.53	XXX	A+
93930-TC	Upper extremity study	0.00	3.77	3.77	0.31	4.08	4.08	$147.69	$147.69	XXX	A+
93931	Upper extremity study	0.31	2.62	2.62	0.22	3.15	3.15	$114.03	$114.03	XXX	A+
93931-26	Upper extremity study	0.31	0.11	0.11	0.02	0.44	0.44	$15.93	$15.93	XXX	A+
93931-TC	Upper extremity study	0.00	2.51	2.51	0.20	2.71	2.71	$98.10	$98.10	XXX	A+
93965	Extremity study	0.35	1.17	1.17	0.12	1.64	1.64	$59.37	$59.37	XXX	A+
93965-26	Extremity study	0.35	0.13	0.13	0.02	0.50	0.50	$18.10	$18.10	XXX	A+
93965-TC	Extremity study	0.00	1.04	1.04	0.10	1.14	1.14	$41.27	$41.27	XXX	A+
93970	Extremity study	0.68	4.16	4.16	0.38	5.22	5.22	$188.96	$188.96	XXX	A+
93970-26	Extremity study	0.68	0.24	0.24	0.05	0.97	0.97	$35.11	$35.11	XXX	A+
93970-TC	Extremity study	0.00	3.92	3.92	0.33	4.25	4.25	$153.85	$153.85	XXX	A+
93971	Extremity study	0.45	2.77	2.77	0.25	3.47	3.47	$125.61	$125.61	XXX	A+
93971-26	Extremity study	0.45	0.16	0.16	0.03	0.64	0.64	$23.17	$23.17	XXX	A+
93971-TC	Extremity study	0.00	2.61	2.61	0.22	2.83	2.83	$102.44	$102.44	XXX	A+
93975	Vascular study	1.80	5.10	5.10	0.47	7.37	7.37	$266.79	$266.79	XXX	A+
93975-26	Vascular study	1.80	0.64	0.64	0.11	2.55	2.55	$92.31	$92.31	XXX	A+
93975-TC	Vascular study	0.00	4.46	4.46	0.36	4.82	4.82	$174.48	$174.48	XXX	A+
93976	Vascular study	1.21	3.41	3.41	0.31	4.93	4.93	$178.46	$178.46	XXX	A+

* **M** = multiple surgery adjustment applies
Me = multiple endoscopy rules may apply
B = bilateral surgery adjustment applies
A = assistant-at-surgery restriction

A+ = assistant-at-surgery restriction unless medical necessity established with documentation
C = cosurgeons payable
C+ = cosurgeons payable if medical necessity established with documentation

T = team surgeons permitted
T+ = team surgeons payable if medical necessity established with documentation
§ = indicates services that are not covered by Medicare.

413   CPT five-digit codes, two-digit numeric modifiers, and descriptions only are © 2001 American Medical Association

Medicare RBRVS: The Physicians' Guide

Relative value units

CPT Code and Modifier	Description	Work RVU	Non Facility Practice Expense RVU	Facility Practice Expense RVU	PLI RVU	Total Non Facility RVUs	Medicare Payment Non Facility	Total Facility RVUs	Medicare Payment Facility	Global Period	Payment Policy Indicators*
93976-26	Vascular study	1.21	0.43	0.43	0.06	1.70	$61.54	1.70	$61.54	XXX	A+
93976-TC	Vascular study	0.00	2.98	2.98	0.25	3.23	$116.92	3.23	$116.92	XXX	A+
93978	Vascular study	0.65	3.88	3.88	0.36	4.89	$177.01	4.89	$177.01	XXX	A+
93978-26	Vascular study	0.65	0.23	0.23	0.05	0.93	$33.67	0.93	$33.67	XXX	A+
93978-TC	Vascular study	0.00	3.65	3.65	0.31	3.96	$143.35	3.96	$143.35	XXX	A+
93979	Vascular study	0.44	2.59	2.59	0.24	3.27	$118.37	3.27	$118.37	XXX	A+
93979-26	Vascular study	0.44	0.16	0.16	0.04	0.64	$23.17	0.64	$23.17	XXX	A+
93979-TC	Vascular study	0.00	2.43	2.43	0.20	2.63	$95.20	2.63	$95.20	XXX	A+
93980	Penile vascular study	1.25	3.75	3.75	0.35	5.35	$193.67	5.35	$193.67	XXX	A+
93980-26	Penile vascular study	1.25	0.44	0.44	0.07	1.76	$63.71	1.76	$63.71	XXX	A+
93980-TC	Penile vascular study	0.00	3.31	3.31	0.28	3.59	$129.96	3.59	$129.96	XXX	A+
93981	Penile vascular study	0.44	3.21	3.21	0.28	3.93	$142.26	3.93	$142.26	XXX	A+
93981-26	Penile vascular study	0.44	0.15	0.15	0.02	0.61	$22.08	0.61	$22.08	XXX	A+
93981-TC	Penile vascular study	0.00	3.06	3.06	0.26	3.32	$120.18	3.32	$120.18	XXX	A+
93990	Doppler flow testing	0.25	2.46	2.46	0.21	2.92	$105.70	2.92	$105.70	XXX	A+
93990-26	Doppler flow testing	0.25	0.09	0.09	0.02	0.36	$13.03	0.36	$13.03	XXX	A+
93990-TC	Doppler flow testing	0.00	2.37	2.37	0.19	2.56	$92.67	2.56	$92.67	XXX	A+
Medicine: Pulmonary											
94010	Breathing capacity test	0.17	0.82	0.82	0.03	1.02	$36.92	1.02	$36.92	XXX	A+
94010-26	Breathing capacity test	0.17	0.06	0.06	0.01	0.24	$8.69	0.24	$8.69	XXX	A+
94010-TC	Breathing capacity test	0.00	0.76	0.76	0.02	0.78	$28.24	0.78	$28.24	XXX	A+
94014	Patient recorded spirometry	0.52	0.46	0.46	0.03	1.01	$36.56	1.01	$36.56	XXX	A+
94015	Patient recorded spirometry	0.00	0.29	0.29	0.01	0.30	$10.86	0.30	$10.86	XXX	A+
94016	Review patient spirometry	0.52	0.17	0.17	0.02	0.71	$25.70	0.71	$25.70	XXX	A+
94060	Evaluation of wheezing	0.31	1.36	1.36	0.06	1.73	$62.62	1.73	$62.62	XXX	A+
94060-26	Evaluation of wheezing	0.31	0.10	0.10	0.01	0.42	$15.20	0.42	$15.20	XXX	A+
94060-TC	Evaluation of wheezing	0.00	1.26	1.26	0.05	1.31	$47.42	1.31	$47.42	XXX	A+

Code	Description							
94070	Evaluation of wheezing	0.60	3.38	3.38	0.10	4.08	$147.69	$147.69	4.08	XXX	A+
94070-26	Evaluation of wheezing	0.60	0.19	0.19	0.02	0.81	$29.32	$29.32	0.81	XXX	A+
94070-TC	Evaluation of wheezing	0.00	3.19	3.19	0.08	3.27	$118.37	$118.37	3.27	XXX	A+
94150 §	Vital capacity test	0.07	0.63	0.63	0.02	0.72	$26.06	$26.06	0.72	XXX	
94150-26 §	Vital capacity test	0.07	0.03	0.03	0.01	0.11	$3.98	$3.98	0.11	XXX	
94150-TC §	Vital capacity test	0.00	0.60	0.60	0.01	0.61	$22.08	$22.08	0.61	XXX	
94200	Lung function test (MBC/MVV)	0.11	0.33	0.33	0.03	0.47	$17.01	$17.01	0.47	XXX	A+
94200-26	Lung function test (MBC/MVV)	0.11	0.04	0.04	0.01	0.16	$5.79	$5.79	0.16	XXX	A+
94200-TC	Lung function test (MBC/MVV)	0.00	0.29	0.29	0.02	0.31	$11.22	$11.22	0.31	XXX	A+
94240	Residual lung capacity	0.26	1.26	1.26	0.05	1.57	$56.83	$56.83	1.57	XXX	A+
94240-26	Residual lung capacity	0.26	0.08	0.08	0.01	0.35	$12.67	$12.67	0.35	XXX	A+
94240-TC	Residual lung capacity	0.00	1.18	1.18	0.04	1.22	$44.16	$44.16	1.22	XXX	A+
94250	Expired gas collection	0.11	0.61	0.61	0.02	0.74	$26.79	$26.79	0.74	XXX	A+
94250-26	Expired gas collection	0.11	0.04	0.04	0.01	0.16	$5.79	$5.79	0.16	XXX	A+
94250-TC	Expired gas collection	0.00	0.57	0.57	0.01	0.58	$21.00	$21.00	0.58	XXX	A+
94260	Thoracic gas volume	0.13	0.38	0.38	0.04	0.55	$19.91	$19.91	0.55	XXX	A+
94260-26	Thoracic gas volume	0.13	0.04	0.04	0.01	0.18	$6.52	$6.52	0.18	XXX	A+
94260-TC	Thoracic gas volume	0.00	0.34	0.34	0.03	0.37	$13.39	$13.39	0.37	XXX	A+
94350	Lung nitrogen washout curve	0.26	1.01	1.01	0.04	1.31	$47.42	$47.42	1.31	XXX	A+
94350-26	Lung nitrogen washout curve	0.26	0.08	0.08	0.01	0.35	$12.67	$12.67	0.35	XXX	A+
94350-TC	Lung nitrogen washout curve	0.00	0.93	0.93	0.03	0.96	$34.75	$34.75	0.96	XXX	A+
94360	Measure airflow resistance	0.26	0.50	0.50	0.06	0.82	$29.68	$29.68	0.82	XXX	A+
94360-26	Measure airflow resistance	0.26	0.08	0.08	0.01	0.35	$12.67	$12.67	0.35	XXX	A+
94360-TC	Measure airflow resistance	0.00	0.42	0.42	0.05	0.47	$17.01	$17.01	0.47	XXX	A+
94370	Breath airway closing volume	0.26	2.03	2.03	0.03	2.32	$83.98	$83.98	2.32	XXX	A+
94370-26	Breath airway closing volume	0.26	0.08	0.08	0.01	0.35	$12.67	$12.67	0.35	XXX	A+
94370-TC	Breath airway closing volume	0.00	1.95	1.95	0.02	1.97	$71.31	$71.31	1.97	XXX	A+
94375	Respiratory flow volume loop	0.31	0.46	0.46	0.03	0.80	$28.96	$28.96	0.80	XXX	A+

*M = multiple surgery adjustment applies
Me = multiple endoscopy rules may apply
B = bilateral surgery adjustment applies
A = assistant-at-surgery restriction

A+ = assistant-at-surgery restriction unless medical necessity established with documentation
C = cosurgeons payable
C+ = cosurgeons payable if medical necessity established with documentation

T = team surgeons permitted
T+ = team surgeons payable if medical necessity established with documentation
§ = indicates services that are not covered by Medicare.

415 CPT five-digit codes, two-digit numeric modifiers, and descriptions only are © 2001 American Medical Association

Medicare RBRVS: The Physicians' Guide

Relative value units

CPT Code and Modifier	Description	Work RVU	Non Facility Practice Expense RVU	Facility Practice Expense RVU	PLI RVU	Total Non Facility RVUs	Medicare Payment Non Facility	Total Facility RVUs	Medicare Payment Facility	Global Period	Payment Policy Indicators*
94375-26	Respiratory flow volume loop	0.31	0.10	0.10	0.01	0.42	$15.20	0.42	$15.20	XXX	A+
94375-TC	Respiratory flow volume loop	0.00	0.36	0.36	0.02	0.38	$13.76	0.38	$13.76	XXX	A+
94400	CO2 breathing response curve	0.40	0.70	0.70	0.06	1.16	$41.99	1.16	$41.99	XXX	A+
94400-26	CO2 breathing response curve	0.40	0.13	0.13	0.01	0.54	$19.55	0.54	$19.55	XXX	A+
94400-TC	CO2 breathing response curve	0.00	0.57	0.57	0.05	0.62	$22.44	0.62	$22.44	XXX	A+
94450	Hypoxia response curve	0.40	0.85	0.85	0.04	1.29	$46.70	1.29	$46.70	XXX	A+
94450-26	Hypoxia response curve	0.40	0.12	0.12	0.02	0.54	$19.55	0.54	$19.55	XXX	A+
94450-TC	Hypoxia response curve	0.00	0.73	0.73	0.02	0.75	$27.15	0.75	$27.15	XXX	A+
94620	Pulmonary stress test/simple	0.64	1.66	1.66	0.10	2.40	$86.88	2.40	$86.88	XXX	A+
94620-26	Pulmonary stress test/simple	0.64	0.21	0.21	0.02	0.87	$31.49	0.87	$31.49	XXX	A+
94620-TC	Pulmonary stress test/simple	0.00	1.45	1.45	0.08	1.53	$55.38	1.53	$55.38	XXX	A+
94621	Pulm stress test/complex	1.42	1.25	1.25	0.13	2.80	$101.36	2.80	$101.36	XXX	A+
94621-26	Pulm stress test/complex	1.42	0.47	0.47	0.05	1.94	$70.23	1.94	$70.23	XXX	A+
94621-TC	Pulm stress test/complex	0.00	0.78	0.78	0.08	0.86	$31.13	0.86	$31.13	XXX	A+
94640	Airway inhalation treatment	0.00	0.74	0.74	0.02	0.76	$27.51	0.76	$27.51	XXX	A+
94642	Aerosol inhalation treatment	0.00	0.00	0.00	0.00	0.00	$0.00	0.00	$0.00	XXX	A+
94650	Pressure breathing (IPPB)	0.00	0.67	0.67	0.02	0.69	$24.98	0.69	$24.98	XXX	A+
94651	Pressure breathing (IPPB)	0.00	0.62	0.62	0.02	0.64	$23.17	0.64	$23.17	XXX	A+
94652	Pressure breathing (IPPB)	0.00	0.77	0.77	0.06	0.83	$30.05	0.83	$30.05	XXX	A+
94656	Initial ventilator mgmt	1.22	NA	0.33	0.06	NA	NA	1.61	$58.28	XXX	A+
94657	Continued ventilator mgmt	0.83	NA	0.26	0.03	NA	NA	1.12	$40.54	XXX	A+
94660	Pos airway pressure, CPAP	0.76	0.67	0.24	0.03	1.46	$52.85	1.03	$37.29	XXX	A+
94662	Neg press ventilation, cnp	0.76	NA	0.24	0.02	NA	NA	1.02	$36.92	XXX	A+
94664	Aerosol or vapor inhalations	0.00	0.53	0.53	0.03	0.56	$20.27	0.56	$20.27	XXX	A+
94665	Aerosol or vapor inhalations	0.00	0.53	0.53	0.04	0.57	$20.63	0.57	$20.63	XXX	A+
94667	Chest wall manipulation	0.00	1.01	1.01	0.04	1.05	$38.01	1.05	$38.01	XXX	A+
94668	Chest wall manipulation	0.00	0.75	0.75	0.02	0.77	$27.87	0.77	$27.87	XXX	A+

Code	Description							
94680	Exhaled air analysis, o2	0.26	1.17	1.17	0.06	1.49	$53.94	1.49	$53.94	XXX	A+
94680-26	Exhaled air analysis, o2	0.26	0.09	0.09	0.01	0.36	$13.03	0.36	$13.03	XXX	A+
94680-TC	Exhaled air analysis, o2	0.00	1.08	1.08	0.05	1.13	$40.91	1.13	$40.91	XXX	A+
94681	Exhaled air analysis, o2/co2	0.20	1.32	1.32	0.11	1.63	$59.00	1.63	$59.00	XXX	A+
94681-26	Exhaled air analysis, o2/co2	0.20	0.07	0.07	0.01	0.28	$10.14	0.28	$10.14	XXX	A+
94681-TC	Exhaled air analysis, o2/co2	0.00	1.25	1.25	0.10	1.35	$48.87	1.35	$48.87	XXX	A+
94690	Exhaled air analysis	0.07	1.59	1.59	0.04	1.70	$61.54	1.70	$61.54	XXX	A+
94690-26	Exhaled air analysis	0.07	0.02	0.02	0.01	0.10	$3.62	0.10	$3.62	XXX	A+
94690-TC	Exhaled air analysis	0.00	1.57	1.57	0.03	1.60	$57.92	1.60	$57.92	XXX	A+
94720	Monoxide diffusing capacity	0.26	1.32	1.32	0.06	1.64	$59.37	1.64	$59.37	XXX	A+
94720-26	Monoxide diffusing capacity	0.26	0.08	0.08	0.01	0.35	$12.67	0.35	$12.67	XXX	A+
94720-TC	Monoxide diffusing capacity	0.00	1.24	1.24	0.05	1.29	$46.70	1.29	$46.70	XXX	A+
94725	Membrane diffusion capacity	0.26	0.71	0.71	0.11	1.08	$39.10	1.08	$39.10	XXX	A+
94725-26	Membrane diffusion capacity	0.26	0.08	0.08	0.01	0.35	$12.67	0.35	$12.67	XXX	A+
94725-TC	Membrane diffusion capacity	0.00	0.63	0.63	0.10	0.73	$26.43	0.73	$26.43	XXX	A+
94750	Pulmonary compliance study	0.23	1.06	1.06	0.04	1.33	$48.14	1.33	$48.14	XXX	A+
94750-26	Pulmonary compliance study	0.23	0.07	0.07	0.01	0.31	$11.22	0.31	$11.22	XXX	A+
94750-TC	Pulmonary compliance study	0.00	0.99	0.99	0.03	1.02	$36.92	1.02	$36.92	XXX	A+
94760	Measure blood oxygen level	0.00	0.10	0.10	0.02	0.12	$4.34	0.12	$4.34	XXX	A+
94761	Measure blood oxygen level	0.00	0.14	0.14	0.05	0.19	$6.88	0.19	$6.88	XXX	A+
94762	Measure blood oxygen level	0.00	0.74	0.74	0.08	0.82	$29.68	0.82	$29.68	XXX	A+
94770	Exhaled carbon dioxide test	0.15	0.91	0.91	0.07	1.13	$40.91	1.13	$40.91	XXX	A+
94770-26	Exhaled carbon dioxide test	0.15	0.04	0.04	0.01	0.20	$7.24	0.20	$7.24	XXX	A+
94770-TC	Exhaled carbon dioxide test	0.00	0.87	0.87	0.06	0.93	$33.67	0.93	$33.67	XXX	A+
94772	Breath recording, infant	0.00	0.00	0.00	0.00	0.00	$0.00	0.00	$0.00	XXX	A+
94772-26	Breath recording, infant	0.00	0.00	0.00	0.00	0.00	$0.00	0.00	$0.00	XXX	A+
94772-TC	Breath recording, infant	0.00	0.00	0.00	0.00	0.00	$0.00	0.00	$0.00	XXX	A+

* **M** = multiple surgery adjustment applies
Me = multiple endoscopy rules may apply
B = bilateral surgery adjustment applies
A = assistant-at-surgery restriction

A+ = assistant-at-surgery restriction unless medical necessity established with documentation
C = cosurgeons payable
C+ = cosurgeons payable if medical necessity established with documentation

T = team surgeons permitted
T+ = team surgeons payable if medical necessity established with documentation
S = indicates services that are not covered by Medicare.

CPT five-digit codes, two-digit numeric modifiers, and descriptions only are © 2001 American Medical Association

Medicare RBRVS: The Physicians' Guide

Relative value units

CPT Code and Modifier	Description	Work RVU	Non Facility Practice Expense RVU	Facility Practice Expense RVU	PLI RVU	Total Non Facility RVUs	Medicare Payment Non Facility	Total Facility RVUs	Medicare Payment Facility	Global Period	Payment Policy Indicators*
94799	Pulmonary service/procedure	0.00	0.00	0.00	0.00	0.00	$0.00	0.00	$0.00	XXX	A+
94799-26	Pulmonary service/procedure	0.00	0.00	0.00	0.00	0.00	$0.00	0.00	$0.00	XXX	A+
94799-TC	Pulmonary service/procedure	0.00	0.00	0.00	0.00	0.00	$0.00	0.00	$0.00	XXX	A+
Medicine: Allergy and clinical immunology											
95004	Allergy skin tests	0.00	0.09	0.09	0.01	0.10	$3.62	0.10	$3.62	XXX	A+
95010	Sensitivity skin tests	0.15	0.45	0.07	0.01	0.61	$22.08	0.23	$8.33	XXX	A+
95015	Sensitivity skin tests	0.15	0.39	0.06	0.01	0.55	$19.91	0.22	$7.96	XXX	A+
95024	Allergy skin tests	0.00	0.14	0.14	0.01	0.15	$5.43	0.15	$5.43	XXX	A+
95027	Skin end point titration	0.00	0.14	0.14	0.01	0.15	$5.43	0.15	$5.43	XXX	A+
95028	Allergy skin tests	0.00	0.22	0.22	0.01	0.23	$8.33	0.23	$8.33	XXX	A+
95044	Allergy patch tests	0.00	0.19	0.19	0.01	0.20	$7.24	0.20	$7.24	XXX	A+
95052	Photo patch test	0.00	0.24	0.24	0.01	0.25	$9.05	0.25	$9.05	XXX	A+
95056	Photosensitivity tests	0.00	0.17	0.17	0.01	0.18	$6.52	0.18	$6.52	XXX	A+
95060	Eye allergy tests	0.00	0.33	0.33	0.02	0.35	$12.67	0.35	$12.67	XXX	A+
95065	Nose allergy test	0.00	0.19	0.19	0.01	0.20	$7.24	0.20	$7.24	XXX	A+
95070	Bronchial allergy tests	0.00	2.17	2.17	0.02	2.19	$79.28	2.19	$79.28	XXX	A+
95071	Bronchial allergy tests	0.00	2.77	2.77	0.02	2.79	$101.00	2.79	$101.00	XXX	A+
95075	Ingestion challenge test	0.95	0.80	0.43	0.03	1.78	$64.43	1.41	$51.04	XXX	A+
95078	Provocative testing	0.00	0.24	0.24	0.02	0.26	$9.41	0.26	$9.41	XXX	A+
95115	Immunotherapy, one injection	0.00	0.37	0.37	0.02	0.39	$14.12	0.39	$14.12	000	A+
95117	Immunotherapy injections	0.00	0.48	0.48	0.02	0.50	$18.10	0.50	$18.10	000	A+
95144	Antigen therapy services	0.06	0.25	0.03	0.01	0.32	$11.58	0.10	$3.62	000	A+
95145	Antigen therapy services	0.06	0.47	0.03	0.01	0.54	$19.55	0.10	$3.62	000	A+
95146	Antigen therapy services	0.06	0.62	0.03	0.01	0.69	$24.98	0.10	$3.62	000	A+
95147	Antigen therapy services	0.06	0.91	0.03	0.01	0.98	$35.48	0.10	$3.62	000	A+
95148	Antigen therapy services	0.06	0.81	0.03	0.01	0.88	$31.86	0.10	$3.62	000	A+

Code	Description								
95149	Antigen therapy services	0.06	1.04	0.03	0.01	1.11	$40.18	0.10	$3.62	000	A+
95165	Antigen therapy services	0.06	0.21	0.02	0.01	0.28	$10.14	0.09	$3.26	000	A+
95170	Antigen therapy services	0.06	0.26	0.02	0.01	0.33	$11.95	0.09	$3.26	000	A+
95180	Rapid desensitization	2.01	1.66	0.85	0.04	3.71	$134.30	2.90	$104.98	000	A+
95199	Allergy immunology services	0.00	0.00	0.00	0.00	0.00	$0.00	0.00	$0.00	000	A+

Medicine: Neurology and neuromuscular procedures

Code	Description								
95250	Glucose monitoring, cont	0.00	1.44	1.44	0.01	1.45	$52.49	1.45	$52.49	XXX	A+
95805	Multiple sleep latency test	1.88	5.89	5.89	0.34	8.11	$293.58	8.11	$293.58	XXX	A+
95805-26	Multiple sleep latency test	1.88	0.70	0.70	0.06	2.64	$95.57	2.64	$95.57	XXX	A+
95805-TC	Multiple sleep latency test	0.00	5.19	5.19	0.28	5.47	$198.01	5.47	$198.01	XXX	A+
95806	Sleep study, unattended	1.66	4.31	4.31	0.32	6.29	$227.69	6.29	$227.69	XXX	A+
95806-26	Sleep study, unattended	1.66	0.57	0.57	0.06	2.29	$82.90	2.29	$82.90	XXX	A+
95806-TC	Sleep study, unattended	0.00	3.74	3.74	0.26	4.00	$144.80	4.00	$144.80	XXX	A+
95807	Sleep study, attended	1.66	10.70	10.70	0.40	12.76	$461.90	12.76	$461.90	XXX	A+
95807-26	Sleep study, attended	1.66	0.56	0.56	0.05	2.27	$82.17	2.27	$82.17	XXX	A+
95807-TC	Sleep study, attended	0.00	10.14	10.14	0.35	10.49	$379.73	10.49	$379.73	XXX	A+
95808	Polysomnography, 1-3	2.65	9.54	9.54	0.44	12.63	$457.20	12.63	$457.20	XXX	A+
95808-26	Polysomnography, 1-3	2.65	0.99	0.99	0.09	3.73	$135.02	3.73	$135.02	XXX	A+
95808-TC	Polysomnography, 1-3	0.00	8.55	8.55	0.35	8.90	$322.17	8.90	$322.17	XXX	A+
95810	Polysomnography, 4 or more	3.53	16.92	16.92	0.47	20.92	$757.29	20.92	$757.29	XXX	A+
95810-26	Polysomnography, 4 or more	3.53	1.26	1.26	0.12	4.91	$177.74	4.91	$177.74	XXX	A+
95810-TC	Polysomnography, 4 or more	0.00	15.66	15.66	0.35	16.01	$579.55	16.01	$579.55	XXX	A+
95811	Polysomnography w/cpap	3.80	17.19	17.19	0.49	21.48	$777.56	21.48	$777.56	XXX	A+
95811-26	Polysomnography w/cpap	3.80	1.34	1.34	0.13	5.27	$190.77	5.27	$190.77	XXX	A+
95811-TC	Polysomnography w/cpap	0.00	15.85	15.85	0.36	16.21	$586.79	16.21	$586.79	XXX	A+
95812	Electroencephalogram (EEG)	1.08	3.96	3.96	0.13	5.17	$187.15	5.17	$187.15	XXX	A+
95812-26	Electroencephalogram (EEG)	1.08	0.48	0.48	0.04	1.60	$57.92	1.60	$57.92	XXX	A+

* **M** = multiple surgery adjustment applies
Me = multiple endoscopy rules may apply
B = bilateral surgery adjustment applies
A = assistant-at-surgery restriction

A+ = assistant-at-surgery restriction unless medical necessity established with documentation
C = cosurgeons payable
C+ = cosurgeons payable if medical necessity established with documentation

T = team surgeons permitted
T+ = team surgeons payable if medical necessity established with documentation
$ = indicates services that are not covered by Medicare.

Medicare RBRVS: The Physicians' Guide

Relative value units

CPT Code and Modifier	Description	Work RVU	Non Facility Practice Expense RVU	Facility Practice Expense RVU	PLI RVU	Total Non Facility RVUs	Medicare Payment Non Facility	Total Facility RVUs	Medicare Payment Facility	Global Period	Payment Policy Indicators*
95812-TC	Electroencephalogram (EEG)	0.00	3.48	3.48	0.09	3.57	$129.23	3.57	$129.23	XXX	A+
95813	Electroencephalogram (EEG)	1.73	5.53	5.53	0.15	7.41	$268.24	7.41	$268.24	XXX	A+
95813-26	Electroencephalogram (EEG)	1.73	0.73	0.73	0.06	2.52	$91.22	2.52	$91.22	XXX	A+
95813-TC	Electroencephalogram (EEG)	0.00	4.80	4.80	0.09	4.89	$177.01	4.89	$177.01	XXX	A+
95816	Electroencephalogram (EEG)	1.08	3.42	3.42	0.12	4.62	$167.24	4.62	$167.24	XXX	A+
95816-26	Electroencephalogram (EEG)	1.08	0.49	0.49	0.04	1.61	$58.28	1.61	$58.28	XXX	A+
95816-TC	Electroencephalogram (EEG)	0.00	2.93	2.93	0.08	3.01	$108.96	3.01	$108.96	XXX	A+
95819	Electroencephalogram (EEG)	1.08	4.34	4.34	0.12	5.54	$200.54	5.54	$200.54	XXX	A+
95819-26	Electroencephalogram (EEG)	1.08	0.49	0.49	0.04	1.61	$58.28	1.61	$58.28	XXX	A+
95819-TC	Electroencephalogram (EEG)	0.00	3.85	3.85	0.08	3.93	$142.26	3.93	$142.26	XXX	A+
95822	Sleep electroencephalogram	1.08	1.78	1.78	0.15	3.01	$108.96	3.01	$108.96	XXX	A+
95822-26	Sleep electroencephalogram	1.08	0.49	0.49	0.04	1.61	$58.28	1.61	$58.28	XXX	A+
95822-TC	Sleep electroencephalogram	0.00	1.29	1.29	0.11	1.40	$50.68	1.40	$50.68	XXX	A+
95824 §	Electroencephalography	0.00	0.00	0.00	0.00	0.00	$0.00	0.00	$0.00	XXX	A+
95824-26	Electroencephalography	0.74	0.30	0.30	0.05	1.09	$39.46	1.09	$39.46	ZZZ	A+
95824-TC §	Electroencephalography	0.00	0.00	0.00	0.00	0.00	$0.00	0.00	$0.00	XXX	A+
95827	Night electroencephalogram	1.08	2.64	2.64	0.15	3.87	$140.09	3.87	$140.09	XXX	A+
95827-26	Night electroencephalogram	1.08	0.46	0.46	0.03	1.57	$56.83	1.57	$56.83	XXX	A+
95827-TC	Night electroencephalogram	0.00	2.18	2.18	0.12	2.30	$83.26	2.30	$83.26	XXX	A+
95829	Surgery electrocorticogram	6.21	31.39	31.39	0.33	37.93	$1,373.04	37.93	$1,373.04	XXX	A+
95829-26	Surgery electrocorticogram	6.21	2.90	2.90	0.31	9.42	$341.00	9.42	$341.00	XXX	A+
95829-TC	Surgery electrocorticogram	0.00	28.49	28.49	0.02	28.51	$1,032.04	28.51	$1,032.04	XXX	A+
95830	Insert electrodes for EEG	1.70	3.76	0.78	0.07	5.53	$200.18	2.55	$92.31	XXX	A+
95831	Limb muscle testing, manual	0.28	0.52	0.12	0.01	0.81	$29.32	0.41	$14.84	XXX	A+
95832	Hand muscle testing, manual	0.29	0.48	0.11	0.01	0.78	$28.24	0.41	$14.84	XXX	A+
95833	Body muscle testing, manual	0.47	0.54	0.24	0.01	1.02	$36.92	0.72	$26.06	XXX	A+

Code	Description								
95834	Body muscle testing, manual	0.60	0.59	0.28	0.02	1.21	$43.80	0.90	$32.58	XXX	A+
95851	Range of motion measurements	0.16	0.55	0.08	0.01	0.72	$26.06	0.25	$9.05	XXX	A+
95852	Range of motion measurements	0.11	0.49	0.05	0.01	0.61	$22.08	0.17	$6.15	XXX	A+
95857	Tensilon test	0.53	0.66	0.24	0.02	1.21	$43.80	0.79	$28.60	XXX	A+
95858	Tensilon test & myogram	1.56	1.10	1.10	0.07	2.73	$98.82	2.73	$98.82	XXX	A+
95858-26	Tensilon test & myogram	1.56	0.72	0.72	0.04	2.32	$83.98	2.32	$83.98	XXX	A+
95858-TC	Tensilon test & myogram	0.00	0.38	0.38	0.03	0.41	$14.84	0.41	$14.84	XXX	A+
95860	Muscle test, one limb	0.96	1.18	1.18	0.05	2.19	$79.28	2.19	$79.28	XXX	A+
95860-26	Muscle test, one limb	0.96	0.45	0.45	0.03	1.44	$52.13	1.44	$52.13	XXX	A+
95860-TC	Muscle test, one limb	0.00	0.73	0.73	0.02	0.75	$27.15	0.75	$27.15	XXX	A+
95861	Muscle test, two limbs	1.54	1.42	1.42	0.10	3.06	$110.77	3.06	$110.77	XXX	A+
95861-26	Muscle test, two limbs	1.54	0.72	0.72	0.05	2.31	$83.62	2.31	$83.62	XXX	A+
95861-TC	Muscle test, two limbs	0.00	0.70	0.70	0.05	0.75	$27.15	0.75	$27.15	XXX	A+
95863	Muscle test, 3 limbs	1.87	1.76	1.76	0.11	3.74	$135.39	3.74	$135.39	XXX	A+
95863-26	Muscle test, 3 limbs	1.87	0.87	0.87	0.06	2.80	$101.36	2.80	$101.36	XXX	A+
95863-TC	Muscle test, 3 limbs	0.00	0.89	0.89	0.05	0.94	$34.03	0.94	$34.03	XXX	A+
95864	Muscle test, 4 limbs	1.99	2.62	2.62	0.16	4.77	$172.67	4.77	$172.67	XXX	A+
95864-26	Muscle test, 4 limbs	1.99	0.93	0.93	0.06	2.98	$107.87	2.98	$107.87	XXX	A+
95864-TC	Muscle test, 4 limbs	0.00	1.69	1.69	0.10	1.79	$64.80	1.79	$64.80	XXX	A+
95867	Muscle test, head or neck	0.79	0.92	0.92	0.06	1.77	$64.07	1.77	$64.07	XXX	A+
95867-26	Muscle test, head or neck	0.79	0.37	0.37	0.03	1.19	$43.08	1.19	$43.08	XXX	A+
95867-TC	Muscle test, head or neck	0.00	0.55	0.55	0.03	0.58	$21.00	0.58	$21.00	XXX	A+
95868	Muscle test, head or neck	1.18	1.23	1.23	0.08	2.49	$90.14	2.49	$90.14	XXX	A+
95868-26	Muscle test, head or neck	1.18	0.57	0.57	0.04	1.79	$64.80	1.79	$64.80	XXX	A+
95868-TC	Muscle test, head or neck	0.00	0.66	0.66	0.04	0.70	$25.34	0.70	$25.34	XXX	A+
95869	Muscle test, thor paraspinal	0.37	0.37	0.37	0.03	0.77	$27.87	0.77	$27.87	XXX	A+
95869-26	Muscle test, thor paraspinal	0.37	0.17	0.17	0.01	0.55	$19.91	0.55	$19.91	XXX	A+

* **M** = multiple surgery adjustment applies
Me = multiple endoscopy rules may apply
B = bilateral surgery adjustment applies
A = assistant-at-surgery restriction

A+ = assistant-at-surgery restriction unless medical necessity established with documentation
C = cosurgeons payable
C+ = cosurgeons payable if medical necessity established with documentation

T = team surgeons permitted
T+ = team surgeons payable if medical necessity established with documentation
$ = indicates services that are not covered by Medicare.

CPT five-digit codes, two-digit numeric modifiers, and descriptions only are © 2001 American Medical Association

Medicare RBRVS: The Physicians' Guide

Relative value units

CPT Code and Modifier	Description	Work RVU	Non Facility Practice Expense RVU	Facility Practice Expense RVU	PLI RVU	Total Non Facility RVUs	Medicare Payment Non Facility	Total Facility RVUs	Medicare Payment Facility	Global Period	Payment Policy Indicators*
95869-TC	Muscle test, thor paraspinal	0.00	0.20	0.20	0.02	0.22	$7.96	0.22	$7.96	XXX	A+
95870	Muscle test, nonparaspinal	0.37	0.37	0.37	0.03	0.77	$27.87	0.77	$27.87	XXX	A+
95870-26	Muscle test, nonparaspinal	0.37	0.17	0.17	0.01	0.55	$19.91	0.55	$19.91	XXX	A+
95870-TC	Muscle test, nonparaspinal	0.00	0.20	0.20	0.02	0.22	$7.96	0.22	$7.96	XXX	A+
95872	Muscle test, one fiber	1.50	1.25	1.25	0.08	2.83	$102.44	2.83	$102.44	XXX	A+
95872-26	Muscle test, one fiber	1.50	0.68	0.68	0.04	2.22	$80.36	2.22	$80.36	XXX	A+
95872-TC	Muscle test, one fiber	0.00	0.57	0.57	0.04	0.61	$22.08	0.61	$22.08	XXX	A+
95875	Limb exercise test	1.10	1.38	1.38	0.09	2.57	$93.03	2.57	$93.03	XXX	A+
95875-26	Limb exercise test	1.10	0.49	0.49	0.04	1.63	$59.00	1.63	$59.00	XXX	A+
95875-TC	Limb exercise test	0.00	0.89	0.89	0.05	0.94	$34.03	0.94	$34.03	XXX	A+
95900	Motor nerve conduction test	0.42	0.73	0.73	0.03	1.18	$42.72	1.18	$42.72	XXX	A+
95900-26	Motor nerve conduction test	0.42	0.20	0.20	0.01	0.63	$22.81	0.63	$22.81	XXX	A+
95900-TC	Motor nerve conduction test	0.00	0.53	0.53	0.02	0.55	$19.91	0.55	$19.91	XXX	A+
95903	Motor nerve conduction test	0.60	0.51	0.51	0.04	1.15	$41.63	1.15	$41.63	XXX	A+
95903-26	Motor nerve conduction test	0.60	0.27	0.27	0.02	0.89	$32.22	0.89	$32.22	XXX	A+
95903-TC	Motor nerve conduction test	0.00	0.24	0.24	0.02	0.26	$9.41	0.26	$9.41	XXX	A+
95904	Sense nerve conduction test	0.34	0.64	0.64	0.03	1.01	$36.56	1.01	$36.56	XXX	A+
95904-26	Sense nerve conduction test	0.34	0.16	0.16	0.01	0.51	$18.46	0.51	$18.46	XXX	A+
95904-TC	Sense nerve conduction test	0.00	0.48	0.48	0.02	0.50	$18.10	0.50	$18.10	XXX	A+
95920	Intraop nerve test add-on	2.11	2.23	2.23	0.20	4.54	$164.34	4.54	$164.34	ZZZ	A+
95920-26	Intraop nerve test add-on	2.11	0.99	0.99	0.14	3.24	$117.29	3.24	$117.29	ZZZ	A+
95920-TC	Intraop nerve test add-on	0.00	1.24	1.24	0.06	1.30	$47.06	1.30	$47.06	ZZZ	A+
95921	Autonomic nerv function test	0.90	0.70	0.70	0.05	1.65	$59.73	1.65	$59.73	XXX	A+
95921-26	Autonomic nerv function test	0.90	0.34	0.34	0.03	1.27	$45.97	1.27	$45.97	XXX	A+
95921-TC	Autonomic nerv function test	0.00	0.36	0.36	0.02	0.38	$13.76	0.38	$13.76	XXX	A+
95922	Autonomic nerv function test	0.96	0.79	0.79	0.05	1.80	$65.16	1.80	$65.16	XXX	A+

Code	Description							
95922-26	Autonomic nerv function test	0.96	0.43	0.43	0.03	1.42	$51.40	$51.40	1.42	XXX	A+
95922-TC	Autonomic nerv function test	0.00	0.36	0.36	0.02	0.38	$13.76	$13.76	0.38	XXX	A+
95923	Autonomic nerv function test	0.90	2.57	2.57	0.05	3.52	$127.42	$127.42	3.52	XXX	A+
95923-26	Autonomic nerv function test	0.90	0.40	0.40	0.03	1.33	$48.14	$48.14	1.33	XXX	A+
95923-TC	Autonomic nerv function test	0.00	2.17	2.17	0.02	2.19	$79.28	$79.28	2.19	XXX	A+
95925	Somatosensory testing	0.54	1.10	1.10	0.07	1.71	$61.90	$61.90	1.71	XXX	A+
95925-26	Somatosensory testing	0.54	0.24	0.24	0.02	0.80	$28.96	$28.96	0.80	XXX	A+
95925-TC	Somatosensory testing	0.00	0.86	0.86	0.05	0.91	$32.94	$32.94	0.91	XXX	A+
95926	Somatosensory testing	0.54	1.11	1.11	0.07	1.72	$62.26	$62.26	1.72	XXX	A+
95926-26	Somatosensory testing	0.54	0.25	0.25	0.02	0.81	$29.32	$29.32	0.81	XXX	A+
95926-TC	Somatosensory testing	0.00	0.86	0.86	0.05	0.91	$32.94	$32.94	0.91	XXX	A+
95927	Somatosensory testing	0.54	1.13	1.13	0.08	1.75	$63.35	$63.35	1.75	XXX	A+
95927-26	Somatosensory testing	0.54	0.27	0.27	0.03	0.84	$30.41	$30.41	0.84	XXX	A+
95927-TC	Somatosensory testing	0.00	0.86	0.86	0.05	0.91	$32.94	$32.94	0.91	XXX	A+
95930	Visual evoked potential test	0.35	0.84	0.84	0.02	1.21	$43.80	$43.80	1.21	XXX	A+
95930-26	Visual evoked potential test	0.35	0.16	0.16	0.01	0.52	$18.82	$18.82	0.52	XXX	A+
95930-TC	Visual evoked potential test	0.00	0.68	0.68	0.01	0.69	$24.98	$24.98	0.69	XXX	A+
95933	Blink reflex test	0.59	1.01	1.01	0.07	1.67	$60.45	$60.45	1.67	XXX	A+
95933-26	Blink reflex test	0.59	0.27	0.27	0.02	0.88	$31.86	$31.86	0.88	XXX	A+
95933-TC	Blink reflex test	0.00	0.74	0.74	0.05	0.79	$28.60	$28.60	0.79	XXX	A+
95934	H-reflex test	0.51	0.44	0.44	0.04	0.99	$35.84	$35.84	0.99	XXX	B A+
95934-26	H-reflex test	0.51	0.24	0.24	0.02	0.77	$27.87	$27.87	0.77	XXX	B A+
95934-TC	H-reflex test	0.00	0.20	0.20	0.02	0.22	$7.96	$7.96	0.22	XXX	B A+
95936	H-reflex test	0.55	0.45	0.45	0.04	1.04	$37.65	$37.65	1.04	XXX	B A+
95936-26	H-reflex test	0.55	0.25	0.25	0.02	0.82	$29.68	$29.68	0.82	XXX	B A+
95936-TC	H-reflex test	0.00	0.20	0.20	0.02	0.22	$7.96	$7.96	0.22	XXX	B A+
95937	Neuromuscular junction test	0.65	0.60	0.60	0.04	1.29	$46.70	$46.70	1.29	XXX	A+

* **M** = multiple surgery adjustment applies
Me = multiple endoscopy rules may apply
B = bilateral surgery adjustment applies
A = assistant-at-surgery restriction

A+ = assistant-at-surgery restriction unless medical necessity established with documentation
C = cosurgeons payable
C+ = cosurgeons payable if medical necessity established with documentation

T = team surgeons permitted
T+ = team surgeons payable if medical necessity established with documentation
$ = indicates services that are not covered by Medicare.

423 CPT five-digit codes, two-digit numeric modifiers, and descriptions only are © 2001 American Medical Association

Medicare RBRVS: The Physicians' Guide

Relative value units

CPT Code and Modifier	Description	Work RVU	Non Facility Practice Expense RVU	Facility Practice Expense RVU	PLI RVU	Total Non Facility RVUs	Medicare Payment Non Facility	Total Facility RVUs	Medicare Payment Facility	Global Period	Payment Policy Indicators*
95937-26	Neuromuscular junction test	0.65	0.28	0.28	0.02	0.95	$34.39	0.95	$34.39	XXX	A+
95937-TC	Neuromuscular junction test	0.00	0.32	0.32	0.02	0.34	$12.31	0.34	$12.31	XXX	A+
95950	Ambulatory eeg monitoring	1.51	4.93	4.93	0.44	6.88	$249.05	6.88	$249.05	XXX	A+
95950-26	Ambulatory eeg monitoring	1.51	0.70	0.70	0.08	2.29	$82.90	2.29	$82.90	XXX	A+
95950-TC	Ambulatory eeg monitoring	0.00	4.23	4.23	0.36	4.59	$166.15	4.59	$166.15	XXX	A+
95951	EEG monitoring/videorecord	6.00	39.72	NA	0.09	45.81	$1,658.29	NA	NA	XXX	A+
95951-26	EEG monitoring/videorecord	6.00	2.72	2.72	0.20	8.92	$322.90	8.92	$322.90	XXX	A+
95951-TC	EEG monitoring/videorecord	0.00	37.00	NA	0.38	37.38	$1,353.13	NA	NA	XXX	A+
95953	EEG monitoring/computer	3.08	7.39	7.39	0.46	10.93	$395.66	10.93	$395.66	XXX	A+
95953-26	EEG monitoring/computer	3.08	1.38	1.38	0.10	4.56	$165.07	4.56	$165.07	XXX	A+
95953-TC	EEG monitoring/computer	0.00	6.01	6.01	0.36	6.37	$230.59	6.37	$230.59	XXX	A+
95954	EEG monitoring/giving drugs	2.45	4.43	4.43	0.15	7.03	$254.48	7.03	$254.48	XXX	A+
95954-26	EEG monitoring/giving drugs	2.45	1.07	1.07	0.10	3.62	$131.04	3.62	$131.04	XXX	A+
95954-TC	EEG monitoring/giving drugs	0.00	3.36	3.36	0.05	3.41	$123.44	3.41	$123.44	XXX	A+
95955	EEG during surgery	1.01	2.26	2.26	0.19	3.46	$125.25	3.46	$125.25	XXX	A+
95955-26	EEG during surgery	1.01	0.40	0.40	0.05	1.46	$52.85	1.46	$52.85	XXX	A+
95955-TC	EEG during surgery	0.00	1.86	1.86	0.14	2.00	$72.40	2.00	$72.40	XXX	A+
95956	Eeg monitoring, cable/radio	3.08	12.39	12.39	0.47	15.94	$577.02	15.94	$577.02	XXX	A+
95956-26	Eeg monitoring, cable/radio	3.08	1.35	1.35	0.11	4.54	$164.34	4.54	$164.34	XXX	A+
95956-TC	Eeg monitoring, cable/radio	0.00	11.04	11.04	0.36	11.40	$412.67	11.40	$412.67	XXX	A+
95957	EEG digital analysis	1.98	2.52	2.52	0.17	4.67	$169.05	4.67	$169.05	XXX	A+
95957-26	EEG digital analysis	1.98	0.90	0.90	0.07	2.95	$106.79	2.95	$106.79	XXX	A+
95957-TC	EEG digital analysis	0.00	1.62	1.62	0.10	1.72	$62.26	1.72	$62.26	XXX	A+
95958	EEG monitoring/function test	4.25	3.51	3.51	0.29	8.05	$291.40	8.05	$291.40	XXX	A+
95958-26	EEG monitoring/function test	4.25	1.86	1.86	0.18	6.29	$227.69	6.29	$227.69	XXX	A+
95958-TC	EEG monitoring/function test	0.00	1.65	1.65	0.11	1.76	$63.71	1.76	$63.71	XXX	A+

Code	Description								
95961	Electrode stimulation, brain	2.97	2.67	0.24	5.88	$212.85	5.88	$212.85	XXX	A+
95961-26	Electrode stimulation, brain	2.97	1.43	0.18	4.58	$165.79	4.58	$165.79	XXX	A+
95961-TC	Electrode stimulation, brain	0.00	1.24	0.06	1.30	$47.06	1.30	$47.06	XXX	A+
95962	Electrode stim, brain add-on	3.21	2.72	0.23	6.16	$222.99	6.16	$222.99	ZZZ	A+
95962-26	Electrode stim, brain add-on	3.21	1.48	0.17	4.86	$175.93	4.86	$175.93	ZZZ	A+
95962-TC	Electrode stim, brain add-on	0.00	1.24	0.06	1.30	$47.06	1.30	$47.06	ZZZ	A+
95965	Meg, spontaneous	0.00	0.00	0.00	0.00	$0.00	0.00	$0.00	XXX	A+
95965-26	Meg, spontaneous	8.00	3.19	0.20	11.39	$412.31	11.39	$412.31	XXX	A+
95965-TC	Meg, spontaneous	0.00	0.00	0.00	0.00	$0.00	0.00	$0.00	XXX	A+
95966	Meg, evoked, single	0.00	0.00	0.00	0.00	$0.00	0.00	$0.00	XXX	A+
95966-26	Meg, evoked, single	4.00	1.60	0.18	5.78	$209.23	5.78	$209.23	XXX	A+
95966-TC	Meg, evoked, single	0.00	0.00	0.00	0.00	$0.00	0.00	$0.00	XXX	A+
95967	Meg, evoked, each addl	0.00	0.00	0.00	0.00	$0.00	0.00	$0.00	ZZZ	A+
95967-26	Meg, evoked, each addl	3.50	1.40	0.17	5.07	$183.53	5.07	$183.53	ZZZ	A+
95967-TC	Meg, evoked, each addl	0.00	0.00	0.00	0.00	$0.00	0.00	$0.00	ZZZ	A+
95970	Analyze neurostim, no prog	0.45	0.18	0.03	0.66	$23.89	0.64	$23.17	XXX	A+
95971	Analyze neurostim, simple	0.78	0.28	0.06	1.12	$40.54	1.08	$39.10	XXX	A+
95972	Analyze neurostim, complex	1.50	0.62	0.17	2.29	$82.90	2.18	$78.91	XXX	A+
95973	Analyze neurostim, complex	0.92	0.42	0.07	1.41	$51.04	1.35	$48.87	XXX	A+
95974	Cranial neurostim, complex	3.00	1.37	0.15	4.52	$163.62	4.52	$163.62	XXX	A+
95975	Cranial neurostim, complex	1.70	0.78	0.07	2.55	$92.31	2.55	$92.31	XXX	A+
95999	Neurological procedure	0.00	0.00	0.00	0.00	$0.00	0.00	$0.00	XXX	A+
96000	Motion analysis, video/3d	1.80	NA	0.02	NA	NA	2.54	$91.95	XXX	A+
96001	Motion test w/ft press meas	2.15	NA	0.02	NA	NA	3.03	$109.68	XXX	A+
96002	Dynamic surface emg	0.41	NA	0.02	NA	NA	0.59	$21.36	XXX	A+
96003	Dynamic fine wire emg	0.37	NA	0.03	NA	NA	0.55	$19.91	XXX	A+
96004	Phys review of motion tests	1.80	0.72	0.08	2.60	$94.12	2.60	$94.12	XXX	A+

* **M** = multiple surgery adjustment applies
Me = multiple endoscopy rules may apply
B = bilateral surgery adjustment applies
A = assistant-at-surgery restriction

A+ = assistant-at-surgery restriction unless medical necessity established with documentation
C = cosurgeons payable
C+ = cosurgeons payable if medical necessity established with documentation

T = team surgeons permitted
T+ = team surgeons payable if medical necessity established with documentation
$ = indicates services that are not covered by Medicare.

CPT five-digit codes, two-digit numeric modifiers, and descriptions only are © 2001 American Medical Association

Medicare RBRVS: The Physicians' Guide

Relative value units

CPT Code and Modifier	Description	Work RVU	Non Facility Practice Expense RVU	Facility Practice Expense RVU	PLI RVU	Total Non Facility RVUs	Medicare Payment Non Facility	Total Facility RVUs	Medicare Payment Facility	Global Period	Payment Policy Indicators*
Medicine: Mental status, speech testing											
96100	Psychological testing	0.00	1.67	1.67	0.15	1.82	$65.88	1.82	$65.88	XXX	A+
96105	Assessment of aphasia	0.00	1.67	1.67	0.15	1.82	$65.88	1.82	$65.88	XXX	A+
96110	Developmental test, lim	0.00	0.00	0.00	0.00	0.00	$0.00	0.00	$0.00	XXX	A+
96111	Developmental test, extend	0.00	1.67	1.67	0.15	1.82	$65.88	1.82	$65.88	XXX	A+
96115	Neurobehavior status exam	0.00	1.67	1.67	0.15	1.82	$65.88	1.82	$65.88	XXX	A+
96117	Neuropsych test battery	0.00	1.67	1.67	0.15	1.82	$65.88	1.82	$65.88	XXX	A+
96150	Assess hlth/behave, init	0.50	0.21	0.20	0.02	0.73	$26.43	0.72	$26.06	XXX	A+
96151	Assess hlth/behave, subseq	0.48	0.21	0.19	0.02	0.71	$25.70	0.69	$24.98	XXX	A+
96152	Intervene hlth/behave, indiv	0.46	0.20	0.18	0.02	0.68	$24.62	0.66	$23.89	XXX	A+
96153	Intervene hlth/behave, group	0.10	0.04	0.04	0.01	0.15	$5.43	0.15	$5.43	XXX	A+
96154	Interv hlth/behav, fam w/pt	0.45	0.19	0.18	0.02	0.66	$23.89	0.65	$23.53	XXX	A+
96155	Interv hlth/behav fam no pt	0.44	0.18	0.18	0.02	0.64	$23.17	0.64	$23.17	XXX	A+
Medicine: Chemotherapy administration											
96400	Chemotherapy, sc/im	0.00	0.13	0.13	0.01	0.14	$5.07	0.14	$5.07	XXX	A+
96405	Intralesional chemo admin	0.52	1.88	0.24	0.02	2.42	$87.60	0.78	$28.24	000	A M
96406	Intralesional chemo admin	0.80	2.94	0.41	0.02	3.76	$136.11	1.23	$44.53	000	A M
96408	Chemotherapy, push technique	0.00	0.92	0.92	0.05	0.97	$35.11	0.97	$35.11	XXX	A+
96410	Chemotherapy infusion method	0.00	1.47	1.47	0.07	1.54	$55.75	1.54	$55.75	XXX	A+
96412	Chemo, infuse method add-on	0.00	1.09	1.09	0.06	1.15	$41.63	1.15	$41.63	ZZZ	A+
96414	Chemo, infuse method add-on	0.00	1.27	1.27	0.07	1.34	$48.51	1.34	$48.51	XXX	A+
96420	Chemotherapy, push technique	0.00	1.18	1.18	0.07	1.25	$45.25	1.25	$45.25	XXX	A+
96422	Chemotherapy infusion method	0.00	1.17	1.17	0.07	1.24	$44.89	1.24	$44.89	XXX	A+
96423	Chemo, infuse method add-on	0.00	0.46	0.46	0.02	0.48	$17.38	0.48	$17.38	ZZZ	A+
96425	Chemotherapy infusion method	0.00	1.36	1.36	0.07	1.43	$51.76	1.43	$51.76	XXX	A+

Code	Description							
96440	Chemotherapy, intracavitary	2.37	7.99	1.06	0.12	10.48	3.55	$128.51	000	A+
96445	Chemotherapy, intracavitary	2.20	8.74	1.08	0.07	11.01	3.35	$121.27	000	A+
96450	Chemotherapy, into CNS	1.89	6.79	0.95	0.06	8.74	2.90	$104.98	000	A+
96520	Pump refilling, maintenance	0.00	0.84	0.84	0.05	0.89	0.89	$32.22	XXX	A+
96530	Pump refilling, maintenance	0.00	1.01	1.01	0.05	1.06	1.06	$38.37	XXX	A+
96542	Chemotherapy injection	1.42	4.70	0.55	0.05	6.17	2.02	$223.35	XXX	A+
96549	Chemotherapy, unspecified	0.00	0.00	0.00	0.00	0.00	0.00	$0.00	XXX	A+
96567	Photodynamic tx, skin	0.00	1.63	1.63	0.03	1.66	1.66	$60.09	XXX	A+
96570	Photodynamic tx, 30 min	1.10	0.46	0.38	0.04	1.60	1.52	$55.02	ZZZ	A
96571	Photodynamic tx, addl 15 min	0.55	0.22	0.20	0.02	0.79	0.77	$27.87	ZZZ	A

Medicine: Special dermatological procedures

96900	Ultraviolet light therapy	0.00	0.45	0.45	0.02	0.47	0.47	$17.01	XXX	A+
96902 §	Trichogram	0.41	0.25	0.16	0.01	0.67	0.58	$21.00	XXX	
96910	Photochemotherapy with UV-B	0.00	1.37	1.37	0.03	1.40	1.40	$50.68	XXX	A+
96912	Photochemotherapy with UV-A	0.00	1.54	1.54	0.04	1.58	1.58	$57.19	XXX	A+
96913	Photochemotherapy, UV-A or B	0.00	2.26	2.26	0.08	2.34	2.34	$84.71	XXX	A+
96999	Dermatological procedure	0.00	0.00	0.00	0.00	0.00	0.00	$0.00	XXX	A+

Medicine: Physical medicine and rehabilitation

97001	Pt evaluation	1.20	0.56	0.37	0.10	1.86	1.67	$67.33	XXX	A+
97002	Pt re-evaluation	0.60	0.35	0.27	0.04	0.99	0.91	$35.84	XXX	A+
97003	Ot evaluation	1.20	0.69	0.32	0.05	1.94	1.57	$70.23	XXX	A+
97004	Ot re-evaluation	0.60	0.69	0.12	0.02	1.31	0.74	$47.42	XXX	A+
97010 §	Hot or cold packs therapy	0.06	0.04	0.04	0.01	0.11	0.11	$3.98	XXX	
97012	Mechanical traction therapy	0.25	0.11	0.11	0.01	0.37	0.37	$13.39	XXX	A+
97014	Electric stimulation therapy	0.18	0.19	0.19	0.01	0.38	0.38	$13.76	XXX	A+
97016	Vasopneumatic device therapy	0.18	0.14	0.14	0.01	0.33	0.33	$11.95	XXX	A+
97018	Paraffin bath therapy	0.06	0.12	0.12	0.01	0.19	0.19	$6.88	XXX	A+

* **M** = multiple surgery adjustment applies
Me = multiple endoscopy rules may apply
B = bilateral surgery adjustment applies
A = assistant-at-surgery restriction

A+ = assistant-at-surgery restriction unless medical necessity established with documentation
C = cosurgeons payable
C+ = cosurgeons payable if medical necessity established with documentation

T = team surgeons permitted
T+ = team surgeons payable if medical necessity established with documentation
§ = indicates services that are not covered by Medicare.

Medicare RBRVS: The Physicians' Guide

Relative value units

CPT Code and Modifier	Description	Work RVU	Non Facility Practice Expense RVU	Facility Practice Expense RVU	PLI RVU	Total Non Facility RVUs	Medicare Payment Non Facility	Total Facility RVUs	Medicare Payment Facility	Global Period	Payment Policy Indicators*
97020	Microwave therapy	0.06	0.05	0.05	0.01	0.12	$4.34	0.12	$4.34	XXX	A+
97022	Whirlpool therapy	0.17	0.26	0.26	0.01	0.44	$15.93	0.44	$15.93	XXX	A+
97024	Diathermy treatment	0.06	0.05	0.05	0.01	0.12	$4.34	0.12	$4.34	XXX	A+
97026	Infrared therapy	0.06	0.05	0.05	0.01	0.12	$4.34	0.12	$4.34	XXX	A+
97028	Ultraviolet therapy	0.08	0.06	0.06	0.01	0.15	$5.43	0.15	$5.43	XXX	A+
97032	Electrical stimulation	0.25	0.21	0.21	0.01	0.47	$17.01	0.47	$17.01	XXX	A+
97033	Electric current therapy	0.26	0.12	0.12	0.02	0.40	$14.48	0.40	$14.48	XXX	A+
97034	Contrast bath therapy	0.21	0.14	0.14	0.01	0.36	$13.03	0.36	$13.03	XXX	A+
97035	Ultrasound therapy	0.21	0.08	0.08	0.01	0.30	$10.86	0.30	$10.86	XXX	A+
97036	Hydrotherapy	0.28	0.34	0.34	0.01	0.63	$22.81	0.63	$22.81	XXX	A+
97039	Physical therapy treatment	0.20	0.07	0.07	0.01	0.28	$10.14	0.28	$10.14	XXX	A+
97110	Therapeutic exercises	0.45	0.25	0.25	0.03	0.73	$26.43	0.73	$26.43	XXX	A+
97112	Neuromuscular reeducation	0.45	0.29	0.29	0.02	0.76	$27.51	0.76	$27.51	XXX	A+
97113	Aquatic therapy/exercises	0.44	0.33	0.33	0.03	0.80	$28.96	0.80	$28.96	XXX	A+
97116	Gait training therapy	0.40	0.21	0.21	0.02	0.63	$22.81	0.63	$22.81	XXX	A+
97124	Massage therapy	0.35	0.21	0.21	0.01	0.57	$20.63	0.57	$20.63	XXX	A+
97139	Physical medicine procedure	0.21	0.21	0.21	0.01	0.43	$15.57	0.43	$15.57	XXX	A+
97140	Manual therapy	0.43	0.23	0.23	0.02	0.68	$24.62	0.68	$24.62	XXX	A+
97150	Group therapeutic procedures	0.27	0.20	0.20	0.02	0.49	$17.74	0.49	$17.74	XXX	A+
97504	Orthotic training	0.45	0.25	0.25	0.03	0.73	$26.43	0.73	$26.43	XXX	A+
97520	Prosthetic training	0.45	0.21	0.21	0.02	0.68	$24.62	0.68	$24.62	XXX	A+
97530	Therapeutic activities	0.44	0.45	0.45	0.02	0.91	$32.94	0.91	$32.94	XXX	A+
97532	Cognitive skills development	0.44	0.17	0.17	0.01	0.62	$22.44	0.62	$22.44	XXX	A+
97533	Sensory integration	0.44	0.21	0.21	0.01	0.66	$23.89	0.66	$23.89	XXX	A+
97535	Self care mngment training	0.45	0.35	0.35	0.02	0.82	$29.68	0.82	$29.68	XXX	A+

Code	Description								
97537	Community/work reintegration	0.45	0.20	0.01	0.66	$23.89	0.66	$23.89	XXX	A+
97542	Wheelchair mngment training	0.45	0.22	0.01	0.68	$24.62	0.68	$24.62	XXX	A+
97545	Work hardening	0.00	0.00	0.00	0.00	$0.00	0.00	$0.00	XXX	A+
97546	Work hardening add-on	0.00	0.00	0.00	0.00	$0.00	0.00	$0.00	ZZZ	A+
97601	Wound(s) care, selective	0.50	1.90	0.04	2.44	$88.33	2.44	$88.33	XXX	
97703	Prosthetic checkout	0.25	0.44	0.02	0.71	$25.70	0.71	$25.70	XXX	A+
97750	Physical performance test	0.45	0.24	0.02	0.71	$25.70	0.71	$25.70	XXX	A+
97799	Physical medicine procedure	0.00	0.00	0.00	0.00	$0.00	0.00	$0.00	XXX	A+
97802	Medical nutrition, indiv, in	0.00	0.45	0.01	0.46	$16.65	0.46	$16.65	XXX	A+
97803	Med nutrition, indiv, subseq	0.00	0.45	0.01	0.46	$16.65	0.46	$16.65	XXX	A+
97804	Medical nutrition, group	0.00	0.17	0.01	0.18	$6.52	0.18	$6.52	XXX	A+

Medicine: Osteopathic manipulative treatment

Code	Description								
98925	Osteopathic manipulation	0.45	0.38	0.01	0.84	$30.41	0.60	$21.72	000	A+
98926	Osteopathic manipulation	0.65	0.44	0.02	1.11	$40.18	0.92	$33.30	000	A+
98927	Osteopathic manipulation	0.87	0.52	0.03	1.42	$51.40	1.21	$43.80	000	A+
98928	Osteopathic manipulation	1.03	0.59	0.03	1.65	$59.73	1.44	$52.13	000	A+
98929	Osteopathic manipulation	1.19	0.65	0.04	1.88	$68.05	1.62	$58.64	000	A+
98940	Chiropractic manipulation	0.45	0.25	0.01	0.71	$25.70	0.59	$21.36	000	A+
98941	Chiropractic manipulation	0.65	0.31	0.02	0.98	$35.48	0.86	$31.13	000	A+
98942	Chiropractic manipulation	0.87	0.37	0.03	1.27	$45.97	1.15	$41.63	000	A+
98943 §	Chiropractic manipulation	0.40	0.34	0.01	0.75	$27.15	0.57	$20.63	XXX	

Medicine: Special services and reports

Code	Description								
99082	Unusual physician travel	0.00	0.00	0.00	0.00	$0.00	0.00	$0.00	XXX	A+
99141 §	Sedation, iv/im or inhalant	0.80	2.12	0.04	2.96	$107.15	1.23	$44.53	XXX	
99142 §	Sedation, oral/rectal/nasal	0.60	1.24	0.03	1.87	$67.69	0.94	$34.03	XXX	
99170	Anogenital exam, child	1.75	2.02	0.07	3.84	$139.00	2.37	$85.79	000	A M
99175	Induction of vomiting	0.00	1.32	0.08	1.40	$50.68	1.40	$50.68	XXX	A+

*M = multiple surgery adjustment applies
Me = multiple endoscopy rules may apply
B = bilateral surgery adjustment applies
A = assistant-at-surgery restriction

A+ = assistant-at-surgery restriction unless medical necessity established with documentation
C = cosurgeons payable
C+ = cosurgeons payable if medical necessity established with documentation

T = team surgeons permitted
T+ = team surgeons payable if medical necessity established with documentation
§ = indicates services that are not covered by Medicare.

CPT five-digit codes, two-digit numeric modifiers, and descriptions only are © 2001 American Medical Association

Medicare RBRVS: The Physicians' Guide

Relative value units

CPT Code and Modifier	Description	Work RVU	Non Facility Practice Expense RVU	Facility Practice Expense RVU	PLI RVU	Total Non Facility RVUs	Medicare Payment Non Facility	Total Facility RVUs	Medicare Payment Facility	Global Period	Payment Policy Indicators*
99183	Hyperbaric oxygen therapy	2.34	NA	0.77	0.12	NA	NA	3.23	$116.92	XXX	A+
99185	Regional hypothermia	0.00	0.61	0.61	0.03	0.64	$23.17	0.64	$23.17	XXX	A+
99186	Total body hypothermia	0.00	1.69	1.69	0.37	2.06	$74.57	2.06	$74.57	XXX	A+
99195	Phlebotomy	0.00	0.42	0.42	0.02	0.44	$15.93	0.44	$15.93	XXX	A+
99199	Special service/proc/report	0.00	0.00	0.00	0.00	0.00	$0.00	0.00	$0.00	XXX	A+

Evaluation and Management: Office or other outpatient services

CPT Code and Modifier	Description	Work RVU	Non Facility Practice Expense RVU	Facility Practice Expense RVU	PLI RVU	Total Non Facility RVUs	Medicare Payment Non Facility	Total Facility RVUs	Medicare Payment Facility	Global Period	Payment Policy Indicators*
99201	Office/outpatient visit, new	0.45	0.47	0.16	0.02	0.94	$34.03	0.63	$22.81	XXX	A+
99202	Office/outpatient visit, new	0.88	0.77	0.33	0.05	1.70	$61.54	1.26	$45.61	XXX	A+
99203	Office/outpatient visit, new	1.34	1.12	0.50	0.08	2.54	$91.95	1.92	$69.50	XXX	A+
99204	Office/outpatient visit, new	2.00	1.51	0.74	0.10	3.61	$130.68	2.84	$102.81	XXX	A+
99205	Office/outpatient visit, new	2.67	1.80	0.98	0.12	4.59	$166.15	3.77	$136.47	XXX	A+
99211	Office/outpatient visit, est	0.17	0.38	0.06	0.01	0.56	$20.27	0.24	$8.69	XXX	A+
99212	Office/outpatient visit, est	0.45	0.53	0.17	0.02	1.00	$36.20	0.64	$23.17	XXX	A+
99213	Office/outpatient visit, est	0.67	0.69	0.24	0.03	1.39	$50.32	0.94	$34.03	XXX	A+
99214	Office/outpatient visit, est	1.10	1.04	0.41	0.04	2.18	$78.91	1.55	$56.11	XXX	A+
99215	Office/outpatient visit, est	1.77	1.36	0.66	0.07	3.20	$115.84	2.50	$90.50	XXX	A+

Evaluation and Management: Hospital observation services

CPT Code and Modifier	Description	Work RVU	Non Facility Practice Expense RVU	Facility Practice Expense RVU	PLI RVU	Total Non Facility RVUs	Medicare Payment Non Facility	Total Facility RVUs	Medicare Payment Facility	Global Period	Payment Policy Indicators*
99217	Observation care discharge	1.28	NA	0.45	0.05	NA	NA	1.78	$64.43	XXX	A+
99218	Observation care	1.28	NA	0.45	0.05	NA	NA	1.78	$64.43	XXX	A+
99219	Observation care	2.14	NA	0.75	0.08	NA	NA	2.97	$107.51	XXX	A+
99220	Observation care	2.99	NA	1.06	0.11	NA	NA	4.16	$150.59	XXX	A+

Evaluation and Management: Hospital inpatient services

CPT Code and Modifier	Description	Work RVU	Non Facility Practice Expense RVU	Facility Practice Expense RVU	PLI RVU	Total Non Facility RVUs	Medicare Payment Non Facility	Total Facility RVUs	Medicare Payment Facility	Global Period	Payment Policy Indicators*
99221	Initial hospital care	1.28	NA	0.47	0.05	NA	NA	1.80	$65.16	XXX	A+
99222	Initial hospital care	2.14	NA	0.77	0.08	NA	NA	2.99	$108.24	XXX	A+
99223	Initial hospital care	2.99	NA	1.08	0.10	NA	NA	4.17	$150.95	XXX	A+
99231	Subsequent hospital care	0.64	NA	0.24	0.02	NA	NA	0.90	$32.58	XXX	A+

Code	Description									
99232	Subsequent hospital care	1.06	NA	0.39	0.03	NA	1.48	$53.57	XXX	A+
99233	Subsequent hospital care	1.51	NA	0.55	0.05	NA	2.11	$76.38	XXX	A+
99234	Observ/hosp same date	2.56	NA	0.93	0.11	NA	3.60	$130.32	XXX	A+
99235	Observ/hosp same date	3.42	NA	1.21	0.13	NA	4.76	$172.31	XXX	A+
99236	Observ/hosp same date	4.27	NA	1.49	0.17	NA	5.93	$214.66	XXX	A+
99238	Hospital discharge day	1.28	NA	0.51	0.04	NA	1.83	$66.24	XXX	A+
99239	Hospital discharge day	1.75	NA	0.71	0.05	NA	2.51	$90.86	XXX	A+

Evaluation and Management: Consultations

Code	Description									
99241	Office consultation	0.64	0.62	0.24	0.04	1.30	0.92	$33.30	XXX	A+
99242	Office consultation	1.29	1.03	0.50	0.09	2.41	1.88	$68.05	XXX	A+
99243	Office consultation	1.72	1.38	0.67	0.10	3.20	2.49	$90.14	XXX	A+
99244	Office consultation	2.58	1.83	0.98	0.13	4.54	3.69	$133.58	XXX	A+
99245	Office consultation	3.43	2.29	1.30	0.16	5.88	4.89	$177.01	XXX	A+
99251	Initial inpatient consult	0.66	NA	0.26	0.04	NA	0.96	$34.75	XXX	A+
99252	Initial inpatient consult	1.32	NA	0.53	0.08	NA	1.93	$69.86	XXX	A+
99253	Initial inpatient consult	1.82	NA	0.72	0.09	NA	2.63	$95.20	XXX	A+
99254	Initial inpatient consult	2.64	NA	1.03	0.11	NA	3.78	$136.83	XXX	A+
99255	Initial inpatient consult	3.65	NA	1.41	0.15	NA	5.21	$188.60	XXX	A+
99261	Follow-up inpatient consult	0.42	NA	0.16	0.02	NA	0.60	$21.72	XXX	A+
99262	Follow-up inpatient consult	0.85	NA	0.32	0.03	NA	1.20	$43.44	XXX	A+
99263	Follow-up inpatient consult	1.27	NA	0.48	0.04	NA	1.79	$64.80	XXX	A+
99271	Confirmatory consultation	0.45	0.67	0.17	0.03	1.15	0.65	$23.53	XXX	A+
99272	Confirmatory consultation	0.84	0.89	0.32	0.06	1.79	1.22	$44.16	XXX	A+
99273	Confirmatory consultation	1.19	1.13	0.47	0.07	2.39	1.73	$62.62	XXX	A+
99274	Confirmatory consultation	1.73	1.41	0.68	0.09	3.23	2.50	$90.50	XXX	A+
99275	Confirmatory consultation	2.31	1.68	0.88	0.10	4.09	3.29	$119.10	XXX	A+

* **M** = multiple surgery adjustment applies
   Me = multiple endoscopy rules may apply
   B = bilateral surgery adjustment applies
   A = assistant-at-surgery restriction

A+ = assistant-at-surgery restriction unless medical necessity established with documentation
C = cosurgeons payable
C+ = cosurgeons payable if medical necessity established with documentation

T = team surgeons permitted
T+ = team surgeons payable if medical necessity established with documentation
§ = indicates services that are not covered by Medicare.

431 CPT five-digit codes, two-digit numeric modifiers, and descriptions only are © 2001 American Medical Association

Medicare RBRVS: The Physicians' Guide

Relative value units

CPT Code and Modifier	Description	Work RVU	Non Facility Practice Expense RVU	Facility Practice Expense RVU	PLI RVU	Total Non Facility RVUs	Medicare Payment Non Facility	Total Facility RVUs	Medicare Payment Facility	Global Period	Payment Policy Indicators*
Evaluation and Management: Emergency department services										
99281	Emergency dept visit	0.33	NA	0.09	0.02	NA	NA	0.44	$15.93	XXX	A+
99282	Emergency dept visit	0.55	NA	0.15	0.03	NA	NA	0.73	$26.43	XXX	A+
99283	Emergency dept visit	1.24	NA	0.32	0.08	NA	NA	1.64	$59.37	XXX	A+
99284	Emergency dept visit	1.95	NA	0.49	0.12	NA	NA	2.56	$92.67	XXX	A+
99285	Emergency dept visit	3.06	NA	0.75	0.19	NA	NA	4.00	$144.80	XXX	A+
Evaluation and Management: Critical care services										
99291	Critical care, first hour	4.00	1.63	1.34	0.14	5.77	$208.87	5.48	$198.37	XXX	A+
99292	Critical care, addl 30 min	2.00	0.92	0.66	0.07	2.99	$108.24	2.73	$98.82	ZZZ	A+
Evaluation and Management: Neonatal intensive care										
99295	Neonatal critical care	16.00	NA	4.53	0.70	NA	NA	21.23	$768.51	XXX	A+
99296	Neonatal critical care	8.00	NA	2.58	0.23	NA	NA	10.81	$391.31	XXX	A+
99297	Neonatal critical care	4.00	NA	1.32	0.12	NA	NA	5.44	$196.92	XXX	A+
99298	Neonatal critical care	2.75	NA	0.97	0.10	NA	NA	3.82	$138.28	XXX	A+
Evaluation and Management: Nursing facility services										
99301	Nursing facility care	1.20	0.70	0.42	0.04	1.94	$70.23	1.66	$60.09	XXX	A+
99302	Nursing facility care	1.61	0.98	0.57	0.05	2.64	$95.57	2.23	$80.72	XXX	A+
99303	Nursing facility care	2.01	1.21	0.70	0.06	3.28	$118.73	2.77	$100.27	XXX	A+
99311	Nursing fac care, subseq	0.60	0.49	0.21	0.02	1.11	$40.18	0.83	$30.05	XXX	A+
99312	Nursing fac care, subseq	1.00	0.68	0.35	0.03	1.71	$61.90	1.38	$49.95	XXX	A+
99313	Nursing fac care, subseq	1.42	0.87	0.50	0.04	2.33	$84.34	1.96	$70.95	XXX	A+
99315	Nursing fac discharge day	1.13	0.74	0.40	0.04	1.91	$69.14	1.57	$56.83	XXX	A+
99316	Nursing fac discharge day	1.50	0.95	0.53	0.05	2.50	$90.50	2.08	$75.29	XXX	A+
Evaluation and Management: Domiciliary, rest home (eg, boarding home), or custodial services										
99321	Rest home visit, new patient	0.71	0.49	0.49	0.02	1.22	$44.16	1.22	$44.16	XXX	A+

Code	Description							
99322	Rest home visit, new patient	1.01	0.70	0.70	0.03	1.74	$62.99	XXX	A+
99323	Rest home visit, new patient	1.28	0.93	0.93	0.04	2.25	$81.45	XXX	A+
99331	Rest home visit, est pat	0.60	0.47	0.47	0.02	1.09	$39.46	XXX	A+
99332	Rest home visit, est pat	0.80	0.59	0.59	0.03	1.42	$51.40	XXX	A+
99333	Rest home visit, est pat	1.00	0.73	0.73	0.03	1.76	$63.71	XXX	A+

Evaluation and Management: Home services

99341	Home visit, new patient	1.01	0.56	0.56	0.05	1.62	$58.64	XXX	A+
99342	Home visit, new patient	1.52	0.87	0.87	0.05	2.44	$88.33	XXX	A+
99343	Home visit, new patient	2.27	1.29	1.29	0.07	3.63	$131.40	XXX	A+
99344	Home visit, new patient	3.03	1.57	1.57	0.10	4.70	$170.14	XXX	A+
99345	Home visit, new patient	3.79	1.86	1.86	0.12	5.77	$208.87	XXX	A+
99347	Home visit, est patient	0.76	0.49	0.49	0.03	1.28	$46.33	XXX	A+
99348	Home visit, est patient	1.26	0.74	0.74	0.04	2.04	$73.85	XXX	A+
99349	Home visit, est patient	2.02	1.08	1.08	0.06	3.16	$114.39	XXX	A+
99350	Home visit, est patient	3.03	1.47	1.47	0.10	4.60	$166.52	XXX	A+

Evaluation and Management: Prolonged services

99354	Prolonged service, office	1.77	1.46	0.66	0.06	3.29	$119.10	ZZZ	A+
99355	Prolonged service, office	1.77	1.24	0.65	0.06	3.07	$111.13	ZZZ	A+
99356	Prolonged service, inpatient	1.71	NA	0.61	0.06	NA	NA	ZZZ	A+
99357	Prolonged service, inpatient	1.71	NA	0.63	0.06	NA	NA	ZZZ	A+

Evaluation and Management: Care plan oversight services

99374	§ Home health care supervision	1.10	1.47	0.44	0.04	2.61	$94.48	XXX	
99377	§ Hospice care supervision	1.10	1.47	0.44	0.04	2.61	$94.48	XXX	
99379	§ Nursing fac care supervision	1.10	1.47	0.44	0.03	2.60	$94.12	XXX	
99380	§ Nursing fac care supervision	1.73	1.72	0.69	0.05	3.50	$126.70	XXX	

Evaluation and Management: Preventive medicine services

99381	§ Prev visit, new, infant	1.19	1.50	0.48	0.04	2.73	$98.82	XXX	

* **M** = multiple surgery adjustment applies
Me = multiple endoscopy rules may apply
B = bilateral surgery adjustment applies
A = assistant-at-surgery restriction

A+ = assistant-at-surgery restriction unless medical necessity established with documentation
C = cosurgeons payable
C+ = cosurgeons payable if medical necessity established with documentation

T = team surgeons permitted
T+ = team surgeons payable if medical necessity established with documentation
§ = indicates services that are not covered by Medicare.

433 CPT five-digit codes, two-digit numeric modifiers, and descriptions only are © 2001 American Medical Association

Medicare RBRVS: The Physicians' Guide

Relative value units

CPT Code and Modifier	Description	Work RVU	Non Facility Practice Expense RVU	Facility Practice Expense RVU	PLI RVU	Total Non Facility RVUs	Medicare Payment Non Facility	Total Facility RVUs	Medicare Payment Facility	Global Period	Payment Policy Indicators*
99382 §	Prev visit, new, age 1-4	1.36	1.54	0.54	0.04	2.94	$106.43	1.94	$70.23	XXX	
99383 §	Prev visit, new, age 5-11	1.36	1.48	0.54	0.04	2.88	$104.25	1.94	$70.23	XXX	
99384 §	Prev visit, new, age 12-17	1.53	1.55	0.61	0.05	3.13	$113.30	2.19	$79.28	XXX	
99385 §	Prev visit, new, age 18-39	1.53	1.55	0.61	0.05	3.13	$113.30	2.19	$79.28	XXX	
99386 §	Prev visit, new, age 40-64	1.88	1.74	0.75	0.06	3.68	$133.21	2.69	$97.38	XXX	
99387 §	Prev visit, new, age 65 & over	2.06	1.87	0.82	0.06	3.99	$144.43	2.94	$106.43	XXX	
99391 §	Prev visit, est, infant	1.02	1.02	0.41	0.03	2.07	$74.93	1.46	$52.85	XXX	
99392 §	Prev visit, est, age 1-4	1.19	1.09	0.48	0.04	2.32	$83.98	1.71	$61.90	XXX	
99393 §	Prev visit, est, age 5-11	1.19	1.06	0.48	0.04	2.29	$82.90	1.71	$61.90	XXX	
99394 §	Prev visit, est, age 12-17	1.36	1.15	0.54	0.04	2.55	$92.31	1.94	$70.23	XXX	
99395 §	Prev visit, est, age 18-39	1.36	1.18	0.54	0.04	2.58	$93.39	1.94	$70.23	XXX	
99396 §	Prev visit, est, age 40-64	1.53	1.27	0.61	0.05	2.85	$103.17	2.19	$79.28	XXX	
99397 §	Prev visit, est, 65 & over	1.71	1.37	0.68	0.05	3.13	$113.30	2.44	$88.33	XXX	
99401 §	Preventive counseling, indiv	0.48	0.62	0.19	0.01	1.11	$40.18	0.68	$24.62	XXX	
99402 §	Preventive counseling, indiv	0.98	0.86	0.39	0.02	1.86	$67.33	1.39	$50.32	XXX	
99403 §	Preventive counseling, indiv	1.46	1.10	0.58	0.03	2.59	$93.76	2.07	$74.93	XXX	
99404 §	Preventive counseling, indiv	1.95	1.35	0.78	0.04	3.34	$120.91	2.77	$100.27	XXX	
99411 §	Preventive counseling, group	0.15	0.18	0.06	0.01	0.34	$12.31	0.22	$7.96	XXX	
99412 §	Preventive counseling, group	0.25	0.24	0.10	0.01	0.50	$18.10	0.36	$13.03	XXX	
Evaluation and Management: Newborn care											
99431	Initial care, normal newborn	1.17	NA	0.39	0.04	NA	NA	1.60	$57.92	XXX	A+
99432	Newborn care, not in hosp	1.26	1.12	0.50	0.06	2.44	$88.33	1.82	$65.88	XXX	A+
99433	Normal newborn care/hospital	0.62	NA	0.21	0.02	NA	NA	0.85	$30.77	XXX	A+
99435	Newborn discharge day hosp	1.50	NA	0.54	0.05	NA	NA	2.09	$75.66	XXX	A+
99436	Attendance, birth	1.50	0.50	0.50	0.05	2.05	$74.21	2.05	$74.21	XXX	A+
99440	Newborn resuscitation	2.93	NA	1.17	0.11	NA	NA	4.21	$152.40	XXX	A+

Evaluation and Management: Special evaluation and management services

99455	Disability examination	0.00	0.00	0.00	0.00	$0.00	$0.00	XXX	A+
99456	Disability examination	0.00	0.00	0.00	0.00	$0.00	$0.00	XXX	A+

Evaluation and Management: Other evaluation and management services

99499	Unlisted e&m service	0.00	0.00	0.00	0.00	$0.00	$0.00	XXX	A+

* **M** = multiple surgery adjustment applies
Me = multiple endoscopy rules may apply
B = bilateral surgery adjustment applies
A = assistant-at-surgery restriction

A+ = assistant-at-surgery restriction unless medical necessity established with documentation
C = cosurgeons payable
C+ = cosurgeons payable if medical necessity established with documentation

T = team surgeons permitted
T+ = team surgeons payable if medical necessity established with documentation
$ = indicates services that are not covered by Medicare.

435   CPT five-digit codes, two-digit numeric modifiers, and descriptions only are © 2001 American Medical Association

Medicare RBRVS: The Physicians' Guide

Relative value units

HCPCS Code and Modifier	Description	Work RVU	Non Facility Practice Expense RVU	Facility Practice Expense RVU	PLI RVU	Total Non Facility RVUs	Medicare Payment Non Facility	Total Facility RVUs	Medicare Payment Facility	Global Period	Payment Policy Indicators*
Alpha-numeric coded services (level 2)											
A4890	Repair/maint cont hemo equip	0.00	0.00	0.00	0.00	0.00	$0.00	0.00	$0.00	XXX	A+
D0150	Comprehensve oral evaluation	0.00	0.00	0.00	0.00	0.00	$0.00	0.00	$0.00	YYY	A+
D0240	Intraoral occlusal film	0.00	0.00	0.00	0.00	0.00	$0.00	0.00	$0.00	YYY	A+
D0250	Extraoral first film	0.00	0.00	0.00	0.00	0.00	$0.00	0.00	$0.00	YYY	A+
D0260	Extraoral ea additional film	0.00	0.00	0.00	0.00	0.00	$0.00	0.00	$0.00	YYY	A+
D0270	Dental bitewing single film	0.00	0.00	0.00	0.00	0.00	$0.00	0.00	$0.00	YYY	A+
D0272	Dental bitewings two films	0.00	0.00	0.00	0.00	0.00	$0.00	0.00	$0.00	YYY	A+
D0274	Dental bitewings four films	0.00	0.00	0.00	0.00	0.00	$0.00	0.00	$0.00	YYY	A+
D0277	Vert bitewings-sev to eight	0.00	0.00	0.00	0.00	0.00	$0.00	0.00	$0.00	XXX	
D0460	Pulp vitality test	0.00	0.00	0.00	0.00	0.00	$0.00	0.00	$0.00	YYY	A+
D0472	Gross exam, prep & report	0.00	0.00	0.00	0.00	0.00	$0.00	0.00	$0.00	XXX	
D0473	Micro exam, prep & report	0.00	0.00	0.00	0.00	0.00	$0.00	0.00	$0.00	XXX	
D0474	Micro w exam of surg margins	0.00	0.00	0.00	0.00	0.00	$0.00	0.00	$0.00	XXX	
D0480	Cytopath smear prep & report	0.00	0.00	0.00	0.00	0.00	$0.00	0.00	$0.00	XXX	
D0501	Histopathologic examinations	0.00	0.00	0.00	0.00	0.00	$0.00	0.00	$0.00	YYY	A+
D0502	Other oral pathology procedu	0.00	0.00	0.00	0.00	0.00	$0.00	0.00	$0.00	YYY	A+
D0999	Unspecified diagnostic proce	0.00	0.00	0.00	0.00	0.00	$0.00	0.00	$0.00	YYY	A+
D1510	Space maintainer fxd unilat	0.00	0.00	0.00	0.00	0.00	$0.00	0.00	$0.00	YYY	A+
D1515	Fixed bilat space maintainer	0.00	0.00	0.00	0.00	0.00	$0.00	0.00	$0.00	YYY	A+
D1520	Remove unilat space maintain	0.00	0.00	0.00	0.00	0.00	$0.00	0.00	$0.00	YYY	A+
D1525	Remove bilat space maintain	0.00	0.00	0.00	0.00	0.00	$0.00	0.00	$0.00	YYY	A+
D1550	Recement space maintainer	0.00	0.00	0.00	0.00	0.00	$0.00	0.00	$0.00	YYY	A+
D2970	Temporary- fractured tooth	0.00	0.00	0.00	0.00	0.00	$0.00	0.00	$0.00	YYY	A+
D2999	Dental unspec restorative pr	0.00	0.00	0.00	0.00	0.00	$0.00	0.00	$0.00	YYY	A+
D3460	Endodontic endosseous implan	0.00	0.00	0.00	0.00	0.00	$0.00	0.00	$0.00	YYY	A+
D3999	Endodontic procedure	0.00	0.00	0.00	0.00	0.00	$0.00	0.00	$0.00	YYY	A+

Code	Description						
D4260	Osseous surgery per quadrant	0.00	0.00	0.00	$0.00	YYY	A+
D4263	Bone replce graft first site	0.00	0.00	0.00	$0.00	YYY	A+
D4264	Bone replce graft each add	0.00	0.00	0.00	$0.00	YYY	A+
D4268	Surgical revision procedure	0.00	0.00	0.00	$0.00	XXX	
D4270	Pedicle soft tissue graft pr	0.00	0.00	0.00	$0.00	YYY	A+
D4271	Free soft tissue graft proc	0.00	0.00	0.00	$0.00	YYY	A+
D4273	Subepithelial tissue graft	0.00	0.00	0.00	$0.00	YYY	A+
D4355	Full mouth debridement	0.00	0.00	0.00	$0.00	YYY	A+
D4381	Localized chemo delivery	0.00	0.00	0.00	$0.00	YYY	A+
D5911	Facial moulage sectional	0.00	0.00	0.00	$0.00	YYY	A+
D5912	Facial moulage complete	0.00	0.00	0.00	$0.00	YYY	A+
D5951	Feeding aid	0.00	0.00	0.00	$0.00	YYY	A+
D5983	Radiation applicator	0.00	0.00	0.00	$0.00	YYY	A+
D5984	Radiation shield	0.00	0.00	0.00	$0.00	YYY	A+
D5985	Radiation cone locator	0.00	0.00	0.00	$0.00	YYY	A+
D5987	Commissure splint	0.00	0.00	0.00	$0.00	YYY	A+
D6920	Dental connector bar	0.00	0.00	0.00	$0.00	YYY	A+
D7110	Oral surgery single tooth	0.00	0.00	0.00	$0.00	YYY	A+
D7120	Each add tooth extraction	0.00	0.00	0.00	$0.00	YYY	A+
D7130	Tooth root removal	0.00	0.00	0.00	$0.00	YYY	A+
D7210	Rem imp tooth w mucoper flp	0.00	0.00	0.00	$0.00	YYY	A+
D7220	Impact tooth remov soft tiss	0.00	0.00	0.00	$0.00	YYY	A+
D7230	Impact tooth remov part bony	0.00	0.00	0.00	$0.00	YYY	A+
D7240	Impact tooth remov comp bony	0.00	0.00	0.00	$0.00	YYY	A+
D7241	Impact tooth rem bony w/comp	0.00	0.00	0.00	$0.00	YYY	A+
D7250	Tooth root removal	0.00	0.00	0.00	$0.00	YYY	A+
D7260	Oral antral fistula closure	0.00	0.00	0.00	$0.00	YYY	A+
D7291	Transseptal fiberotomy	0.00	0.00	0.00	$0.00	YYY	A+

* M = multiple surgery adjustment applies
Me = multiple endoscopy rules may apply
B = bilateral surgery adjustment applies
A = assistant-at-surgery restriction

A+ = assistant-at-surgery restriction unless medical necessity established with documentation
C = cosurgeons payable
C+ = cosurgeons payable if medical necessity established with documentation

T = team surgeons permitted
T+ = team surgeons payable if medical necessity established with documentation
§ = indicates services that are not covered by Medicare.

CPT five-digit codes, two-digit numeric modifiers, and descriptions only are © 2001 American Medical Association

Medicare RBRVS: The Physicians' Guide

Relative value units

HCPCS Code and Modifier	Description	Work RVU	Non Facility Practice Expense RVU	Facility Practice Expense RVU	PLI RVU	Total Non Facility RVUs	Medicare Payment Non Facility	Total Facility RVUs	Medicare Payment Facility	Global Period	Payment Policy Indicators*
D7940	Reshaping bone orthognathic	0.00	0.00	0.00	0.00	0.00	$0.00	0.00	$0.00	YYY	A+
D9110	Tx dental pain minor proc	0.00	0.00	0.00	0.00	0.00	$0.00	0.00	$0.00	YYY	A+
D9230	Analgesia	0.00	0.00	0.00	0.00	0.00	$0.00	0.00	$0.00	YYY	A+
D9248	Sedation (non-iv)	0.00	0.00	0.00	0.00	0.00	$0.00	0.00	$0.00	XXX	
D9630	Other drugs/medicaments	0.00	0.00	0.00	0.00	0.00	$0.00	0.00	$0.00	YYY	A+
D9930	Treatment of complications	0.00	0.00	0.00	0.00	0.00	$0.00	0.00	$0.00	YYY	A+
D9940	Dental occlusal guard	0.00	0.00	0.00	0.00	0.00	$0.00	0.00	$0.00	YYY	A+
D9950	Occlusion analysis	0.00	0.00	0.00	0.00	0.00	$0.00	0.00	$0.00	YYY	A+
D9951	Limited occlusal adjustment	0.00	0.00	0.00	0.00	0.00	$0.00	0.00	$0.00	YYY	A+
D9952	Complete occlusal adjustment	0.00	0.00	0.00	0.00	0.00	$0.00	0.00	$0.00	YYY	A+
G0002	Temporary urinary catheter	0.50	3.32	0.17	0.03	3.85	$139.37	0.70	$25.34	000	M A
G0004	ECG transm phys review & int	0.52	7.10	7.10	0.45	8.07	$292.13	8.07	$292.13	XXX	A+
G0005	ECG 24 hour recording	0.00	1.18	1.18	0.07	1.25	$45.25	1.25	$45.25	XXX	A+
G0006	ECG transmission & analysis	0.00	5.71	5.71	0.36	6.07	$219.73	6.07	$219.73	XXX	A+
G0007	ECG phy review & interpret	0.52	0.21	0.21	0.02	0.75	$27.15	0.75	$27.15	XXX	A+
G0015	Post symptom ECG tracing	0.00	5.71	5.71	0.36	6.07	$219.73	6.07	$219.73	XXX	A+
G0030	PET imaging prev PET single	0.00	0.00	0.00	0.00	0.00	$0.00	0.00	$0.00	XXX	A+
G0030-26	PET imaging prev PET single	1.50	0.52	0.52	0.04	2.06	$74.57	2.06	$74.57	XXX	A+
G0030-TC	PET imaging prev PET single	0.00	0.00	0.00	0.00	0.00	$0.00	0.00	$0.00	XXX	A+
G0031	PET imaging prev PET multple	0.00	0.00	0.00	0.00	0.00	$0.00	0.00	$0.00	XXX	A+
G0031-26	PET imaging prev PET multple	1.87	0.70	0.70	0.06	2.63	$95.20	2.63	$95.20	XXX	A+
G0031-TC	PET imaging prev PET multple	0.00	0.00	0.00	0.00	0.00	$0.00	0.00	$0.00	XXX	A+
G0032	PET follow SPECT 78464 singl	0.00	0.00	0.00	0.00	0.00	$0.00	0.00	$0.00	XXX	A+
G0032-26	PET follow SPECT 78464 singl	1.50	0.52	0.52	0.05	2.07	$74.93	2.07	$74.93	XXX	A+
G0032-TC	PET follow SPECT 78464 singl	0.00	0.00	0.00	0.00	0.00	$0.00	0.00	$0.00	XXX	A+
G0033	PET follow SPECT 78464 mult	0.00	0.00	0.00	0.00	0.00	$0.00	0.00	$0.00	XXX	A+
G0033-26	PET follow SPECT 78464 mult	1.87	0.70	0.70	0.06	2.63	$95.20	2.63	$95.20	XXX	A+

Code	Description								
G0033-TC	PET follow SPECT 78464 mult	0.00	0.00	0.00	0.00	0.00	$0.00	XXX	A+
G0034	PET follow SPECT 76865 singl	0.00	0.00	0.00	0.00	0.00	$0.00	XXX	A+
G0034-26	PET follow SPECT 76865 singl	1.50	0.52	0.05	2.07	$74.93	$74.93	XXX	A+
G0034-TC	PET follow SPECT 76865 singl	0.00	0.00	0.00	0.00	0.00	$0.00	XXX	A+
G0035	PET follow SPECT 78465 mult	0.00	0.00	0.00	0.00	0.00	$0.00	XXX	A+
G0035-26	PET follow SPECT 78465 mult	1.87	0.70	0.06	2.63	$95.20	$95.20	XXX	A+
G0035-TC	PET follow SPECT 78465 mult	0.00	0.00	0.00	0.00	0.00	$0.00	XXX	A+
G0036	PET follow cornry angio sing	0.00	0.00	0.00	0.00	0.00	$0.00	XXX	A+
G0036-26	PET follow cornry angio sing	1.50	0.52	0.04	2.06	$74.57	$74.57	XXX	A+
G0036-TC	PET follow cornry angio sing	0.00	0.00	0.00	0.00	0.00	$0.00	XXX	A+
G0037	PET follow cornry angio mult	0.00	0.00	0.00	0.00	0.00	$0.00	XXX	A+
G0037-26	PET follow cornry angio mult	1.87	0.70	0.06	2.63	$95.20	$95.20	XXX	A+
G0037-TC	PET follow cornry angio mult	0.00	0.00	0.00	0.00	0.00	$0.00	XXX	A+
G0038	PET follow myocard perf sing	0.00	0.00	0.00	0.00	0.00	$0.00	XXX	A+
G0038-26	PET follow myocard perf sing	1.50	0.52	0.04	2.06	$74.57	$74.57	XXX	A+
G0038-TC	PET follow myocard perf sing	0.00	0.00	0.00	0.00	0.00	$0.00	XXX	A+
G0039	PET follow myocard perf mult	0.00	0.00	0.00	0.00	0.00	$0.00	XXX	A+
G0039-26	PET follow myocard perf mult	1.87	0.70	0.07	2.64	$95.57	$95.57	XXX	A+
G0039-TC	PET follow myocard perf mult	0.00	0.00	0.00	0.00	0.00	$0.00	XXX	A+
G0040	PET follow stress echo singl	0.00	0.00	0.00	0.00	0.00	$0.00	XXX	A+
G0040-26	PET follow stress echo singl	1.50	0.52	0.04	2.06	$74.57	$74.57	XXX	A+
G0040-TC	PET follow stress echo singl	0.00	0.00	0.00	0.00	0.00	$0.00	XXX	A+
G0041	PET follow stress echo mult	0.00	0.00	0.00	0.00	0.00	$0.00	XXX	A+
G0041-26	PET follow stress echo mult	1.87	0.70	0.05	2.62	$94.84	$94.84	XXX	A+
G0041-TC	PET follow stress echo mult	0.00	0.00	0.00	0.00	0.00	$0.00	XXX	A+
G0042	PET follow ventriculogm sing	0.00	0.00	0.00	0.00	0.00	$0.00	XXX	A+
G0042-26	PET follow ventriculogm sing	1.50	0.52	0.04	2.06	$74.57	$74.57	XXX	A+
G0042-TC	PET follow ventriculogm sing	0.00	0.00	0.00	0.00	0.00	$0.00	XXX	A+

* **M** = multiple surgery adjustment applies
Me = multiple endoscopy rules may apply
B = bilateral surgery adjustment applies
A = assistant-at-surgery restriction

A+ = assistant-at-surgery restriction unless medical necessity established with documentation
C = cosurgeons payable
C+ = cosurgeons payable if medical necessity established with documentation

T = team surgeons permitted
T+ = team surgeons payable if medical necessity established with documentation
§ = indicates services that are not covered by Medicare.

CPT five-digit codes, two-digit numeric modifiers, and descriptions only are © 2001 American Medical Association

Medicare RBRVS: The Physicians' Guide

Relative value units

HCPCS Code and Modifier	Description	Work RVU	Non Facility Practice Expense RVU	Facility Practice Expense RVU	PLI RVU	Total Non Facility RVUs	Medicare Payment Non Facility	Total Facility RVUs	Medicare Payment Facility	Global Period	Payment Policy Indicators*
G0043	PET follow ventriculogm mult	0.00	0.00	0.00	0.00	0.00	$0.00	0.00	$0.00	XXX	A+
G0043-26	PET follow ventriculogm mult	1.87	0.70	0.70	0.06	2.63	$95.20	2.63	$95.20	XXX	A+
G0043-TC	PET follow ventriculogm mult	0.00	0.00	0.00	0.00	0.00	$0.00	0.00	$0.00	XXX	A+
G0044	PET following rest ECG singl	0.00	0.00	0.00	0.00	0.00	$0.00	0.00	$0.00	XXX	A+
G0044-26	PET following rest ECG singl	1.50	0.52	0.52	0.04	2.06	$74.57	2.06	$74.57	XXX	A+
G0044-TC	PET following rest ECG singl	0.00	0.00	0.00	0.00	0.00	$0.00	0.00	$0.00	XXX	A+
G0045	PET following rest ECG mult	0.00	0.00	0.00	0.00	0.00	$0.00	0.00	$0.00	XXX	A+
G0045-26	PET following rest ECG mult	1.87	0.70	0.70	0.06	2.63	$95.20	2.63	$95.20	XXX	A+
G0045-TC	PET following rest ECG mult	0.00	0.00	0.00	0.00	0.00	$0.00	0.00	$0.00	XXX	A+
G0046	PET follow stress ECG singl	0.00	0.00	0.00	0.00	0.00	$0.00	0.00	$0.00	XXX	A+
G0046-26	PET follow stress ECG singl	1.50	0.52	0.52	0.04	2.06	$74.57	2.06	$74.57	XXX	A+
G0046-TC	PET follow stress ECG singl	0.00	0.00	0.00	0.00	0.00	$0.00	0.00	$0.00	XXX	A+
G0047	PET follow stress ECG mult	0.00	0.00	0.00	0.00	0.00	$0.00	0.00	$0.00	XXX	A+
G0047-26	PET follow stress ECG mult	1.87	0.70	0.70	0.06	2.63	$95.20	2.63	$95.20	XXX	A+
G0047-TC	PET follow stress ECG mult	0.00	0.00	0.00	0.00	0.00	$0.00	0.00	$0.00	XXX	A+
G0050	Residual urine by ultrasound	0.00	0.81	0.81	0.04	0.85	$30.77	0.85	$30.77	XXX	A+
G0101	CA screen;pelvic/breast exam	0.45	0.52	0.18	0.01	0.98	$35.48	0.64	$23.17	XXX	A+
G0102	Prostate ca screening; dre	0.17	0.38	0.06	0.01	0.56	$20.27	0.24	$8.69	XXX	
G0104	CA screen;flexi sigmoidscope	0.96	1.92	0.53	0.05	2.93	$106.06	1.54	$55.75	000	M A
G0105	Colorectal scrn; hi risk ind	3.70	8.79	1.77	0.20	12.69	$459.37	5.67	$205.25	000	M A
G0106	Colon CA screen;barium enema	0.99	2.47	2.47	0.15	3.61	$130.68	3.61	$130.68	XXX	A+
G0106	Colon CA screen;barium enema	0.99	2.47	2.47	0.15	3.61	$130.68	3.61	$130.68	XXX	A+
G0106	Colon CA screen;barium enema	0.99	2.47	2.47	0.15	3.61	$130.68	3.61	$130.68	XXX	A+
G0106-26	Colon CA screen;barium enema	0.99	0.35	0.35	0.04	1.38	$49.95	1.38	$49.95	XXX	A+
G0106-26	Colon CA screen;barium enema	0.99	0.35	0.35	0.04	1.38	$49.95	1.38	$49.95	XXX	A+
G0106-26	Colon CA screen;barium enema	0.99	0.35	0.35	0.04	1.38	$49.95	1.38	$49.95	XXX	A+
G0106-TC	Colon CA screen;barium enema	0.00	2.12	2.12	0.11	2.23	$80.72	2.23	$80.72	XXX	A+

Code	Description								
G0106-TC	Colon CA screen;barium enema	0.00	2.12	2.12	0.11	2.23	$80.72	2.23	$80.72	XXX	A+
G0106-TC	Colon CA screen;barium enema	0.00	2.12	2.12	0.11	2.23	$80.72	2.23	$80.72	XXX	A+
G0108	Diab manage trn per indiv	0.00	1.64	1.64	0.01	1.65	$59.73	1.65	$59.73	XXX	A+
G0109	Diab manage trn ind/group	0.00	0.96	0.96	0.01	0.97	$35.11	0.97	$35.11	XXX	A+
G0110	Nett pulm-rehab educ; ind	0.90	0.67	0.36	0.03	1.60	$57.92	1.29	$46.70	XXX	A+
G0111	Nett pulm-rehab educ; group	0.27	0.29	0.11	0.01	0.57	$20.63	0.39	$14.12	XXX	A+
G0112	Nett;nutrition guid, initial	1.72	1.24	0.69	0.05	3.01	$108.96	2.46	$89.05	XXX	A+
G0113	Nett;nutrition guid, subseqnt	1.29	0.97	0.51	0.04	2.30	$83.26	1.84	$66.61	XXX	A+
G0114	Nett; psychosocial consult	1.20	0.49	0.48	0.03	1.72	$62.26	1.71	$61.90	XXX	A+
G0115	Nett; psychological testing	1.20	0.57	0.48	0.04	1.81	$65.52	1.72	$62.26	XXX	A+
G0116	Nett; psychosocial counsel	1.11	0.69	0.44	0.04	1.84	$66.61	1.59	$57.56	XXX	A+
G0117	Glaucoma scrn hgh risk direc	0.45	0.97	0.22	0.02	1.44	$52.13	0.69	$24.98	XXX	A+
G0118	Glaucoma scrn hgh risk direc	0.17	0.84	0.08	0.01	1.02	$36.92	0.26	$9.41	XXX	A+
G0120	Colon ca scrn; barium enema	0.99	2.47	2.47	0.15	3.61	$130.68	3.61	$130.68	XXX	A+
G0120	Colon ca scrn; barium enema	0.99	2.47	2.47	0.15	3.61	$130.68	3.61	$130.68	XXX	A+
G0120	Colon ca scrn; barium enema	0.99	2.47	2.47	0.15	3.61	$130.68	3.61	$130.68	XXX	A+
G0120-26	Colon ca scrn; barium enema	0.99	0.35	0.35	0.04	1.38	$49.95	1.38	$49.95	XXX	A+
G0120-26	Colon ca scrn; barium enema	0.99	0.35	0.35	0.04	1.38	$49.95	1.38	$49.95	XXX	A+
G0120-26	Colon ca scrn; barium enema	0.99	0.35	0.35	0.04	1.38	$49.95	1.38	$49.95	XXX	A+
G0120-TC	Colon ca scrn; barium enema	0.00	2.12	2.12	0.11	2.23	$80.72	2.23	$80.72	XXX	A+
G0120-TC	Colon ca scrn; barium enema	0.00	2.12	2.12	0.11	2.23	$80.72	2.23	$80.72	XXX	A+
G0120-TC	Colon ca scrn; barium enema	0.00	2.12	2.12	0.11	2.23	$80.72	2.23	$80.72	XXX	A+
G0121	Colon ca scrn not hi rsk ind	3.70	8.79	1.77	0.20	12.69	$459.37	5.67	$205.25	000	A M
G0124	Screen c/v thin layer by MD	0.42	0.19	0.19	0.01	0.62	$22.44	0.62	$22.44	XXX	A+
G0125	PET img WhBD sgl pulm ring	1.50	56.10	56.10	2.00	59.60	$2,157.47	59.60	$2,157.47	XXX	A+
G0125	PET img WhBD sgl pulm ring	1.50	56.10	56.10	2.00	59.60	$2,157.47	59.60	$2,157.47	XXX	A+
G0125	PET img WhBD sgl pulm ring	1.50	56.10	56.10	2.00	59.60	$2,157.47	59.60	$2,157.47	XXX	A+
G0125-26	PET img WhBD sgl pulm ring	1.50	0.52	0.52	0.05	2.07	$74.93	2.07	$74.93	XXX	A+

* **M** = multiple surgery adjustment applies
Me = multiple endoscopy rules may apply
B = bilateral surgery adjustment applies
A = assistant-at-surgery restriction

A+ = assistant-at-surgery restriction unless medical necessity established with documentation
C = cosurgeons payable
C+ = cosurgeons payable if medical necessity established with documentation

T = team surgeons permitted
T+ = team surgeons payable if medical necessity established with documentation
$ = indicates services that are not covered by Medicare.

CPT five-digit codes, two-digit numeric modifiers, and descriptions only are © 2001 American Medical Association

Medicare RBRVS: The Physicians' Guide

Relative value units

HCPCS Code and Modifier	Description	Work RVU	Non Facility Practice Expense RVU	Facility Practice Expense RVU	PLI RVU	Total Non Facility RVUs	Medicare Payment Non Facility	Total Facility RVUs	Medicare Payment Facility	Global Period	Payment Policy Indicators*
G0125-26	PET img WhBD sgl pulm ring	1.50	0.52	0.52	0.05	2.07	$74.93	2.07	$74.93	XXX	A+
G0125-26	PET img WhBD sgl pulm ring	1.50	0.52	0.52	0.05	2.07	$74.93	2.07	$74.93	XXX	A+
G0125-TC	PET img WhBD sgl pulm ring	0.00	55.58	55.58	1.95	57.53	$2,082.54	57.53	$2,082.54	XXX	A+
G0125-TC	PET img WhBD sgl pulm ring	0.00	55.58	55.58	1.95	57.53	$2,082.54	57.53	$2,082.54	XXX	A+
G0125-TC	PET img WhBD sgl pulm ring	0.00	55.58	55.58	1.95	57.53	$2,082.54	57.53	$2,082.54	XXX	A+
G0127	Trim nail(s)	0.17	0.26	0.07	0.01	0.44	$15.93	0.25	$9.05	000	M A
G0128	CORF skilled nursing service	0.08	0.03	0.03	0.01	0.12	$4.34	0.12	$4.34	XXX	A+
G0130	Single energy x-ray study	0.22	0.90	0.90	0.05	1.17	$42.35	1.17	$42.35	XXX	A+
G0130-26	Single energy x-ray study	0.22	0.11	0.11	0.01	0.34	$12.31	0.34	$12.31	XXX	A+
G0130-TC	Single energy x-ray study	0.00	0.79	0.79	0.04	0.83	$30.05	0.83	$30.05	XXX	A+
G0131	CT scan, bone density study	0.25	3.18	3.18	0.14	3.57	$129.23	3.57	$129.23	XXX	A+
G0131-26	CT scan, bone density study	0.25	0.13	0.13	0.01	0.39	$14.12	0.39	$14.12	XXX	A+
G0131-TC	CT scan, bone density study	0.00	3.05	3.05	0.13	3.18	$115.11	3.18	$115.11	XXX	A+
G0132	CT scan, bone density study	0.22	0.90	0.90	0.05	1.17	$42.35	1.17	$42.35	XXX	A+
G0132-26	CT scan, bone density study	0.22	0.11	0.11	0.01	0.34	$12.31	0.34	$12.31	XXX	A+
G0132-TC	CT scan, bone density study	0.00	0.79	0.79	0.04	0.83	$30.05	0.83	$30.05	XXX	A+
G0141	Scr c/v cyto,autosys and md	0.42	0.19	0.19	0.01	0.62	$22.44	0.62	$22.44	XXX	A+
G0166	Extrnl counterpulse, per tx	0.07	4.17	0.03	0.01	4.25	$153.85	0.11	$3.98	XXX	A+
G0168	Wound closure by adhesive	0.45	2.33	0.19	0.01	2.79	$101.00	0.65	$23.53	000	M A
G0179	MD recertification HHA PT	0.45	1.21	1.21	0.01	1.67	$60.45	1.67	$60.45	XXX	A+
G0180	MD certification HHA patient	0.67	1.29	1.29	0.02	1.98	$71.67	1.98	$71.67	XXX	A+
G0181	Home health care supervision	1.73	1.57	1.57	0.06	3.36	$121.63	3.36	$121.63	XXX	A+
G0182	Hospice care supervision	1.73	1.97	1.97	0.06	3.76	$136.11	3.76	$136.11	XXX	A+
G0195	Clinicalevalswallowingfunct	1.50	1.95	0.76	0.07	3.52	$127.42	2.33	$84.34	XXX	A+
G0196	Evalofswallowingwithradioopa	1.50	1.95	0.76	0.07	3.52	$127.42	2.33	$84.34	XXX	A+
G0197	Evalofptforprescipspeechdevi	1.35	2.11	0.75	0.04	3.50	$126.70	2.14	$77.47	XXX	A+
G0198	Patientadapation&trainforspe	0.99	1.14	0.58	0.03	2.16	$78.19	1.60	$57.92	XXX	A+

Code	Description							
G0199	Reevaluationofpatientusespec	1.01	1.92	0.56	0.03	2.96	$107.15	1.60	$57.92	XXX	A+
G0200	Evalofpatientprescipofvoicep	1.35	2.11	0.75	0.04	3.50	$126.70	2.14	$77.47	XXX	A+
G0201	Modifortraininginusevoicepro	0.99	1.14	0.58	0.03	2.16	$78.19	1.60	$57.92	XXX	A+
G0202	Screeningmammographydigital	0.70	2.70	2.70	0.09	3.49	$126.34	3.49	$126.34	XXX	A+
G0202	Screeningmammographydigital	0.70	2.70	2.70	0.09	3.49	$126.34	3.49	$126.34	XXX	A+
G0202	Screeningmammographydigital	0.70	2.70	2.70	0.09	3.49	$126.34	3.49	$126.34	XXX	A+
G0202-26	Screeningmammographydigital	0.70	0.28	0.28	0.03	1.01	$36.56	1.01	$36.56	XXX	A+
G0202-26	Screeningmammographydigital	0.70	0.28	0.28	0.03	1.01	$36.56	1.01	$36.56	XXX	A+
G0202-26	Screeningmammographydigital	0.70	0.28	0.28	0.03	1.01	$36.56	1.01	$36.56	XXX	A+
G0202-TC	Screeningmammographydigital	0.00	2.42	2.42	0.06	2.48	$89.77	2.48	$89.77	XXX	A+
G0202-TC	Screeningmammographydigital	0.00	2.42	2.42	0.06	2.48	$89.77	2.48	$89.77	XXX	A+
G0202-TC	Screeningmammographydigital	0.00	2.42	2.42	0.06	2.48	$89.77	2.48	$89.77	XXX	A+
G0204	Diagnosticmammographydigital	0.87	2.73	2.73	0.09	3.69	$133.58	3.69	$133.58	XXX	A+
G0204	Diagnosticmammographydigital	0.87	2.73	2.73	0.09	3.69	$133.58	3.69	$133.58	XXX	A+
G0204	Diagnosticmammographydigital	0.87	2.73	2.73	0.09	3.69	$133.58	3.69	$133.58	XXX	A+
G0204-26	Diagnosticmammographydigital	0.87	0.35	0.35	0.03	1.25	$45.25	1.25	$45.25	XXX	A+
G0204-26	Diagnosticmammographydigital	0.87	0.35	0.35	0.03	1.25	$45.25	1.25	$45.25	XXX	A+
G0204-26	Diagnosticmammographydigital	0.87	0.35	0.35	0.03	1.25	$45.25	1.25	$45.25	XXX	A+
G0204-TC	Diagnosticmammographydigital	0.00	2.38	2.38	0.06	2.44	$88.33	2.44	$88.33	XXX	A+
G0204-TC	Diagnosticmammographydigital	0.00	2.38	2.38	0.06	2.44	$88.33	2.44	$88.33	XXX	A+
G0204-TC	Diagnosticmammographydigital	0.00	2.38	2.38	0.06	2.44	$88.33	2.44	$88.33	XXX	A+
G0206	Diagnosticmammographydigital	0.70	2.20	2.20	0.08	2.98	$107.87	2.98	$107.87	XXX	A+
G0206	Diagnosticmammographydigital	0.70	2.20	2.20	0.08	2.98	$107.87	2.98	$107.87	XXX	A+
G0206	Diagnosticmammographydigital	0.70	2.20	2.20	0.08	2.98	$107.87	2.98	$107.87	XXX	A+
G0206-26	Diagnosticmammographydigital	0.70	0.28	0.28	0.03	1.01	$36.56	1.01	$36.56	XXX	A+
G0206-26	Diagnosticmammographydigital	0.70	0.28	0.28	0.03	1.01	$36.56	1.01	$36.56	XXX	A+
G0206-26	Diagnosticmammographydigital	0.70	0.28	0.28	0.03	1.01	$36.56	1.01	$36.56	XXX	A+
G0206-TC	Diagnosticmammographydigital	0.00	1.92	1.92	0.05	1.97	$71.31	1.97	$71.31	XXX	A+

* **M** = multiple surgery adjustment applies
Me = multiple endoscopy rules may apply
B = bilateral surgery adjustment applies
A = assistant-at-surgery restriction

A+ = assistant-at-surgery restriction unless medical necessity established with documentation
C = cosurgeons payable
C+ = cosurgeons payable if medical necessity established with documentation

T = team surgeons permitted
T+ = team surgeons payable if medical necessity established with documentation
$ = indicates services that are not covered by Medicare.

CPT five-digit codes, two-digit numeric modifiers, and descriptions only are © 2001 American Medical Association

Medicare RBRVS: The Physicians' Guide

Relative value units

HCPCS Code and Modifier	Description	Work RVU	Non Facility Practice Expense RVU	Facility Practice Expense RVU	PLI RVU	Total Non Facility RVUs	Medicare Payment Non Facility	Total Facility RVUs	Medicare Payment Facility	Global Period	Payment Policy Indicators*
G0206-TC	Diagnosticmammographydigital	0.00	1.92	1.92	0.05	1.97	$71.31	1.97	$71.31	XXX	A+
G0206-TC	Diagnosticmammographydigital	0.00	1.92	1.92	0.05	1.97	$71.31	1.97	$71.31	XXX	A+
G0210	PET img WhBD ring dxlung ca	0.00	0.00	0.00	0.00	0.00	$0.00	0.00	$0.00	XXX	A+
G0210-26	PET img WhBD ring dxlung ca	1.50	0.60	0.60	0.04	2.14	$77.47	2.14	$77.47	XXX	A+
G0210-TC	PET img WhBD ring dxlung ca	0.00	0.00	0.00	0.00	0.00	$0.00	0.00	$0.00	XXX	A+
G0211	PET img WhBD ring init lung	0.00	0.00	0.00	0.00	0.00	$0.00	0.00	$0.00	XXX	A+
G0211-26	PET img WhBD ring init lung	1.50	0.60	0.60	0.04	2.14	$77.47	2.14	$77.47	XXX	A+
G0211-TC	PET img WhBD ring init lung	0.00	0.00	0.00	0.00	0.00	$0.00	0.00	$0.00	XXX	A+
G0212	PET img WhBD ring restag lun	0.00	0.00	0.00	0.00	0.00	$0.00	0.00	$0.00	XXX	A+
G0212-26	PET img WhBD ring restag lun	1.50	0.60	0.60	0.04	2.14	$77.47	2.14	$77.47	XXX	A+
G0212-TC	PET img WhBD ring restag lun	0.00	0.00	0.00	0.00	0.00	$0.00	0.00	$0.00	XXX	A+
G0213	PET img WhBD ring dx colorec	0.00	0.00	0.00	0.00	0.00	$0.00	0.00	$0.00	XXX	A+
G0213-26	PET img WhBD ring dx colorec	1.50	0.60	0.60	0.04	2.14	$77.47	2.14	$77.47	XXX	A+
G0213-TC	PET img WhBD ring dx colorec	0.00	0.00	0.00	0.00	0.00	$0.00	0.00	$0.00	XXX	A+
G0214	PET img WhBD ring init colre	0.00	0.00	0.00	0.00	0.00	$0.00	0.00	$0.00	XXX	A+
G0214-26	PET img WhBD ring init colre	1.50	0.60	0.60	0.04	2.14	$77.47	2.14	$77.47	XXX	A+
G0214-TC	PET img WhBD ring init colre	0.00	0.00	0.00	0.00	0.00	$0.00	0.00	$0.00	XXX	A+
G0215	PETimg whbd restag col	0.00	0.00	0.00	0.00	0.00	$0.00	0.00	$0.00	XXX	A+
G0215-26	PETimg whbd restag col	1.50	0.60	0.60	0.04	2.14	$77.47	2.14	$77.47	XXX	A+
G0215-TC	PETimg whbd restag col	0.00	0.00	0.00	0.00	0.00	$0.00	0.00	$0.00	XXX	A+
G0216	PET img WhBD ring dx melanom	0.00	0.00	0.00	0.00	0.00	$0.00	0.00	$0.00	XXX	A+
G0216-26	PET img WhBD ring dx melanom	1.50	0.60	0.60	0.04	2.14	$77.47	2.14	$77.47	XXX	A+
G0216-TC	PET img WhBD ring dx melanom	0.00	0.00	0.00	0.00	0.00	$0.00	0.00	$0.00	XXX	A+
G0217	PET img WhBD ring init melan	0.00	0.00	0.00	0.00	0.00	$0.00	0.00	$0.00	XXX	A+
G0217-26	PET img WhBD ring init melan	1.50	0.60	0.60	0.04	2.14	$77.47	2.14	$77.47	XXX	A+
G0217-TC	PET img WhBD ring init melan	0.00	0.00	0.00	0.00	0.00	$0.00	0.00	$0.00	XXX	A+
G0218	PET img WhBD ring restag mel	0.00	0.00	0.00	0.00	0.00	$0.00	0.00	$0.00	XXX	A+

G0218-26	PET img WhBD ring restag mel	1.50	0.60	0.04	2.14	$77.47	2.14	$77.47	XXX	A+
G0218-TC	PET img WhBD ring restag mel	0.00	0.00	0.00	0.00	$0.00	0.00	$0.00	XXX	A+
G0220	PET img WhBD ring dx lymphom	0.00	0.00	0.00	0.00	$0.00	0.00	$0.00	XXX	A+
G0220-26	PET img WhBD ring dx lymphom	1.50	0.60	0.04	2.14	$77.47	2.14	$77.47	XXX	A+
G0220-TC	PET img WhBD ring dx lymphom	0.00	0.00	0.00	0.00	$0.00	0.00	$0.00	XXX	A+
G0221	PET img WhBD ring init lymph	0.00	0.00	0.00	0.00	$0.00	0.00	$0.00	XXX	A+
G0221-26	PET img WhBD ring init lymph	1.50	0.60	0.04	2.14	$77.47	2.14	$77.47	XXX	A+
G0221-TC	PET img WhBD ring init lymph	0.00	0.00	0.00	0.00	$0.00	0.00	$0.00	XXX	A+
G0222	PET img WhBD ring resta lymp	0.00	0.00	0.00	0.00	$0.00	0.00	$0.00	XXX	A+
G0222-26	PET img WhBD ring resta lymp	1.50	0.60	0.04	2.14	$77.47	2.14	$77.47	XXX	A+
G0222-TC	PET img WhBD ring resta lymp	0.00	0.00	0.00	0.00	$0.00	0.00	$0.00	XXX	A+
G0223	PET img WhBD reg ring dx hea	0.00	0.00	0.00	0.00	$0.00	0.00	$0.00	XXX	A+
G0223-26	PET img WhBD reg ring dx hea	1.50	0.60	0.04	2.14	$77.47	2.14	$77.47	XXX	A+
G0223-TC	PET img WhBD reg ring dx hea	0.00	0.00	0.00	0.00	$0.00	0.00	$0.00	XXX	A+
G0224	PETing WhBD reg ring ini hea	0.00	0.00	0.00	0.00	$0.00	0.00	$0.00	XXX	A+
G0224-26	PETing WhBD reg ring ini hea	1.50	0.60	0.04	2.14	$77.47	2.14	$77.47	XXX	A+
G0224-TC	PETing WhBD reg ring ini hea	0.00	0.00	0.00	0.00	$0.00	0.00	$0.00	XXX	A+
G0225	PET img WhBD ring restag hea	0.00	0.00	0.00	0.00	$0.00	0.00	$0.00	XXX	A+
G0225-26	PET img WhBD ring restag hea	1.50	0.60	0.04	2.14	$77.47	2.14	$77.47	XXX	A+
G0225-TC	PET img WhBD ring restag hea	0.00	0.00	0.00	0.00	$0.00	0.00	$0.00	XXX	A+
G0226	PET img WhBD dx esopha	0.00	0.00	0.00	0.00	$0.00	0.00	$0.00	XXX	A+
G0226-26	PET img WhBD dx esophag	1.50	0.60	0.04	2.14	$77.47	2.14	$77.47	XXX	A+
G0226-TC	PET img WhBD dx esophag	0.00	0.00	0.00	0.00	$0.00	0.00	$0.00	XXX	A+
G0227	PET img whbd ini esopha	0.00	0.00	0.00	0.00	$0.00	0.00	$0.00	XXX	A+
G0227-26	PET img whbd ini esopha	1.50	0.60	0.04	2.14	$77.47	2.14	$77.47	XXX	A+
G0227-TC	PET img whbd ini esopha	0.00	0.00	0.00	0.00	$0.00	0.00	$0.00	XXX	A+
G0228	PET img WhBD ring restg esop	0.00	0.00	0.00	0.00	$0.00	0.00	$0.00	XXX	A+
G0228-26	PET img WhBD ring restg esop	1.50	0.60	0.04	2.14	$77.47	2.14	$77.47	XXX	A+

* **M** = multiple surgery adjustment applies
Me = multiple endoscopy rules may apply
B = bilateral surgery adjustment applies
A = assistant-at-surgery restriction

A+ = assistant-at-surgery restriction unless medical necessity established with documentation
C = cosurgeons payable
C+ = cosurgeons payable if medical necessity established with documentation

T = team surgeons permitted
T+ = team surgeons payable if medical necessity established with documentation
$ = indicates services that are not covered by Medicare.

CPT five-digit codes, two-digit numeric modifiers, and descriptions only are © 2001 American Medical Association

Medicare RBRVS: The Physicians' Guide

Relative value units

HCPCS Code and Modifier	Description	Work RVU	Non Facility Practice Expense RVU	Facility Practice Expense RVU	PLI RVU	Total Non Facility RVUs	Medicare Payment Non Facility	Total Facility RVUs	Medicare Payment Facility	Global Period	Payment Policy Indicators*
G0228-TC	PET img WhBD ring restg esop	0.00	0.00	0.00	0.00	0.00	$0.00	0.00	$0.00	XXX	A+
G0229	PET img metabolic brain ring	0.00	0.00	0.00	0.00	0.00	$0.00	0.00	$0.00	XXX	A+
G0229-26	PET img metabolic brain ring	1.50	0.60	0.60	0.04	2.14	$77.47	2.14	$77.47	XXX	A+
G0229-TC	PET img metabolic brain ring	0.00	0.00	0.00	0.00	0.00	$0.00	0.00	$0.00	XXX	A+
G0230	PET myocard viability ring	0.00	0.00	0.00	0.00	0.00	$0.00	0.00	$0.00	XXX	A+
G0230-26	PET myocard viability ring	1.50	0.60	0.60	0.04	2.14	$77.47	2.14	$77.47	XXX	A+
G0230-TC	PET myocard viability ring	0.00	0.00	0.00	0.00	0.00	$0.00	0.00	$0.00	XXX	A+
G0231	PET WhBD colorec; gamma cam	0.00	0.00	0.00	0.00	0.00	$0.00	0.00	$0.00	XXX	A+
G0231-26	PET WhBD colorec; gamma cam	1.50	0.60	0.60	0.04	2.14	$77.47	2.14	$77.47	XXX	A+
G0231-TC	PET WhBD colorec; gamma cam	0.00	0.00	0.00	0.00	0.00	$0.00	0.00	$0.00	XXX	A+
G0232	PET WhBD lymphoma; gamma cam	0.00	0.00	0.00	0.00	0.00	$0.00	0.00	$0.00	XXX	A+
G0232-26	PET WhBD lymphoma; gamma cam	1.50	0.60	0.60	0.04	2.14	$77.47	2.14	$77.47	XXX	A+
G0232-TC	PET WhBD lymphoma; gamma cam	0.00	0.00	0.00	0.00	0.00	$0.00	0.00	$0.00	XXX	A+
G0233	PET WhBD melanoma; gamma cam	0.00	0.00	0.00	0.00	0.00	$0.00	0.00	$0.00	XXX	A+
G0233-26	PET WhBD melanoma; gamma cam	1.50	0.60	0.60	0.04	2.14	$77.47	2.14	$77.47	XXX	A+
G0233-TC	PET WhBD melanoma; gamma cam	0.00	0.00	0.00	0.00	0.00	$0.00	0.00	$0.00	XXX	A+
G0234	PET WhBD pulm nod; gamma cam	0.00	0.00	0.00	0.00	0.00	$0.00	0.00	$0.00	XXX	A+
G0234-26	PET WhBD pulm nod; gamma cam	1.50	0.60	0.60	0.04	2.14	$77.47	2.14	$77.47	XXX	A+
G0234-TC	PET WhBD pulm nod; gamma cam	0.00	0.00	0.00	0.00	0.00	$0.00	0.00	$0.00	XXX	A+
G0236	digital film convert diag ma	0.06	0.41	NA	0.02	0.49	$17.74	NA	NA	ZZZ	A+
G0236-26	digital film convert diag ma	0.06	0.02	0.02	0.01	0.09	$3.26	0.09	$3.26	ZZZ	A+
G0236-TC	digital film convert diag ma	0.00	0.39	NA	0.01	0.40	$14.48	NA	NA	ZZZ	A+
G0237	Therapeutic procd strg endur	0.00	0.45	0.45	0.02	0.47	$17.01	0.47	$17.01	XXX	A+
G0240	Critic care by MD transport	4.00	1.60	1.60	0.14	5.74	$207.78	5.74	$207.78	XXX	A+
G0241	Each additional 30 minutes	2.00	0.80	0.80	0.07	2.87	$103.89	2.87	$103.89	ZZZ	A+
J3370	Vancomycin hcl injeciton	0.00	0.00	0.00	0.00	0.00	$0.00	0.00	$0.00	XXX	A+
M0064	Visit for drug monitoring	0.37	0.25	0.12	0.01	0.63	$22.81	0.50	$18.10	XXX	A+

P3001	Screening pap smear by phys	0.42	0.19	0.19	0.01	0.62	$22.44	0.62	$22.44	XXX	A+
Q0035	Cardiokymography	0.17	0.44	0.44	0.03	0.64	$23.17	0.64	$23.17	XXX	A+
Q0035	Cardiokymography	0.17	0.44	0.44	0.03	0.64	$23.17	0.64	$23.17	XXX	A+
Q0035	Cardiokymography	0.17	0.44	0.44	0.03	0.64	$23.17	0.64	$23.17	XXX	A+
Q0035-26	Cardiokymography	0.17	0.07	0.07	0.01	0.25	$9.05	0.25	$9.05	XXX	A+
Q0035-26	Cardiokymography	0.17	0.07	0.07	0.01	0.25	$9.05	0.25	$9.05	XXX	A+
Q0035-26	Cardiokymography	0.17	0.07	0.07	0.01	0.25	$9.05	0.25	$9.05	XXX	A+
Q0035-TC	Cardiokymography	0.00	0.37	0.37	0.02	0.39	$14.12	0.39	$14.12	XXX	A+
Q0035-TC	Cardiokymography	0.00	0.37	0.37	0.02	0.39	$14.12	0.39	$14.12	XXX	A+
Q0035-TC	Cardiokymography	0.00	0.37	0.37	0.02	0.39	$14.12	0.39	$14.12	XXX	A+
Q0091	Obtaining screen pap smear	0.37	0.68	0.15	0.01	1.06	$38.37	0.53	$19.19	XXX	A+
Q0092	Set up port xray equipment	0.00	0.30	0.30	0.01	0.31	$11.22	0.31	$11.22	XXX	A+
V5299	Hearing service	0.00	0.00	0.00	0.00	0.00	$0.00	0.00	$0.00	XXX	A+
V5362	Speech screening	0.00	0.00	0.00	0.00	0.00	$0.00	0.00	$0.00	XXX	A+
V5363	Language screening	0.00	0.00	0.00	0.00	0.00	$0.00	0.00	$0.00	XXX	A+
V5364	Dysphagia screening	0.00	0.00	0.00	0.00	0.00	$0.00	0.00	$0.00	XXX	A+

*M = multiple surgery adjustment applies
Me = multiple endoscopy rules may apply
B = bilateral surgery adjustment applies
A = assistant-at-surgery restriction

A+ = assistant-at-surgery restriction unless medical necessity established with documentation
C = cosurgeons payable
C+ = cosurgeons payable if medical necessity established with documentation

T = team surgeons permitted
T+ = team surgeons payable if medical necessity established with documentation
S = indicates services that are not covered by Medicare.

447 CPT five-digit codes, two-digit numeric modifiers, and descriptions only are © 2001 American Medical Association

List of Geographic Practice Cost Indices for Each Medicare Locality

These lists present the geographic practice cost indices (GPCIs) for 2002 for each Medicare payment locality. Because each component of the Medicare payment schedule (physician work, practice costs, and professional liability insurance) is adjusted for geographic cost differences, there are three GPCI values for each locality.

Chapter 7 discusses the GPCIs in detail. In addition, Chapters 8 and 10 explain how the GPCIs are combined with the RVUs and conversion factor to calculate the full payment schedule amount for each service in a locality.

GPCIs

Geographic Practice Cost Indices by State and Locality, 2002

Carrier Number	Locality Number	Locality Number	Work GPCI	Practice Cost GPCI	PLI GPCI
00510	00	**Alabama**	0.978	0.870	0.807
00831	01	**Alaska**	1.064	1.172	1.223
00832	00	**Arizona**	0.994	0.978	1.111
00520	13	**Arkansas**	0.953	0.847	0.340
		California			
02050	26	Anaheim/Santa Ana, CA	1.037	1.184	0.955
02050	18	Los Angeles, CA	1.056	1.139	0.955
31140	03	Marin/Napa/Solano, CA	1.015	1.248	0.687
31140	07	Oakland/Berkeley, CA	1.041	1.235	0.687
31140	05	San Francisco, CA	1.068	1.458	0.687
31140	06	San Mateo, CA	1.048	1.432	0.687
31140	09	Santa Clara, CA	1.063	1.380	0.639
02050	17	Ventura, CA	1.028	1.125	0.783
02050	99	Rest of California*	1.007	1.034	0.748
31140	99	Rest of California*	1.007	1.034	0.748
00824	01	**Colorado**	0.985	0.992	0.840
10230	00	**Connecticut**	1.050	1.156	0.966
00902	01	**Delaware**	1.019	1.035	0.712
00903	01	**DC + MD/VA Suburbs**	1.050	1.166	0.909
		Florida			
00590	03	Fort Lauderdale, FL	0.996	1.018	1.877
00590	04	Miami, FL	1.015	1.052	2.528
00590	99	Rest of Florida	0.975	0.946	1.265
		Georgia			
00511	01	Atlanta, GA	1.006	1.059	0.935
00511	99	Rest of Georgia	0.970	0.892	0.935
00833	01	**Hawaii/Guam**	0.997	1.124	0.834
05130	00	**Idaho**	0.960	0.881	0.497
		Illinois			
00952	16	Chicago, IL	1.028	1.092	1.797
00952	12	East St. Louis, IL	0.988	0.924	1.691
00952	15	Suburban Chicago, IL	1.006	1.071	1.645

GPCIs

Geographic Practice Cost Indices by State and Locality, 2002

Carrier Number	Locality Number	Locality Number	Work GPCI	Practice Cost GPCI	PLI GPCI
00952	99	Rest of Illinois	0.964	0.889	1.157
00630	00	**Indiana**	0.981	0.922	0.481
00826	00	**Iowa**	0.959	0.876	0.596
00650	00	**Kansas***	0.963	0.895	0.756
00740	04	**Kansas***	0.963	0.895	0.756
00660	00	**Kentucky**	0.970	0.866	0.877
		Louisiana			
00528	01	New Orleans, LA	0.998	0.945	1.283
00528	99	Rest of Louisiana	0.968	0.870	1.073
		Maine			
31142	03	Southern Maine	0.979	0.999	0.666
31142	99	Rest of Maine	0.961	0.910	0.666
		Maryland			
00901	01	Baltimore/Surr. Cntys, MD	1.021	1.038	0.916
00901	99	Rest of Maryland	0.984	0.972	0.774
		Massachusetts			
31143	01	Metropolitan Boston	1.041	1.239	0.784
31143	99	Rest of Massachusetts	1.010	1.129	0.784
		Michigan			
00953	01	Detroit, MI	1.043	1.038	2.738
00953	99	Rest of Michigan	0.997	0.938	1.571
10240	00	**Minnesota**	0.990	0.974	0.452
10250	00	**Mississippi**	0.957	0.837	0.779
		Missouri			
00740	02	Metropolitan Kansas City, MO	0.988	0.967	0.846
00523	01	Metropolitan St. Louis, MO	0.994	0.938	0.846
00740	99	Rest of Missouri*	0.946	0.825	0.793
00523	99	Rest of Missouri*	0.946	0.825	0.793
00751	01	**Montana**	0.950	0.876	0.727
00655	00	**Nebraska**	0.948	0.877	0.430
00834	00	**Nevada**	1.005	1.039	1.209
31144	40	**New Hampshire**	0.986	1.030	0.825
		New Jersey			

GPCIs

Geographic Practice Cost Indices by State and Locality, 2002

Carrier Number	Locality Number	Locality Number	Work GPCI	Practice Cost GPCI	PLI GPCI
00805	01	Northern NJ	1.058	1.193	0.860
00805	99	Rest of New Jersey	1.029	1.110	0.860
00521	05	**New Mexico**	0.973	0.900	0.902
		New York			
00803	01	Manhattan, NY	1.094	1.351	1.668
00803	02	NYC Suburbs/Long I., NY	1.068	1.251	1.952
00803	03	Poughkpsie/N NYC Suburbs, NY	1.011	1.075	1.275
14330	04	Queens, NY	1.058	1.228	1.871
00801	99	Rest of New York	0.998	0.944	0.764
05535	00	**North Carolina**	0.970	0.931	0.595
00820	01	**North Dakota**	0.950	0.880	0.657
16360	00	**Ohio**	0.988	0.944	0.957
00522	00	**Oklahoma**	0.968	0.876	0.444
		Oregon			
00835	01	Portland, OR	0.996	1.049	0.436
00835	99	Rest of Oregon	0.961	0.933	0.436
		Pennsylvania			
00865	01	Metropolitan Philadelphia,	1.023	1.092	1.413
00865	99	Rest of Pennsylvania	0.989	0.929	0.774
00973	20	**Puerto Rico**	0.881	0.712	0.275
00870	01	**Rhode Island**	1.017	1.065	0.883
00880	01	**South Carolina**	0.974	0.904	0.279
00820	02	**South Dakota**	0.935	0.878	0.406
05440	35	**Tennessee**	0.975	0.900	0.592
		Texas			
00900	31	Austin, TX	0.986	0.996	0.859
00900	20	Beaumont, TX	0.992	0.890	1.338
00900	09	Brazoria, TX	0.992	0.978	1.338
00900	11	Dallas, TX	1.010	1.065	0.931
00900	28	Fort Worth, TX	0.987	0.981	0.931
00900	15	Galveston, TX	0.988	0.969	1.338
00900	18	Houston, TX	1.020	1.007	1.336
00900	99	Rest of Texas	0.966	0.880	0.956
00910	09	**Utah**	0.976	0.941	0.644

GPCIs

Geographic Practice Cost Indices by State and Locality, 2002

Carrier Number	Locality Number	Locality Number	Work GPCI	Practice Cost GPCI	PLI GPCI
31145	50	**Vermont**	0.973	0.986	0.539
00973	50	**Virgin Islands**	0.965	1.023	1.002
10490	00	**Virginia**	0.984	0.938	0.500
		Washington			
00836	02	Seattle (King Cnty), WA	1.005	1.100	0.788
00836	99	Rest of Washington	0.981	0.972	0.788
16510	16	**West Virginia**	0.963	0.850	1.378
00951	00	**Wisconsin**	0.981	0.929	0.939
00825	21	**Wyoming**	0.967	0.895	1.005

*Payment locality is serviced by two carriers.

RVUs for Anesthesiology Services

Anesthesiologists' services had been compensated according to a "relative value guide" prior to implementing the Medicare payment schedule. This approach has continued with some modifications. Medicare payments for anesthesiology services are based on the ASA Relative Value Guide with some of the basic units adjusted by CMS. There are about 250 ASA codes that correspond to the anesthesia services for over 4,000 surgical, endoscopic and radiological procedures. Each service is assigned a base unit. The base unit reflects the complexity of the service and includes work provided before and after reportable anesthesia time. The base units also cover usual preoperative and postoperative visits, administering fluids and blood that are part of the anesthesia care, and monitoring procedures.

Because the base units reflect all but the time required for the procedure, they are added to a time factor for each service an anesthesiologist provides. Under the 1991 *Final Rule,* anesthesia time starts when the physician begins to prepare the patient for induction and ends when the patient is placed under postoperative supervision when the anesthesiologist is no longer in attendance. Time for each procedure is divided into 15 minute increments and is assigned a unit value of one and are added to the base units. The time units account for the time from continuous hands on care to transfer of the patient to post anesthesia care personnel. Currently each 15 minutes of time is equal to one time unit according to CMS. The sum of the base and time units are then multiplied by the anesthesiology conversion factor to arrive at the final payment for each service. The current anesthesiology conversion factor is $17.26.

Because the RBRVS payment system continues to use the uniform relative value guide, CMS did not need to rescale the guide to conform with the RBRVS, but only needed to establish a separate conversion factor for anesthesiology that would appropriately integrate payments for these services with payments for services on the Harvard scale. To compute this conversion factor, CMS determined the difference between the average payment under the old base and time unit system and the average payment that would result from using Harvard work RVUs for 19 anesthesia services surveyed by Harvard. The 1992 anesthesiology conversion factor represented a reduction of 42% in the work component of anesthesiology services, but an overall reduction from the 1991 conversion factor of 29% across all components. The anesthesia work RVUs for 1997 were increased by 22.76% as a result of the 5-year review, which translated into a 15.95% increase in the anesthesia conversion factor.

Comparing ASA Values to RBRVS Values

Comparing ASA values to physician work values is not a straightforward process. In the Medicare RBRVS, physician relative values are comprised of three components:

physician work, practice expense and professional liability insurance and are calculated for each code. In the Anesthesia Medicare Payment Schedule, physician work, practice expense, and professional liability insurance components are calculated as a fraction of each anesthesia unit and applied globally across all anesthesia codes. Therefore, the ASA base units include all three components. To begin to place the ASA values on the same scale as the physician work relative values, the ASA base units must be combined with standard time units and then reduced by a percentage that reflects the practice expense and PLI components in the ASA values. For 2002, the percentage of the anesthesia units allocated to physician work is .7790 and is set by CMS and updated annually. Thus, for every anesthesia procedure, the fraction of the total base and time units attributed to physician work is fixed, and the calculated physician work for a given anesthesia code varies with the total base and time units of the procedure.

It is necessary to include physician time and adjust the units to reflect only the work portion of the units in order to compare ASA values on the same scale as the RBRVS. The current formula (published by HCFA in the 1994 *Federal Register*) for converting ASA values on the same scale as physician relative values is as follows:

Formula 1: *Anesthesia units × (Anesthesia CF/Fee schedule CF) × .7790 (Anesthesia work fraction) = RVUs.*

The following table lists the base units for approximately 250 anesthesia services.

Anesthesiology Base Units

Code	2002 Base Units	*Descriptor*
00100	5	Anesthesia for procedures on salivary glands, including biopsy
00102	6	Anesthesia for procedures on plastic repair of cleft lip
00103	5	Anesthesia for reconstructive procedures of eyelid (eg, blepharoplasty, ptosis surgery)
00104	4	Anesthesia for electroconvulsive therapy
00120	5	Anesthesia for procedures on external, middle, and inner ear including biopsy; not otherwise specified
00124	4	Anesthesia for procedures on external, middle, and inner ear including biopsy; otoscopy
00126	4	Anesthesia for procedures on external, middle, and inner ear including biopsy; tympanotomy
00140	5	Anesthesia for procedures on eye; not otherwise specified
00142	4	Anesthesia for procedures on eye; lens surgery
00144	6	Anesthesia for procedures on eye; corneal transplant
00145	6	Anesthesia for procedures on eye; vitreoretinal surgery
00147	4	Anesthesia for procedures on eye; iridectomy
00148	4	Anesthesia for procedures on eye; ophthalmoscopy
00160	5	Anesthesia for procedures on nose and accessory sinuses; not otherwise specified
00162	7	Anesthesia for procedures on nose and accessory sinuses; radical surgery
00164	4	Anesthesia for procedures on nose and accessory sinuses; biopsy, soft tissue
00170	5	Anesthesia for intraoral procedures, including biopsy; not otherwise specified
00172	6	Anesthesia for intraoral procedures, including biopsy; repair of cleft palate
00174	6	Anesthesia for intraoral procedures, including biopsy; excision of retropharyngeal tumor
00176	7	Anesthesia for intraoral procedures, including biopsy; radical surgery
00190	5	Anesthesia for procedures on facial bones or skull; not otherwise specified
00192	7	Anesthesia for procedures on facial bones or skull; radical surgery (including prognathism)
00210	11	Anesthesia for intracranial procedures; not otherwise specified
00212	5	Anesthesia for intracranial procedures; subdural taps
00214	9	Anesthesia for intracranial procedures; burr holes, including ventriculography
00215	9	Anesthesia for intracranial procedures; cranioplasty or elevation of depressed skull fracture, extradural (simple or compound)
00216	15	Anesthesia for intracranial procedures; vascular procedures
00218	13	Anesthesia for intracranial procedures; procedures in sitting position
00220	10	Anesthesia for intracranial procedures; cerebrospinal fluid shunting procedures
00222	6	Anesthesia for intracranial procedures; electrocoagulation of intracranial nerve
00300	5	Anesthesia for all procedures on the integumentary system, muscles and nerves of head, neck, and posterior trunk, not otherwise specified

CPT five-digit codes, two-digit numeric modifiers, and descriptions only are copyright 2001 American Medical Association

Anesthesiology Base Units

Code	2002 Base Units	*Descriptor*
00320	6	Anesthesia for all procedures on esophagus, thyroid, larynx, trachea and lymphatic system of neck; not otherwise specified
00322	3	Anesthesia for all procedures on esophagus, thyroid, larynx, trachea and lymphatic system of neck; needle biopsy of thyroid
00350	10	Anesthesia for procedures on major vessels of neck; not otherwise specified
00352	5	Anesthesia for procedures on major vessels of neck; simple ligation
00400	3	Anesthesia for procedures on the integumentary system on the extremities, anterior trunk and perineum; not otherwise specified
00402	5	Anesthesia for procedures on the integumentary system on the extremities, anterior trunk and perineum; reconstructive procedures on breast (eg, reduction or augmentation mammoplasty, muscle flaps)
00404	5	Anesthesia for procedures on the integumentary system on the extremities, anterior trunk and perineum; radical or modified radical procedures on breast
00406	13	Anesthesia for procedures on the integumentary system on the extremities, anterior trunk and perineum; radical or modified radical procedures on breast with internal mammary node dissection
00410	4	Anesthesia for procedures on the integumentary system on the extremities, anterior trunk and perineum; electrical conversion of arrhythmias
00450	5	Anesthesia for procedures on clavicle and scapula; not otherwise specified
00452	6	Anesthesia for procedures on clavicle and scapula; radical surgery
00454	3	Anesthesia for procedures on clavicle and scapula; biopsy of clavicle
00470	6	Anesthesia for partial rib resection; not otherwise specified
00472	10	Anesthesia for partial rib resection; thoracoplasty (any type)
00474	13	Anesthesia for partial rib resection; radical procedures (eg, pectus excavatum)
00500	15	Anesthesia for all procedures on esophagus
00520	6	Anesthesia for closed chest procedures; (including bronchoscopy) not otherwise specified
00522	4	Anesthesia for closed chest procedures; needle biopsy of pleura
00524	4	Anesthesia for closed chest procedures; pneumocentesis
00528	8	Anesthesia for closed chest procedures; mediastinoscopy and diagnostic thoracoscopy
00530	4	Anesthesia for permanent transvenous pacemaker insertion
00532	4	Anesthesia for access to central venous circulation
00534	7	Anesthesia for transvenous insertion or replacement of pacing cardioverter-defibrillator
00537	7	Anesthesia for cardiac electrophysiologic procedures including radiofrequency ablation
00540	13	Anesthesia for thoracotomy procedures involving lungs, pleura, diaphragm, and mediastinum (including surgical thoracoscopy); not otherwise specified
00542	15	Anesthesia for thoracotomy procedures involving lungs, pleura, diaphragm, and mediastinum (including surgical thoracoscopy); decortication

CPT five-digit codes, two-digit numeric modifiers, and descriptions only are copyright 2001 American Medical Association

Anesthesiology Base Units

Code	2002 Base Units	Descriptor
00544	15	Anesthesia for thoracotomy procedures involving lungs, pleura, diaphragm, and mediastinum (including surgical thoracoscopy); pleurectomy
00546	15	Anesthesia for thoracotomy procedures involving lungs, pleura, diaphragm, and mediastinum (including surgical thoracoscopy); pulmonary resection with thoracoplasty
00548	15	Anesthesia for thoracotomy procedures involving lungs, pleura, diaphragm, and mediastinum (including surgical thoracoscopy); intrathoracic procedures on the trachea and bronchi
00550	10	Anesthesia for sternal debridement
00560	15	Anesthesia for procedures on heart, pericardial sac, and great vessels of chest; without pump oxygenator
00562	20	Anesthesia for procedures on heart, pericardial sac, and great vessels of chest; with pump oxygenator
00563	25	Anesthesia for procedures on heart, pericardial sac, and great vessels of chest; with pump oxygenator with hypothermic circulatory arrest
00566	25	Anesthesia for direct coronary artery bypass grafting without pump oxygenator
00580	20	Anesthesia for heart transplant or heart/lung transplant
00600	10	Anesthesia for procedures on cervical spine and cord; not otherwise specified
00604	13	Anesthesia for procedures on cervical spine and cord; procedures with patient in the sitting position
00620	10	Anesthesia for procedures on thoracic spine and cord; not otherwise specified
00622	13	Anesthesia for procedures on thoracic spine and cord; thoracolumbar sympathectomy
00630	8	Anesthesia for procedures in lumbar region; not otherwise specified
00632	7	Anesthesia for procedures in lumbar region; lumbar sympathectomy
00634	10	Anesthesia for procedures in lumbar region; chemonucleolysis
00635	4	Anesthesia for procedures in lumbar region; diagnostic or therapeutic lumbar puncture
00670	13	Anesthesia for extensive spine and spinal cord procedures (eg, spinal instrumentation or vascular procedures)
00700	3	Anesthesia for procedures on upper anterior abdominal wall; not otherwise specified
00702	4	Anesthesia for procedures on upper anterior abdominal wall; percutaneous liver biopsy
00730	5	Anesthesia for procedures on upper posterior abdominal wall
00740	5	Anesthesia for upper gastrointestinal endoscopic procedures, endoscope introduced proximal to duodenum
00750	4	Anesthesia for hernia repairs in upper abdomen; not otherwise specified
00752	6	Anesthesia for hernia repairs in upper abdomen; lumbar and ventral (incisional) hernias and/or wound dehiscence
00754	7	Anesthesia for hernia repairs in upper abdomen; omphalocele
00756	7	Anesthesia for hernia repairs in upper abdomen; transabdominal repair of diaphragmatic hernia
00770	15	Anesthesia for all procedures on major abdominal blood vessels

CPT five-digit codes, two-digit numeric modifiers, and descriptions only are copyright 2001 American Medical Association

Anesthesiology Base Units

Code	2002 Base Units	Descriptor
00790	7	Anesthesia for intraperitoneal procedures in upper abdomen including laparoscopy; not otherwise specified
00792	13	Anesthesia for intraperitoneal procedures in upper abdomen including laparoscopy; partial hepatectomy or management of liver hemorrhage (excluding liver biopsy)
00794	8	Anesthesia for intraperitoneal procedures in upper abdomen including laparoscopy; pancreatectomy, partial or total (eg, Whipple procedure)
00796	30	Anesthesia for intraperitoneal procedures in upper abdomen including laparoscopy; liver transplant (recipient)
00797	8	Anesthesia for intraperitoneal procedures in upper abdomen including laparoscopy; gastric restrictive procedure for morbid obesity
00800	3	Anesthesia for procedures on lower anterior abdominal wall; not otherwise specified
00802	5	Anesthesia for procedures on lower anterior abdominal wall; panniculectomy
00810	6	Anesthesia for lower intestinal endoscopic procedures, endoscope introduced distal to duodenum
00820	5	Anesthesia for procedures on lower posterior abdominal wall
00830	4	Anesthesia for hernia repairs in lower abdomen; not otherwise specified
00832	6	Anesthesia for hernia repairs in lower abdomen; ventral and incisional hernias
00840	6	Anesthesia for intraperitoneal procedures in lower abdomen including laparoscopy; not otherwise specified
00842	4	Anesthesia for intraperitoneal procedures in lower abdomen including laparoscopy; amniocentesis
00844	7	Anesthesia for intraperitoneal procedures in lower abdomen including laparoscopy; abdominoperineal resection
00846	8	Anesthesia for intraperitoneal procedures in lower abdomen including laparoscopy; radical hysterectomy
00848	8	Anesthesia for intraperitoneal procedures in lower abdomen including laparoscopy; pelvic exenteration
00851	6	Anesthesia for intraperitoneal procedures in lower abdomen including laparoscopy; tubal ligation/transection
00860	6	Anesthesia for extraperitoneal procedures in lower abdomen, including urinary tract; not otherwise specified
00862	7	Anesthesia for extraperitoneal procedures in lower abdomen, including urinary tract; renal procedures, including upper 1/3 of ureter, or donor nephrectomy
00864	8	Anesthesia for extraperitoneal procedures in lower abdomen, including urinary tract; total cystectomy
00865	7	Anesthesia for extraperitoneal procedures in lower abdomen, including urinary tract; radical prostatectomy (suprapubic, retropubic)
00866	10	Anesthesia for extraperitoneal procedures in lower abdomen, including urinary tract; adrenalectomy

CPT five-digit codes, two-digit numeric modifiers, and descriptions only are copyright 2001 American Medical Association

Anesthesiology Base Units

Code	2002 Base Units	*Descriptor*
00868	10	Anesthesia for extraperitoneal procedures in lower abdomen, including urinary tract; renal transplant (recipient)
00869	3	Anesthesia for extraperitoneal procedures in lower abdomen, including urinary tract; vasectomy, unilateral/bilateral
00870	5	Anesthesia for extraperitoneal procedures in lower abdomen, including urinary tract; cystolithotomy
00872	7	Anesthesia for lithotripsy, extracorporeal shock wave; with water bath
00873	5	Anesthesia for lithotripsy, extracorporeal shock wave; without water bath
00880	15	Anesthesia for procedures on major lower abdominal vessels; not otherwise specified
00882	10	Anesthesia for procedures on major lower abdominal vessels; inferior vena cava ligation
00902	4	Anesthesia for; anorectal procedure
00904	7	Anesthesia for; radical perineal procedure
00906	4	Anesthesia for; vulvectomy
00908	6	Anesthesia for; perineal prostatectomy
00910	3	Anesthesia for transurethral procedures (including urethrocystoscopy); not otherwise specified
00912	5	Anesthesia for transurethral procedures (including urethrocystoscopy); transurethral resection of bladder tumor(s)
00914	5	Anesthesia for transurethral procedures (including urethrocystoscopy); transurethral resection of prostate
00916	5	Anesthesia for transurethral procedures (including urethrocystoscopy); post-transurethral resection bleeding
00918	5	Anesthesia for transurethral procedures (including urethrocystoscopy); with fragmentation, manipulation and/or removal of ureteral calculus
00920	3	Anesthesia for procedures on male genitalia (including open urethral procedures); not otherwise specified
00922	6	Anesthesia for procedures on male genitalia (including open urethral procedures); seminal vesicles
00924	4	Anesthesia for procedures on male genitalia (including open urethral procedures); undescended testis, unilateral or bilateral
00926	4	Anesthesia for procedures on male genitalia (including open urethral procedures); radical orchiectomy, inguinal
00928	6	Anesthesia for procedures on male genitalia (including open urethral procedures); radical orchiectomy, abdominal
00930	4	Anesthesia for procedures on male genitalia (including open urethral procedures); orchiopexy, unilateral or bilateral
00932	4	Anesthesia for procedures on male genitalia (including open urethral procedures); complete amputation of penis
00934	6	Anesthesia for procedures on male genitalia (including open urethral procedures); radical amputation of penis with bilateral inguinal lymphadenectomy

CPT five-digit codes, two-digit numeric modifiers, and descriptions only are copyright 2001 American Medical Association

Anesthesiology Base Units

Code	2002 Base Units	*Descriptor*
00936	8	Anesthesia for procedures on male genitalia (including open urethral procedures); radical amputation of penis with bilateral inguinal and iliac lymphadenectomy
00938	4	Anesthesia for procedures on male genitalia (including open urethral procedures); insertion of penile prosthesis (perineal approach)
00940	3	Anesthesia for vaginal procedures (including biopsy of labia, vagina, cervix or endometrium); not otherwise specified
00942	4	Anesthesia for vaginal procedures (including biopsy of labia, vagina, cervix or endometrium); colpotomy, vaginectomy, colporrhaphy, and open urethral procedures
00944	6	Anesthesia for vaginal procedures (including biopsy of labia, vagina, cervix or endometrium); vaginal hysterectomy
00948	4	Anesthesia for vaginal procedures (including biopsy of labia, vagina, cervix or endometrium); cervical cerclage
00950	5	Anesthesia for vaginal procedures (including biopsy of labia, vagina, cervix or endometrium); culdoscopy
00952	4	Anesthesia for vaginal procedures (including biopsy of labia, vagina, cervix or endometrium); hysteroscopy and/or hysterosalpingography
01112	5	Anesthesia for bone marrow aspiration and/or biopsy, anterior or posterior iliac crest
01120	6	Anesthesia for procedures on bony pelvis
01130	3	Anesthesia for body cast application or revision
01140	15	Anesthesia for interpelviabdominal (hindquarter) amputation
01150	8	Anesthesia for radical procedures for tumor of pelvis, except hindquarter amputation
01160	4	Anesthesia for closed procedures involving symphysis pubis or sacroiliac joint
01170	8	Anesthesia for open procedures involving symphysis pubis or sacroiliac joint
01180	3	Anesthesia for obturator neurectomy; extrapelvic
01190	4	Anesthesia for obturator neurectomy; intrapelvic
01200	4	Anesthesia for all closed procedures involving hip joint
01202	4	Anesthesia for arthroscopic procedures of hip joint
01210	6	Anesthesia for open procedures involving hip joint; not otherwise specified
01212	10	Anesthesia for open procedures involving hip joint; hip disarticulation
01214	10	Anesthesia for open procedures involving hip joint; total hip arthroplasty
01215	10	Anesthesia for open procedures involving hip joint; revision of total hip arthroplasty
01220	4	Anesthesia for all closed procedures involving upper 2/3 of femur
01230	6	Anesthesia for open procedures involving upper 2/3 of femur; not otherwise specified
01232	5	Anesthesia for open procedures involving upper 2/3 of femur; amputation
01234	8	Anesthesia for open procedures involving upper 2/3 of femur; radical resection
01250	4	Anesthesia for all procedures on nerves, muscles, tendons, fascia, and bursae of upper leg

CPT five-digit codes, two-digit numeric modifiers, and descriptions only are copyright 2001 American Medical Association

Anesthesiology Base Units

Code	2002 Base Units	Descriptor
01260	3	Anesthesia for all procedures involving veins of upper leg, including exploration
01270	8	Anesthesia for procedures involving arteries of upper leg, including bypass graft; not otherwise specified
01272	4	Anesthesia for procedures involving arteries of upper leg, including bypass graft; femoral artery ligation
01274	6	Anesthesia for procedures involving arteries of upper leg, including bypass graft; femoral artery embolectomy
01320	4	Anesthesia for all procedures on nerves, muscles, tendons, fascia, and bursae of knee and/or popliteal area
01340	4	Anesthesia for all closed procedures on lower 1/3 of femur
01360	5	Anesthesia for all open procedures on lower 1/3 of femur
01380	3	Anesthesia for all closed procedures on knee joint
01382	3	Anesthesia for arthroscopic procedures of knee joint
01390	3	Anesthesia for all closed procedures on upper ends of tibia, fibula, and/or patella
01392	4	Anesthesia for all open procedures on upper ends of tibia, fibula, and/or patella
01400	4	Anesthesia for open procedures on knee joint; not otherwise specified
01402	7	Anesthesia for open procedures on knee joint; total knee arthroplasty
01404	5	Anesthesia for open procedures on knee joint; disarticulation at knee
01420	3	Anesthesia for all cast applications, removal, or repair involving knee joint
01430	3	Anesthesia for procedures on veins of knee and popliteal area; not otherwise specified
01432	5	Anesthesia for procedures on veins of knee and popliteal area; arteriovenous fistula
01440	5	Anesthesia for procedures on arteries of knee and popliteal area; not otherwise specified
01442	8	Anesthesia for procedures on arteries of knee and popliteal area; popliteal thromboendarterectomy, with or without patch graft
01444	8	Anesthesia for procedures on arteries of knee and popliteal area; popliteal excision and graft or repair for occlusion or aneurysm
01462	3	Anesthesia for all closed procedures on lower leg, ankle, and foot
01464	3	Anesthesia for arthroscopic procedures of ankle joint
01470	3	Anesthesia for procedures on nerves, muscles, tendons, and fascia of lower leg, ankle, and foot; not otherwise specified
01472	5	Anesthesia for procedures on nerves, muscles, tendons, and fascia of lower leg, ankle, and foot; repair of ruptured Achilles tendon, with or without graft
01474	5	Anesthesia for procedures on nerves, muscles, tendons, and fascia of lower leg, ankle, and foot; gastrocnemius recession (eg, Strayer procedure)
01480	3	Anesthesia for open procedures on bones of lower leg, ankle, and foot; not otherwise specified
01482	4	Anesthesia for open procedures on bones of lower leg, ankle, and foot; radical resection (including below knee amputation)

CPT five-digit codes, two-digit numeric modifiers, and descriptions only are copyright 2001 American Medical Association

Anesthesiology Base Units

Code	2002 Base Units	*Descriptor*
01484	4	Anesthesia for open procedures on bones of lower leg, ankle, and foot; osteotomy or osteoplasty of tibia and/or fibula
01486	7	Anesthesia for open procedures on bones of lower leg, ankle, and foot; total ankle replacement
01490	3	Anesthesia for lower leg cast application, removal, or repair
01500	8	Anesthesia for procedures on arteries of lower leg, including bypass graft; not otherwise specified
01502	6	Anesthesia for procedures on arteries of lower leg, including bypass graft; embolectomy, direct or with catheter
01520	3	Anesthesia for procedures on veins of lower leg; not otherwise specified
01522	5	Anesthesia for procedures on veins of lower leg; venous thrombectomy, direct or with catheter
01610	5	Anesthesia for all procedures on nerves, muscles, tendons, fascia, and bursae of shoulder and axilla
01620	4	Anesthesia for all closed procedures on humeral head and neck, sternoclavicular joint, acromioclavicular joint, and shoulder joint
01622	4	Anesthesia for arthroscopic procedures of shoulder joint
01630	5	Anesthesia for open procedures on humeral head and neck, sternoclavicular joint, acromioclavicular joint, and shoulder joint; not otherwise specified
01632	6	Anesthesia for open procedures on humeral head and neck, sternoclavicular joint, acromioclavicular joint, and shoulder joint; radical resection
01634	9	Anesthesia for open procedures on humeral head and neck, sternoclavicular joint, acromioclavicular joint, and shoulder joint; shoulder disarticulation
01636	15	Anesthesia for open procedures on humeral head and neck, sternoclavicular joint, acromioclavicular joint, and shoulder joint; interthoracoscapular (forequarter) amputation
01638	10	Anesthesia for open procedures on humeral head and neck, sternoclavicular joint, acromioclavicular joint, and shoulder joint; total shoulder replacement
01650	6	Anesthesia for procedures on arteries of shoulder and axilla; not otherwise specified
01652	10	Anesthesia for procedures on arteries of shoulder and axilla; axillary-brachial aneurysm
01654	8	Anesthesia for procedures on arteries of shoulder and axilla; bypass graft
01656	10	Anesthesia for procedures on arteries of shoulder and axilla; axillary-femoral bypass graft
01670	4	Anesthesia for all procedures on veins of shoulder and axilla
01680	3	Anesthesia for shoulder cast application, removal or repair; not otherwise specified
01682	4	Anesthesia for shoulder cast application, removal or repair; shoulder spica
01710	3	Anesthesia for procedures on nerves, muscles, tendons, fascia, and bursae of upper arm and elbow; not otherwise specified
01712	5	Anesthesia for procedures on nerves, muscles, tendons, fascia, and bursae of upper arm and elbow; tenotomy, elbow to shoulder, open
01714	5	Anesthesia for procedures on nerves, muscles, tendons, fascia, and bursae of upper arm and elbow; tenoplasty, elbow to shoulder

CPT five-digit codes, two-digit numeric modifiers, and descriptions only are copyright 2001 American Medical Association

Anesthesiology Base Units

Code	2002 Base Units	Descriptor
01716	5	Anesthesia for procedures on nerves, muscles, tendons, fascia, and bursae of upper arm and elbow; tenodesis, rupture of long tendon of biceps
01730	3	Anesthesia for all closed procedures on humerus and elbow
01732	3	Anesthesia for arthroscopic procedures of elbow joint
01740	4	Anesthesia for open procedures on humerus and elbow; not otherwise specified
01742	5	Anesthesia for open procedures on humerus and elbow; osteotomy of humerus
01744	5	Anesthesia for open procedures on humerus and elbow; repair of nonunion or malunion of humerus
01756	6	Anesthesia for open procedures on humerus and elbow; radical procedures
01758	5	Anesthesia for open procedures on humerus and elbow; excision of cyst or tumor of humerus
01760	7	Anesthesia for open procedures on humerus and elbow; total elbow replacement
01770	8	Anesthesia for procedures on arteries of upper arm and elbow; not otherwise specified
01772	6	Anesthesia for procedures on arteries of upper arm and elbow; embolectomy
01780	3	Anesthesia for procedures on veins of upper arm and elbow; not otherwise specified
01782	4	Anesthesia for procedures on veins of upper arm and elbow; phleborrhaphy
01810	3	Anesthesia for all procedures on nerves, muscles, tendons, fascia, and bursae of forearm, wrist, and hand
01820	3	Anesthesia for all closed procedures on radius, ulna, wrist, or hand bones
01830	3	Anesthesia for open procedures on radius, ulna, wrist, or hand bones; not otherwise specified
01832	6	Anesthesia for open procedures on radius, ulna, wrist, or hand bones; total wrist replacement
01840	6	Anesthesia for procedures on arteries of forearm, wrist, and hand; not otherwise specified
01842	6	Anesthesia for procedures on arteries of forearm, wrist, and hand; embolectomy
01844	6	Anesthesia for vascular shunt, or shunt revision, any type (eg, dialysis)
01850	3	Anesthesia for procedures on veins of forearm, wrist, and hand; not otherwise specified
01852	4	Anesthesia for procedures on veins of forearm, wrist, and hand; phleborrhaphy
01860	3	Anesthesia for forearm, wrist, or hand cast application, removal, or repair
01905	5	Anesthesia for myelography, diskography, vertebroplasty
01916	5	Anesthesia for diagnostic arteriography/venography
01920	7	Anesthesia for cardiac catheterization including coronary angiography and ventriculography (not to include Swan-Ganz catheter)
01922	7	Anesthesia for non-invasive imaging or radiation therapy
01924	5	Anesthesia for therapeutic interventional radiologic procedures involving the arterial system; not otherwise specified
01925	7	Anesthesia for therapeutic interventional radiologic procedures involving the arterial system; carotid or coronary

CPT five-digit codes, two-digit numeric modifiers, and descriptions only are copyright 2001 American Medical Association

Anesthesiology Base Units

Code	2002 Base Units	*Descriptor*
01926	8	Anesthesia for therapeutic interventional radiologic procedures involving the arterial system; intracranial, intracardiac, or aortic
01930	5	Anesthesia for therapeutic interventional radiologic procedures involving the venous/lymphatic system (not to include access to the central circulation); not otherwise specified
01931	7	Anesthesia for therapeutic interventional radiologic procedures involving the venous/lymphatic system (not to include access to the central circulation); intrahepatic or portal circulation (eg, transcutaneous porto-caval shunt (TIPS))
01932	6	Anesthesia for therapeutic interventional radiologic procedures involving the venous/lymphatic system (not to include access to the central circulation); intrathoracic or jugular
01933	7	Anesthesia for therapeutic interventional radiologic procedures involving the venous/lymphatic system (not to include access to the central circulation); intracranial
01951	3	Anesthesia for second and third degree burn excision or debridement with or without skin grafting, any site, for total body surface area (TBSA) treated during anesthesia and surgery; less than four percent total body surface area
01952	5	Anesthesia for second and third degree burn excision or debridement with or without skin grafting, any site, for total body surface area (TBSA) treated during anesthesia and surgery; between four and nine percent of total body surface area
01953	1	Anesthesia for second and third degree burn excision or debridement with or without skin grafting, any site, for total body surface area (TBSA) treated during anesthesia and surgery; each additional nine percent total body surface area or part thereof (Li
01960	5	Anesthesia for; vaginal delivery only
01961	7	Anesthesia for; cesarean delivery only
01962	8	Anesthesia for; urgent hysterectomy following delivery
01963	8	Anesthesia for; cesarean hysterectomy without any labor analgesia/anesthesia care
01964	4	Anesthesia for; abortion procedures
01967	5	Neuraxial labor analgesia/anesthesia for planned vaginal delivery (this includes any repeat subarachnoid needle placement and drug injection and/or any necessary replacement of an epidural catheter during labor)
01968	2	Cesarean delivery following neuraxial labor analgesia/anesthesia (List separately in addition to code for primary procedure)
01969	5	Cesarean hysterectomy following neuraxial labor analgesia/anesthesia (List separately in addition to code for primary procedure)
01990	7	Physiological support for harvesting of organ(s) from brain-dead patient
01995	5	Regional intravenous administration of local anesthetic agent or other medication (upper or lower extremity)
01996	3	Daily management of epidural or subarachnoid drug administration
01999	0	Unlisted anesthesia procedure(s)

CPT five-digit codes, two-digit numeric modifiers, and descriptions only are copyright 2001 American Medical Association

Appendixes

Appendix A
Glossary of Terms

actual charge — The physician's billed or submitted charge, which is the amount Medicare will pay if it is lower than the Medicare payment schedule amount.

AMA/Specialty Society RVS Update Committee (RUC) — The RUC was established by the AMA and national medical specialty societies in 1991 and makes annual recommendations to the Centers for Medicare and Medicaid Services (CMS) on the work relative value units (RVUs) to be assigned to new and revised Current Procedural Terminology (CPT) codes as they are adopted by the AMA CPT Editorial Panel.

approved amount — The full Medicare payment amount that a physician or other provider is allowed to receive for a service provided to a Medicare beneficiary; the Medicare program pays 80% and the patient the remaining 20%. Payments to physicians who do not participate in Medicare are calculated based on 95% of the payment schedule; the physician's charges are limited to 115% of this amount.

assignment — When a physician accepts the Medicare approved amount (including the 80% Medicare payment and 20% patient copayment) as payment in full, it is called "accepting assignment." The physician submits a claim to Medicare directly and collects only the appropriate deductible and the 20% copayment from the patient.

balance bill — That portion of a physician's charge exceeding the Medicare approved amount, which is billed to the patient. When a physician balance bills, the patient is responsible for the amount of the physician's charge that exceeds the Medicare approved amount up to the limiting charge, as well as the 20% copayment. Only nonparticipating physicians may balance bill their Medicare patients.

Balanced Budget Act of 1997 — Legislation signed by President Clinton on August 5, 1997, significantly changing the Medicare program. The legislation created a Medicare+Choice program that expanded beneficiaries' health plan options; extended Medicare coverage to some preventive medicine services; and changed the system for annual updates to physician payments. Chapter 1 summarizes key provisions of the legislation.

baseline adjustment — A 6.5% reduction to the conversion factor to maintain budget neutrality that was adopted in the 1991 *Final Rule* to account for volume increases due to patient demand, physician responses to the RBRVS payment system, and other factors projected by the Centers for Medicare and Medicaid Services (CMS). This adjustment replaced an initial 10% "behavioral offset" proposed in the *Notice of Proposed Rulemaking (NPRM)* that reflected anticipated increases in physician services. The CMS adopted the term "baseline adjustment due to concerns of the AMA and others that the term "behavioral offset" was misleading. Such offsets are again included in the budget neutrality adjustments in 1999.

behavioral offset — A reduction in the conversion factor proposed in the *Notice of Proposed Rulemaking (NPRM)* to compensate for the Centers for Medicare and Medicaid Services (CMS) assumption that physicians would increase the volume of services in response to decreases in payment. The NPRM included a 10% volume or "behavioral" offset in 1992 payments, but it was replaced in the 1991 Final Rule with a 6.5% baseline adjustment to maintain budget neutrality during the full transition period. Behavioral offsets also were applied to the conversion factors in 1997 (–0.9%), 1998 (–0.1%), 1999 (–0.28%), 2000 (–0.12%), 2001 (–.20%), and 2002 (–.18%).

budget neutrality — A provision of the Omnibus Budget Reconciliation Act of 1989 (OBRA 89), the legislation creating the Medicare RBRVS payment system, that required 1992 expenditures to neither increase nor decrease from what they would have been under a continuation of customary, prevailing, and reasonable (CPR). A similar limitation continues to apply, specifying that changes in the relative value units (RVUs) resulting from changes in medical practice, coding, new data, or addition of new services may not cause Part B expenditures to differ by more than $20 million from the spending level that would occur in the absence of these adjustments.

The CMS has applied a budget neutrality adjustment each year since implementation of the RBRVS payment system, although its form has varied. In 1996 and 1998, the conversion factors were adjusted downward to achieve budget neutrality. Two separate adjustments were applied in 1997, to the conversion factors and to the work RVUs. In all other years, the adjuster was applied to the relative values for all three components, work, practice expense, and professional liability insurance (PLI). This year, the adjustments are applied to the conversion factor.

carrier — A private contractor to the Centers for Medicare and Medicaid Services (CMS) that administers claims processing and payment for Medicare Part B services.

Centers for Medicare and Medicaid Services (CMS) — Formerly the agency within the Department of Health and Human Services (HHS) that administers the Medicare program.

conversion factor (CF) — The factor that transforms the geographically adjusted relative value for a service into a dollar amount under the physician payment schedule. The current conversion factor for 2002 is $36.1992.

Current Procedural Terminology® (CPT®) — System for coding physician services developed by the American Medical Association to file claims with Medicare and other third-party payers; level 3 of the Healthcare Common Procedure Coding System (HCPCS).

customary charge — The physician's median charge for a service that is based on data collected during the July-June period preceding the current calendar year. One of the factors considered in determining a physician's Medicare payment under the "customary, prevailing, and reasonable" (CPR) system.

customary, prevailing, and reasonable (CPR) — The payment system used to determine physician payment under the Medicare program prior to implementation of the Medicare resource-based relative value scale (RBRVS) payment system on January 1, 1992. The CPR system paid the lowest of the physician's actual charge for a service, that physician's customary charge, or the prevailing charge in the locality. Due to diversity in physicians' charges for the same services, the CPR system allowed for wide variation in Medicare payment levels across specialties and geographic areas. The CPR system is described in Chapter 1.

deductible — A specified amount of covered medical expenses a beneficiary must pay before receiving benefits. Medicare Part B has an annual deductible of $100 in 2002.

Department of Health and Human Services (HHS) — Department within the US government that is responsible for administering health and social welfare programs.

evaluation and management (E/M) services — Patient evaluation and management services that a physician provides during a patient's office, hospital, or other visit or consultation. New codes for visits and consultations, developed by the AMA CPT Editorial Panel and adopted by Health Care Financing Administration (CMS) for implementation under the Medicare program beginning January 1, 1992, improved the coding uniformity for these services, and their appropriateness for use in an RBRVS-based payment schedule. The E/M codes, described in Chapter 10, utilize a more precise method of describing services. This method is based primarily on type of history, examination, and medical decision making.

Final Notice — A portion of the November 25, 1992, *Federal Register* containing a summary of the comments received on the 1991 "interim" relative values, a description of the Health Care Financing Administration (CMS) refinement methodology, and a table of the resulting 1993 relative values for physician services.

Final Rule — A portion of the *Federal Register* that contains a summary of the final regulations for implementing the Medicare RBRVS payment schedule for a particular year. It generally includes updated relative value units for all physician services payable under the payment schedule, revised payment rules, analyses of comments on the previous proposed rule and CMS's response, updated geographic practice cost indexes, and an impact analysis of the new rules on physicians and beneficiaries.

five-year review — A review process mandated by OBRA 89 requiring CMS to conduct a review of all work relative values no less often than every 5 years. Activities for this first 5-year review were initiated in 1995 and included work RVUs for all codes on the 1995 RBRVS payment schedule. Final RVUs were published by CMS in the 1996 *Final Rule,* effective for the 1997 Medicare relative value scale (RVS). The second five-year review began in 2000, with changes to be implemented in 2002. The AMA/Specialty Society RVS Update Committee (RUC) plays a key role in both review processes.

geographic adjustment factor (GAF) — The adjustment made to a service included in the resource-based relative value scale (RBRVS) to account for geographic cost differences across Medicare localities, which are based on the geographic practice cost indexes (GPCIs).

geographic practice cost index (GPCI) — An index reflecting differences across geographic areas in physicians' resource costs relative to the national average: cost of living, practice costs, and professional liability insurance (PLI). Three distinct GPCIs are used to calculate the payment schedule amount for a service in a Medicare locality. The list of GPCIs is contained in Part 5.

global charge — The sum of the professional component and technical component of a procedure when provided and billed by the same physician. This is further described in Chapter 11.

global service — A payment concept defined by Medicare as a surgical "package" that includes all intraoperative and follow-up services, as well as some preoperative services, associated with the surgery for which the surgeon receives a single payment. The initial evaluation or consultation is excluded from the global package under the Medicare payment schedule. This term is further described in Chapter 11.

Healthcare Common Procedure Coding System (HCPCS) — Coding system, required for billing Medicare, that is based on Current Procedural Terminology (CPT) but supplemented with additional codes for nonphysician services.

health professional shortage areas (HPSAs) — Urban or rural areas identified by the Public Health Service (PHS) as medically underserved. The PHS may also designate population groups and public nonprofit medical facilities as medically underserved. Physicians in designated HPSAs who furnish covered services to Medicare patients receive a 10% bonus payment in addition to the payment schedule amount.

limiting charge — Statutory limit on the amount a nonparticipating physician can charge for services to Medicare patients. The limiting charge replaced the maximum allowable actual charge (MAAC), effective January 1, 1991. The limiting charge in 1993 and subsequent years is 115% of the Medicare approved amount for nonparticipating physicians. This term is further described in Chapter 9.

locality — Geographic areas defined by CMS and used to establish payment amounts for physician services. The CMS fundamentally revised the methodology for establishing localities effective for 1997 payments, reducing the number to 89 from 211. The new methodology increased the number of statewide localities and generally combined others into counties and groups of counties.

maximum allowable actual charge (MAAC) — Under the customary, prevailing, and reasonable (CPR) system, a limit on the amount nonparticipating physicians could charge their Medicare patients above the Medicare approved amount. The MAACs were different for each physician because they were based on the individual physician's customary charges. During a transition period from January 1, 1991, through December 31, 1992, MAACs were phased out and replaced by limiting charges.

Medicare economic index (MEI) — An index introduced in 1976 that is intended to measure the annual growth in physicians' practice costs and general inflation in the cost of operating a medical practice. Under the Medicare payment schedule, the MEI is a factor in updating the conversion factor. Under the customary, prevailing, and reasonable (CPR) payment system, the MEI was a limitation on increases in a physician's prevailing charges.

Medicare payment schedule — A payment schedule adopted by the Centers for Medicare and Medicaid Services (CMS) for payment of physician services effective January 1, 1992, replacing the customary, prevailing, and reasonable (CPR) system. This payment schedule is based on the resource costs of physician work, practice overhead, and professional liability insurance, with adjustments for differences in geographic practice costs. The payment schedule for a service includes both the 80% that Medicare pays and the patient's 20% copayment.

Medicare, Medicaid, and SCHIP Benefits Improvement and Protection Act of 2000 (BIPA) — Legislation enacted on December 21, 2000, provides for revisions to policies applicable to the physician payment schedule. This legislation created Medicare coverage changes for several services, including: enhancements to screening mammography, pelvic examinations, colonoscopy, and telehealth; new coverage for screening for glaucoma; new coverage for medical nutrition therapy performed by registered dietitians and nutrition professionals.

Medicare volume performance standard (MVPS) — A spending goal for Medicare Part B services prior to 1998. It was established either by Congress, based upon recommendations submitted by the Department of Health and Human services (HHS) and Physician Payment Review Commission (PPRC) or by a statutory default formula, if Congress chose not to act. The MVPS was intended to encompass all factors contributing to the growth in Medicare spending for physicians' services, including changes in payment levels, size and age composition of Medicare patients, technology, utilization patterns, and access to care.

A conversion factor update default formula became automatically effective if Congress failed to act by October 31 of each year. It was linked to changes in the medical economic index (MEI) as adjusted for the amount by which actual expenditures the preceding year were greater or less than the MVPS-established goals.

Medicare Payment Advisory Commission (MedPAC) — A new commission created by the Balanced Budget Act of 1997, to advise Congress on Medicare payment policies and other issues affecting Medicare and the broader health system. It merges the roles of the Physician Payment Review Commission (PPRC) and the Prospective Payment Assessment Commission, which previously provided Congress with analysis and advice on policy issues affecting Medicare Parts B and A, respectively.

model fee schedule — A payment schedule the Centers for Medicare and Medicaid Services (CMS) developed in 1990, as required in OBRA 89. The narrative portion of the model fee schedule included the statutory requirements of OBRA 89 as well as technical and policy issues not prescribed by statute; preliminary estimates of the relative values for approximately 1400 services studied under Phase I of the Harvard study; and preliminary geographic practice cost indexes (GPCIs) for all Medicare localities.

nonparticipating physician — A physician who has not signed a participation agreement with Medicare and, therefore, is not obligated to accept the Medicare approved amount as payment in full for all cases. Their Medicare patients are billed directly, including the balance of the charge that is not covered by the Medicare approved amount, but this balance cannot exceed the limiting charge. Nonparticipating physicians may still accept assignment on a case-by-case basis.

Notice of Proposed Rulemaking (NPRM) — The proposed rules to implement the Medicare payment schedule and relative values for 4000 services studied under Phase II of the Harvard study; published by Medicare for public comment on June 5, 1991.

OBRA 89 (Omnibus Budget Reconciliation Act of 1989) — The congressional legislation creating Medicare physician payment reform that provided for a payment schedule based on a resource-based relative value scale (RBRVS), which included three components: physician work, practice expense, and professional liability insurance (PLI) costs.

OBRA 93 — The congressional legislation that included a number of revisions to Medicare physician payment under the RBRVS. These provisions include the elimination of payment reductions for "new" physicians, the repeal of the ban on payment for interpretation of ECGs, and several changes to the default payment update and MVPS.

participating physician — A physician who has signed a participation agreement with Medicare; the physician is bound by the agreement to accept assignment on all Medicare claims for the calendar year.

Physician Payment Review Commission (PPRC) — An advisory body created by Congress in 1986 to recommend Medicare reforms in physician payment methods. The PPRC's charge was broadened to include recommendations for health system reforms to the private as well as public sectors. Its functions were subsumed by a new Medicare Payment Advisory Commission (MedPAC), which was created under the Balanced Budget Act of 1997. MedPAC merges the roles of the PPRC and the Prospective Payment Assessment Commission.

physician work — The physician's individual effort in providing a service, which includes time, technical difficulty of the procedure, severity of patient's condition, and the physical and mental effort required to provide the service; one of three resource cost components included in the formula for computing payment amounts under the Medicare payment schedule.

practice expense — The cost of physician practice overhead, including rent, staff salaries and benefits, medical equipment, and supplies; one of three resource cost components included in the formula for computing Medicare payment schedule amounts.

prevailing charge — One of the factors under the CPR system used to determine physician payment for a particular service. The prevailing charge for a service was an amount set high enough to cover the full customary charges of the physicians in a locality whose billings accounted for at least 75% of the charges for that service. Increases in prevailing charges were capped by increases in the Medicare economic index (MEI).

primary care services — The CMS restricts its definition of primary care services to the following: Office or other outpatient services (99201–99215); Emergency department services (99281–99285); Nursing facility services (99301–99313); Domiciliary, rest home, or custodial care services (99321–99333); Home services (99341–99355); Eye exam, new patient (92002–92004); Prolonged services, office (99354–99355); Care plan oversight services (99375); and End-stage renal disease (ESRD) services (90935–90947).

professional component — In coding for physician services, that portion of the service that denotes the physician's work and associated overhead and professional liability insurance (PLI) costs.

professional liability insurance (PLI) — Insurance to protect a physician against professional liability; one of three resource cost components included in the formula developed by CMS for computing Medicare payment schedule amounts.

relative value scale (RVS) — An index of physicians' services ranked according to "value," with value defined according to the basis for the scale. In a charge-based RVS, services are ranked according to the average fee for the service or some other charge basis. A resource-based RVS ranks services according to the relative costs of the resources required to provide them.

relative value unit (RVU) — The unit of measure for the Medicare resource-based relative value scale. The RVUs must be multiplied by a dollar conversion factor to become payment amounts.

resource-based practice expense — A methodology for determining practice expense relative values based on physicians' practice overhead costs, including rent, staff salaries, and medical equipment and supplies. The Balanced Budget Act of 1997 contains provisions mandating development of resource-based practice expense relative values to be fully implemented on January 1, 2002.

resource-based relative value scale (RBRVS) — A relative value scale based on the resource costs of providing physician services; adopted in OBRA 89 as the basis for physician payment for Medicare Part B services effective January 1, 1992. The relative value of each service is the sum of relative value units (RVUs) representing physician work, practice expense, and professional liability insurance (PLI) adjusted for each locality by a geographic adjustment factor and converted into dollar payment amounts by a conversion factor.

Social Security Act Amendments of 1994 — Technical corrections legislation adopted by Congress that contains a number of provisions relative to the Medicare RBRVS. These provisions include development of resource-based practice expense relative values, CMS authority to enforce balance billing requirements, study of needed data refinements to update the geographic practice cost indexes (GPCIs), and development and refinement of relative values for the full range of pediatric services.

specialty differential — Under the customary, prevailing, and reasonable (CPR) system, some Medicare carriers paid different amounts to physicians, according to specialty, for providing the same service. The OBRA 89 required that such payment differentials be eliminated.

sustainable growth rate (SGR) — A new system for determining annual conversion factor updates that replaced the Medicare volume performance standard (MVPS) system, under provisions of the Balanced Budget Act of 1997. The SGR bases the update on volume growth in real per capita gross domestic product (GDP). Similar to the MVPS, the SGR reflects changes in inflation, Medicare beneficiary enrollment, real GDP, and spending due to legislative and regulatory requirements. It does not rely on historical patterns of growth in volume and intensity of physician services, however, as did the MVPS; rather, it uses projected growth in real GDP per capita. The SGR is constructed so that projected spending will match growth targets by the end of each year. The 2002 estimated SGR is 5.6%.

technical component — In coding for physician services, the portion of a service or procedure that includes cost of equipment, supplies, and technician salary. Payment for the technical component of a service is composed of relative values for practice expense and professional liability insurance (PLI).

transition asymmetry — The effect of payments for evaluation and management (E/M) services increasing at a faster rate than payments for other services decrease during the 1992 through 1995 transition to the full payment schedule, causing total outlays in 1992 to exceed what they would have been had the CPR system been retained. To allow payments for services during the transition period to increase and decrease at about the same rate and maintain budget neutrality, Centers for Medicare and Medicaid Services (CMS) made a one-time 5.5% reduction to the adjusted historical payment basis (AHPB).

transition offset — To maintain budget neutrality during the transition to the full payment schedule, given the transition asymmetry, a 5.5% adjustment was adopted in the 1991 *Final Rule* and applied to the adjusted historical payment basis (AHPB) instead of the conversion factor, as proposed in the *Notice of Proposed Rulemaking (NPRM)*. By applying this adjustment to the AHPBs, permanent cuts to the conversion factor were prevented.

Appendix B
Directory of Resources

This directory includes the names, addresses, and phone numbers of national organizations, medical societies, Medicare Part B carriers, and Centers for Medicare and Medicaid Services (CMS) regional offices. Such information changes over time. For example, Medicare Part B carriers occasionally change their field office locations and Medicare contracts with new carriers from time to time. The CMS regional offices should be able to provide updated contact information in such cases.

American Medical Association

Physicians with general questions or seeking up-to-date coding information should use the address and telephone numbers listed below.

American Medical Association
515 N State Street
Chicago, IL 60610
312 464-5000

Member Service Center
(for AMA members only)
800 262-3211

CPT® Information Services

CPT Information Services—a fee-for service subscription resource—gives you the coding answers you need by phone, fax or mail. Five convenient subscription packages let you select the level of service you need. As an added benefit, AMA members receive their first four inquiries free. Call 800 621-8335

Medicare Payment Review Commission (MedPAC)

Physicians may write or telephone MedPAC to obtain copies of its reports.

Medicare Payment Advisory Commission
1730 K Street, NW, Suite 800,
Washington, DC 20006
202 653-7220
202 653-7238 Fax

Medical Societies

State medical associations and national medical specialty societies can offer assistance on Medicare physician payment questions. Many societies have well-established liaisons with Medicare insurance carriers. Medical society staff thus may have firsthand information about how to approach the problems that physicians may experience. The following list contains addresses and general telephone numbers of state and national specialty societies. Physicians should request that their inquiries be routed to the appropriate knowledgeable staff person.

State Medical Societies

Alabama
Medical Association of the State of Alabama
Cary J. Kuhlmann, Executive Director
19 S Jackson Street
Montgomery, AL 36102-1900
334 954-2500
334 269-5200 (Fax)
Website: www.MASALINK.org

Alaska
Alaska State Medical Association
James J. Jordan, Executive Director
4107 Laurel Street
Anchorage, AK 99508
907 562-0304
907 561-2063 (Fax)
Society E-mail address:
 ASMA@alaska.net

Arizona
Arizona Medical Association
Chic Older, Executive Vice President
810 W Bethany Home Road
Phoenix, AZ 85013
602 246-8901
602 242-6283 (Fax)
chicolder@azmedassn.org
 (E-mail)

Arkansas
Arkansas Medical Society
Kenneth L. LaMastus, CAE, Executive Vice President
10 Corporate Hill Drive,
 Suite 300
Little Rock, AR 72205
501 224-8967
501 224-6489 (Fax)
ams@arkmed.org (E-mail)
Website: www.arkmed.org

California
California Medical Association
John C. Lewin, MD, Executive Vice President/CEO
1201 J Street
Sacramento, CA 95914-2906
916-551-2020
916-551-2027 (Fax)
jlewin@calmed.org (E-mail)
Website: www.cmanet.org

Colorado
Colorado Medical Society
Sandra L. Maloney, Executive Director
7351 Lowry Boulevard
Denver, CO 80230
720 859-1001
720 859-7509 (Fax)
sandi@maloney@cms.org (E-mail)
Website: www.cms.org

Connecticut
Connecticut State Medical Society
Timothy B. Norbeck, Executive Director
160 St Ronan Street
New Haven, CT 06511
203 865-0587
203 865-4997 (Fax)
tnorbeck@csms.org (E-mail)
Website: www.csms.org

Delaware
Medical Society of Delaware
Mark A. Meister, Sr, Executive Director
131 Continental Drive, Ste. 405
Newark, DE 19713
302 658-7596
302 658-9669 (Fax)
mam@medsocdel.org (E-mail)
Internet address:
 www.medsocdel.org
Society E-mail address:
info-msd@medsocdel.org

District of Columbia
Medical Society of the District of Columbia
K. Edward Shanbacker, Executive Director
2175 K Street NW, Suite 200
Washington, DC 20037-1809
202 466-1800
202 452-1542 (Fax)
shanback@msdc.org (E-mail)
Internet address: www.msdc.org

Florida
Florida Medical Association, Inc.
Sandra B. Mortham, Executive Vice President/CEO
113 E College Street
Tallahassee, FL 32301
850 224-6496
850 224-6627 (Fax)
smortham@medone.org (E-mail)
Society E-mail address:
 info@medone.org
Website: www.fmaonline.org

Georgia
Medical Association of Georgia
David Cook, Interim Executive Director
1330 W Peachtree Street NW,
 Suite 500
Atlanta, GA 30309-2904
404 876-7535
404 881-5021 (Fax)
Website: www.mag.org

Guam
Guam Medical Society
Executive Director
C/o Guam Medical Hospital
850 Gov. Carlos Camacho Road
Tamuning, GU 96911
671 649-5801
guammedicalsociety@usa.net
 (E-Mail)
Website:
 www.guammedicalsociety.com

Hawaii
Hawaii Medical Association
Stephanie Aveiro, Executive Director
1360 S Beretania Street,
 Suite 100
Honolulu, HI 96814
808 536-7702
808 528-2376 (Fax)
stephanie-aveiro@hma-assn.org
 (E-mail)
Society E-mail address:
 www.hma-assn.org

Idaho
Idaho Medical Association
Robert K. Seehusen,
 Chief Executive Officer
305 W Jefferson
Boise, ID 83702
208 344-7888
208 344-7903 (Fax)
Society E-mail address:
 mail@idmed.org
Website: www.idmed.org

Illinois
Illinois State Medical Society
Alexander R. Lerner, Executive Vice President/CEO
20 N Michigan Avenue, Suite 700
Chicago, IL 60602
312 782-1654
312 782-2023 (Fax)
Internet address: www.isms.org

Indiana
Indiana State Medical Association
Richard R. King, JD, Executive Director
322 Canal Walk, Canal Level
Indianapolis, IN 46202-3252
317 261-2060
317 261-2076 (Fax)
Rking@ismanet.org (E-mail)
Internet address:
 www.ismanet.org

Iowa
Iowa Medical Society
Michael D. Abrams, Executive Vice President
1001 Grand Avenue
W Des Moines, IA 50265
515 223-1401
515 223-8420 (Fax)
mdabrams@iowamedicalsociety.org
 (E-mail)
Internet address:
 www.iowamedicalsociety.org

Kansas
Kansas Medical Society
Jerry Slaughter, Executive Director
623 SW 10th Avenue
Topeka, KS 66612
785 235-2383
785 235-5114 (Fax)
jslaughter@kmsonline.org
 (E-mail)
Website: www.kmsonline.org

Kentucky
Kentucky Medical Association
William T. Applegate, Executive Vice President
4965 US Highway 42, Suite 2000
Louisville, KY 40222-6301
502 426-6200
502 426-6877 (Fax)
wta@kyma.org (E-mail)
Society E-mail address:
 member@kyma.org
Website: www.kyma.org

Louisiana
Louisiana State Medical Society
David L. Tarver, Executive Vice President
6767 Perkins Road
Baton Rouge, LA 70808
225 763-8500
225 763-6122 (Fax)
Website: www.lsms.org

Maine
Maine Medical Association
Gordon H. Smith, Esq
 Executive Vice President
Association Drive
Manchester, ME 04351
207 622-3374
207 622-3332 (Fax)
gsmith@ctel.net (E-mail)
Website: www.mainemed.com

Maryland
MedChi, The Maryland State Medical Society
T. Michael Preston, Executive Director
1211 Cathedral Street
Baltimore, MD 21201
410 539-0872
410 547-0915 (Fax)
michael@mail.medchi.org (E-mail)
Website: www.medchi.org

Massachusetts
Massachusetts Medical Society
Corinne Broderick, Acting Executive Vice President
860 Winter Street
Waltham, MA 02451-1411
781 893-4610
781 893-9136 (Fax)
Website: www.massmed.org
Society E-mail address: info@massmed.org

Michigan
Michigan State Medical Society
William E. Madigan, Executive Director
120 W Saginaw
East Lansing, MI 48826-0950
517 337-1351
517 337-2490 (Fax)
wmadigan@msms.org (E-mail)
Internet address: www.msms.org

Minnesota
Minnesota Medical Association
Paul S. Sanders, MD, Chief, CEO
3433 Broadway Street, NE
Suite 300
Minneapolis, MN 55413-1760
612 378-1875
612 378-3875 (Fax)
psanders@mnmed.org (E-mail)
Website: www.mnmed.org

Mississippi
Mississippi State Medical Association
William F. Roberts, Executive Director
408 W Parkway Place
Ridgeland, MS 39157
601 853-6733
601 853-6746 (Fax)
msmaonline.com (E-mail)
Website: www.msmaonline.com

Missouri
Missouri State Medical Association
C. C. Swarens, Executive Vice President
113 Madison Street
Jefferson City, MO 65102
573 636-5151
573 636-8552 (Fax)
cswarens@msma.org (E-mail)
Internet address: www.msma.org

Montana
Montana Medical Association
G. Brian Zins, Executive Vice President/CEO
2021 Eleventh Avenue, Suite 1
Helena, MT 59601-4890
406 443-4000
406 443-4042 (Fax)
brianmma@uswest.net (E-mail)
Website: www.mmaoffice.com
Society E-mail address: mmaoffice.com

Nebraska
Nebraska Medical Association
Sandra Johnson, Executive Director
233 S 13th Street, Suite 1512
Lincoln, NE 68508-2091
402 474-4472
402 474-2198 (Fax)
Internet address: www.nebmed.org
Society E-mail address: nma@inetnebr.com

Nevada
Nevada State Medical Association
Lawrence P. Matheis, Executive Director
3660 Baker Lane, Suite 101
Reno, NV 89509
775 825-6788
775 825-3202 (Fax)
lmatheis@nsmadocs.org (E-mail)
Society E-mail address: nsma@nsmadocs.org
Website: www.nsmadoc.org

New Hampshire
New Hampshire Medical Society
Palmer P. Jones, Executive Vice President
7 N State Street
Concord, NH 03301-4018
603 224-1909
603 226-2432 (Fax)
nhmsppj@aol.com (E-mail)
Internet address: www.nhms.org
Society E-mail address: nhmed@aol.com

New Jersey
Medical Society of New Jersey
Vincent A. Maressa, Executive Director
2 Princess Road
Lawrenceville, NJ 08648-2302
609 896-1766
609 896-0674 (Fax)
vamaress@msnj.org (E-mail)
Internet address: www.msnj.org

New Mexico
New Mexico Medical Society
G. Randy Marshall, Executive Director
7770 Jefferson NE, Suite 400
Albuquerque, NM 87109
505 828-0237
505 828-0336 (Fax)
Internet address: www.nmms.org/ nmms
Society E-mail address: nmms@nmms.org

New York
Medical Society of the State of New York
Charles N. Aswad, MD, Executive Vice President
420 Lakeville Road, PO Box 5404
Lake Success, NY 11042-5404
516 488-6100
516 488-6136 (Fax)
caswad@mssny.org (E-mail)
Internet address: www.mssny.org
Society E-mail address: ccaplan@mssny.org

North Carolina
North Carolina Medical Society
Robert W. Seligson, CAE Executive Vice President
222 N Person Street
Raleigh, NC 27611-7167
919 833-3836, Ext 133
919 833-2023 (Fax)
rseligson@ncmedsoc.org (E-mail)
Website: www.ncmedsoc.org
Society E-mail address: ncms@ncmedsoc.org

North Dakota
North Dakota Medical Association
Bruce T. Levi, Executive Director
1025 N Third Street
PO Box 1198
Bismarck, ND 58502-1198
701 223-9475
701 223-9476 (Fax)
Blevi@ndmed.com (E-mail)
Society E-mail address: staff@ndmed.com

Ohio
Ohio State Medical Association
D. Brent Mulgrew, Executive Director
3401 Mill Run Drive
Hilliard, OH 43026
614 527-6762
614 527-6763 (Fax)
bmulgrew@osma.org (E-mail)
Internet address: www.osma.org
Society E-mail address: osma@osma.org

Oklahoma
Oklahoma State Medical Association
Brian O. Foy, Executive Director
601 NW Grand Boulevard
Oklahoma City, OK 73118
405 843-9571
405 842-1834 (Fax)
foy@osmaonline.org (E-mail)
Internet address: www.osmaonline.org
Society E-mail address: osma@osmaonline.org

Oregon
Oregon Medical Association
Robert L. Dernedde, CAE, Executive Director
5210 SW Corbett Street
Portland, OR 97201
503 226-1555
503 241-7148 (Fax)
rdernedde@ormedassoc.org (E-mail)
Website: www.ormedassoc.org
Society E-mail address: oma@ormedassoc.org

Pennsylvania
Pennsylvania Medical Society
Roger F. Mecum, Executive Director
777 E Park Drive
Harrisburg, PA 17105-8820
717 558-7750
717 558-7840 (Fax)
rmecum@pamedsoc.org (E-mail)
Internet address: www.pamedsoc.org
Society E-mail address: stat@pamedsoc.org

Puerto Rico
Puerto Rico Medical Association
Rafael Alicea-Alicea, Executive Director
1305 Fernandez Juncos Avenue
Stop 19, PO Box 9387
San Juan, PR 00908-9387
787 721-6969
787 722-1191 (Fax)
Website:
www.home.coqui.net/ asocmed
Society E-mail address:
asocmed@coqui.net

Rhode Island
Rhode Island Medical Society
Newell E. Warde, PhD, Executive Director
106 Francis Street
Providence, RI 02903
401 331-3207
401 751-8050 (Fax)
Society E-mail address:
RIMS@ids.net

South Carolina
South Carolina Medical Association
William F. Mahon, Chief Executive Officer
PO Box 11188, 3210 Fernandina Road
Columbia, SC 29211
803 798-6207 Ext 224
803 772-6783 (Fax)
bill@scmanet.org (E-mail)
Internet address:
www.scmanet.org
Society E-mail address:
contact@scmanet.org

South Dakota
South Dakota State Medical Association
L. Paul Jensen, CEO
1323 S Minnesota Avenue
Sioux Falls, SD 57105
605 336-1965
605 336-0270 (Fax)
Website:
www.usd.edu/med/ sdsm

Tennessee
Tennessee Medical Association
Donald H. Alexander, Chief Executive Officer
2301 21st Avenue, S,
PO Box 120909
Nashville, TN 37212-0909
615 385-2100
615 385-3319 (Fax)
dona@tma.medwire.org (E-mail)
Website: www.medwire.org
Society E-mail address:
info@tma.medwire.org

Texas
Texas Medical Association
Louis J. Goodman, PhD, CAE, Executive Vice President/CEO
401 W 15th Street
Austin, TX 78701-1680
512 370-1300
512 370-1633 (Fax)
lou_g@texmed.org (E-mail)
Internet address:
www.texmed.org
Society E-mail address:
info@texmed.org

Utah
Utah Medical Association
J. Leon Sorenson, Executive Vice President
540 E 500 South
Salt Lake City, UT 84102
801 355-7477
801 532-1550 (Fax)
leon@utahmed.org (E-mail)
Internet address:
www.utahmed.org
Society E-mail address:
uma@utahmed.org

Vermont
Vermont Medical Society
Karen N. Meyer, Executive Vice President
P.O. Box 1457
Montpelier, VT 05602
802 223-7898
802 223-1201 (Fax)
kmeyer@vtmd.org (E-mail)

Virgin Islands
Virgin Islands Medical Society
Cora L. E. Christian, MD, MPH, Executive Secretary/ Treasurer
PO Box 5986 Sunny Isle
St Croix, VI 00823-5986
340 712-2400
340 712-2449 (Fax)
christian@hovensa.com (E-mail)

Virginia
Medical Society of Virginia
Paul L. Kitchen, Executive Vice President
4205 Dover Road
Richmond, VA 23221-3267
804 353-2721
804 355-6189 (Fax)
pkitchen@msv.org (E-mail)
Website: www.msv.org
Society E-mail address:
bcimino@msv.org

Washington
Washington State Medical Association
Thomas J. Curry, Executive Director/CEO
2033 6th Avenue, Suite 1100
L. Paul Jensen, CEO
Seattle, WA 98121
206 441-9762
206 441-5863 (Fax)
tjc@wsma.org (E-mail)
Internet address: www.wsma.org
Society E-mail address:
wsma@wsma.org

West Virginia
West Virginia State Medical Association
Evan H. Jenkins, Executive Director
4037 MacCorkle Avenue, SE
Charleston, WV 25304
304 925-0342
304 925-0345 (Fax)
evan@wvsma.com (E-mail)
Society E-mail address:
wvsma@aol.com
Website: www.@wvsma.com

Wisconsin
State Medical Society of Wisconsin
John E. Patchett, JD, Executive Vice President
330 E. Lakeside Street,
PO Box 1109
Madison, WI 53701-1109
608 257-6781
608 283-5406 (Fax)
JohnP@wismed.org (E-mail)
Website: www.wismed.com

Wyoming
Wyoming Medical Society
Wendy P. Curran, Executive Director
1920 Evans, PO Box 4009
Cheyenne, WY 82001
307 635-2424
307 632-1973 (Fax)
wcurran@wyomed.org (E-mail)
Internet address:
www.wyomed.org
Society E-mail address:
info@wyomed.org

National Medical Specialty and Other Societies

Aerospace Medical Association
Russell B. Rayman, MD, Executive Director
320 S Henry Street
Alexandria, VA 22314-3579
703 739-2240 x103
703 739-9652 (Fax)
rrayman@asma.org (E-mail)

American Academy of Allergy, Asthma, and Immunology
Lynda J. Patterson, CAE, Associate Executive Vice President
611 E Wells Street
Milwaukee, WI 53202-3889
414 272-6071
414 272-6070 (Fax)
lpatterson@aaaai.org (E-mail)
Internet address: www.aaaai.org
Society E-mail address:
info@aaaai.org

American Academy of Child and Adolescent Psychiatry
Virginia Q. Anthony, Executive Director
3615 Wisconsin Avenue NW
Washington, DC 20016
202 966-7300
202 966-2037 (Fax)
vqanthony@aacap.org (E-mail)
Internet address: www.aacap.org

American Academy of Cosmetic Surgery
Jeff Knezovich, Executive Vice President
737 N Michigan Avenue,
Suite 820
Chicago, IL 60611
312 981-6760
312 981-6687 (Fax)
jknezovich@cosmeticsurgery.org (E-mail)
Society E-mail address:
infor@cosmeticsurgery.org

American Academy of Dermatology
Tim Conway, Executive Director
930 N Meacham Road
Schaumburg, IL 60173-4965
847 240-1002
847 330-1123 (Fax)
tconway@aad.org (E-mail)
Internet address: www.aad.org

American Academy of Facial Plastic and Reconstructive Surgery
Stephen C. Duffy, Executive Vice President
310 S Henry Street
Alexandria, VA 22314
703 299-9291
703 299-8284 (Fax)
scduffy@aafprs.org (E-mail)
Internet address: www.aafprs.org
Society E-mail address:
mail@aafprs.org

American Academy of Family Physicians
Douglas Henley, MD, Executive Vice President
11400 Tomahawk Creek Parkway
Leawood, KS 66211
800 274-2237 x5100
913 906-6000 (Fax)
dhenley@aafp.org (E-mail)
Internet address: www.aafp.org

American Academy of Insurance Medicine
Charles Jones, MD, Secretary/Treasurer
ING — Security Life of Denver
1290 Broadway, 15th Floor
Denver, CO 80203
303 860-2049
303 813-2049 (Fax)
charles_jones@mindspring.com (E-mail)
Internet address:
www.aaimedicine.org

American Academy of Neurology
Catherine Rydell, Executive Director
1080 Montreal Avenue
St Paul, MN 55116-2325
651 695-1940
651 695-2791 (Fax)
crydell@aan.com (E-mail)
Internet address: www.aan.com

American Academy of Ophthalmology
H. Dunbar Hoskins, Jr, MD, Executive Vice President
655 Beach Street
San Francisco, CA 94109-7424
415 561-8500
415 561-8526 (Fax)
dhoskins@aao.org (E-mail)
Internet address: www.eyenet.org

American Academy of Orthopaedic Surgeons
William W. Tipton, Jr, MD, Executive Vice President
6300 N River Road
Rosemont, IL 60018-4262
847 823-7186
847 823-7208 (Fax)
tipton@aaos.org (E-mail)
Internet address: www.aaos.org

American Academy of Otolaryngic Allergy
Jami Lucas, Executive Director
1990 M Street, NW, Suite 680
Washington, DC 20036
202 955-5010
202 955-5016 (Fax)
Internet address:
www.allergy-ent.org
Society E-mail address:
aaoa@aaoaf.org

American Academy of Otolaryngology — Head and Neck Surgery, Inc
G. Holt, MD, MPH, Executive Vice President
1 Prince Street
Alexandria, VA 22314-3357
703 836-4444
703 519-1553 (Fax)
grholt@entnet.org (E-mail)
Internet address: www.entnet.org

American Academy of Pain Medicine
Jeffrey W. Engle, CMP, Executive Director
4700 W Lake Avenue
Glenview, IL 60025-1485
847 375-4731
847 375-6331 (Fax)
Internet address:
www.painmed.org
Society E-mail address:
aapm@amctec.com

American Academy of Pediatrics
Joe M. Sanders, Jr, MD, Executive Director
141 NW Point Boulevard
Elk Grove Village, IL 60007
847 228-5005
847 228-5027 (Fax)
jsanders@aap.org (E-mail)
Internet address: www.aap.org

American Academy of Physical Medicine and Rehabilitation
Ronald A. Henrichs, CAE, Executive Director
One IBM Plaza, Suite 2500
Chicago, IL 60611-3604
312 464-9700
312 464-0227 (Fax)
rhenrichs@aapmr.org (E-mail)
Internet address: www.aapmr.org

American Academy of Sleep Medicine
Jerome Barrett, Executive Director
6301 Bandel Road, Suite 101
Rochester, MN 55901
507 287-6006
507 287-6008 (Fax)
jbarrett@aasmnet.org (E-mail)
Internet address:
www.aasmnet.org

American Association for Thoracic Surgery
William T. Maloney, Executive Director
13 Elm Street
Manchester, MA 01944
978 526-8330
978 526-4018 (Fax)
Internet address: www.aats.org
Society E-mail address:
aats@prri.com

American Association for Vascular Surgery
David Cloud, Executive Director
13 Elm Street
Manchester, MA 01944-1314
978 526-8330
978 526-4018 (Fax)
Internet address:
www.vascsurg.org

American Association of Clinical Endocrinologists
Donald Jones, CEO
1000 Riverside Avenue, Suite 205
Jacksonville, FL 32204
904 353-7878
904 353-8185 (Fax)
Society E-mail address:
info@aace.com
Internet address: www.aace.com

American Association of Clinical Urologists, Inc
Wendy J. Weiser, Executive Director
1111 N Plaza Drive, Suite 550
Schaumburg, IL 60173-4950
847 517-1050
847 517-7229 (Fax)
Wendy@WJWEISER.com (E-mail)

American Association of Electrodiagnostic Medicine
Shirlyn A. Adkins, JD, Executive Director
421 First Avenue SW, Suite 300 East
Rochester, MN 55902
507 288-0100
507 288-1225 (Fax)
Internet address: www.aaem.net
Society E-mail address:
aaem@aaem.net

American Association of Gynecologic Laparoscopists
Linda Michels, Executive Director
13021 E Florence Avenue
Santa Fe Springs, CA 90670
800 554-2245
562 946-0073 (Fax)
lmichels@aagl.com (E-mail)
Internet address: www.aagl.com

American Association of Hip and Knee Surgeons
Julie Kahlfeldt, Executive Director
6300 N. River Road, Suite 727
Rosemont, IL 60018-4226
847-384-4216
847-823-4921 (Fax)
kahlfeldt@aaos.org

American Association of Neurological Surgeons
Tom Marshall, Executive Director
5550 Meadowbrook Drive
Rolling Meadows, IL 60008
847 378-0500
847 378-0647 (Fax)
Internet address: www.aans.org

American Association of Plastic Surgeons
Thomas F. Fise, Executive Secretary
4900B South 31st Street
Arlington, VA 22206-1656
703 820-7400
703 931-4520 (Fax)
cd005258@mindspring.com (E-mail)
Internet address:
www.aaps1921.org

American Association of Public Health Physicians
Shri Deep, MD, Acting Executive Manager
AAPHP - PMB 1720
PO Box 2430
Pensacola, FL 32513-2430
412-422-9351
630 604-3256 (Fax)
aaphp@iname.com (E-mail)
Internet address: www.aaphp.org

American Clinical Neurophysiology Society
Jacquelyn T. Coleman, CAE, Executive Director
PO Box 30, 1 Regency Drive
Bloomfield, CT 06002
860 243-3977
860 286-0787 (Fax)
jcoleman@acns.org (E-mail)
Internet address: www.acns.org

American College of Allergy, Asthma, and Immunology
James R. Slawny, Executive Director
85 W Algonquin Road, Suite 550
Arlington Heights, IL 60005
847 427-1200
847 427-1294 (Fax)
jamesslawny@acaai.org
Internet address: www.allergy.mcg.edu
Society E-mail address: mail@acaai.org

American College of Cardiology
Christine W. McEntee, Executive Vice President
9111 Old Georgetown Road
Bethesda, MD 20814
301 897-2691
301 897-9745 (Fax)
cmcentee@acc.org (E-mail)
Internet address: www.acc.org
Society E-mail address: exec@acc.org

American College of Chest Physicians
Alvin Lever, Executive Vice President and CEO
3300 Dundee Road
Northbrook, IL 60062-2348
847 498-8300
847 498-5460 (Fax)
alever@chestnet.org (E-mail)
Internet address: www.chestnet.org

American College of Emergency Physicians
Colin C. Rorrie, Jr, PhD, CAE, Executive Director
PO Box 619911
Dallas, TX 75261-9911
972 550-0911
972 580-2816 (Fax)
crorrie@acep.org (E-mail)
Internet address: www.acep.org

American College of Gastroenterology
Thomas F. Fise, Executive Director
4900B S 31st Street
Arlington, VA 22206-1656
703 820-7400
703 931-4520 (Fax)
Internet address: www.acg.gi.org

American College of Medical Genetics
Michael Watson, PhD, Executive Director
9650 Rockville Pike
Bethesda, MD 20814-3998
301 530-7127
301 571-1895 (Fax)
Internet address: www.faseb.org/genetics/acmg

American College of Medical Quality
Bridget J. Brodie, Executive Vice President
4334 Montgomery Avenue, 2nd Floor
Bethesda, MD 20814
301 913-9149
301 913-9142 (Fax)
Internet address: www.acmq.org
Society E-mail address: acmq@aol.com

American College of Nuclear Medicine
Robert Powell, Executive Director
PO Box 175
Landisville, PA 17538-0175
717 898-5008
717 898-2555 (Fax)
Rpowell2248@aol.com (E-mail)
Internet address: www.acnucmed.org

American College of Nuclear Physicians
William Bertera, Executive Director
1850 Samuel Morse Drive
Reston, VA 20190
703 708-9000, Ext. 1240
703 708-9015 (Fax)
Wbertera@snm.org (E-mail)
Internet address: www.acnp.com

American College of Obstetricians and Gynecologists
Ralph W. Hale, MD, Executive Vice President
409 12th Street SW
Washington, DC 20024-2188
202 863-2525
202 863-1643 (Fax)
rhale@acog.org (E-mail)
Internet address: www.acog.org

American College of Occupational and Environmental Medicine
Barry Eisenberg, Executive Director
1114 N Arlington Heights Road
Arlington Heights, IL 60004-4770
847 818-1800
847 818-9289 (Fax)
Internet address: www.acoem.org

American College of Physician Executives
Roger S. Schenke, Executive Vice President
4890 W Kennedy Boulevard, Suite 200
Tampa, FL 33609
813 287-2000
813 287-8993 (Fax)
rschenke@acpe.org (E-mail)
Internet address: www.acpe.org

American College of Physicians/American Society of Internal Medicine
Walter J. McDonald, MD, FACP, Executive Vice President
190 N Independence Mall West
Philadelphia, PA 19106-1572
215 351-2800
215 351-2829 (Fax)
wmcdonald@mail.acponline.org (E-mail)
Internet address: www.acponline.org

American College of Preventive Medicine
Jordan H. Richland, MPA, Executive Director
1307 New York Avenue, NW, Ste. 200
Washington, DC 20035
202 466-2044
202 466-2662 (Fax)
jhr@acpm.org (E-mail)
Internet address: www.acpm.org
Society E-mail address: info@acpm.org

American College of Radiation Oncology
Catherine Carey, Executive Director
820 Jorie Boulevard
Oak Brook, IL 60521
630 368-7896
630 571-7837 (Fax)
carey@rsna.org (E-mail)
Internet address: www.acro.org

American College of Radiology
John J. Curry, Executive Director
1891 Preston White Drive
Reston, VA 20191-4397
703 648-8902
800 832-9227 (Fax)
johnc@acr.org (E-mail)
Internet address: www.acr.org

American College of Rheumatology
Mark Andrejeski, Executive Vice President
1800 Century Place, Suite 250
Atlanta, GA 30345
404 633-3777
404 633-1870 (Fax)
mandrejeski@rheumatology.org (E-mail)
Internet address: www.rheumatology.org
Society E-mail address: acr@rheumatology.org

American College of Surgeons
Thomas Russell, MD, Executive Director
633 N St Clair Street
Chicago, IL 60611-3211
312 202-5000
312 202-5001 (Fax)
trussell@facs.org (E-mail)
Internet address: www.facs.org

American Gastroenterological Association
Robert B. Greenberg, JD, Executive Vice President
7910 Woodmont Avenue, Suite 700
Bethesda, MD 20814
301 654-2055
301 654-5920 (Fax)
rgreenberg@gastro.org (E-mail)
Internet address: www.gastro.org

American Geriatrics Society
Linda H. Barondess, Executive Vice President
Empire State Building
350 Fifth Avenue, Suite 801
New York, NY 10118
212 308-1414
212 832-8646 (Fax)
Internet address:
 www.americangeriatrics.org
Society E-mail address:
 info.amger@
 americangeriatrics.org

American Institute of Ultrasound in Medicine
Carmine M. Valente, PhD, CAE, Executive Director
14750 Sweitzer Lane, Suite 100
Laurel, MD 20707-5906
301 498-4100
301 498-4450 (Fax)
cvalente@aium.org (E-mail)
Internet address: www.aium.org

American Medical Directors Association
Lorraine Tarnove, Executive Director
10480 Little Patuxent Parkway, Suite 760
Columbia, MD 21044
410 740-9743
410 740-4572 (Fax)
ltarnove@amda.org (E-mail)
Internet address: www.amda.com

American Medical Group Association
Donald W. Fisher, PhD, Chief Executive Officer
1422 Duke Street
Alexandria, VA 22314-3430
703 838-0033
703 548-1890 (Fax)
dfisher@amga.org (E-mail)
Internet address:
 www.amga.org/amga

American Medical Women's Association
Eileen McGrath, JD, Executive Director
801 N Fairfax Street, Suite 400
Alexandria, VA 22314
703 838-0500
703 549-3864 (Fax)
emcgrath@amwa-doc.org (E-mail)
Internet address:
 www.amwa-doc.org
Society E-mail address:
 info@amwa-doc.org

American Orthopaedic Association
Thomas Stautzenbach, Executive Director
6300 N River Road, Suite 505
Rosemont, IL 60018-4263
847 318-7330
847 318-7339 (Fax)
stautzenbach@aoassn.org (E-mail)
Internet address: www.aoassn.org

American Orthopaedic Foot and Ankle Society
Richard Cantrall, Executive Director
2517 Eastlake Avenue, East, Ste. 200
Seattle, WA 98102
206 223-1120
206 223-1178 (Fax)
Website: aofas@aofas.org

American Osteopathic Association
John B. Crosby, JD, Executive Director
142 E Ontario Street
Chicago, IL 60611
312 202-8001
312 202-8208 (Fax)
jcrosby@aoa-net.org (E-mail)
Internet address:
 www.aoa-net.org

American Pediatric Surgical Association
Robert Arensman, Secretary
Children's Memorial Hospital
2300 Children's Plaza #115
Chicago, IL 60614
773-880-4340
773-880-8383 (Fax)
rarensman@
 childrensmemorial.org (E-mail)
Internet address:
 www.ped-surg.org

American Psychiatric Association
Steve Mirin, MD, Medical Director
1400 K Street NW
Washington, DC 20005
202 682-6833
202 682-6353 (Fax)
smirin@psych.org (E-mail)
Internet address: www.psych.org

American Roentgen Ray Society
Susan Cappitelli, Executive Director
44211 Slatestone Court
Leesburg, VA 20176
703 729-3353
703 729-4839 (Fax)
Website: www.arrs.org

American Society for Aesthetic Plastic Surgery, Inc.
Robert Stanton, Executive Director
11081 Winners Circle, Suite 200
Los Alamitos, CA 90720-2813
562 799-2356
562 799-1098 (Fax)
bob@surgery.org (E-mail)
Internet address:
 www.surgery.org

American Society for Dermatologic Surgery, Inc
Katherine Svedman, Executive Director
930 N Meacham Road
Schaumburg, IL 60173-6016
847 249-1429
847 330-1135 (Fax)
Internet address:
 www.asds_net.org

American Society for Gastrointestinal Endoscopy
David Cloud, Executive Director
13 Elm Street
Manchester, MA 01944-1314
978 526-8330
978 526-4018 (Fax)
Internet address: www.asge.org
Society E-mail address:
 asge@shore.net

American Society for Reproductive Medicine
J. Benjamin Younger, MD, Executive Director
1209 Montgomery Highway
Birmingham, AL 35216-2809
205 978-5000
205 978-5005 (Fax)
younger@asrm.org (E-mail)
Internet address: www.asrm.org
Society E-mail address:
 asrm@asrm.org

American Society for Surgery of the Hand
Mark Anderson, Executive Director
6300 N River Road, Suite 600
Rosemont, IL 60018-4256
847 384-8300
847 384-1435 (Fax)
manderson@hand-surg.com (E-mail)
Internet address:
 www.hand-surg.org
Society E-mail address:
 info@hand-surg.com

American Society for Therapeutic Radiology and Oncology
Frank J. Malouff, Executive Director
12500 Fair Lakes Circle, Suite 375
Fairfax, VA 22033-3882
703 502-1550
703 502-7852 (Fax)
frankm@astro.org (E-mail)
Internet address: www.astro.org

American Society of Abdominal Surgeons
Louis F. Alfano, MD, Executive Secretary
675 Main Street
Melrose, MA 02176-3195
781 665-6102
781 665-4127 (Fax)
Internet address:
 www.abdominalsurg.org
Society E-mail address:
 office@abdominalsurg.org

American Society of Addiction Medicine
James Callahan, PhD, DPA, Executive Vice President
4601 N Park Avenue, Upper Arcade, #101
Chevy Chase, MD 20815-4520
301 656-3920
301 656-3815 (Fax)
jcall@asam.org (E-mail)
Internet address: www.asam.org
Society E-mail address:
 email@asam.org

American Society of Anesthesiologists
Glenn W. Johnson, Executive Director
520 N Northwest Highway
Park Ridge, IL 60068-2573
847 825-5586
847 825-1692 (Fax)
g.johnson@ASAhq.org (E-mail)

Internet address: www.asahq.org
Society E-mail address:
mail@asahq.org

American Society of Bariatric Physicians
Beth Little, Interim Executive Director
5453 E Evans Place
Denver, CO 80222-5234
303-770-2526 (X14)
303-779-4834 (Fax)

American Society of Cataract and Refractive Surgery
David Karcher, Executive Director
4000 Legato Road, Suite 850
Fairfax, VA 22033
703 591-2220
703 591-0614 (Fax)
dkarcher@ascrs.org (E-mail)
Internet address: www.ascrs.org
Society E-mail address:
Ascrs@ascrs.org

American Society of Clinical Oncology
Charles Balch, MD, Executive Vice President/CEO
1900 Duke Street, Ste. 200
Alexandria, VA 22314
703 299-0180
703 299-1044 (Fax)
balchc@asco.org (E-mail)
Internet address: www.asco.org
Society E-mail address:
info@asco.org

American Society of Clinical Pathologists
Anna Graham, MD, Interim Executive Vice President
2100 W Harrison Street, Suite 313N
Chicago, IL 60612-3798
312 738-1336 Ext 4885
312 738-9798 (Fax)
Society E-mail address:
info@ascp.org
Internet address: www.ascp.org

American Society of Colon and Rectal Surgeons
James R. Slawny, Executive Director
85 W Algonquin Road, Suite 550
Arlington Heights, IL 60005
847 290-9184
847 290-9203 (Fax)
jamesslawny@acaai.org (E-mail)
Internet address: www.fascrs.org
Society E-mail address:
ascrs@aol.org

American Society of Cytopathology
Elizabeth Jenkins, Executive Administrator
400 W 9th Street, Suite 201
Wilmington, DE 19801
302 429-8802
302 429-8807 (Fax)
Internet address:
www.cytopathology.org
Society E-mail address:
asc@cytopathology.org

American Society of General Surgeons
L. Jack Carow III, Executive Director
2122 Grove
Glenview, IL 60025
847 998-4570
847 998-4577 (Fax)
Internet address:
www.theasgs.org
Society E-mail address:
asgs-info@theasgs.org

American Society of Hematology
Martha L. Liggett, JD, Executive Director
1900 M Street, NW, Suite 200
Washington, DC 20036
202 776-0544
202 776-0545 (Fax)
martha_liggett@dc.sba.com
Internet address:
www.hematology.org
Society E-mail address:
ash@sba.com

American Society of Maxillofacial Surgeons
Thomas Fise, Executive Director
4900 B South 31st Street
Arlington, VA 22206-1656
703 820-7400
703 931-4520 (Fax)
cd005258@mindspring.org (E-mail)

American Society of Neuroimaging
Linda J. Wilkerson, Executive Director
5841 Cedar Lake Road, Suite 204
Minneapolis, MN 55416
952 545-6291
952 545-6073 (Fax)
jgantenberg@asnr.org (E-mail)
Internet address: www.asna.org

American Society of Neuroradiology
James B. Gantenberg, CHE, Executive Director/CEO
2210 Midwest Road, Suite 207
Oak Brook, IL 60521
630 574-0220 x224
630 574-0661 (Fax)
Website: www.asnr.org

American Society of Ophthalmic Plastic and Reconstructive Surgery, Inc
Barbara Beatty, Executive Director
1133 W Morse Boulevard, #201
Winter Park, FL 32789
407 647-8839
407 629-2502 (Fax)
barbara@crowsegal.com (E-mail)
Internet address: www.asoprs.org

American Society of Plastic and Reconstructive Surgeons, Inc
Lousanne Lofgren, Interim Manangement Team
444 E Algonquin Road
Arlington Heights, IL 60005
847 228-9900, X328
847 228-9131 (Fax)
Website: www.plasticsurgery.org

American Thoracic Society
Carl Booberg, Executive Director
1740 Broadway
New York, NY 10019-4374
212 315-8621
212 315-6498 (Fax)
cbooberg@thoracic.org (E-mail)
Internet address:
www.thoracic.org

American Urological Association
G. James Gallagher, Executive Director
1120 N Charles Street
Baltimore, MD 21201-5559
410 727-1100
410 223-6407 (Fax)
jgallagh@auanet.org (E-mail)
Internet address: www.auanet.org

Association of Military Surgeons of the United States
RADM Frederic G. Sanford, USN MC Ret, Executive Director
9320 Old Georgetown Road
Bethesda, MD 20814-1653
301 897-8800 Ext 11
301 530-5446 (Fax)
freds@amsus.org (E-mail)
Internet address: www.amsus.org
Society E-mail address:
amsus@amsus.org

Association of University Radiologists
Josette Szalko, Account Executive
820 Jorie Boulevard
Oak Brook, IL 60523
630 368-3730
630 571-7837 (Fax)
szalko@rsna.org (E-mail)
Society E-mail address:
aur@rsna.org

Contact Lens Association of Ophthalmogists
John Massare, Director
721 Papwoth Avenue, Suite 206
Metairie, LA 70005
504 835-3937
504 833-5884 (Fax)
jmassare@clao.org (E-mail)
Internet address: www.clao.org
Society E-mail address:
eyes@clao.org

College of American Pathologists
Nikki Norris, Executive Vice President
325 Waukegan Road
Northfield, IL 60093-2750
847 832-7500
847 832-8151 (Fax)
Internet address: www.cap.org

Congress of Neurological Surgeons
Mark N. Hadley, MD, Secretary
10 North Martingale Road, Ste. 190
Schaumburg, IL 60173
847-240-2500
847-240-0804 (Fax)
Website: www.neurosurgery.org

International College of Surgeons-US Section
Nick Rebel, Executive Director
1516 N Lake Shore Drive
Chicago, IL 60610
312 787-6274
312 787-9289 (Fax)
Internet address: www.ics-us.org
Society E-mail address:
icsus@ics-us.org

National Association of Medical Examiners
Michael A. Graham, MD, Secretary Treasurer
1402 S Grand Boulevard, Room C305
St Louis, MO 63104
314 577-8298
314 268-5124 (Fax)
grahamma@slu.edu (E-mail)
Internet address:
www.thename.org
Society E-mail address:
randazdd@slu.edu

National Medical Association
Lorraine Cole, PhD, Executive Director
1012 10th Street NW
Washington, DC 20001
202 347-1895
202 898-2510 (Fax)
dwanda@nmanet.org (E-mail)

North American Spine Society
Eric J. Muehlbauer, BA, Executive Director
22 Calendar Court, 2nd Floor
LaGrange, IL 60525
708 588-8080
708 588-1080 (Fax)
muehlbauer@spine.org (E-mail)
Internet address: www.spine.org

Radiological Society of North America, Inc
Dave Fellers, CAE, Executive Director
820 Jorie Boulevard
Oak Brook, IL 60523
630 571-2670
630 590-7221 (Fax)
Fellers@rsna.org (E-Mail)
Internet address: www.rsna.org

Renal Physicians Association
Dale Singer, MHA, Executive Director
4701 Randolph Road, Suite 102
Rockville, MD 20852
301 468-3515
301 468-3511 (Fax)
dsinger@renalmd.org (E-mail)
Society E-mail address:
Rpa@renalmed.org

Society for Investigative Dermatology
Angela Welsh, Administrative Director
820 W Superior Avenue, Ste 340
Cleveland, OH 44113-1800
216 579-9300
216 579-9333 (Fax)
sid@sidnet.org (E-mail)
Internet address: www.sidnet.org

Society of American Gastrointestinal Endoscopic Surgeons
Sallie Matthews, Executive Director
2716 Ocean Park Boulevard, Suite 3000
Santa Monica, CA 90405
310 314-2404
310 314-2585 (Fax)
sagesmail@aol.com (E-mail)
Internet address: www.sages.org

Society of Cardiovascular and Interventional Radiology
Paul Pomerantz, Executive Director
10201 Lee Highway, Suite 500
Fairfax, VA 22030
703 691-1805
703 691-1855 (Fax)
Internet address: www.scvir.org

Society of Critical Care Medicine
David Martin, Executive Vice President/CEO
701 Lee Street
Des Plaines, IL 60016
847-827-6869
847-827-6886 (Fax)
Internet address: www.sccm.org

Society of Medical Consultants to the Armed Forces
Margo Cabrero, Executive Director
c/o 5 Southern Way
Fredericksburg, VA 22406
301 295-1243
504 361-2589 (Fax)
smcaf@usuhs.mil (E-mail)

Society of Nuclear Medicine
William J. Bertera, Executive Director
1850 Samuel Morse Drive
Reston, VA 20190
703 708-9000 ext 246
703 708-9020 (Fax)
wbertera@snm.org (E-mail)
Internet address: www.snm.org

The Endocrine Society
Scott Hunt, Executive Director
4350 E West Highway, Ste 500
Bethesda, MD 20814-4426
301 941-0200, Ext 205
301 941-0259 (Fax)
shunt@endo-society.org (E-mail)
Internet address:
www.endo-society.org
Society E-mail address:
endostaff@endo-society.org

Society of Thoracic Surgeons
Michael G. Thompson, PhD, Executive Director
401 N Michigan Avenue, 24th Floor
Chicago, IL 60611-4267
312 644-6610
312 527-6635 (Fax)
michael_thompson@SBA.com (E-mail)
Internet address: www.sts.org

The Triological Society
Patrick Brookhouser, MD, Executive Secretary
555 N 30th Street
Omaha, NE 68131
402 498-6666
402 498-6357 (Fax)
binderup@boystown.org (E-mail)
Society E-mail address:
triolog@boystown.org

The Vitreous Society
Gerry Lewis, Administrator
10525 Ford Street, PO Box 1170
Mendocino, CA 95460
707 937-5800
707 937-5809 (Fax)
gerrylewis@aol.com (E-mail)

United States and Canadian Academy of Pathology
Fred Silva, MD, Secretary-Treasurer/Executive Director
3643 Walton Way Extension, Building 6
Augusta, GA 30909
706 733-7550
706 733-8033 (Fax)
iap@uscap.usa.com (E-mail)

Medicare Part B Carriers

Listed below are Medicare Part B carriers according to state. Physicians may need to contact their carrier for more specific information on payment policies and procedures than that provided in the *Physicians' Guide*. Such requests can be made over the telephone using the numbers provided below, although in some instances physicians may find that a written communication provides important documentation if a dispute with a carrier should arise.

The number of insurance companies contracting with Medicare for Part B claims processing has declined over the past few years as a number of companies have chosen not to renew their Medicare contracts. As a result, a single carrier may process claims from a number of different states.

Effective October 1, 1997, all claims processing and other carrier functions performed by Aetna Life Insurance Company will be transferred to other contractors, as indicated below. In addition, carrier services will be split between two contractors in the following states: Alaska, Arizona, Hawaii, Nevada, Oregon, and Washington. Blue Cross and Blue Shield of North Dakota will process physician claims for these states, while other carrier services, including medical review, fraud and abuse, and Medicare secondary payer, will be performed by Transamerica Occidental Life Insurance Company. The Health Insurance Portability and Accountability Act of 1996 allows the separation of payment integrity functions from other carrier services.

Alabama
Blue Cross/Blue Shield
of Alabama
(800) 292-8855
(205) 220-2100
www.cahabcgba.com

Alaska
Noridian Mutual Insurance
Company
Provider # (701) 282-1100
www.noridian.com/medweb

Arizona
Noridian Mutual Insurance
Company
Provider # (701) 282-1100
www.noridian.com/medweb

Arkansas
Arkansas Blue Cross/Blue Shield
A Mutual Insurance Company
(800) 482-5525
Provider # (501) 378-2000
www.tlwhite@arkbluecross.com

California
Tansamerica Occidental Life Ins.
Counties of Los Angeles,
Orange, San Diego, Ventura,
Imperial, San Luis Obispo, and
Santa Barbara
(800) 675-2266
Provider # (866) 502-9054
Rest of state: Natl. Heritage
Ins. Co.
(800) 952-8627
Provider # (530) 634-7000
NHICMEDICARE@EDS.COM

Colorado
Noridian Mutual Insurance
Company
Provider # (701) 282-1100
www.noridian.com/medweb

Connecticut
Blue Cross/Blue Shield of Florida,
Inc.
(877) 847-4992
Provider # (866) 454-9007
www.medicare-link.com

Delaware
Trail Blazer Health Enterprise,
LLC
(800) 444-4606
Provider # (972) 766-6900

District of Columbia
Trail Blazer Health Enterprise,
LLC
(800) 444-4606
Provider # (972) 766-6900

Florida
Blue Cross/Blue Shield of Florida
(877) 847-4992
(866) 454-9007
www.medicare.gov

Georgia
Blue Cross/Blue Shield of
Alabama
(800) 299-8855
Provider # (205) 220-2100
www.cahabagba.com

Hawaii
Noridan Mutual Insurance
Company
Provider # (701) 282-1100
www.noridian.com/medweb

Idaho
Connecticut General Life
Insurance
CIGNA
Provider # (615) 782-4571
www.cigna.com

Illinois
Wisconsin Physicians Services
(800) 642-6930
TDD (800) 535-6152
Provider # (608) 221-4711
Wps00951@madison.tds.net

Indiana
AdminaStar Federal
(800) 622-4792 or
Provider # (317) 841-4400

Iowa
Noridian Mutual Insurance
Provider # (701) 282-1100
www.noridian.com/medweb

Kansas
Blue Cross/Blue Shield
of Kansas
(800) 432-3531
Provider # (785) 291-7000
Bc.medicare@bcbsks.com

Kentucky
AdminaStar Federal, Inc.
(800) 999-7608
Provider # (317) 841-4400
www.AdminaStar.com

Louisiana
Arkansas Blue Cross/Blue Shield
(800) 462-9666
Provider # (501) 378-2000

Maine
National Heritage Insurance Co
(800) 492-0919
Provider # (530) 634-7000
NHICMEDICARE@EDS.COM

Maryland
Trail Blazer Health Enterprise,
LLC
(800) 444-4606
Provider # (972) 766-6900

Massachusetts
National Heritage Insurance Co
(800) 882-1228
Provider # (530) 634-7000
NHICMEDICARE@EDS.COM

Michigan
Wisconsin Physicians Services
(800) 482-4045
Provider # (608) 221-4711
Wps00951@madison.tds.net

Minnesota
Wisconsin Physicians Service
Insurance Corporation
Provider # (608) 221-4711
www.wps00951@madison.tds.net

Mississippi
A Division of Blue Cross/Blue
Shield of Alabama
Provider # (205) 220-2100
www.cahabagba.com

Missouri
Blue Cross/Blue Shield of Kansas
(Western Missouri)
(800) 892-5900
Provider # (785) 291-7000
bc.medicare@bcbsks.com
Arkansas Blue Cross/Blue Shield
A Mutual Insurance Company
(Eastern Missouri)
Provider # (501) 378-2000
bc.medicare@bcbsks.com

Montana
Blue Cross/Blue Shield
of Montana
(800) 332-6146
(406) 442-9968

Nebraska
Blue Cross/Blue Shield of Kansas
(800) 633-1113
Provider # (785) 291-7000
www.bc.medicare@bcbsks.com

Nevada
Noridian Mutual Insurance
  Company
Provider # (701) 282-1100
www.bsbsnd.com/medweb

New Hampshire
National Heritage Insurance Co
(800) 447-1142
Provider # (530) 634-7000
NHICMEDICARE@EDS.COM

New Jersey
Empire Blue Cross and Blue
  Shield
(800) 462-9306
Provider # (914) 248-2852
www.empiremedicareservices.com

New Mexico
Arkansas Blue Cross/Blue Shield
A Mutual Insurance Company
(800) 423-2925
Provider # (501) 378-2000
www.tlwhite@arkbluecross.com

New York
Empire BC/BS: Bronx,
  Columbia, Delaware, Dutchess,
  Greene, Kings, Nassau, New
  York, Orange, Putnam,
  Richmond, Rockland, Suffolk,
  Sullivan, Ulster and
  Westchester
(800) 442-8430
Provider # (914) 248-2852
Group Health Incorporated
(646) 458-6600
Healthnow New York, Inc.
Provider # (716) 887-6900
bcbswny@ix.netcom.com

North Carolina
CIGNA
(800) 672-3071
(615) 782-4445

North Dakota
Noridian Mutual Insurance Co.
Provider # (701) 282-1100
www.noridian.com/medweb

Ohio
Nationwide Mutual Insurance Co
(800) 282-0530 or
(614) 277-0287
Provider # (614) 277-1199
www.nationwide-medicare.com

Oklahoma
Arkansas Blue Cross/Blue Shield
(800) 522-9079
Provider # (501) 378-2000
www.oknmmedicare.com

Oregon
Noridian Mutual Insurance
Provider # (701) 282-1100
www.noridian.com/medweb

Pennsylvania
Pennsylvania Blue Shield
  Highmark, Inc
(800) 382-1275
(800) 452-8086TTY
Provider # (717) 763-3151
hgsa@hgsa.com

Puerto Rico
Triple-S, Inc
(787) 749-4949
(787) 749-4083

Rhode Island
Blue Cross/Blue Shield of Rhode
  Island
(800) 662-5170
(401) 861-2273
401 459-1709
888 239-3356TTY

South Carolina
Blue Cross/Blue Shield
  of South Carolina
Provider # (803) 788-0222

South Dakota
Noridian Mutual Insurance
  Company
Provider # (701) 282-1100
www.noridian.com/medweb

Tennessee
CIGNA Medicare
800 342-8900
Provider # (615) 244-5600
www.cigna.com

Texas
Trail Blazer
800 444-4606
Provider # (972) 766-6900

Utah
Regence Blue Shield of Utah
800 274-2290
801 481-6196
Provider # (801) 333-2000

Vermont
National Heritage Insurance
  Compamy
Provider # (530) 634-7000
NHICMEDICARE@EDS.COM

Virginia
Trail Blazer
800 444-4606
Provider # (972) 766-6900

Washington
Noridian Mutual Insurance
  Company
Provider # (701) 282-1100
www.noridian.com/medweb

West Virginia
Nationwide Mutual Insurance
800 848-0106
800 542-5250TTY

Wisconsin
WPS 800 944-0051
608 221-3330
800 828-2837TTY
Provider # (608) 221-4711
wps00951@madison.tds.net

Wyoming
Noridian Mutual Insurance
  Company
Provider # (701) 282-1100
www.noridian.com/medweb

Centers for Medicare and Medicaid Services (CMS) Regional Offices

In situations where the appropriate medical society liaison or a Medicare carrier is unable to provide adequate information, questions can be directed to the appropriate CMS regional office. This listing provides addresses and phone numbers of the 10 CMS regional offices across the country.

Region I - Boston
Connecticut, Maine, Massachusetts, New Hampshire, Rhode Island, and Vermont
Associate Regional Administrator, HCFA Program Operations, John F. Kennedy Federal Building, Government Center, Room 2325
Boston, MA 02203-0033
617 565-1232

Region II - New York
New Jersey, New York, Puerto Rico and Virgin Islands
Associate Regional Administrator, HCFA Program Operations, 26 Federal Plaza, Room 3811
New York, NY 10278-0063
212 264-3657

Region III - Philadelphia
Delaware, District of Columbia, Maryland, Pennsylvania, Virginia, and West Virginia
Associate Regional Administrator, HCFA Program Operations, Suite 216, The Public Ledger Building, 150 S Independence Mall West, Philadelphia, PA 19106
215 861-4140

Region IV - Atlanta
Alabama, Florida, Georgia, Kentucky, Mississippi, North Carolina, South Carolina, and Tennessee
Associate Regional Administrator, HCFA Program Operations, Atlanta Federal Center, 61 Forsyth Street SW, Suite 4T20, Atlanta, GA 30303-8909
404 562-7200

Region V - Chicago
Indiana, Illinois, Michigan, Minnesota, Ohio, and Wisconsin
Associate Regional Administrator, HCFA Program Operations, 233 N. Michigan Ave., Ste. 600
Chicago, IL 60601
312 886-6432

Region VI - Dallas
Arkansas, Louisiana, Oklahoma, New Mexico, and Texas
Associate Regional Administrator, HCFA Program Operations, 1301 Young Street, 8th Floor
Dallas, TX 75202
214 767-6423

Region VII - Kansas City
Iowa, Kansas, Missouri, and Nebraska
Associate Regional Administrator, HCFA Program Operations, Richard Bolling Federal Building, 601 E 12th Street, Rm 235, Kansas City, MO 64106-2808
816 426-2866

Region VIII - Denver
Colorado, Montana, North Dakota, South Dakota, Wyoming, and Utah
Associate Regional Administrator, HCFA Program Operations, Federal Office Building, 1961 Stout Street, Room 522, Denver, CO 80294-3538
303 844-4024

Region IX - San Francisco
Arizona, California, Nevada, Commonwealth of Northern Mairianas Islands, Guam, Hawaii, and American Samoa
Associate Regional Administrator, HCFA Program Operations, 75 Hawthorne Street, 4th and 5th Floors, San Francisco, CA 94105-3903
415 744-3501

Region X - Seattle
Alaska, Idaho, Oregon, and Washington
Associate Regional Administrator, HCFA Program Operations, 2201 Sixth Avenue, MS/RX-40, Seattle, WA 98121-2500
206 615-2354

Appendix C
Temporary Codes—Splints and Casts

The following temporary Q codes have been established for the supplies used by physicians and other practitioners to create splints and casts used for reduction of fractures and dislocations. Beginning in 2001, the casting supplies were removed from the practice expenses for all HCPCS codes, including the CPT codes for fracture management and for casts and splints. For settings in which CPT codes are used to pay for services which include the provision for a cast or splint, new temporary codes are being established to pay physicians and other practitioners for the supplies used in creating casts. The work and practice expenses involved in the creation of the cast or splint should continue to be coded using the appropriate CPT code. The use of the new temporary codes will replace less specific coding for the casting and splinting supplies.

Payment amounts for splints and casts are currently made in accordance with the reasonable charge payment methodology. The charge data required for calculating these codes does not exist. Therefore, the customary, prevailing, and inflation-indexed charge amounts for 2002 have been gap-filled using payment amounts based on current retail pricing information, and an inflationary index charge. Year 2002 payment for these select items are listed below.

Code	Description	2002 Payment
A4565	Slings	$6.30
Q4001	Cast supplies, body cast adult, with or without head, plaster	$35.89
Q4002	Cast supplies, body cast adult, with or without head, fiberglass	$135.65
Q4003	Cast supplies, application of shoulder cast, adult (11 years +), plaster	$25.78
Q4004	Cast supplies, application of shoulder cast, adult (11 years +), fiberglass	$89.25
Q4005	Cast supplies, long arm cast, adult (11 years +), plaster	$9.50
Q4006	Cast supplies, long arm cast, adult (11 years +), fiberglass	$21.42
Q4007	Cast supplies, long arm cast, pediatric (0-10 years), plaster	$4.76
Q4008	Cast supplies, long arm cast, pediatric (0-10 years), fiberglass	$10.71
Q4009	Cast supplies, short arm cast, adult (11 years +), plaster	$6.34
Q4010	Cast supplies, short arm cast, adult (11 years +), fiberglass	$14.28
Q4011	Cast supplies, short arm cast, pediatric (0-10 years), plaster	$3.17
Q4012	Cast supplies, short arm cast, pediatric (0-10 years), fiberglass	$7.14
Q4013	Cast supplies, gauntlet cast (includes lower forearm and hand), adult (11 years +), plaster	$11.54
Q4014	Cast supplies, gauntlet cast (includes lower forearm and hand), adult (11 years +), fiberglass	$19.48
Q4015	Cast supplies, gauntlet cast (includes lower forearm and hand, pediatric (0-10 years), plaster	$5.77
Q4016	Cast supplies, gauntlet cast (includes lower forearm and hand), pediatric (0-10 years), fiberglass	$9.74
Q4017	Cast supplies, long arm splint, adult (11 years +), plaster	$6.68
Q4018	Cast supplies, long arm splint, adult (11 years +), fiberglass	$10.65
Q4019	Cast supplies, long arm splint, pediatric (0-10 years), plaster	$3.34
Q4020	Cast supplies, long arm splint, pediatric (0-10 years), fiberglass	$5.33
Q4021	Cast supplies, short arm splint, adult (11 years +), plaster	$4.94
Q4022	Cast supplies, short arm splint, adult (11 years +), fiberglass	$8.92
Q4023	Cast supplies, short arm splint, pediatric (0-10 years), plaster	$2.48
Q4024	Cast supplies, short arm splint, pediatric (0-10 years), fiberglass	$4.46
Q4025	Cast supplies, hip spica (one or both legs), adult (11 years +), plaster	$27.72
Q4026	Cast supplies, hip spica (one or both legs), adult (11 years +), fiberglass	$86.53
Q4027	Cast supplies, hip spica (one or both legs), pediatric (0-10 years), plaster	$13.86

Code	Description	2002 Payment
Q4028	Cast supplies, hip spica (one or both legs), pediatric (0-10 years), fiberglass	$43.27
Q4029	Cast supplies, long leg cast, adult (11 years +), plaster	$21.19
Q4030	Cast supplies, long leg cast, adult (11 years +), fiberglass	$55.78
Q4031	Cast supplies, long leg cast, pediatric (0-10 years), plaster	$10.60
Q4032	Cast supplies, long leg cast, pediatric (0-10 years), fiberglass	$27.89
Q4033	Cast supplies, long leg cylinder cast, adult (11 years +), plaster	$19.76
Q4034	Cast supplies, long leg cylinder cast, adult (11 years +), fiberglass	$49.17
Q4035	Cast supplies, long leg cylinder cast, pediatric (0-10 years), plaster	$9.89
Q4036	Cast supplies, long leg cylinder cast, pediatric (0-10 years), fiberglass	$24.59
Q4037	Cast supplies, short leg cast, adult (11 years +), plaster	$12.06
Q4038	Cast supplies, short leg cast, adult (11 years +), fiberglass	$30.21
Q4039	Cast supplies, short leg cast, pediatric (0-10 years), plaster	$6.04
Q4040	Cast supplies, short leg cast, pediatric (0-10 years), fiberglass	$15.11
Q4041	Cast supplies, long leg splint, adult (11 years +), plaster	$14.66
Q4042	Cast supplies, long leg splint, adult (11 years +), fiberglass	$25.03
Q4043	Cast supplies, long leg splint, pediatric (0-10 years), plaster	$7.33
Q4044	Cast supplies, long leg splint, pediatric (0-10 years), fiberglass	$12.52
Q4045	Cast supplies, short leg splint, adult (11 years +), plaster	$8.51
Q4046	Cast supplies, short leg splint, adult (11 years +), fiberglass	$13.69
Q4047	Cast supplies, short leg splint, pediatric (0-10 years), plaster	$4.25
Q4048	Cast supplies, short leg splint, pediatric (0-10 years), fiberglass	$6.85
Q4049	Finger splint, static	$1.55
Q4050	Cast supplies, for unlisted types and material of casts	See Below
Q4051	Splint supplies, miscellaneous (includes thermoplastics, strapping, fasteners, padding and other supplies)	See Below

Codes listed above (except codes Q4050 and Q4051) are only to be used for splints and casts used to reduce a fracture or dislocation. Payment for claims for miscellaneous splints and casts (Q4050 and Q4051) is determined by the carrier based upon their individual consideration for each item.

Codes A4570, A4580, A4590, L2101, L2104, L2122, and L2124 which were previously used for billing of splints and casts were invalid for Medicare use effective July 1, 2001, for carrier processed claims and October 1, 2001, for intermediary processed claims.

To assist the physician and practitioner in the selection of the correct code for the cast and splinting supplies, the following crosswalk provides guidance as to which supply codes are applicable for the various types of casts described by Level I or CPT codes.

Level I	Level II
29000	Q4001 or Q4002
29010	Q4001 or Q4002
29015	Q4001 or Q4002
29020	Q4001 or Q4002
29025	Q4001 or Q4002
29035	Q4001 or Q4002
29040	Q4001 or Q4002
29044	Q4001 or Q4002
29046	Q4001 or Q4002
29049	Q4050
29055	Q4003 or Q4004
29058	Q4003
29065	Q4005 through Q4008
29075	Q4009 through Q4012
29085	Q4013 through Q4016

Level I	Level II
29105	Q4017 through Q4020
29125	Q4021 through Q4024
29126	Q4021 through Q4024
29130	Q4049
29131	Q4051
29305	Q4025 through Q4028
29325	Q4025 through Q4028
29345	Q4029 through Q4032
29355	Q4029 through Q4032
29365	Q4033 through Q4036
29405	Q4037 through Q4040
29425	Q4037 through Q4040
29435	Q4037 through Q4040
29440	Q4050
29445	Q4037 through Q4040
29450	Q4035, Q4036, Q4039, or Q4040
29505	Q4041 through Q4044
29515	Q4045 through Q4048

Index

A

Abuse
  AMA views on, 100
  new legislative initiatives to detect, 99-100
Adjusted historical payment basis. See AHPB
Administrative Subcommittee of RUC, 30
Advisory Committee of RUC, 29
AEP (Annual Election Period), 10
Agency for Health Care Policy Research, 11
AHPB (adjusted historical payment basis), 16
Allergen immunotherapy, codes for, 98
AMA (American Medical Association), 12
  advocacy efforts, 103-104
  and charge-based RVS, 5
  and Medicare, 4
  legislative and regulatory activity, 18-19
  position on fee-for-service, 124
  position on Medicare physician payments, 124
  views on GPCIs, 55
AMA Councils on Medical Service and Legislation, 8
AMA Physician Masterfile, 109
AMA's Center for Health Policy Research, GPCI evaluation by, 56
AMA's CPT coding system, 26
AMA's House of Delegates, 8, 18
AMA's recommendations on Harvard study, 9
AMA/Specialty Society RVS Update Committee (RUC), 29, 73
  Administrative Subcommittee of, 30
  Advisory Committee, 29
  Facilitation Committees of 30
  Practice Expense Advisory Committee of, 30
  Practice Expense Subcommittee of, 30
  Research Subcommittee of, 30
  structure and process of, 29-31
American Association of Retired Persons, 13
American Medical Association. See AMA
American National Standard Institute. See ANSI
Anesthesia services by nonanesthesiologist, 98
Annual Election Period. See AEP
ANSI (American National Standard Institute), 109
Antigen services, 91
Approved amount, 4
Aspen Systems Corporation, 99
Assignment acceptance, 66, 67
Assistants-at-surgery, payment to, 80
Audiologist, codes for, 92

B

Balance bill, 4
Balance billing, 9, 65, 110
  limits on, 14-15
  monitoring by CMS of, 67
Balanced Budget Act of 1997. See BBA of 1997
Balanced Budget Refinement Act of 1999. See BBRA of 1999
BBA (Balanced Budget Act) of 1997, 10, 11, 14, 15, 19, 21, 50, 70, 71, 86, 87, 90, 100, 111
BBRA (Balanced Budget Refinement Act) of 1999, 71, 72
Budget neutrality, 74
  adjustments, 15
Bulletin of the American College of Surgeons, 8
Bundling services, 4

C

CACs (Carrier Advisory Committees), 104
California Medical Association, 4
California Relative Value Studies. See CRVS
Capitation-based system, 4
Carrier Advisory Committees. See CACs
Carrier medical directors. See CMDs
CCPC (Correct Coding Policy Committee), 79
Centers for Medicare and Medicaid Services. See CMS
Certified registered nurse anesthetists, payment for. See CRNAs
Charge-based RVS, 4
  and AMA, 5
Chemotherapy management, separate payment for, 91
Chiropractors, codes for, 91
CLCCP (Comprehensive Limiting Charge Compliance Program), 67
Clinical consultation services, 88
Clinical Laboratory Improvement Act, 89
Clinical laboratory services, 88
  interpretation, 89
Clinical nurse specialist. See CNS
Clinical Practice Expert Panel. See CPEP
Clinical Practice Expert Panel Technical Expert Group. See TEG
Clinical psychologist, payment for, 93
Clinical social workers. See CSWs
CMDs (carrier medical directors), 7, 74
CMS (Centers for Medicare and Medicaid Services), 5, 6, 12, 67, 71
CMS/Aspen clinical examples, 99
CMS-funded RBRVS study, 7
CMS methodology for assigning practice expense RVUs, 36, 39
  SMS data used in, 44

CMS revisions, 20
CMS's Correct Coding Initiative (CCI), 100
CMS's global surgical policy, 77
CNS (clinical nurse specialist), coverage of, 92
Colorectal cancer screening coverage, 101
　reporting and payment, 101
Complications following surgery, 78
Comprehensive Limiting Charge Compliance Program.
　See CLCCP
Consolidated Consulting Group, Inc., 8, 27
Consolidated Omnibus Budget Reconciliation Act of 1985, 6
Consultation by surgeon, 77
Conversion factors, 74
　establishing using RBRVS, 113
Coordinated care plan, 10-11
Copayments, 111
Correct Coding Policy Committee. *See* CCPC
Cost-of-living GPCIs, 54-55
CPEP (Clinical Practice Expert Panel), 40
CPR (customary, prevailing, and reasonable) charges, 2-3, 4
　balance billing under, 13
　geographic variation in, 107
　governmental options for change, 6
　options for change to, 3-4
　problems with, 3
CPR system and RBRVS, 20
CPT (Current Procedural Terminology), 29
CPT 1987, 26
CPT 1992, 26, 28
CPT 1997, 33
CPT 1998, 93, 94
CPT coding system, 26
CPT Editorial Panel, 18, 93, 94, 99
CPT modifiers, 80-84
　modifier -22, 82
　modifier -24, 80
　modifier -25, 80-81, 97, 107
　modifier -26, 89
　modifier -50, 81-82
　modifier -51, 81
　modifier -52, 82
　modifier -53, 81
　modifier -54, 83
　modifier -55, 83
　modifier -56, 83
　modifier -57, 82
　modifier -58, 82
　modifier -59, 81
　modifier -60, 82
　modifier -62, 83-84
　modifier -66, 83-84
　modifier -78, 82
　modifier -79, 82
　modifier -80, 83
　modifier -81, 83
　modifier -82, 83
　multiple, 84
　not affecting payment levels, 84
CPT system, 7
CPT-4 codes, rebundling of, 79
Critical care, codes for, 97
CRNAs (certified registered nurse anesthetists), payment
　　for, 92-93
Cross-specialty process for RVS, 26-27
CRVS (California Relative Value Studies), 4
CSWs (clinical social workers), payment for, 93
Current Procedural Terminology. *See* CPT
Current Procedural Terminology system. *See* CPT system
Customary, prevailing, and reasonable charges.
　　See CPR charges

D

Dear Doctor letter, 66, 110
Deductibles, 111
Diagnosis related groups. *See* DRGs
Diagnostic tests
　criteria for, 86-87
　coverage conditions for, 87
　purchased, 87-88
DME (durable medical equipment), payment for, 89
DME prosthetics, orthotics, supplies. *See* DMEPOS
DME regional carriers. *See* DMERC
DMEPOS (DME prosthetics, orthotics, supplies), 89
DMERC (DME regional carriers), 89
*Documentation Guidelines for Evaluation and Management
　　Services,* 102
DRGs (diagnosis related groups), 3, 5
　hospital system, 4
　physician system, 4
Drugs, Part B coverage of, 90-91
Durable medical equipment. *See* DME

E

Electronic claims processing, 108
Electronic data interchange, 108-110
Electronic formats, standardized, 109
Emergency department services, codes for, 97
Emergency/management (E/M) codes under physician
　　payment schedule
　background of, 93-99
　refinements to, 94
　reporting, 94-95
　reporting issues for, 95-98
Endoscopic procedures, multiple, 79-80
EOMB (Explanation of Medicare Benefits), 67, 100, 110
Evaluating GPCIs, 56
Evaluation and Management Documentation Guidelines,
　　98-99
Expenditure targets, 9
Explanation of Medicare Benefits. *See* EOMB

F
Facilitation Committees of RUC, 30
Federal Hospital Insurance Trust Fund, 100
Federal Register, 7
Federal Register (1998), 92
Federal Trade Commission. *See* FTC
Fee-for-service, AMA position on, 124
Fee-for-service options for Medicare, 6, 8
Fee-for-service payment systems, 4, 9, 10
   in Medicare+Choice plans, 10
   private, 10
   traditional, 10
Fees, discussing with patients, 111
Final Notice (1992), 28, 29, 88
Final Rule (1991), 17, 18, 28, 86, 88, 89
   assistants-at-surgery in, 80
   global surgical package in, 77
   practice expense data used to assign RVUs in, 36
Final Rule (1993), 31
Final Rule (1994), 29, 32
Final Rule (1995), 84, 88, 92, 103
Final Rule (1996), 85
Final Rule (1999), 29, 32, 50
Final Rule (2000), 46, 97, 98
Final Rule (2001), 34
Five-year review by RUC
   recommendations of, 33-34
   scope of, 32-33
Fraud
   AMA views on, 100
   new legislative initiatives to detect, 99-100
FTC (Federal Trade Commission), 4, 5

G
GAF (geographic adjustment factor), 55-56
   payment localities and, 57
GAO (General Accounting Office), 42
GDP (Gross Domestic Product), 71
General Accounting Office. *See* GAO
Geographic adjustment, OBRA 89
   provision for, 53-54
Geographic adjustment factor. *See* GAF
Geographic adjustments for RBRVS, 14
Geographic cost indexes, 14
Geographic payment variations under RBRVS, 107
Geographic practice cost indexes. *See* GPCIs
Glaucoma screening coverage for, 102
Global surgical package
   defining, 77
   under RBRVS, 107
Global surgical period, duration of, 79
Global surgical services, 34-35
GPCI (geographic practice cost indexes), 19, 51, 54-56, 66
   AMA views on, 55
   cost-of-living, 54-55

   PLI, 55
   practice expense, 56
   updating, 75
Gross Domestic Product. *See* GDP

H
Harvard RBRVS study, 4-5, 6-8, 9, 25, 83
   Phase I, 7, 8, 13
   Phase II, 7, 13
   Phase III, 7, 25
   Phase IV, 25
   physician work RVUs in, 77
   review of Phase I, 27-28
   value estimates for services in Phase I, 25
   value estimates for services in Phase II, 25
Harvard University School of Public Health, 5
HCPAC (Health Care Professionals Advisory Committee), 30
HCPAC review board, 30
Health and Human Services. *See* HHS
Health Care Financing Administration, 5
Health Care Fraud and Abuse Control Account, 99
Health Care Professionals Advisory Committee. *See* HCPAC
Health Insurance Portability and Accountability Act of 1996. *See* HIPAA
Health maintenance organization. *See* HMO
Health Professional Shortage Areas. *See* HPSAs
HHS (Health and Human Services), 6, 17
HIPAA (Health Insurance Portability and Accountability Act) of 1996, 99, 108, 109
Historical payment basis for service, 16
HMO (health maintenance organization), Medicare, 3
HMO-based system, 4
HMOs in Medicare+Choice plans, 10
HMOs for Medicare, 6
Home visits, codes for, 95
Hospital DRG system, 4
HPSAs (Health Professional Shortage Areas), 57-58
   criteria for, 57-58

I
Incident-to services, 21
   coverage of, 89-90
Incomplete claims, 108
Initial evaluation by surgeon, 77
Injections, payment for, 90
Intraoperative services by surgeon, 77
Intraservice work, 25-26

J
Journal of the American Medical Association (JAMA), 8

K
Kyl-Archer Bill, *See* Medicare Beneficiary Freedom to Contract Act

L

Law, changes in with OBRA 89, 17-19
LCER (Limiting Charge Exception Report), 67, 110
Legislation, payment policy changes through, 100-102
Legislative activity by AMA, 18-19
Limited license practitioners, payment schedule for, 91
Limiting Charge Exception Report, *See* LCER
Limiting charges under RBRVS, 107
Lock-in of Medicare elections, 10
LOCM (nonionic contrast material), 86

M

MAACs (maximum allowable actual charges), 13, 14, 66, 110
Major surgical procedures, 7
Malpractice GPCI, 55
Mammography screening coverage, 100-101
Mandatory assignment, 4, 9
Manual Therapy Techniques Workgroup, 92
Maximum allowable actual charges. *See* MAAC
Medical Economic Index, 51
Medical nutrition therapy. *See* MNT
Medical Savings Account. *See* MSA
Medicare
  HMOs for, 6
  nonparticipation in, 110-111
  participation in, 110
Medicare approved amount, 4
Medicare Beneficiary Freedom to Contract Act, 112
Medicare bonus payment for HPSAs, 57-58
Medicare carriers, 3
Medicare conversion factor updates, 70-73
Medicare Economic Index. *See* MEI
Medicare HMO, 20
Medicare Part A, 20
Medicare Part B, 2, 8, 20-21, 84
  claims, 3
  clinical laboratory services and, 88
  expenditures, 5
Medicare Part C, 10
Medicare Participating Physician/Supplier Agreement, 66, 110
Medicare Payment Advisory Commission. *See* MedPAC
Medicare payment localities, 56-58
  AMA views on, 57
  payment impacts on new, 57
Medicare payment schedule, 59-64
  formula for calculating, 59-60
Medicare payment system
  calculating for nonparticipating physicians, 63-64
  determining impact on individual physician practices, 61-62
Medicare payments, increased PLI expenses reflected in, 51

Medicare physician payment, 2
  AMA position on, 124
Medicare physician payment system, 9
  prescription for changing, 12
Medicare Preservation and Restoration Act, 112
Medicare proposed practice expense methodology
  legislation revising, 42
  opposition to, 41-42
Medicare RBRVS, 2, 52
  payment system, 66
Medicare RVS (1992) refinement process, 28-29
Medicare Volume Performance Standard. *See* MVPS
Medicare+Choice, 10-11
Medigap, 66, 108
MedPAC (Medicare Payment Advisory Commission), 11, 50
  recommendations to revise SGR, 72
MEI (Medicare Economic Index), 3, 5, 15, 70
  changes measured by, 70
MFS (Model Fee Schedule), 17
Microcosting, 40
Minor surgery, 79-80
MNT (medical nutrition therapy) 93, 102
  coverage of, 102
Model Fee Schedule. *See* MFS
MSA (Medical Savings Account)
  demonstration project, 11
  in Medicare+Choice plans, 10
MVPS (Medicare Volume Performance Standard), 13, 15, 70
  conversion factor updates before 1998, 71
  update process, 9

N

National Bipartisan Commission on the Future of Medicare, 11
National payer identifier. *See* PAYERID
National provider identifier. *See* NPI
National Standard Format, 109
National standard RBRVS, establishing fees through, 112
National Study of Resource-Based Relative Value Scales for Physician Services, Harvard, 5
National survey of physician work, 26
New England Journal of Medicine, 8
Nonincisional procedures, 79-80
Nonionic contrast material. *See* LOCM
Nonparticipation in Medicare, 110-111
Nonphysicians, payment for, 91-93
Notice of Proposed Rule Making. See NPRM
NPI (national provider identifier), 109
NPRM (Notice of Proposed Rule Making), 17, 28
  AMA's position on, 17-18
NPs (nurse practitioners), coverage of, 92
Nurse midwives, payment for, 93
Nurse practitioners. *See* NPs

O

OBRA (Omnibus Budget Reconciliation Act) 86, 7
OBRA 89, 12-17, 19, 29, 59, 71
   physician payment reform provisions, 13
   provision for geographic adjustment, 53-54
   transition methods, 16
OBRA 89 method of assigning practice expense RVUs, 36, 39
   concerns with, 39-40
   revisions to, 40
OBRA 90, 17, 75
   five-year review required by, 32-35
   RUC's role in review, 32
OBRA 93, 9, 17, 19, 70, 71
Observation Care Services, codes for, 98
Occupational therapists, codes for, 92
OEP (Open Enrollment Period), 10
Office management practices, evaluation of, 107-108
Office of Technology Assessment, 6
Ohio Medicine, 8
Omnibus Budget Reconciliation Act. *See* OBRA
Open Enrollment Period. *See* OEP
Outlier, 5

P

Packaging services, 4
Panel E&M Workgroup, 99
PAR (Physician Participation Program), 4, 65-67
Participating Physician Program, 15
Participation in Medicare, 110
PAs (physician assistants), payment for, 92
Pathology services, 88
PAYERID (national payer identifier), 109
Payment policy changes through legislation, 100-102
Payment policy changes under RBRVS, 102-103
Payment policy indicators, list of, 126
Payment schedule, list of, 126
PEAC (Practice Expense Advisory Committee), 47, 48
   of RUC, 30
Pelvic examination, coverage of, 101
Performance adjustment, 70
Performance standard factor, 71
Phase I Harvard RBRVS study, 7, 13
   AMA policy on, 8-9
   AMA's reaction to, 8
   reaction to completion of, 8-9
   reviews of, 27-28
   value estimates for services in, 25
Phase II Harvard RBRVS study, 7, 13
   value estimates for services in, 25
Phase III Harvard RBRVS study, 7, 25
Phase IV Harvard RBRVS study, 25
Physical therapists, codes for, 92

Physician assistants. *See* PAs
Physician charges, using RBRVS to establish, 112-113
Physician DRG system, 4, 6
Physician Participation Program. *See* PAR
Physician Payment Review Commission. *See* PPRC
Physician Payment Task Force, 8
Physician payment under RBRVS, 106-107
Physician work
   defining, 25-26
   national survey of, 26
Physicians
   payment for new, 84
   payment for provider-based, 84-85
   payment for teaching, 84-85
PLI (professional liability insurance), 9
   relative values, 49
PLI components of RBRVS, adjustment of, 54
PLI GPCI, 55
PLI RVUs
   combining work, practice expense, and, 52
   data used to assign charge based, 49-50
   steps in CMS's calculation of, 50-51
Postoperative consultations by nonsurgeons, 96-97
Postoperative pain management, 78-79
Postoperative services by surgeon, 78
Postservice work, 25-26, 27
PPOs (Preferred Provider Organizations) in Medicare+Choice plans, 10
PPRC (Physician Payment Review Commission), 12, 39, 40, 50, 66, 67, 71
   establishing, 6
   evaluation of Harvard study Phase I, 27
   recommendations on Harvard study, 9
PPS (prospective pricing system), 5
Practice expense, combining work, PLI RVUs, and, 52
Practice Expense Advisory Committee. *See* PEAC
Practice expense GPCIs, 56
Practice Expense Subcommittee of RUC, 30
Practice management audit, 107-108
Practicing Physician Advisory council, 104
Preferred Provider Organizations. *See* (PPOs)
Preoperative medical clearance by primary care physician, 96
Preoperative visits by surgeon, 77
Preservice work, 25-26, 27
Preventive Medicine Services codes, 96
Private contracting, 11
Private contracts with Medicare patients, 111-112
Private fee-for-service plan, 10
Private Health Plan Option, 6
   for Medicare, 6
Professional component modifiers, 85-86
Professional liability insurance. *See* PLI

Prospective Payment Assessment Commission, 11
Prospective pricing, 2
Prospective pricing system. *See* PPS
Provider-based physicians, payment for, 84-85
Provider-sponsored organization. *See* PSO
PSO (provider-sponsored organization), 10
    in Medicare+Choice plans, 10
Psychotherapy, payment for, 98
Pulse oximetry, codes for, 98

R

Radiology services, separate fee schedule for, 85-86
RBRVS (Resource-Based Relative Value Scales), 4
    AMA proposal to develop, 5
    based on Harvard study, 13-14
    coding system in, 26
    establishing fees through national standard, 112
    geographic adjustments for, 14
    government's interest in, 5-6
    payment schedule, 2
    physician payment schedule, 2
    physician payment system and CPR, 20
    physician payment under, 106-107
RBRVS-based physician payment system, 2
RBRVS study, AMA's role in, 7-8
RBRVS survey results, 114-123
    adoption of RBRVS among four payer types, 118-119
    adoption rate of RBRVS, all payers, 115
    characteristics of respondents, 115
    conclusions of survey, 123-124
    conversion factors used, 116, 117-118
    conversion factors used by four payer types, 119
    design of, 114
    factors influencing adoption of RBRVS, 122
    opinion of RBRVS, 121-122
    other uses of RBRVS, 123
    payment policies among four payer types, 120
    product line application of RBRVS, 119
    use of RBRVS among four payer types, 119-121
    use of RBRVS by all payers, 116-118
Reagan administration, 6
Registered dietitians, benefits for, 93
Regulations, changes in with OBRA 89, 17-19
Regulatory activity by AMA, 18-19
Relative value scale. *See* RVS
Relative value unit. *See* RVU
Relative values, updating, 73-74
Research Subcommittee of RUC, 30
Resource-based methodology (1999), 42-44
    steps in, 42-44
Resource-based PLI relative values, 50-52
    BBA and, 50

Resource based practice expense relative values
    refinement of, 46-48
    RUC role in refinement, 47-48
    transition period for, 46
Resource-based practice expenses, 40-46
    developing methodology for, 40-41
Resource-Based Relative Value Scales. *See* RBRVS
Risk-sharing in HMOs, 6
Routine physical exam, 95-96
RUC (RVS Update Committee)
    future plans of, 35
    process to develop relative value recommendations, 30-31
RUC's role in five-year reviews of relative values, 32
RVS (relative value scale), 3, 4
    basis for, 4-5
RVS Update Committee. *See* RUC
RVU (relative value unit), 15
    1992 refinement of evaluation and management codes, 28
    assigning to nonsurveyed services, 27
    list of, 126
    work, 25

S

SGR (sustainable growth rate), 70
    MedPAC recommendations to revise, 72
SGR-BBRA, 72-73
SGR methodology, 11
SGR system, 71-72
    flaws in, 72
SMS (Socioeconomic Monitoring System), AMA's, 41
Social Security Amendments Act of 1994, 32, 108, 110
Socioeconomic Monitoring System. *See* SMS
Special Election Period, 10
Speech-language pathologist, codes for, 92
Standardization of payment schedule, 16-17
Supplemental benefits, 108
Supplies, payment for, 89
Sustainable growth rate. *See* SGR

T

TCGs (Technical Consulting Groups), 7, 25
Teaching physicians, payment for, 84-85
Technical component modifiers, 85-86
Technical Consulting Groups. *See* TCGs
TEG (Clinical Practice Expert Panel Technical Expert Group), 40
Telephone consultations, payment for, 84
Total work period, 26
Travel, payment for, 84

U

UCR (usual, customary, and reasonable) system, 3
Unique Physician Identification Number. *See* UPIN
UPIN (Unique Physician Identification Number), 109
Usual, customary, and reasonable. *See* UCR

V

Vaccinations, coverage of, 90-91
   evaluating the, 56
   impact of revised, 55-56
   variation in the, 55
Ventilator management same day as E/M service, codes for, 98

W

Work, combining practice expense, PLI RVUs, and, 52
Work relative values, updating, 31-32
Work RVUs for Medicare noncovered services, 29

X

X-ray, portable, payment policy for, 86

Comprehensive Coding Resources...
From the Publisher of CPT®

The American Medical Association, the source of CPT codes, offers so many ways to help health care professionals code more accurately and efficiently. Whether you are new to CPT coding or are a veteran coder, stay up-to-date with the CPT references that simplify the coding process.

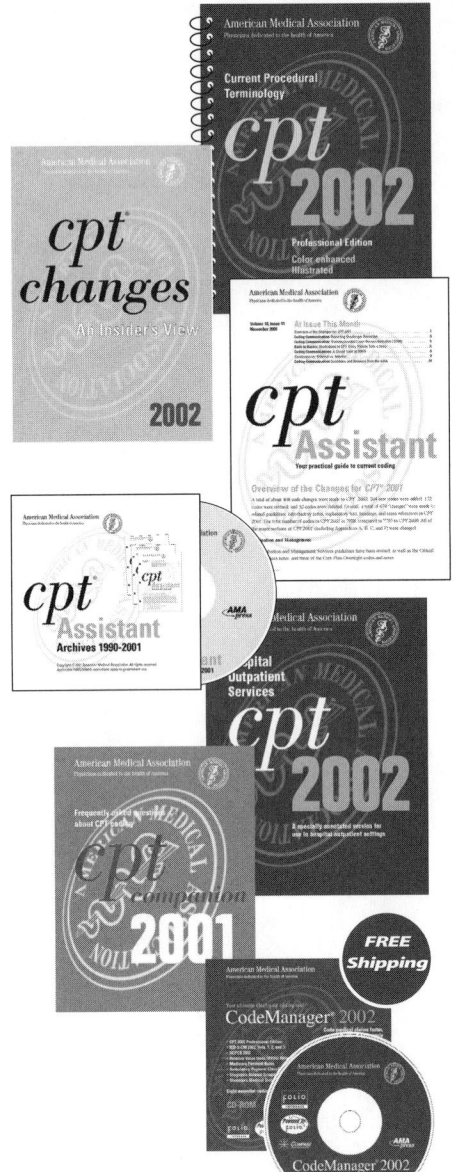

CPT 2002 Professional Edition – The code book designed for the professional coder! The AMA's most comprehensive coding resource in spiral-bound format. Contains more than 700 code changes and the new Category III "Emerging Technology" subsection. Includes illustrations, color-coded keys, and references to the AMA's *CPT Assistant* newsletter and *CPT Changes* publications.
EP054102BMP   Price: $74.95   AMA Member Price: $64.95

CPT Changes 2002: An Insider's View – A reference tool for understanding each of the more than 700 code changes found in CPT 2002. Every new, revised, or deleted code is listed along with a detailed rationale for the change.
OP512902BMP   Price: $49.95   AMA Member Price: $39.95

CPT Assistant – A monthly newsletter that brings you the kind of coding information you need to keep your claims running smoothly. Articles include timely coding information, case studies, clinical vignettes, coding scenarios, and answers to tough coding questions.
CA500900BMP   Price: $169.00 (One-Year)   AMA Member Price: $115.00 (One-Year)

CPT Assistant Archives 1990-2001 – A complete digital library of the AMA's CPT coding newsletter from 1990 through 2001 on one easy-to-use fully searchable CD-ROM. Annual updates are available.
OP510001BMP   Price: $235.00 (Single User)   AMA Member Price: $185.00 (Single User)

CPT 2002 for Hospital Outpatient Services – A specially annotated version of CPT containing the most recent instructional information released by HCFA regarding hospital use of CPT in Medicare.
OP055002BMP   Price: $56.95

CPT Companion – The most comprehensive source of frequently asked questions and answers regarding CPT codes. An excellent source of examples, discussion points, and exam questions for the classroom!
OP083101BMP   Price: $49.95   AMA Member Price: $39.95

CodeManager 2002 – The ultimate coders' resource, providing eight essential coding tools on one CD-ROM. This easy-to-learn software package puts the most up-to-date versions of the most widely used medical coding references at your fingertips. Three updates per year are included to keep you current.
OP081702BMP   Price: $464.00 (Single User)   AMA Member Price: $364.00 (Single User)

Call **800 621-8335** to order or request a catalog of all our coding and reimbursement, practice management, and reference products.
Or visit us online at **www.amapress.org**.

Prices do not include shipping & handling, or state sales tax if applicable. Visa, MasterCard, and Amex/Optima accepted. CPT is a registered trademark of the American Medical Association.

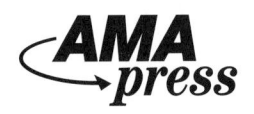

American Medical Association
Physicians dedicated to the health of America

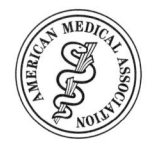

AMA press

CPT Assistant...
your monthly coding advisor

You know how critical it is to have the "hot" coding information first... to receive coding commentaries that give you insight behind confusing coding issues... obtain tips and interpretations that are accurate and reliable and save you time and unnecessary errors in determining the right codes.

CPT Assistant is the only coding newsletter that can offer you the rationale behind the codes. And, only *CPT Assistant* is published by the source of CPT codes – The American Medical Association.

▼ *Practical advice you can use.*
Find articles written by the industry's top coding specialists and the latest information on new codes and how to interpret them.

▼ *Timely articles keep you current.*
Every issue features articles designed to demystify certain codes and give you the latest trends and developments in coding.

▼ *Clinical vignettes.*
Through detailed case studies we'll demonstrate the practical application of codes.

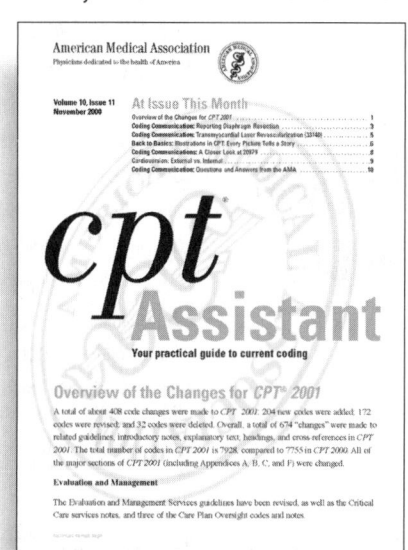

▼ *Coding communication.*
Discover timely information on codes and trends in the industry.

▼ *Questions and answers.* Your direct link to the coding experts at the AMA. Find the answers to the questions professional coders ask most often.

▼ *Anatomical illustrations, charts, and graphs for quick reference.*

CPT Assistant is a must for users of *CPT Professional*. The arrow symbol " ⊃ " found next to various codes in *CPT Professional*, directs you to the exact issue of *CPT Assistant* that contains further information on that code.

Subscribe today and save 15% off your newsletter subscription.
You must mention priority code BMP to receive the discounted price.

Order #: CA500900BMP

Price: ~~$299.00~~ $254.15/two-years
Price: ~~$169.00~~ $143.65/one-year

AMA Member Price: ~~$205.00~~ $174.25/two-year
AMA Member Price: ~~$115.00~~ $97.75/one-year

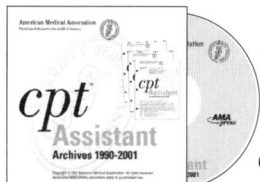

A complete digital library of *CPT Assistant* is available on CD-ROM – from its inception in 1990 through 2001. Just point and click and you're instantly in touch with the actual *CPT Assistant* articles referenced in *CPT Professional*. Coming March 2002.

Order # OP511302BMP (single user) Price: $235.00 AMA Member Price: $185.00

Call 800-621-8335 Today to Order or Order Online at *www.amapress.org*

Prices do not include shipping & handling, or state sales tax if applicable. Visa, MasterCard, and Amex/Optima accepted.
CPT is a registered trademark of the American Medical Association.

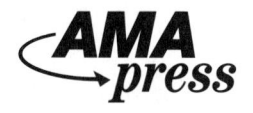

American Medical Association
Physicians dedicated to the health of America

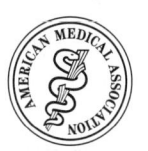

AMA press

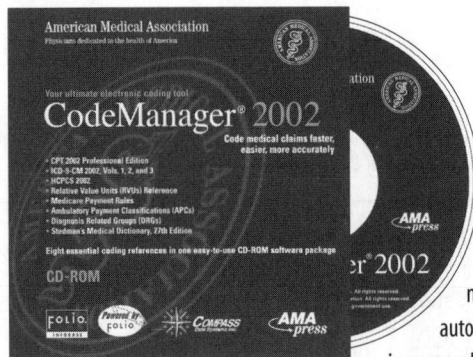

Eight Essential Coding Tools on One CD-ROM

With American Medical Association's *CodeManager*, you can code medical claims more easily and accurately than ever. Just enter a key word or code and all the information you need is right at your fingertips. Full-text descriptions, color-coded symbols and illustrations automatically appear to help you select the code that's most appropriate. And since *CodeManager* is arranged just like the books you've become so familiar with, navigating the system is easy.

This powerful tool gives you:

- The entire text of *CPT Professional 2002*
- *ICD-9-CM 2002*, Volumes 1, 2, and 3
- HCPCS 2002 Level II Codes
- Relative Value Units (RVUs) Reference
- Medicare Payment Rules
- Diagnosis Related Groups (DRGs)
- Ambulatory Payment Classifications (APCs)
- *Stedman's Electronic Medical Dictionary, 27th Edition*

Also included is the entire text of the *National Correct Coding Policy* with comprehensive and component code groupings and mutually exclusive codes, updated quarterly free of charge.

Request your free CD-ROM demo! Call 800-621-8335 and mention NC080902.

Timely updates keep you current

The AMA ensures the information on *CodeManager* remains current throughout the year. In December 2001, you receive the most current CPT and ICD-9-CM codes, DRGs, and *Stedman's Electronic Dictionary* for use during the following year. Then, three quarterly information updates follow to include: *HCPCS 2002*, updated RBRVS RVUs, Medicare Payment Rules, APCs, CMS/Medicare annually updated information, ASC information and National Correct Coding Policy quarterly updates.

Easy-to-install, easy-to-use, and updated regularly, *CodeManager 2002* is your ultimate electronic tool for coding.

1-year subscription (single user) Order#: OP081702BMP
Price: $464.00   AMA Member Price: $364.00

2-year subscription (single user) Order#: OP514802BMP
Price: $703.50   AMA Member Price: $553.50

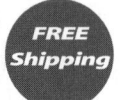

FREE Shipping

Add-on Software Makes CodeManager Even More Powerful!

This software works with or without CodeManager.

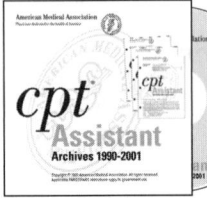

CPT Assistant Archives on CD-ROM 1990-2001

A complete digital library of the AMA's authoritative coding newsletter. Every issue of *CPT Assistant* newsletter – from its inception in 1990 through 2001 on one CD-ROM. Just point and click and your instantly in touch with the actual *CPT Assistant* articles referenced in *CodeManager's CPT Professional* section.

Order#: OP511302BMP (single user)   Price: $235   AMA Member Price: $185

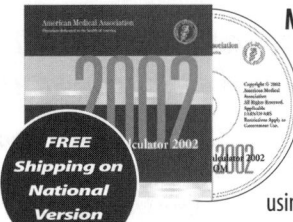

Medicare Fee Calculator CD-ROM 2002

Use your own conversion factor against the RBRVS to display reimbursement amounts for CPT codes for both facility and non-facility, HCPCS codes, and Clinical Lab codes using Physician's, Durable Medical Equipment, and the Clinical Diagnostic Laboratory fee schedules.

Available in local and national versions.

FREE Shipping on National Version

Order#: OP087102BMP (local version, single user)   Price: $95   AMA Member Price: $75
Order#: OP087402BMP (national version, single user)   Price: $254   AMA Member Price: $214

Call for pricing on network versions.

Call 800-621-8335 Today to Order or Order Online at www.amapress.org

Prices do not include shipping & handling, or state sales tax if applicable. Visa, MasterCard, American Express, and Amex/Optima accepted. CPT is a registered trademark of the American Medical Association.

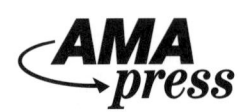

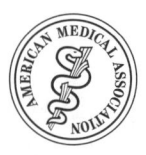

AMA press

American Medical Association
Physicians dedicated to the health of America

Order Your *ICD-9-CM 2002* and *HCPCS 2002* main books from the AMA

AMA Physician ICD-9-CM 2002 Volumes 1 & 2

This best-selling code book provides the most up-to-date information on medical diagnosis coding. Stay current on the new ICD-9-CM code changes that will impact code accuracy and claims submission. Provide your email address when ordering to receive Email Delivered Code Change Special reports. These reports will help you stay current on important code developments and changes.

Spiral Bound Edition
Order #: OP065102BMP
Price: $79.95
AMA Member Price: $69.95

Softbound Edition
Order #: OP065302BMP
Price: $79.95
AMA Member Price: $69.95

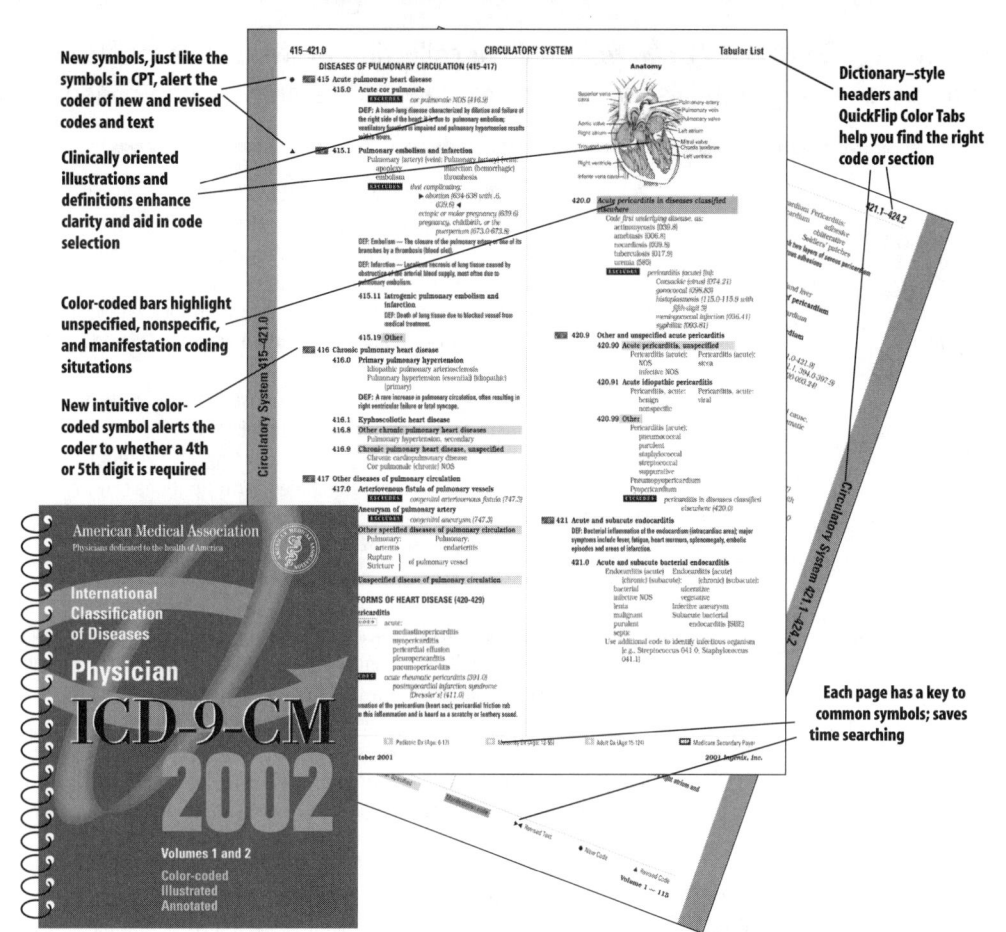

Callouts on sample page:
- New symbols, just like the symbols in CPT, alert the coder of new and revised codes and text
- Clinically oriented illustrations and definitions enhance clarity and aid in code selection
- Color-coded bars highlight unspecified, nonspecific, and manifestation coding situtations
- New intuitive color-coded symbol alerts the coder to whether a 4th or 5th digit is required
- Dictionary–style headers and QuickFlip Color Tabs help you find the right code or section
- Each page has a key to common symbols; saves time searching

AMA HCPCS 2002

Everything You Need From a Single Source.

The AMA's guide to Medicare's National Level II Codes for DME, medical supplies, and drugs. Contains the mandated changes and new codes for 2002.

- Detailed Annotations and Coding Advice make code selection easier and more accurate.
- Enhanced color-coded icons flag codes with special Medicare instructions and coverage issues.
- Modifier Information.
- Improved Medicare Carriers Manual and Coverage Issues Manual Reference.
- Expanded Front Index.
- Payor Appendix.

Softbound
Order #: OP095102BMP   Price: $79.95   AMA Member Price: $69.95

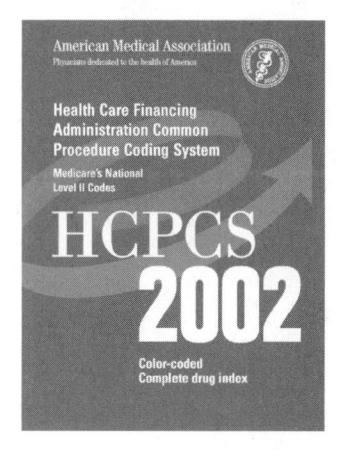

Call 800-621-8335 Today to Order or Order Online at **www.amapress.org**

Prices do not include shipping & handling, or state sales tax if applicable. Visa, MasterCard, and Amex/Optima accepted.
CPT is a registered trademark of the American Medical Association.

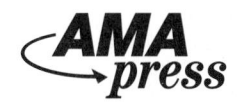

AMA press

American Medical Association
Physicians dedicated to the health of America

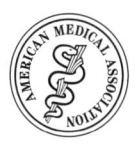

Teach Coding with Confidence
with the AMA's Coding Educational Resources

The *Coding Trainer's Package,* a unique collection of five educational coding resources, is perfect for trainers, coding supervisors, instructors, new coders and veteran coders alike.

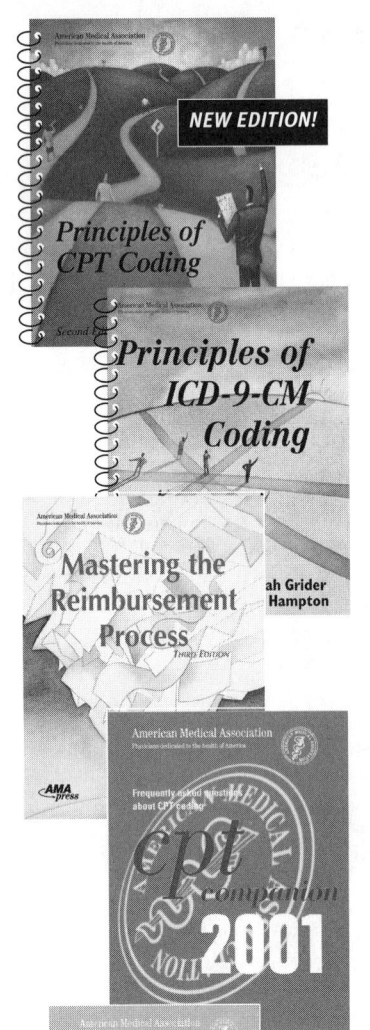

Principles of CPT Coding, Second Edition is a newly revised training and educational tool that covers the basic to intermediate concepts of CPT coding. Chapters include all areas of CPT – from the history and basic coding concepts, to E/M guidelines and medical specialties, to chapters on hospital outpatient reporting and CPT-5. Ample use is made of illustrations, charts and diagrams, coding tips, practical examples and chapter quizzes, all to help facilitate faster learning.
OP501001BMP   Price: $54.95   AMA Member Price: $44.95

Principles of ICD-9-CM Coding is an essential coding textbook designed to help students and professional coders gain a better understanding of ICD-9-CM coding and its relationship to the reimbursement process. *Principles* will help beginning and veteran coders learn how to apply coding conventions, interpret basic coding guidelines for outpatient care, and assign ICD-9-CM codes to the highest level of specificity. Includes chapter learning objectives and section checkpoint exercises, history, coding trivia, tips and clinical examples.
OP065800BMP   Price: $59.95   AMA Member Price: $54.95

Mastering the Reimbursement Process, Third Edition leads the reader to a comprehensive understanding of health insurance, claims submission, and the follow-up necessary to get paid by third-party payers. Revised and updated with 200 new pages, this outstanding text contains significant new material about Medicare program changes, patient confidentiality, sample position descriptions and tips on appeals. Also includes entirely new chapters covering Electronic Data Interchange (EDI), compliance programs and OIG, and privacy, confidentiality and HIPPA.
OP080000BMP   Price: $59.95   AMA Member Price: $54.95

CPT Companion is the most comprehensive source of frequently asked questions and answers regarding CPT codes. Questions are drawn from the volumes of correspondence answered by the AMA each year and the answers have been subjected to careful medical review. An excellent source of examples, discussion points, and exam questions for the classroom!
OP083101BMP   Price: $49.95   AMA Member Price: $39.95

CPT Changes 2002 serves as a reference tool to understanding each of the more than 700 code changes found in *CPT 2002*. Every new, revised and deleted code is listed along with a detailed rationale for the change. References to new, revised and deleted CPT codes, cited in *CPT Changes*, are now included in *CPT Professional*.
OP512902BMP   Price: $49.95   AMA Member Price: $39.95

Order all five with the *Coding Trainer's Package* today and save 15% and more!
Order #: OP506702BMP   Price $224.23   AMA Member Price: $182.58

Call 800 621-8335 or order online at www.amapress.org

Prices do not include shipping & handling, or state sales tax if applicable. Visa, MasterCard, and Amex/Optima accepted. CPT is a registered trademark of the American Medical Association.

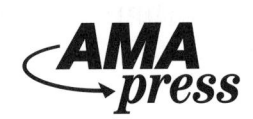

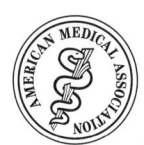

American Medical Association
Physicians dedicated to the health of America

AMA press

Total Health & Safety
for medical practices

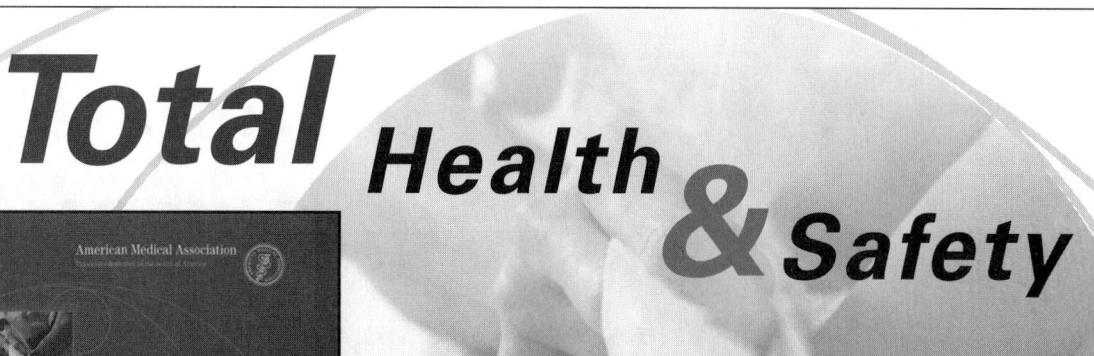

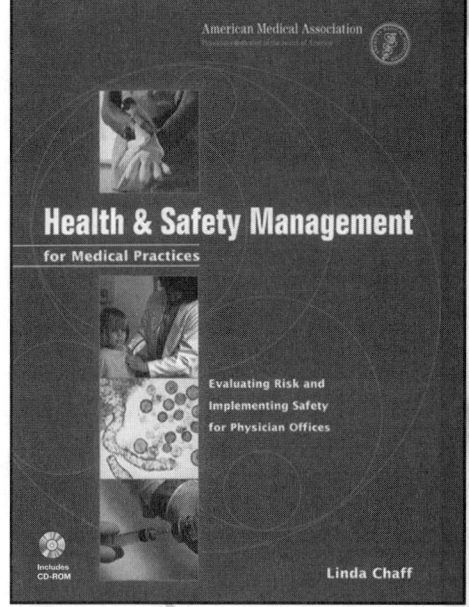

Health care workers are not immune to the threat of occupational injury and illness. Infectious disease transmission, hazardous medical waste, and even carpal tunnel syndrome can make the modern medical practice a dangerous place to work. Medical practitioners need a complete health and safety program to help combat these occupational hazards.

A single-volume reference, *Health and Safety Management for Medical Practices* outlines everything necessary to plan, assess, implement, and maintain a comprehensive safety management program for any physician office practice. It offers concise, authoritative guidance on:

- Setting priorities and preforming a needs assessment
- Developing policies and procedures
- Infection control, personal protective equipment, and ergonomics
- Chemicals, pharmaceuticals, medical equipment, and waste disposal
- Workplace violence, patient safety, and fire prevention

Health and Safety Management for Medical Practices includes guidelines for education and training, creating and using an incident reporting system, as well as the steps necessary for ongoing program evaluation. It also includes a CD-ROM of checklists, training materials, sample policy guidelines, and ready-to-use forms to help practice managers, physician assistants, nurses, and health administration professionals successfully implement their complete health and safety program.

To Order:
Call AMA Press at: 800 621-8335

Visit our secure Web site at:
www.amapress.com

Order #: OP209300BMU
Price: $70.00   AMA member price: $60.00

VISA, MasterCard, American Express and Optima accepted. State sales tax and shipping/handling charges apply. Satisfaction guaranteed or return within 30 days for full refund.

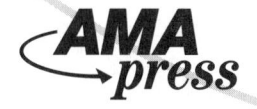

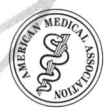

AMA press

American Medical Association
Physicians dedicated to the health of America

Set standards. Achieve results.

Assessing and Improving Practice Operations—A Three Book Series

Essential Support for the "Business" of Your Medical Practice

There's always room for improvement in the operations of any successful medical practice. Assessing and Improving Practice Operations is the ideal resource for the "business" of medicine. Whether you want to build and maintain a professional office staff, implement the highest quality patient contact, or improve your billing systems and procedures, this practical series provides ideal support for strengthening your operations.

This three-book series assists you in identifying opportunities for improvement in the business areas that are critical to a successful medical practice:
- Assessing and Improving Staffing and Organization
- Assessing and Improving Patient Encounters
- Assessing and Improving Billing and Collections

Each volume in this series contains a variety of easy-to-implement evaluation tools and techniques to assess specific practice operations, identify problems, and develop improvement plans. You'll also discover activities to strengthen the physician/administrator team. A convenient diskette of tools and exercises accompanies each book. The Assessing and Improving Practice Operations series provides valuable support for every medical practice.

Order today toll-free!
800 621-8335

...or on the Web, 24/7!
www.ama-assn.org/catalog

Visa, MasterCard, American Express, Optima accepted. Applicable state sales tax and handling added. Satisfaction guaranteed or return within 30 days for a full refund.

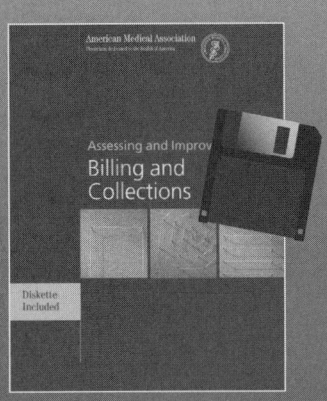

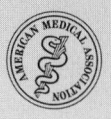

American Medical Association
Physicians dedicated to the health of America

AMA press

Assessing and Improving
Billing and Collections
Order #: OP318600BGB
Price $56.00
AMA Member Price $45.00

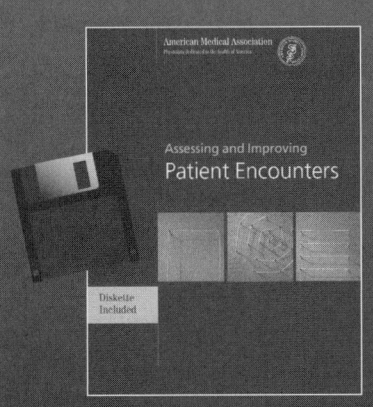

Assessing and Improving
Patient Encounters
Order #: OP318400BGB
Price $56.00
AMA Member Price $45.00

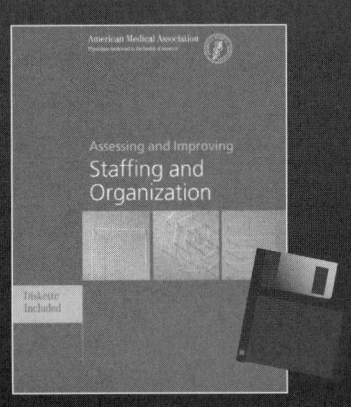

Assessing and Improving Staffing
and Organization
Order #: OP318500BGB
Price $56.00
AMA Member Price $45.00

Assessing and Improving Practice
Operations—A Three Book Series
Order #OP319000BGB
Price $143.00
AMA Member Price $115.00

How to Build Physician Practice Web Sites

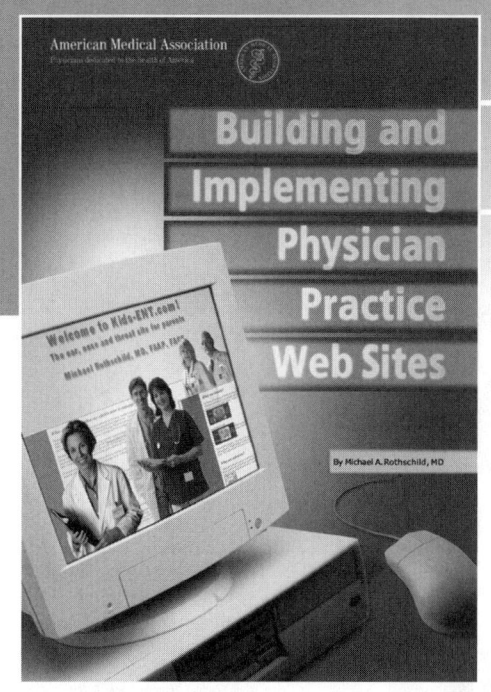

The internet presents incredible opportunities to promote and expand your medical practice. To stay competitive, building a successful web site has become more a necessity than an option. AMA Press now offers all the information you need to create a dynamic, vibrant web site in one valuable resource: *Building and Implementing Physician Practice Web Sites*.

Written by Michael A. Rothschild, MD, an expert in the online marketing of medical practices, this book provides a comprehensive understanding of web site development, including how to:

- Create, design, and post the site
- Avoid common errors in web site creation
- Include the web site as part of an integrated marketing strategy
- Register a domain, and host/promote the site
- Understand the ethical and legal issues regarding "cybermedicine"

To Order:
Call AMA Press at: 800 621-8335
Visit our secure Web site at:
www.amapress.com

Order #: OP318200BMA
Price: $50.00
AMA member price: $45.00

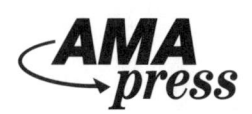

AMA press

VISA, MasterCard, American Express and Optima accepted. State sales tax and shipping/handling charges apply. Satisfaction guaranteed or return within 30 days for full refund.

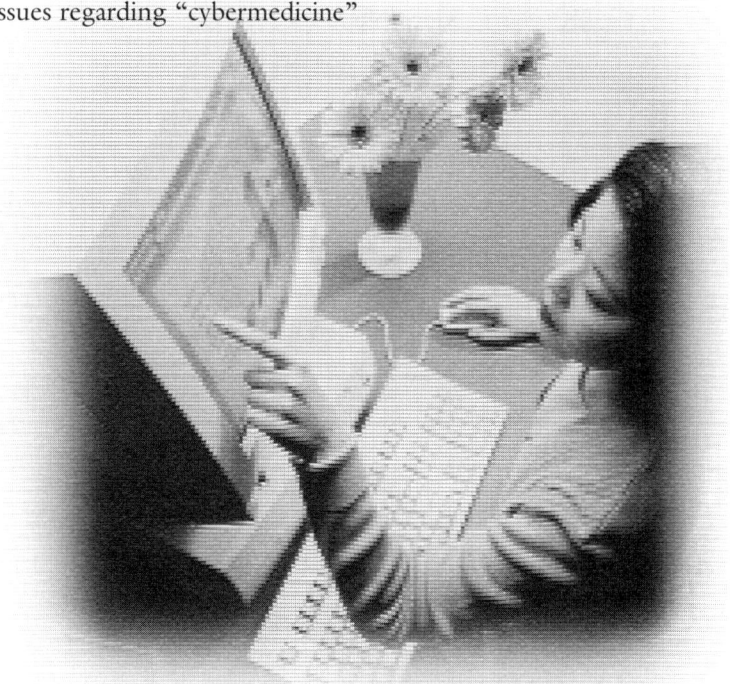

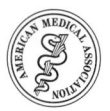

American Medical Association
Physicians dedicated to the health of America

Effective professional correspondence for your practice...

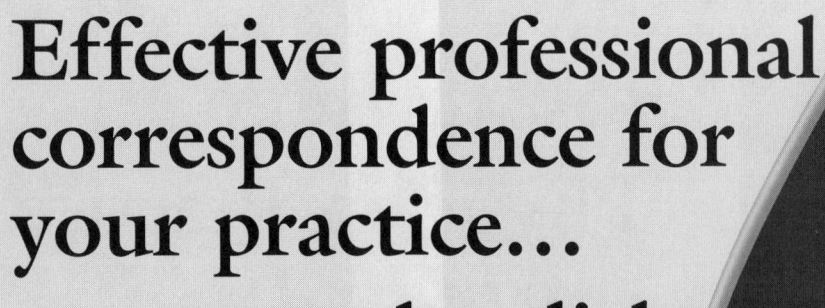

...at the click of a mouse!

Effective communication is critical to running your medical practice, and writing is often the best avenue for communication. Yet, whether you are writing a letter, memorandum or other documents, composing "from scratch" can be a slow and tedious process for busy physicians and their personnel.

The AMA's *Handbook of Physician Office Letters* provides you with an ideal resource for tackling the business and professional writing challenge. This practical and comprehensive resource contains 175 carefully crafted sample letters to patients, suppliers, insurance companies, pharmacists, lawyers and hospitals. Concise models provide "blueprints" for content, tone and format.

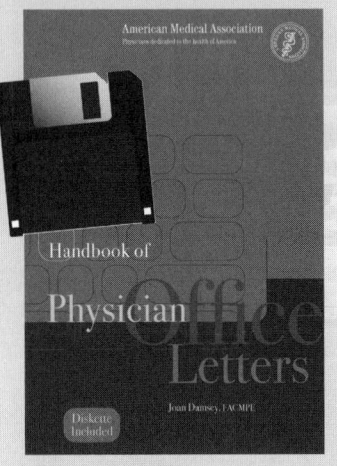

Every letter is also available on a time-saving companion diskette in easy-edit format. *The Handbook of Physician Office Letters* is the medical professional's answer to easy and effective written communication, assisting you in creating professional correspondence that reflects favorably on you and your practice.

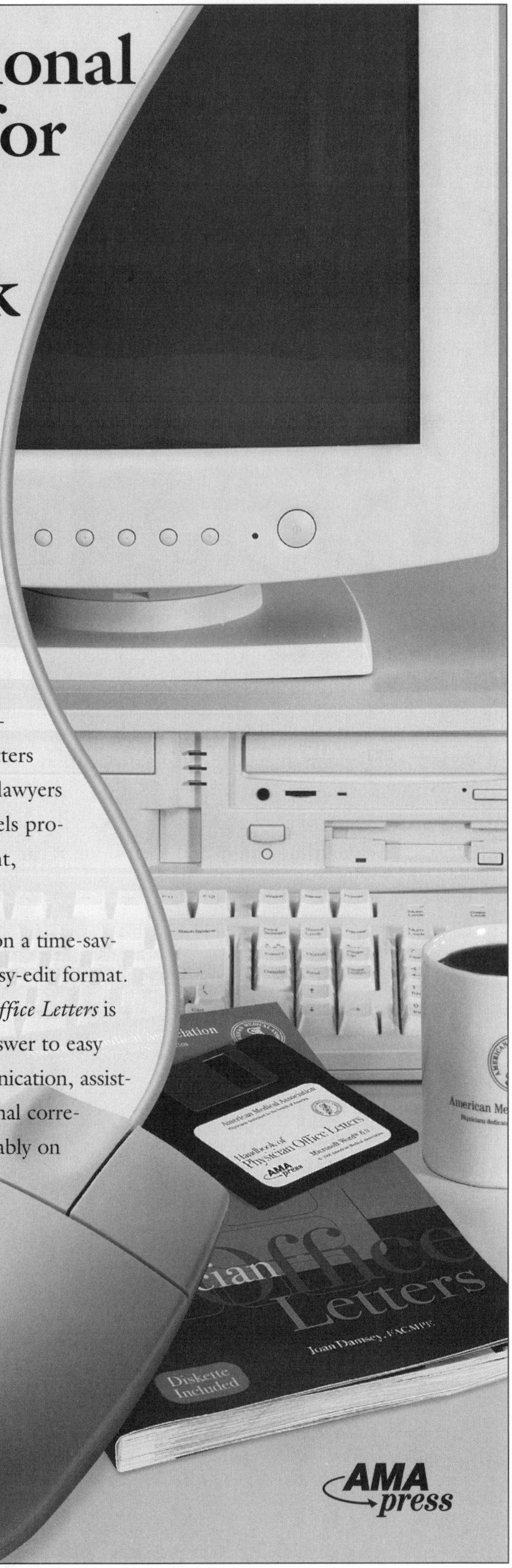

Order #OP318700
Price $60.00
AMA Member Price $50.00

Order Toll Free 800 621 8335 or Online @ www.ama-assn.org/catalog

For fastest service, mention **Priority Code BGE**. MasterCard, VISA, American Express, and Optima accepted. State sales tax and shipping/handling charges apply.

American Medical Association
Physicians dedicated to the health of America

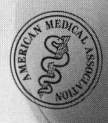

AMA press

Staying Resilient
...in the Face of Stress

Stress has always been a part of the busy physician's life. Unfortunately, physicians and medical organizations today are ill-equipped to handle many of the escalating tensions they face. *The Resilient Physician* teaches how to manage these stress reactions, and how to respond to others when they are stressed.

How can physicians transform the medical workplace into a positive interpersonal culture? Authors Wayne and Mary Sotile employ a model for stress-hardiness called "Effective Emotional Management." Gleaned from over 25 years of research and clinical experience, the "Effective Emotional Management" model explains how to:

- Create a spirit of optimism in times of crisis and conflict.
- Gain skills to better manage emotions at work and home.
- Decrease destructive psychological patterns.
- Improve the ability to balance work, family, and self.
- Transform the workplace by replacing negative coping styles with positive ones.

Managing emotions is a key to staying healthy and building successful medical organizations. *The Resilient Physician* helps unlock the secrets of personal and organizational stress resilience. Order your copy today!

To Order:
Call AMA Press at: 800 621-8335
Visit our secure Web site at:
www.amapress.com

Order #: OP318200BMJ
Price: $30.00
AMA member price: $27.50

VISA, MasterCard, American Express and Optima accepted. State sales tax and shipping/handling charges apply. Satisfaction guaranteed or return within 30 days for full refund.

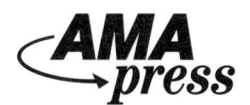

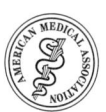

AMA press

American Medical Association
Physicians dedicated to the health of America

Sharing Stories from the Soul

Doctors Speaking about Passion, Resilience, and Hope

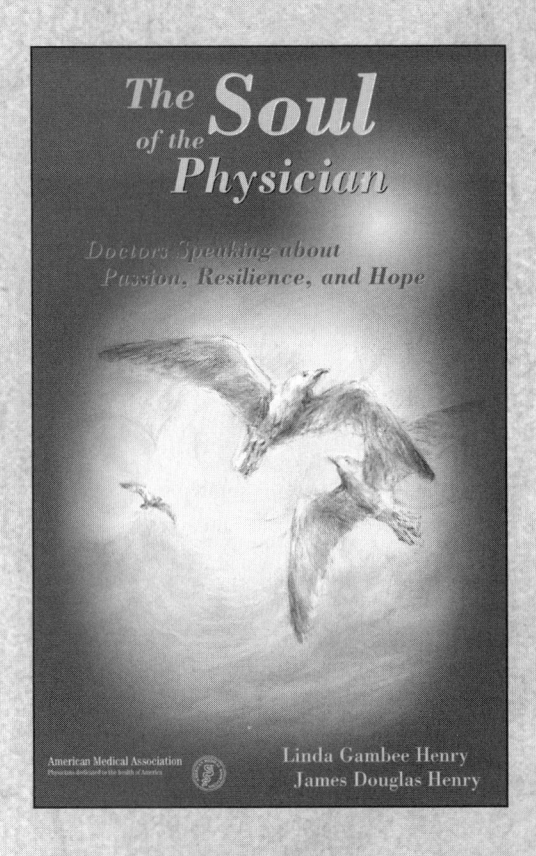

The *Soul of the Physician* provides a powerful message about passion, resilience, and hope. Through face-to-face personal interviews, the authors capture 33 powerful stories of physicians' personal struggles and triumphs—each story as its own complete chapter.

An antidote to professional and personal loneliness, *The Soul of the Physician* comprises stories of physicians speaking what's in their hearts. As physicians struggle to deal with feelings of isolation typical of the profession, they will find these stories help them discover a sense of community with their colleagues.

The Soul of the Physician shares personal messages from physicians of diverse disciplines, and includes a final chapter on taking care of oneself. Emotionally supportive and encouraging, *The Soul of the Physician* will inspire and rejuvenate physicians—mind and soul—as they continue on their own journeys.

AMA press

To Order:
Call AMA Press at: 800 621-8335
Visit our secure Web site at:
www.amapress.com

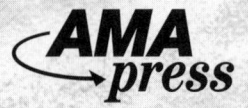

Order #: OP209701BNS
ISBN: 1-57947-244-3
Price: $30.00
AMA member price: $27.50

VISA, MasterCard, American Express and Optima accepted. State sales tax and shipping/handling charges apply. Satisfaction guaranteed or return within 30 days for full refund.

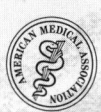

American Medical Association
Physicians dedicated to the health of America

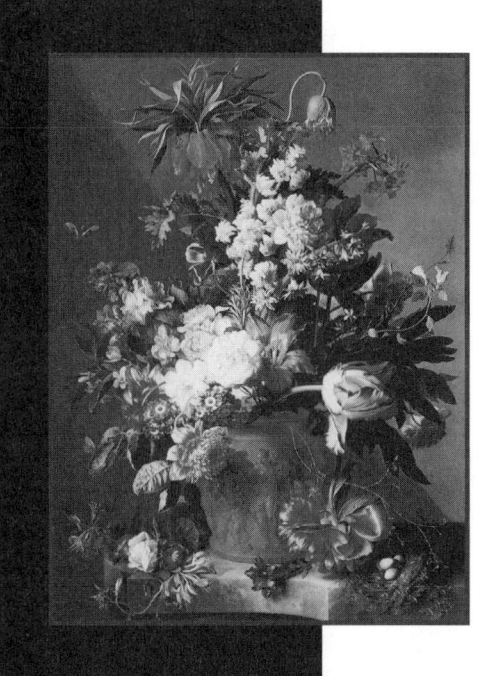

The Art of JAMA II
An Enlightening Conversation Continues

For nearly forty years, the cover of JAMA has featured vibrant color reproductions of paintings from museums around the world. The newest collection of these beautiful covers is now available in an attractive, coffee-table volume—*The Art of JAMA II: Covers and Essays From The Journal of the American Medical Association.*

Opposite each full-page color reproduction is an essay by M. Therese Southgate, MD, that presents unique insights into the work. With her discerning comments, personal reactions, and provocative thoughts she brings the reader into contact with ideas of art and culture expressed in their broadest and yet most particular terms.

The Art of JAMA II offers a well-rounded display of fine art from well-known and lesser-known collections. Portraits, landscapes, still lifes, and abstracts encompass works from the Renaissance to the Moderns. This remarkable new collection will appeal to persons of all ages and backgrounds—physicians and other professionals, teachers and students, artists and art collectors—anyone interested in the world of art.

Handsomely bound and jacketed, *The Art of JAMA II* includes a new preface by the author and two new forewords. A worthy companion to its predecessor—*The Art of JAMA*—this new collection promises to be a cherished addition to anyone's personal library.

Phone orders: 800 621-8335
Secured online orders:
www.amapress.org

The Art of JAMA II
Order#: OP080001BGL
Price: $69.95
AMA Member Price: $64.95

Buy both and save:
The Art of JAMA and *The Art of JAMA II*
Order#: OP210800BGL
Price: $109.95
AMA Member Price: $99.95

VISA, MasterCard, American Express, and Optima accepted. State sales tax and shipping/handling charges apply. Satisfaction guaranteed or return within 30 days for full refund.

The Art of JAMA II presents inspiring works by these and many other notable artists:

- Degas
- Dürer
- Eakins
- Ensor
- Fragonard
- Gorky
- Hals
- Kandinsky
- Manet
- Marin
- Millet
- Miró
- Mondrian
- Monet
- Munch
- Pippin
- Rembrandt
- Renoir
- Toulouse-Lautrec
- Van Huysum
- Velázquez
- Vermeer

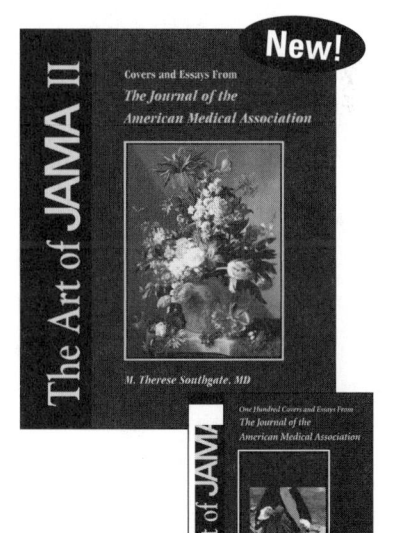

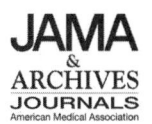

JAMA & ARCHIVES JOURNALS
American Medical Association

AMA press